José Costa

Current Concepts in Gynecologic Pathology: Epithelial Tumors of the Gynecologic Tract

Guest Editor

ROBERT A. SOSLOW, MD

SURGICAL PATHOLOGY CLINICS

surgpath.theclinics.com

Consulting Editor
JOHN R. GOLDBLUM, MD

March 2011 • Volume 4 • Number 1

SAUNDERS an imprint of ELSEVIER, Inc.

W.B. SAUNDERS COMPANY
A Division of Elsevier Inc.

1600 John F. Kennedy Boulevard • Suite 1800 • Philadelphia, Pennsylvania 19103-2899

http://www.surgpath.theclinics.com

SURGICAL PATHOLOGY CLINICS Volume 4, Number 1
March 2011 ISSN 1875-9181, ISBN-13: 978-1-4377-2265-9

Editor: Joanne Husovski

Surgical Pathology Clinics (ISSN 1875-9181) is published quarterly by Elsevier Inc., 360 Park Avenue South, New York, NY 10010. Months of issue are March, June, September, and December. Business and Editorial Office: Elsevier Inc., 1600 John F. Kennedy Blvd., Ste. 1800, Philadelphia, PA 19103-2899. Accounting and Circulation Offices: Elsevier Inc., 3251 Riverport Lane, Maryland Heights, MO 63043. Periodicals postage paid at New York, NY and at additional mailing offices. Subscription prices are $170.00 per year (US individuals), $199.00 per year (US institutions), $84.00 per year (US students/residents), $213.00 per year (Canadian individuals), $225.00 per year (Canadian Institutions), $213.00 per year (foreign individuals), $225.00 per year (foreign institutions), and $104.00 per year (international & Canadian students/residents). Foreign air speed delivery is included in all *Clinics'* subscription prices. All prices are subject to change without notice. **POSTMASTER:** Send address changes to *Surgical Pathology Clinics*, Elsevier, 3251 Riverport Lane, Maryland Heights, MO 63043. Customer Service: 1-800-654-2452 (US). From outside the United States, call 1-314-447-8871. Fax: 1-314-447-8029. E-mail: JournalsCustomerServiceusa@elsevier.com (for print support) and JournalsOnlineSupport-usa@elsevier.com (for online support).

Reprints. For copies of 100 or more, of articles in this publication, please contact the Commercial Reprints Department, Elsevier Inc., 360 Park Avenue South, New York, NY 10010-1710. Tel. (212) 633-3812; Fax: (212) 462-1935; email: reprints@elsevier.com.

Printed in the United States of America.

Contributors

CONSULTING EDITOR

JOHN R. GOLDBLUM, MD
Chairman, Department of Anatomic Pathology;
Professor of Pathology, Cleveland Clinics,
Lerner College of Medicine, Cleveland Clinic,
Cleveland, Ohio

GUEST EDITOR

ROBERT A. SOSLOW, MD
Attending Pathologist and Director
of Gynecologic Pathology, Memorial
Sloan-Kettering Cancer Center, New York,
New York

AUTHORS

NADEEM R. ABU-RUSTUM, MD, FACOG, FACS
Director, Minimally Invasive Surgery;
Director, Resident and Medical Education,
Gynecology Service, Department of Surgery,
Memorial Sloan-Kettering Cancer Center,
New York, New York

OSAMA M. AL-AGHA, MD, FCAP, FRCPC
Fellow, Department of Pathology and
Laboratory Medicine, Vancouver General
Hospital and University of British Columbia,
Vancouver, British Columbia, Canada

RICHARD R. BARAKAT, MD
Ronald O. Perelman Chief of Gynecology,
Division of Gynecology, Department of
Surgery, Memorial Sloan-Kettering Cancer
Center, New York, New York

NADIM BOU-ZGHEIB, MD
The Women's Institute for Gynecologic
Cancer and Special Pelvic Surgery,
Phillipsburg, New Jersey

RUSSELL R. BROADDUS, MD, PhD
Associate Professor, Department
of Pathology, University of Texas M.D.
Anderson Cancer Center, Houston, Texas

DENNIS S. CHI, MD
Deputy Chief, Gynecology Service; Director,
Fellowship Program, Gynecology Service;
Co-Director, Pelvic Reconstructive Surgery,
Department of Surgery, Memorial
Sloan-Kettering Cancer Center,
New York, New York

BOJANA DJORDJEVIC, MD
Assistant Professor, Department of
Pathology and Laboratory Medicine,
University of Ottawa, Ottawa,
Ontario, Canada

KARUNA GARG, MD
Assistant Attending Pathologist, Department
of Pathology, Memorial Sloan-Kettering
Cancer Center, New York, New York

C. BLAKE GILKS, MD, FRCPC
Professor, Department of Pathology and
Laboratory Medicine, Vancouver General
Hospital and University of British Columbia,
Vancouver, British Columbia, Canada

GUANGMING HAN, MD
Memorial Sloan-Kettering Cancer Center,
New York, New York; Clinical Assistant
Professor, Department of Pathology and
Laboratory Medicine, Foothills Medical Centre,
University of Calgary, Alberta, Canada

DAVID HUNTSMAN, MD
Professor, Faculty of Medicine, University of
British Columbia; Genetic Pathologist, British
Columbia Cancer Agency, Department of
Pathology and Laboratory Medicine, University
of British Columbia, Vancouver, British
Columbia, Canada

MARTIN KÖBEL, MD
Assistant Professor, Department of Pathology,
University of Calgary and Calgary Laboratory
Services, Foothills Medical Centre, Calgary,
Alberta, Canada

MARIO M. LEITAO Jr, MD
Assistant Member, Division of Gynecology,
Department of Surgery, Memorial
Sloan-Kettering Cancer Center,
New York, New York

KARA C. LONG, MD
Fellow in Gynecologic Oncology, Gynecology
Service, Department of Surgery, Memorial
Sloan-Kettering Cancer Center, New York,
New York

TERI A. LONGACRE, MD
Professor of Pathology, Department of
Pathology, Stanford University School of
Medicine, Stanford, California

W. GLENN MCCLUGGAGE, FRCPath
Professor, Department of Pathology, Royal
Group of Hospitals Trust, Northern Ireland,
United Kingdom

ANNE M. MILLS, MD
Resident in Pathology, Department
of Pathology, Stanford University,
Stanford, California

ESTHER OLIVA, MD
Associate Professor, Harvard Medical School;
Associate Pathologist, Massachusetts
General Hospital, Boston, Massachusetts

KAY J. PARK, MD
Assistant Attending Pathologist, Department
of Pathology, Memorial Sloan-Kettering
Cancer Center, New York, New York

EDYTA C. PIROG, MD
Department of Pathology, Weill Medical
College of Cornell University, New York,
New York

PATRICIA A. SHAW, MD
Associate Professor, Department of
Laboratory Medicine and Pathobiology,
University of Toronto; Gynecological
Pathologist, Department of Pathology,
University Health Network, Toronto,
Ontario, Canada

DAVID F. SILVER, MD
Director of Gynecologic Oncology,
The Women's Institute for Gynecologic
Cancer and Special Pelvic Surgery,
Phillipsburg, New Jersey

ROBERT A. SOSLOW, MD
Attending Pathologist and Director
of Gynecologic Pathology, Memorial
Sloan-Kettering Cancer Center, New York,
New York

Contents

CERVIX AND VULVA

> This content presents pathology of the cervix and vulva – its diagnosis, staging, treatment, and prognosis. The authors distinguish between the clinical staging of cervical cancer and the surgical staging of vulvar cancer and note advances in surgical, medical, and radiation oncology in the treatment of both cervical and vulvar carcinoma that allow for individualization of patient treatment resulting in improved oncologic outcomes and improved quality of life. Treatment algorithms are presented based on the varying stages at which the cancer is diagnosed.

> This review presents a discussion of the gross and microscopic features, diagnosis, differential diagnosis, and prognosis of neoplastic lesions of the cervix. Biomarkers are discussed for each entity presented – cervical intraepithelial neoplasia, squamous carcinoma, glandular neoplasms, adenocarcinoma in situ, adenosquamous carcinoma, and others.

> Carcinoma of the vulva is an uncommon malignant neoplasm (approximately one-fifth as frequent as cervical cancer) and represents 4% of all genital cancers in women. Approximately two-thirds of cases occur in women older than 60 years, and squamous cell carcinoma is the most common histologic type. Several different subtypes of squamous cell carcinoma have been described in the vulva; however, in terms of etiology, pathogenesis, and histologic features, most carcinomas belong to one of two categories: keratinizing squamous cell carcinomas associated with chronic inflammatory skin disorders, and basaloid or warty carcinomas related to infection with high oncogenic risk human papillomaviruses. Glandular neoplasms of the vulva arise from the vulvar apocrine sweat glands (papillary hidradenoma and Paget disease) or the Bartholin gland and their cause is not known.

CORPUS

> This article focuses on the most important neoplastic epithelial lesions of the uterus, endometrial hyperplasia and carcinoma. The primary management of hyperplastic

lesions and carcinoma is often surgical but nonsurgical options are possible for both, depending on specific patients and tumor characteristics. Many controversies still exist regarding the optimal medical and surgical treatments of hyperplasias and carcinomas of the endometrium. There is a need to more accurately select patients for lymph node sampling or dissection. The role of adjuvant therapies for endometrial carcinomas is still under investigation. This review covers current understanding in the diagnosis and clinical management of endometrial hyperplasias and carcinomas.

In the developed world, endometrial carcinoma is the most common malignant tumor of the female gynecologic tract. Numerous epidemiologic studies indicate that exposure to unopposed estrogen is a significant risk factor for developing endometrial cancer, particularly endometrioid-type endometrial carcinoma; however, a number of other molecular pathways and mechanisms are also important in endometrial cancer. In this review, the authors highlight some of the more interesting molecular pathways in endometrial cancer, such as the PTEN/PI3K/AKT pathway, microsatellite instability, and molecular mediators of epithelial-to-mesenchymal transition.

The distinction between atypical endometrial hyperplasia and well differentiated adenocarcinoma of the endometrium is one of the more difficult differential diagnoses in gynecologic pathology. Different pathologists apply different histologic criteria, often with different individual thresholds for atypical endometrial hyperplasia and grade 1 adenocarcinoma. While some classifications are based on a series of molecular genetic alterations (which may or may not translate into biologically or clinically relevant risk lesions), almost all current diagnostic criteria use a series of histologic features - usually a combination of architecture and cytology - for diagnosing atypical hyperplasia and adenocarcinoma. This article presents evidence-based histologic criteria for atypical endometrial hyperplasia and low grade endometrial carcinoma (both FIGO grade 1 and 2) with emphasis on common and not so common histologic mimics. Grade 3 endometrioid carcinoma is discussed in the Oliva and Soslow article in this publication.

High-grade endometrial carcinomas are a heterogeneous group of clinically aggressive tumors. They include FIGO grade 3 endometrioid carcinoma, serous carcinoma, clear cell carcinoma, undifferentiated carcinoma, and malignant mixed Müllerian tumor (MMMT). Epidemiologic, genetic, biologic prognostic and morphologic differences between these entities are striking in prototypic cases, yet substantial overlap exists and diagnostic criteria and therapeutic approaches that account for the group's diversity are currently insufficient. FIGO grade 3 endometrioid carcinoma demonstrates solid, trabecular or nested growth and may resemble poorly differentiated squamous cell carcinoma. Endometrioid glandular differentiation is usually focally present. Serous carcinoma usually displays papillary architecture but glandular and solid patterns may predominate. Tumor cells typically display diffuse and severe atypia. Clear cell carcinoma should be diagnosed by recognizing characteristic papillary or tubulocystic architecture with cuboidal tumor cells showing atypical but uniform nuclei. Cells with clear cytoplasm are frequently but not always present. On the other hand, clear cells may be encountered in endometrioid and serous carcinomas. Immunohistochemical stains for p53, p16, ER, PR, mib-1, hepatocyte nuclear factor 1β and pan-cytokeratin can be helpful in classifying these high-grade carcinomas. They should be used in concert with thorough morphologic examination, as part of a rational panel of markers and only in specific circumstances. Although these tumors may appear clinically and even morphologically similar, demographic and epidemiologic features as well as patterns of spread and treatment modalities differ.

Women with Lynch syndrome are at considerable risk for developing endometrial carcinoma, but current screening guidelines for detection of Lynch syndrome focus almost exclusively on colorectal carcinoma. Lynch syndrome associated colorectal and endometrial carcinomas have some important differences with implications for screening strategies. These differences are discussed in this review, along with the most effective screening criteria and testing methods for detection of Lynch syndrome in endometrial carcinoma patients.

OVARY, FALLOPIAN TUBE, AND PERITONEUM

Ovarian, fallopian tube and peritoneal carcinomas make up the deadliest group of malignancies of the female genital tract. Ovarian carcinoma is the second most common malignancy of the female reproductive tract in developed countries and the sixth most common cancer diagnosed in women in the United States. While signs and symptoms of ovarian carcinoma related to the mass-effect of advanced disease are relatively common, no reliable signs or symptoms are seen in patients with early ovarian carcinoma. The diagnosis can only be made by surgical removal and pathologic evaluation of a suspicious mass. The authors present an overview of the disease and discussions of genetic predisposition, prevention, screening, and diagnosis of ovarian, fallopian tube and primary peritoneal carcinomas. Details on staging procedures as well as surgical and chemotherapeutic techniques are outlined for the various stages of disease.

This content presents a review of molecular pathology of ovarian cancer. The authors present key molecular features for high-grade and low-grade serous carcinomas, endometrioid carcinomas, clear cell carcinomas, and mucinous carcinomas. Cell lineage, mutation and gene expression, pathway alterations, risk factors, prognostic markers, and treatment targets are discussed.

In this review, ovarian metastatic carcinomas from various sites, as well as other neoplasms secondarily involving the ovary, are discussed. As well as describing the morphology, the value of immunohistochemistry in distinguishing between primary and metastatic neoplasms in the ovary is discussed. While immunohistochemistry has a valuable role to play and is paramount in some cases, the results should be interpreted with caution and with regard to the clinical picture and gross and microscopic pathologic findings.

This review focuses on recent advances in the area of low-grade ovarian serous neoplasia with emphasis on key diagnostic criteria, differential diagnosis, and disease classification based on current understanding of low-grade serous carcinogenesis. Despite considerable controversy surrounding serous tumors of low malignant potential (S-LMP) or borderline tumors, there have been great strides in our understanding of the serous group of borderline and malignant pelvic epithelial neoplasms in the past decade. Most S-LMP have a favorable prognosis, but recurrences and progression to carcinoma occur, sometimes following a protracted clinical course. Pathologic risk factors vary, but the extraovarian implant status is the most important predictor for progressive disease. Progression of S-LMP usually takes the form of low-grade serous carcinoma, although transformation to high-grade carcinoma is occasionally seen. A pelvic S-LMP – low-grade serous carcinoma pathway has been proposed based on global gene expression profiling, shared mutations in KRAS and/or BRAF, and in most cases, the presence of S-LMP in de novo low-grade serous carcinoma. Unlike high-grade serous carcinoma, low-grade serous carcinoma responds poorly to standard platinum-based chemotherapy. Development of more tailored therapy for S-LMP with invasive implants and low-grade serous carcinoma, ideally based on a relative risk model for disease progression, is under active clinical investigation.

The focus of this review is high-grade serous carcinoma (HGSC); for the purposes of this review, the term "pelvic SC" is used for HGSC that could be considered, based on historical definitions, to have arisen from ovary, fallopian tube, or peritoneum. These assignments of primary site are arbitrary and there is evidence that the distal fallopian tube is the site of origin of many pelvic HGSCs. The diagnosis of HGSC can be made readily based on routine histomorphologic examination in most cases; however, a variety of neoplasms can resemble HGSC. Thus, we review the key features of pelvic SC, current concepts of its pathogenesis, histopathological diagnostic criteria, discuss differential diagnosis, and review diagnostic ancillary studies that can be used in practice.

This review covers the group of relatively uncommon nonserous ovarian epithelial tumors. The authors focus on the group's distinctiveness from the much more common serous tumors and show the similarities across entities. Diagnostic criteria that separate the different entities are currently being debated. Particular problems include the reproducible diagnosis of high-grade endometrioid, transitional cell, mixed epithelial and undifferentiated carcinomas. Furthermore, despite recognition that most malignant mucinous tumors involving ovary represent metastases from extraovarian primary sites, many misdiagnoses still occur. The authors discuss their rationale behind their opinions about these problematic topics.

Patricia A. Shaw

Approximately 10% of ovarian cancers are associated with inherited germline mutations, most commonly of the *BRCA1* or *BRCA2* genes. The majority of BRCA1 and BRCA2 cancers are high-grade serous carcinomas diagnosed at an advanced stage, and there are as yet no histologic features that distinguish these tumors from sporadic serous cancers. Many women identified as being at high genetic risk undergo prophylactic salpingo-oophorectomy, and careful histopathological examination of these specimens may identify occult carcinoma, frequently in the distal fallopian tube. In addition, serous cancer precursors, including tubal intraepithelial carcinoma, have been increasingly recognized in distal and fimbrial epithelium. Little has been documented to date of the histopathological features of the cancers associated with the hereditary nonpolyposis colon cancer syndrome, but it appears these ovarian cancers may include a variety of histologic types, and in contrast to the BRCA cancers, are low grade and early stage.

Surgical Pathology Clinics

THE CLINICS ARE NOW AVAILABLE ONLINE!

Access your subscription at:
www.theclinics.com

Gynecologic Pathologists: Physicians at the Crossroads of Diagnosis and Clinical Care

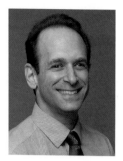

Robert A. Soslow, MD
Guest Editor

Editing this publication was a great joy despite the challenges. It presented many wonderful opportunities: working with compelling subject matter; collaborating with some of the finest pathologists in the world; mentoring younger pathologists (who are also among the finest pathologists around); learning a great deal about gynecologic oncology and pathology; honing editorial skills; and creating work whose scope is broad enough to spark interest in investigative pursuits and sufficiently specific to be of practical value.

In this publication, the reader will find content about clinical gynecologic oncology that provides depth and clinical perspective to the more traditional content focused on diagnostic pathology. I believe strongly that one cannot become an accomplished pathologist without understanding clinical practice in great detail. After all, practicing pathology is not merely an exercise in pattern recognition. Our mandate is not only accurate, meaningful, and relevant diagnosis; rather, it is also our responsibility to provide expert consultation, guiding the surgeons' hands and the oncologists' choice of therapy. We are physicians, not technicians.

Several of the pathology topics are organized in new ways. For example, instead of finding one article about endometrioid carcinoma of the endometrium, the reader will find two articles about endometrial carcinoma—one dealing with hyperplasia and low-grade endometrioid carcinoma, and another about high-grade endometrial carcinomas, including FIGO grade 3 endometrioid carcinoma. This is intended to emphasize biological, clinical, and pathologic similarities across

entities. For the endometrial content, the organization also facilitates discussion of differential diagnosis. There are also three articles devoted to primary ovarian carcinomas and related lesions. High-grade serous carcinoma, by far the most common ovarian carcinoma in North America and Europe, gets its own discussion, but low-grade serous carcinoma and nonserous carcinoma are each covered in separate topic presentations. Assembling the fascinating nonserous tumors into one presentation emphasizes the group's distinctiveness from the other much more common tumors and brings attention to similarities shared by different entities. The content is not meant to be exhaustive, but it features points that pathologists should find helpful in daily practice.

My experience working as a general surgical pathologist and a gynecologic pathologist suggests to me that the current overall state of training in neoplastic gynecologic pathology is not optimal. Of all of the diagnostic services at Memorial Hospital, diagnostic discrepancies uncovered on review of consultation cases appear most frequently on the gynecology service. Learning gynecologic pathology can be difficult: many of the concepts are foreign to general pathologists; terminology can be unfamiliar; and the field is changing quickly. I feel passionately that gynecologic cancer patients be offered the very best care, which necessitates a knowledgeable and engaged pathologist. I sincerely hope this volume inspires its readers and promotes outstanding gynecologic cancer care.

Surgical Pathology 4 (2011) xi–xii
doi:10.1016/j.path.2010.12.013

I'd like to thank all of the outstanding contributors, those whose names appear in the table of contents, and also those whose names you will not find anywhere but here. Thank you to John Goldblum for the invitation to guest edit this work. Marc Rosenblum and Victor Reuter deserve recognition for having established a Department of Pathology staffed by friendly, smart, and dedicated people. We have time, support, and resources to do good diagnostic work and also pursue our academic interests. Kin Kong and Allyne Manzo did excellent work assisting with photography. My colleagues on the Gynecology Disease Management Team have been wonderful teachers and great collaborators and our gynecologic pathology team, including Kay Park, Melissa Murray, Karuna Garg, Deborah DeLair, and Guangming Han, are unmatched. I owe a great debt to my mentors, Richard Kempson and Michael Hendrickson, and many influential people along the way. I also had the pleasure of interacting with Joanne Husovski, the professional, highly capable, and always helpful friendly face of the publisher. I thank my family and friends for encouragement, with special thanks going to my partner of 25 years, Michael Ogborn.

Robert A. Soslow, MD
Department of Pathology
Memorial Sloan-Kettering Cancer Center
1275 York Avenue
New York, NY 10065, USA

E-mail address:
soslowr@MSKCC.ORG

CLINICAL APPROACH TO DIAGNOSIS AND MANAGEMENT OF CANCER OF THE CERVIX AND VULVA

Kara C. Long, MD, Nadeem R. Abu-Rustum, MD*

KEYWORDS

- Cervix cancer • Vulva cancer • Cancer staging • Gynecologic malignancies
- Treatment gynecologic cancer

ABSTRACT

This review presents pathology of the cervix and vulva – its diagnosis, staging, treatment, and prognosis. The authors distinguish between the clinical staging of cervical cancer and the surgical staging of vulvar cancer and note advances in surgical, medical, and radiation oncology in the treatment of both cervical and vulvar carcinoma that allow for individualization of patient treatment resulting in improved oncologic outcomes and improved quality of life. Treatment algorithms are presented based on the varying stages at which the cancer is diagnosed.

Key Features
PATHOLOGIC REPORTING FOR CERVICAL CARCINOMA

Histology

Tumor dimensions

    Gross tumor diameter (for visible lesions)[a]

    Tumor width (especially for superficial lesions)

    Depth of stromal invasion (Reported as a %)[a]

Lymphovascular invasion[a]

Margin status[b]

Lymph node assessment

    Nodal counts

    Nodal status[b]

Parametrial status[b]

[a] Intermediate risk criteria (Sedlis 1999).
[b] High risk criteria (Peters 2000).

CERVIX

EPIDEMIOLOGY AND ETIOLOGY

Cervical cancer is the third most common gynecologic malignancy in the United States following endometrial and ovarian cancer. In 2009, it is predicted that there were 11,270 new cases and 4,070 deaths from cervical cancer alone.[1] The peak age of diagnosis is during the late forties, with almost half of the cases diagnosed in women under age 35. Cervical cancer remains a major cause of morbidity and mortality in developing countries where access to screening tests is limited. In industrialized countries, the incidence of invasive cervical cancer has dramatically decreased since the introduction and popularization of cervical screening cytology techniques [Papanicolaou (pap) smear] during the latter half of the twentieth century. Almost all precancerous and cancerous lesions of the cervix can be

---

Gynecology Service, Department of Surgery, Memorial Sloan-Kettering Cancer Center, 1275 York Avenue, New York, NY 10065, USA
* Corresponding author.
E-mail address: abu-rusn@mskcc.org

Surgical Pathology 4 (2011) 1–16
doi:10.1016/j.path.2010.12.005

attributed to persistent human papillomavirus infections, specifically genotypes 16, 18, 45, 31, 33, 35.[2] Several risk factors have been associated with the development of cervical carcinoma, including[3]:

- Advanced age
- Low socioeconomic status
- Limited access to health care
- Early coitarche
- Large number of sexual partners
- Smoking
- Immunodeficiency states such as human immunodeficiency virus (HIV) infection.

The majority of invasive cervical cancers are squamous cell (80%), followed by adenocarcinoma (20%); other cell types such as small cell are extremely rare.

DIAGNOSIS

Presenting symptoms may include abnormal vaginal bleeding (including post-coital bleeding) or discharge, although many women are asymptomatic and their cancer is detected only during routine screening. Pelvic pain, lower extremity edema, deep vein thrombosis, neuropathic pain, and obstructive renal failure are less common presentations and are associated with advanced disease.

Although invasive cervical cancer may be suspected after inspection and palpation of the cervix, histologic confirmation is essential before proceeding with definitive therapy. All previous diagnostic material should be carefully reviewed and the diagnosis confirmed. Cervical tumors often appear friable and necrotic. Colposcopy with directed cervical biopsy is commonly recommended for the initial evaluation of abnormal or suspicious Pap smears; it is safe and generally well tolerated by most women. Persistent symptoms of abnormal bleeding/discharge, abnormalities on cervical inspection, abnormal cervical cytology including ASCUS with +HPV testing, and in utero exposure to DES are all indications for colposcopy. Lugol's solution and acetic acid can be used to highlight abnormalities in the cervix.

If carcinoma is suspected but the biopsy was not diagnostic, or if cancer was seen but the degree of invasion could not be reliably determined, a diagnostic cervical conization is necessary. This can be accomplished using a loop electrosurgical excision procedure (LEEP) or a cold knife conization (CKC). LEEPs are generally as effective as CKC and have the advantage of low cost, ease of use, and less need for anesthesia; however, the cautery can obscure surgical margins. Diagnostic conization can also be therapeutic if the histology only shows dysplasia, squamous cell carcinoma in situ, or invasive squamous cell carcinoma stage IA1 (with negative margins and no lymphovascular invasion). For more invasive squamous cell cancers, conization alone is not sufficient treatment (**Fig. 1**).

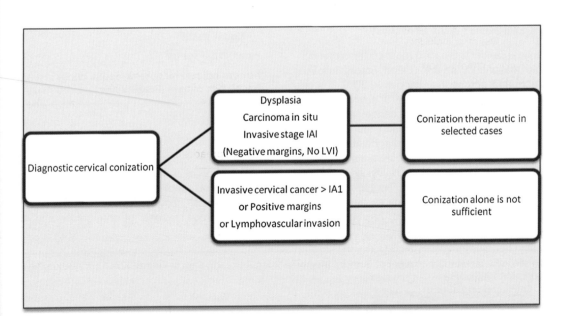

Fig. 1. Cervical Cancer. Pathologic evidence of carcinoma with no visible lesion: proceed to conization.

Pitfalls
IN DIAGNOSIS OF CERVICAL CANCER

! Expert pathologic review is paramount particularly if fertility preservation is an issue

! Large conization may be needed to exclude invasive disease and can clarify the clinical stage in early-stage cases

! MRI may facilitate identifying an endometrial primary verus a cervical primary adenocarcinoma in select cases where the diagnosis is not clear

Diagnostic cervical conization is crucial for accurate staging of preclinical, early invasive cervical cancer [International Federation of Gynecology and Obstetrics (FIGO) stages IA1, IA2, and preclinical IB1 lesions] where the management options and recommendations vary depending on the depth and size of these early lesions. Women with stage IA squamous cell carcinoma may be candidates for more conservative treatment (such as therapeutic conization) compared with those with preclinical (no gross tumor) stage IB1 disease; the differentiation between these two stages is usually not feasible without diagnostic conization.

STAGING

Cervical cancer is staged according to the 2009 FIGO classification (**Box 1**).[4] The staging procedures allowed by FIGO and generally practiced by most physicians include:

Physical examination
Cervical biopsy
Cervical conization (for subclinical tumors)
Chest radiography
Intravenous pyelography
Cystoscopy
Proctoscopy.

The latter three procedures have relatively low yield, are less important in patients with stage IA1 to IB1 disease, and may be omitted based on physician discretion. Barium enema is another staging procedure allowed by FIGO; however, is usually reserved for symptomatic patients or those with locally advanced disease (stage II-IVA). Computed tomography (CT), ultrasonography, magnetic resonance imaging (MRI), lymphangiography, and positron emission tomography (PET) may be used to evaluate tumor spread, and the

Box 1
Cervical cancer staging

Stage I The carcinoma is strictly confined to the cervix

IA Invasive carcinoma which can be diagnosed only by microscopy, with deepest invasion ≤ 5 mm and largest extension not >7 mm

IA1 Measured stromal invasion of ≤ 3.0 mm in depth and ≤ 7.0 mm

IA2 Measured stromal invasion of >3.0 mm and not >5.0 mm with an extension of not >7.0 mm

IB Clinically visible lesions limited to the cervix uteri or preclinical cancers greater than stage IA

IB1 Clinically visible lesion ≤ 4 cm in greatest dimension

IB2 Clinically visible lesion >4 cm in greatest dimension

Stage II Cervical carcinoma invades beyond the uterus, but not to the pelvic wall or to the lower third of the vagina

IIA Without parametrial invasion

IIA1 Clinically visible lesion ≤ 4 cm in greatest dimension

IIA2 Clinically visible lesion >4 cm in greatest dimension

IIB With obvious parametrial invasion

Stage III The tumor extends to the pelvic wall and/or involves the lower third of the vagina and/or causes hydronephrosis or nonfunctioning kidney

Stage IV The carcinoma has extended beyond the true pelvis or has involved (biopsy proven) the mucosa of the bladder or rectum. A bullous edema, as such, does not permit a case to be allotted to stage IV.

IVA Spread of the growth to adjacent organs

IVB Spread to distant organs

information obtained from these tests may modify the treatment plan. Pretreatment MRI and PET scan are the preferred methods used to detect tumor spread in patients with stage IB2 through stage IV tumors, where the risk of regional and distant metastases is increased. Suspicious lesions noted on imaging studies usually require histologic evaluation with fine-needle aspiration or biopsy, particularly if the results would alter the initial treatment plan. HIV testing should be offered to all women diagnosed with cervical cancer, especially young women.[5] The diagnosis of HIV does not usually alter the treatment plan but does allow identification of subjects who may benefit from antiretroviral therapy, which may ultimately improve survival.

TREATMENT

The standard treatment strategies for invasive cervical cancer are radical surgery, radiotherapy, and chemotherapy. For select women, fertility sparing surgery such as radical trachelectomy may also be an option. Radiotherapy may be used for all stages of cervical cancer with certain modifications in dosimetry and technique. Each patient must be evaluated individually and a treatment scheme tailored to achieve the best outcome with the least morbidity.

STAGE IA1 LESIONS

The surgical options for stage IA1 disease (3 mm depth or less of stromal invasion and 7 mm or less width) depend on several factors, including the desire for future fertility, histology, lymphovascular invasion, and cone biopsy margin status. Simple hysterectomy or cervical conization with negative margins (in patients who desire future fertility) are adequate therapy for stage IA1 squamous cell lesions with no lymphatic or vascular invasion.[6] Women with evidence of lymphovascular invasion

Key Features
TREATMENT POINTS FOR CERVICAL CANCER

1. For stage I disease a local procedure (conization, radical trachelectomy, radical hysterectomy) and assessment of nodal status is commonly an acceptable initial surgical approach

2. Assessment of pelvic nodes is important in patients who have greater than 3 mm invasive lesions, gross lesions, or any lymphovascular invasion

3. Fertility may be preserved in many women with stage I disease

4. Resection of parametrial tissue remains an important component of the operation for stage IB1-IIA disease

5. Select stage IB2 and IIB-IVA patients are best treated with chemoradiation

may be at increased risk for metastasis, and the treatment should be modified to address this issue.[5,7,8] In these patients, a modified radical hysterectomy, radical hysterectomy, or radical trachelectomy (sparing of the uterine corpus) with pelvic lymphadenectomy should be considered.[5] If surgical therapy is contraindicated, select patients with stage IA cervical cancer at low risk for nodal metastasis (<3 mm stromal invasion and no lymphovascular invasion) may be treated with intracavitary radiation therapy alone for a total dose of 7000 to 7500 cGy to point A, an imaginary point 2 cm superior and 2 cm lateral to the external cervical os.

Treatment of invasive cervical adenocarcinoma, which constitutes approximately 20% of all cervical cancers, is essentially similar to that of squamous cell carcinomas. However, the management of adenocarcinoma in situ in women who desire future fertility may be more challenging than its squamous cell counterpart, as several retrospective reports have indicated that conservative therapy with cervical conization leaves residual cancer in 30 to 40% of patients even if negative surgical margins were obtained. Nevertheless, conization is the appropriate initial step for documenting in situ or invasive disease. For patients with adenocarcinoma in situ, simple hysterectomy may be the safest treatment.[9–11] The histologic diagnosis of a microinvasive cervical adenocarcinoma is difficult, and treatment recommendations remain controversial. Therefore, cervical adenocarcinoma with any stromal invasion is usually treated with radical hysterectomy and pelvic lymphadenectomy or definitive radiation therapy. Radical trachelectomy with pelvic lymphadenectomy may be suitable only for selected patients who have a strong desire for fertility. Some maintain, however, that microinvasive adenocarcinoma of the cervix is a clinicopathologic entity that appears to have the same prognosis and should be treated in the same way as its squamous cell counterpart (**Fig. 2**).[12]

STAGE IA2 LESIONS

Women with depth of cervical stromal invasion greater than 3 mm and not greater than 5 mm, and extension 7 mm or less (stage IA2) should be offered radical hysterectomy with pelvic lymphadenectomy (**Fig. 3**). Alternatively, these women may be offered a fertility sparing approach (radical trachelectomy with pelvic lymphadenectomy) or a non-surgical approach with radiotherapy (whole pelvis and intracavitary). These recommendations are valid regardless of the presence of lymphovascular invasion, as the risk of metastasis is increased when the depth of stromal invasion exceeds 3 mm. Radical

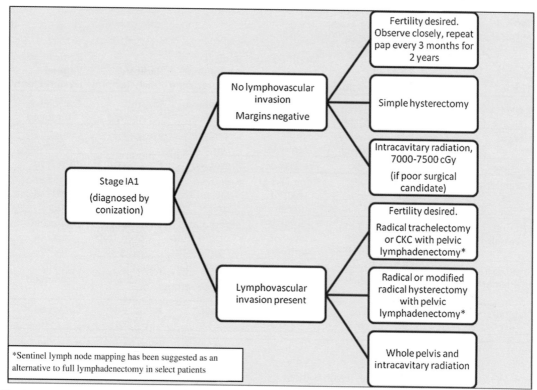

Fig. 2. Cervical Cancer. Stage IA1 diagnosed on conization.

hysterectomy and trachelectomy can be performed with a varied combination of approaches including abdominal, vaginal, laparoscopic, and robotic assisted laparoscopic.[13–18] The main differences between these surgical approaches to early cervical cancer are summarized in **Table 1**.[19–21] Criteria for consideration of a radical trachelectomy include: reproductive age with a strong desire for fertility,

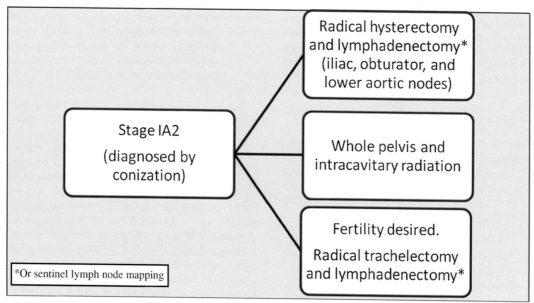

Fig. 3. Cervical Cancer. Stage IA2.

Table 1
Surgical approaches to early-stage cervical cancer

Tissue	Cervical Conization	Total Hysterectomy	Modified Radical Hysterectomy	Radical Abdominal Hysterectomy	Radical Trachelectomy	Radical Vaginal Hysterectomy
Cervix	Partially removed	Completely removed	Completely removed	Completely removed	Mostly removed	Completely removed
Corpus	Preserved	Completely removed	Completely removed	Completely removed	Preserved	Completely removed
Adnexa	Preserved	Preserved	Preserved	Preserved	Preserved	Preserved
Parametria and paracolpos	Preserved	Preserved	Removed at level of ureter	Removed lateral to ureter	Partially removed	Removed at level of ureter
Uterine vessels	Preserved	Ligated at level of internal os	Ligated at level of ureter	Ligated at origin from hypogastric	Ligated at origin from hypogastric	Ligated at level of ureter
Uterosacral ligaments	Preserved	Ligated at uterus	Ligated midway to rectum	Ligated near rectum	Partially removed	Partially removed
Vaginal cuff	Preserved	Removed <1 cm	Removed 1–2 cm	Removed ≥2 cm	Removed 1–2 cm	Removed ≥2 cm

stage IA2 to IB1 disease, up to 4 cm lesion without involvement of the upper endocervical canal, negative regional lymph nodes.[22]

Sentinel lymph node (SLN) mapping is suggested as an adjunct, and in some circumstances, an alternative to traditional lymphadenectomy. SLN mapping allows for ultra-staging of the first draining lymph node, and in theory, elimination of the need for a full lymphadenectomy. This technique may be able to increase the detection of micro-metastases while decreasing the chance of post-operative complications related to full lymphadenectomy, such as lymphedema. Current evidence supporting the use of SLN mapping is promising, however further studies are needed to standardize this approach.

STAGE IB1 LESIONS

Stage IB cervical cancer is categorized into two subgroups: IB1 (≤4 cm) and IB2 (>4 cm). Stage IB1 disease can be adequately treated with comparable cure rates, using radical hysterectomy and pelvic lymphadenectomy or definitive radiotherapy (**Fig. 4**). Advantages of surgery include[20]:

Allowing exploration of the abdomen and pelvis to exclude metastasis
Shorter overall treatment duration
Preservation of ovarian function in premenopausal women

Preservation of vaginal pliability and lubrication
Limited injury to normal tissue
Less risk of bowel fistulas and disturbances in intestinal function
Corrective surgery is more easily performed in nonirradiated tissue without the need for diversion if complications such as urinary tract fistulas occur as a result of treatment
Surgery can be used in a variety of conditions where radiotherapy may not be indicated, such as pyometria, presence of an adnexal mass, pelvic prolapse, altered vaginal anatomy, history of severe pelvic adhesions, inflammatory bowel disease, and presence of a pelvic kidney.

For selected patients who have a strong desire to maintain fertility options, radical trachelectomy appears to have a similar oncologic outcome to radical hysterectomy.[23] After primary surgery, patients at high risk for recurrence can be identified by the presence of positive margins, positive lymph nodes, or positive parametria.[24] Intermediate risk patients can be identified by having 2 out of 3 of the following risk factors: large tumor diameter (≥4 cm), depth of stromal invasion (expressed as superficial, middle, or deep third invasion of cervical wall), positive lymphovascular invasion.[25] It is recommended that these patients be offered adjuvant external beam radiation to decrease their risk of recurrence.

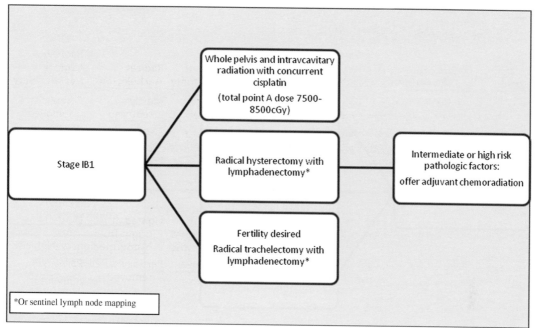

```
                    ┌─────────────────────────┐
                    │ Whole pelvis and intravcavitary │
                    │  radiation with concurrent │
                    │        cisplatin        │
                    │  (total point A dose 7500- │
                    │        8500cGy)         │
                    └─────────────────────────┘

┌──────────────┐    ┌─────────────────────────┐    ┌─────────────────────────┐
│              │    │ Radical hysterectomy with │    │ Intermediate or high risk │
│  Stage IB1   │────│    lymphadenectomy*     │────│     pathologic factors:   │
│              │    │                         │    │ offer adjuvant chemoradiation │
└──────────────┘    └─────────────────────────┘    └─────────────────────────┘

                    ┌─────────────────────────┐
                    │     Fertility desired   │
                    │  Radical trachelectomy with │
                    │     lymphadenectomy*    │
                    └─────────────────────────┘
```

*Or sentinel lymph node mapping

Fig. 4. Cervical Cancer. Stage IB1.

Concerning the role of oophorectomy during radical hysterectomy for cervical cancer, Sutton and colleagues[26] in a Gynecologic Oncology Group study reported on the incidence of ovarian metastases in 990 patients with stage IB cervical carcinoma. Ovarian metastases were noted in 4 of 770 (0.5%) patients with squamous cell carcinoma and 2 of 121 (1.7%) with adenocarcinoma ($P = .19$). No patients with adenosquamous carcinoma or other histology had ovarian metastases. These data suggest no increase in occult ovarian metastases in nonsquamous cell cervical cancers, and ovarian preservation is commonly performed in women younger than 40 years where there is no gross ovarian abnormality and no obvious extracervical metastases at the time of radical hysterectomy.

Alternatively, radiotherapy may be used as primary definitive treatment in almost all women; it is associated with less direct mortality and usually less risk of urinary tract injury. Intracavitary radiation therapy (ICRT) for stage IB cervical cancer is performed with a technique similar to that used for more advanced lesions, using a tandem and two colpostats (Fletcher or Henshkie). The tandem is a metallic hollow curved rod that is inserted into the cervical os to the fundus and the colpostats are two metallic rods, each with a cavity at the tip for radioactive sources, placed on either side of the tandem. Cesium 137 is then loaded in the tandem and two colpostats for brachytherapy. Intracavitary irradiation treats central pelvic disease, whereas external beam irradiation treats the primary tumor and its locoregional draining lymphatic tissue. The combination is associated with better local control and survival than is seen with external beam radiation alone. Interstitial implants are not indicated for stage I lesions. The timing and insertion is similar to that for advanced lesions, however the total dose provided by ICRT may be modified based on tumor size and frequently is less than that for more advanced and bulky lesions with a total dose ranging from 7500 to 8500 cGy to point A.

STAGE IB2 - IIA LESIONS

Tumor size and volume of early stage cervical cancers appear to be independent prognostic factors in several retrospective studies.[27,28] Women with bulky early-stage cervical cancer (larger than 4 cm, stage IB2-IIA) have a significantly higher risk for local and distant metastases and recurrence than those women with earlier stage disease. The optimal treatment for stage IB2 to IIA disease remains controversial. Current options include: primary surgery (radical hysterectomy and lymphadenectomy) followed by adjuvant chemoradiation, neoadjuvant chemotherapy followed by radical hysterectomy (and possibly post-operative radiation), and primary definitive chemo-radiation (**Fig. 5**).

The Gynecologic Oncology Group completed a study of women with bulky stage IB tumors (4 cm or larger in diameter). Patients were

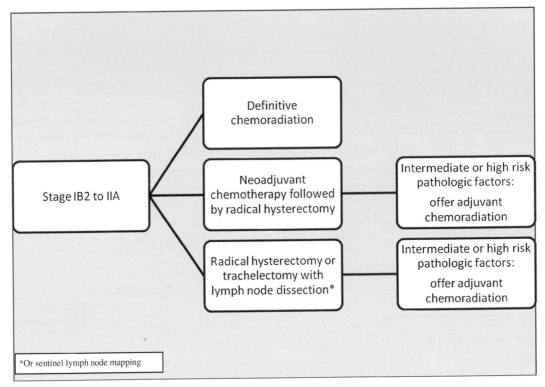

Fig. 5. Cervical Cancer. Stage IB2 to IIA.

randomized to radiation alone or in combination with cisplatin; all subjects subsequently underwent hysterectomy. Irradiation consisted of both external beam and intracavitary irradiation, reaching a dose of 75 cGy to point A (cervical parametrium) and 55 cGy to the lateral pelvis. Cisplatin (40 mg/m^2 weekly for 6 doses) was given during external irradiation. Hysterectomy was done 3 to 6 weeks after irradiation. In the preoperative combined treatment group, the progression free survival and overall survival rates were significantly higher, although there were more hematologic and gastrointestinal side effects. In addition, more patients in the combined group had no detectable cancer in the hysterectomy specimen (52% vs 41%, $P = .004$).[29] The role of hysterectomy following adjuvant therapy is controversial, and many contend that eliminating hysterectomy from the two treatment arms above would not have adversely affected survival for patients with bulky IB disease (larger than 4 cm). The current trend and preferred method is to combine radiotherapy with cisplatin-based chemotherapy for women with stage IB2 through IVA disease.

STAGE IIB - IVA LESIONS

It is recommended that women with stage IIB-IVA cervical cancer be treated initially with definitive chemoradiation. Surgical resection of these locally advanced tumors usually requires extended radical or ultra-radical resection of adjacent organs to secure negative margins; it is rarely if ever indicated as the initial treatment. Radiotherapy consists of a combination of external beam therapy followed by brachytherapy. External beam radiation usually delivers approximately 4500 cGy to the pelvis in 180 cGy daily fractions 5 days per week over 5 weeks to cover the primary tumor and the draining pelvic lymphatics. Brachytherapy, either intracavitary or interstitial, usually follows external beam therapy; this practice permits more central tumor mass reduction and, hopefully, normal reproductive organ anatomy for easier insertion of the implants and better tumor dosimetry. Intracavitary applicators with a tandem and two colpostats or ovoids (Fletcher or Henshkie) are most commonly used; however, interstitial implants (Syed-Neblett template) may be indicated for selected patients with more locally advanced tumors. Brachytherapy usually delivers an additional 4000 cGy to point A in one or two applications at 1- to 2-week intervals; in addition, parametrial boosts with external radiotherapy may be given as indicated. The complete course of radiotherapy is preferably completed within 8 weeks. The total dose prescribed varies depending on the tumor stage and size, but it usually ranges from 8500 cGy to 9000 cGy total dose to point A, keeping the bladder and the rectal dose limited to radiation tolerance. The availability of outpatient high-dose-rate brachytherapy may eliminate the need for hospitalization to deliver low-dose-rate brachytherapy.[30] Concomitant platinum-based chemotherapy with radiotherapy is generally well tolerated by most patients and has been shown to improve survival. Subsequently, it has become the standard of care in the United States (**Fig. 6**).

Three studies from the Gynecologic Oncology Group deserve mention. Morris and colleagues[31] studied women with stage IIB-IVA disease or stage IB or IIA disease with tumors larger than 5 cm or positive pelvic lymph nodes. The women were randomized to groups undergoing pelvic and paraaortic irradiation or pelvic irradiation and a fluorouracil/cisplatin regimen. The radiation dose was 45 Gy. Chemotherapy was given on days 1 through 5 and days 22 through 26. One or two applications of intracavitary radiation and a third cycle of chemotherapy were given. The 5-year survival was better (73% vs 58%, $P = .004$) for the combined-therapy group. In another study, women with stage IIB-IVA disease received external beam radiation and were also randomized into one of three chemotherapy arms.

1. Cisplatin 40 mg/m^2 per week for 6 weeks, or
2. Cisplatin 50 mg/m^2 on days 1 and 29 followed by 5-fluorouracil (5-Fu) 4 g/m^2 on days 1, 29, and hydroxyurea 2 g/m^2 twice weekly for 6 weeks
3. Hydroxyurea 3 g/m^2 twice weekly for 6 weeks.

The group receiving hydroxyurea alone had a lower rate of progression-free survival and a lower overall survival rate.[32] The survival advantage of cisplatin-based chemoradiation in stage IIB-IVA cervical carcinoma is further confirmed by another large, randomized Gynecologic Oncology Group-Southwest Oncology Group trial.[33]

RECURRENCE

Recurrent cervical cancer usually carries a poor prognosis, as no consistently effective salvage therapy is available. Ultra-radical pelvic surgery (pelvic exenteration) and radiotherapy may salvage some patients with isolated pelvic recurrences following primary irradiation or surgery, respectively. In addition, patients with isolated distant metastases in the lung or liver may be candidates for surgical resection provided the pelvis is tumor free. Unfortunately, many patients

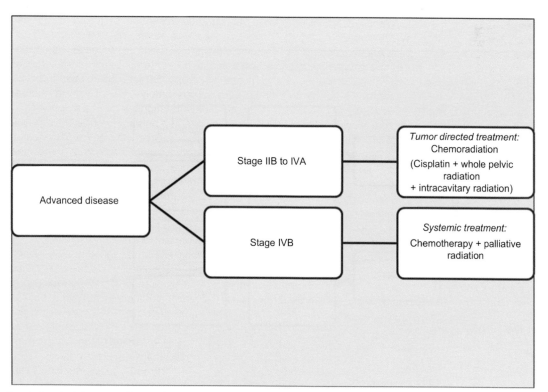

Fig. 6. Cervical Cancer. Advanced disease (Stage IIB to IVB).

with recurrent disease have unresectable cancer in a previously irradiated pelvis or have combined locoregional and distant metastases; these patients are usually treated with salvage cisplatin-based systemic chemotherapy, but have a poor overall outcome (**Fig. 7**).

Optimal candidates for pelvic exenteration are women who:

1. Were previously treated with definitive pelvic irradiation and have a small (<3 cm) localized central pelvic recurrence
2. Have a relatively long disease free interval (over 1 year)
3. Are medically and psychologically fit to undergo major pelvic surgery.

Permanent urinary and fecal diversions are usually needed.[34,35] Preoperative evaluation may include MRI, PET, or CT scans of the abdomen, pelvis, and chest. An exenteration is undertaken only if there is no evidence of distant disease. At the time of exploration, a thorough inspection for intraabdominal metastasis is performed, and a paraaortic lymph node biopsy specimen is sent for frozen section analysis, as are biopsy specimens of any enlarged pelvic lymph nodes. The paravesical and pararectal spaces are opened, and tumor fixation to the pelvic sidewall is assessed. If intra-abdominal, retroperitoneal, or pelvic-wall metastases are noted, the procedure is abandoned, as these patients tend to have a poor survival and should be spared a potentially highly morbid procedure. On the other hand, pelvic exenteration may provide a 5-year survival rate of approximately 30 to 50% in selected women with recurrent cervical cancer who successfully undergo the operation.[34,36] Laparoscopy may provide an alternative to laparotomy for initial assessment of resectability, and it may spare some patients (50%) laparotomy if distant disease is identified. Selected patients are candidates for anterior or posterior exenteration rather than total pelvic exenteration; the decision is made intraoperatively. **Table 2** summarizes the surgical approaches for management of centrally recurrent cervical cancer. Continent urinary diversion with a colonic reservoir and neovaginal reconstruction with myocutaneous flaps provide some patients with improved quality of life after pelvic exenteration. Low rectal reanastomosis following radical pelvic radiotherapy is associated with a high anastomotic leak rate; and, if performed, temporary intestinal diversion may be of benefit.[35]

As our knowledge and skills for treating cervical cancer improve, we should continue to seek the most effective and least morbid treatment modality, and our focus should remain on primary prevention. A proven and cost-effective screening

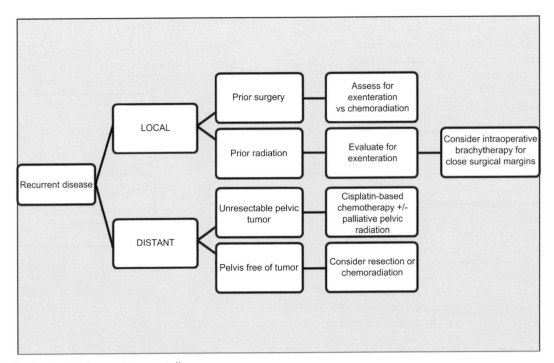

Fig. 7. Cervical Cancer. Recurrent disease.

Table 2
Surgical approaches to centrally recurrent cervical cancer in the pelvis

Tissue Removed	Anterior Exenteration	Posterior Exenteration	Total Exenteration
Bladder	Removed	Preserved	Removed
Vagina	Removed	Removed	Removed
Uterus	Removed	Removed	Removed
Adnexa	Removed	Removed	Removed
Parametria and paracolpos	Removed	Removed	Removed
Rectum	Preserved	Removed	Removed

tool (Pap smear) has been available for decades; and if it is made available on a regular basis to all women, advanced invasive disease may become one of the rarest malignancies in humans.

SUMMARY

Cervical cancer is one of the more common pelvic malignancies, and fortunately the death rate has dropped substantially because of early diagnosis (specifically Pap smear screening). Stage IA1 disease is rarely associated with lymph node metastases and therefore, may be treated conservatively in the appropriate candidate with excellent control rates. Higher stage disease (up to IIA) can be treated with surgery, chemoradiation, or a combination with comparable cure rates. Surgery consists of radical hysterectomy (ie, removal of the cervix, corpus, parametrial tissue, and upper third of the vagina) and node dissection of the iliac, obturator, and lower aortic regions. Sentinel lymph node mapping is an emerging technique that may improve the detection of micrometastases, while decreasing the morbidity of the surgical procedure. Surgery may be accomplished abdominally, vaginally, laparoscopically, or robotically. Radical trachelectomy is also an option in appropriate candidates who have a strong desire to maintain fertility. For patients with stage IIB and higher disease, surgery is rarely performed initially. Rather, external beam radiation and either interstitial or intracavitary irradiation are applied concomitantly with cisplatin based chemotherapy. Following treatment, patients with cervical cancer should have close follow-up on a regular basis. Most persistent or recurrent disease will manifest in the first 2 years after completion of therapy. Follow-up includes cytologic studies and biopsy of abnormal areas every 3 months the first 2 years, then every 6 months for 5 years, then every 6 to 12 months thereafter.

VULVA

EPIDEMIOLOGY AND ETIOLOGY

Vulvar cancer is a rare disease accounting for less than 5% of all gynecologic malignancies. It is estimated that in the year 2009, there will be 3,580 new cases and 900 deaths from vulvar cancer.[1] Vulvar cancer is comprised of a heterogenous group of malignancies, the majority of which are squamous cell carcinoma (86%), followed by basal cell carcinoma, verrucous carcinoma, malignant melanoma, and Paget's disease. They occur most frequently in post-menopausal women with a peak in the 8th decade of life.[37] In younger women with vulvar carcinoma, there tends to be an association with the human papilloma virus (HPV), specifically subtypes 16, 6, and 33.[38] Non-HPV related vulvar malignancies, which

> ### Key Features
> ### PATHOLOGIC REPORTING FOR VULVAR CARCINOMA
>
> Histology
>
> Tumor dimensions
>
>   Gross tumor diameter (for visible lesions)
>
>   Depth of stromal invasion
>
> Lymphovascular invasion
>
> Margin status with measurement of gross and microscopic margin clearance
>
> Lymph node assessment
>
>   Nodal counts
>
>   Nodal status (presence/absence of extracapsular extension)
>
> Presence of concurrent conditions (such as Lichen Sclerosus)

Pitfalls
IN DIAGNOSIS OF VULVAR CANCER

! Biopsy of any suspicious vulvar lesions is warranted. Clinical impression must be confirmed pathologically

! Diagnostic wide local excision of small (<1 cm) lesions is preferred

! Palpation of the groins is inferior to nodal biopsy in detecting metastatic disease

ultimately comprise the majority of invasive squamous carcinomas of the vulva, are commonly associated with chronic inflammatory conditions such as lichen sclerosus and vulvar dystrophy and are more common in older patients.[39] Mutations in tumor suppressor genes such as the *p53* mutation have also been implicated in the pathogenesis of vulvar carcinoma in tumors unassociated with HPV infection.[40] It is believed that the development of vulvar cancer is the result of multiple converging etiologic pathways.[41]

DIAGNOSIS

The most common presenting symptoms of vulvar carcinoma are:

Vulvar pruritus
Irritation
Pain
Vulvar mass
Non-healing lesion.

Enlarged, palpable groin lymph nodes are a rare presenting symptom associated with the presence of advanced disease. The majority of women have had long-term symptoms at the time of diagnosis.

On examination, an ulcerated, fleshy, discolored, or verrucous lesion may be present. When the diagnosis of a vulvar malignancy is suspected, a careful physical examination must be performed with attention to the size, location, and extension of the lesion. Specifically, measurements, assessment for invasion of surrounding structures, and a thorough lymph node examination must be performed. In addition, inspection, appropriate cytologic screening, and colposcopic evaluation of the cervix and vagina are also recommended. To rule out or confirm the diagnosis of malignancy, multiple biopsies from the primary lesion must be obtained, as lesions tend to be multifocal especially in younger patients. Biopsies should include both skin and some underlying connective tissue

so that pathologic depth may be assessed. If advanced stage disease is suspected, or if the primary tumor is large, other diagnostic procedures may be indicated such as: proctoscopy, cystourethroscopy, barium enema, intravenous pyelography, and CT scan. If distant metastases are suspected, fine needle aspiration may be used to confirm malignant spread.

STAGING

Staging of vulvar cancer is determined by assessment of the primary tumor during physical examination, lymph node involvement after surgical excision, and endoscopy in select cases.[42] In

Box 2
Vulvar cancer staging

Stage I Tumor confined to the vulva

IA Lesions ≤2 cm in size, confined to the vulva or perineum and with stromal invasion ≤1.0 mm, no modal metastases

IB Lesions >2 cm in size or with stromal invasion >1.0 mm, confined to the vulva or perineum, with negative nodes

Stage II Tumor of any size with extension to adjacent perineal structures (1/3 lower urethra, 1/3 lower vagina, anus) with negative nodes

Stage III Tumor of any size with or without extension to adjacent perineal structures (1/3 lower urethra, 1/3 lower vagina, anus) with positive inguina-femoral lymph nodes

IIIA (i) With 1 lymph node metastases (≥ 5 mm), or (ii) 1–2 lymph node metastasis(es) (<5 mm)

IIIB (i) With 2 lymph node metastases (≥ 5 mm), or (ii) 3 or more lymph node metastases (<5 mm)

IIIC With positive nodes with extracapsular spread

Stage IV Tumor invades other regional (2/3 upper urethra, 2/3 upper vagina), or distant structures

IVA Tumor invades any of the following:

(i) Upper urethra and/or vaginal mucosa, bladder mucosa, rectal mucosa, or fixed to pelvic bone, or

(ii) Fixed or ulcerated inguina-femoral lymph nodes

IVB Any distant metastases including pelvic lymph nodes

2009, the FIGO Committee on Gynecologic Oncology published a revised staging system for carcinoma of the vulva (**Box 2**). The distance from the epithelial – stromal junction of the adjacent most superficial dermal papilla to the deepest point of invasion is defined as the depth of invasion.[4] Vulvar carcinoma is theorized to spread in 3 ways: local direct growth and extension, lymphatic spread to regional nodes, and hematogenous dissemination. The vulvar lymphatics drain superiorly into the mons and then laterally into the superficial inguinal lymph nodes (between Camper's fascia and the fascia lata) of the ipsilateral groin. These superficial lymph nodes then drain through the cribriform fascia into the deep or femoral lymph nodes (medial to the femoral vein). Lateral lesions tend to reliably drain into the ipsilateral groin, however midline lesions will occasionally drain bilaterally.[43,44]

TREATMENT

As in the treatment of cervical cancer, the treatment of vulvar cancer depends mostly on the stage and extent of the spread of disease (**Fig. 8**).

STAGE I AND II DISEASE

In the case of microinvasive disease, defined as 1 mm or less invasion, wide local excision with a 1 cm tumor free margin is generally sufficient for a long-term cure.[45] In these patients, there is only a minimal risk of lymphatic dissemination (<1%) and therefore surgical evaluation of the groin is unnecessary.[46] For early stage (IB and II) disease, the traditional treatment is radical vulvectomy with bilateral inguinofemoral lymph node dissection. This procedure is generally performed through a "long-horn" or "butterfly" incision with en bloc removal of the entire vulva, dermal lymphatics, and both superficial and deep inguinal lymph nodes. The vast majority of patients (90%) experience excellent long-term survival and local

control after this treatment. However, this procedure is associated with a significant degree of morbidity including loss of normal anatomy and sexual function, a 50% risk of wound breakdown, a 30% risk of groin complications, and a 10 or 15% chance of lymphedema.[47,48] It is for this reason that great efforts have been taken to develop a suitable, less invasive surgical option. Resection of the primary lesion with at least a 1 cm margin combined with a limited groin dissection has been suggested as an alternative to the more radical traditional approach.[49,50]

A solitary, unilateral lesion 2 cm or less in size with stromal invasion 1 mm or less does not require surgical evaluation of the lymph nodes. Multifocal lesions, lesions greater than 2 cm in size, or with greater than 1 mm of stromal invasion require radical excision and ipsilateral lymphadenectomy. In these cases, if the tumor is greater than 2 cm in diameter, greater than 5 mm in depth, or if any positive ipsilateral lymph nodes are detected it is recommended that the patient undergo a contralateral inguinofemoral lymphadenectomy as well. Bilateral inguinofemoral lymphadenectomy is recommended in all patients with midline (within 1 cm) or bilateral lesions.[51] Risk factors for groin node metastases include clinically enlarged nodes, lymphovascular space invasion, tumor grade, age, and depth of invasion.[52] Sentinel lymph node mapping is another technique that can be performed as an alternative to traditional radical lymphadenectomy. The goal of sentinel lymph node mapping is to detect the first draining lymph node from the primary lesion thereby eliminating the need to assess any further lymph nodes. Sentinel lymph node mapping is best suited for physicians experienced with sentinel lymph node evaluation and in patients with unifocal, unilateral lesions smaller than 4 cm in size, who have had no previous vulvar surgery.[53] Adjuvant radiation has been suggested in high risk patients – those with primary tumors 4.1 cm or greater in diameter, positive margins, or lymphovascular space invasion. However, attempts at re-excision should be made if margins are positive after initial surgery.

STAGE III AND IV

Radical surgery such as radical vulvectomy and pelvic exenteration may remain an option for patients with advanced vulvar cancer, however commonly a combined modality approach using surgical resection, radiation, and/or chemotherapy is indicated. Radiation can be used preoperatively in bulky lesions to improve the likelihood of complete surgical resection. After surgical

---

Key Features
TREATMENT POINTS FOR VULVAR CANCER

1. Biopsy and wide local excision are paramount for proper diagnosis

2. The local procedure should aim at obtaining at least a 1 cm negative pathologic margin

3. Assessment of groin nodes is important in patients who have greater than 1 mm invasive lesions

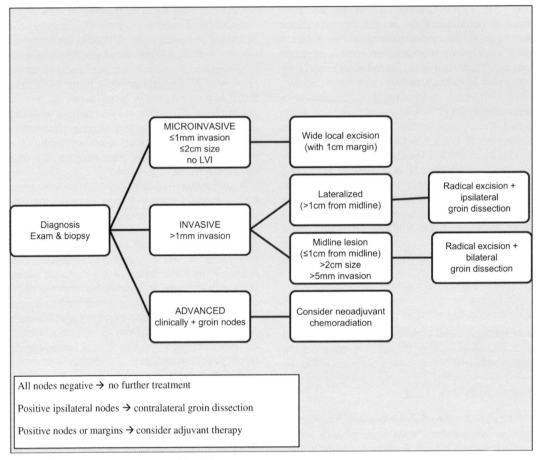

Fig. 8. Vulvar Cancer. Management Algorithm.

resection, some investigators recommend adjuvant radiation in patients with 2 or more microscopically involved lymph nodes, 1 or more macroscopically involved lymph nodes, extracapsular spread, or limited sampling.[54,55] However, all patients with positive lymph nodes or positive margins should be considered for adjuvant therapy. Primary treatment with chemoradiation is an alternative in patients who are poor surgical candidates, have inoperable locally advanced tumors (anorectal or bladder involvement or tumor fixed to bone). However, chemoradiation has significant morbidities and should be considered after surgical options are explored.

RECURRENT DISEASE

Lymph node status, margin status, and depth of invasion are all factors independently associated with the risk of recurrence. Local recurrences can be managed with surgical resection alone. In these cases, if a negative clinical margin can be

obtained up to 75% of patients will be cured.[56] Unfortunately, many patients recur in either the groin or in distant sites and have a much less favorable prognosis. Radiation and systemic chemotherapy are treatment options in these patients.

SUMMARY

Vulvar carcinoma is a rare gynecologic malignancy that mainly affects post-menopausal women. The symptoms often go unreported and delay in diagnosis is one of the most significant obstacles in treatment. Thorough examination including assessment of lymph nodes, as well as multiple biopsies of any suspicious lesions should be promptly performed in any patient with a suspicious lesion. In patients with clinically early disease, radical excision and an individualized approach to limited inguinofemoral lymphadenectomy is the preferred treatment to minimize surgical and psychosexual morbidity and improve detection of lymph node metastases. In more advanced disease, chemoradiation is the recommended primary treatment. Advances in the treatment of vulvar malignancy have allowed for individualization of treatment and a decrease in the overall morbidity of the treatment.

REFERENCES

1. Jemal A, Siegel R, Ward E, et al. Cancer statistics, 2009. CA Cancer J Clin 2009;59(4):225–49.
2. Viscidi RP, Schiffman M, Hildesheim A, et al. Seroreactivity to human papillomavirus (HPV) types 16, 18, or 31 and risk of subsequent HPV infection: results from a population based study in Costa Rica. Cancer Epidemiol Biomarkers Prev 2004;13: 324–7.
3. Jones WB, Shingleton HM, Russell AH, et al. Patterns for invasive cervical cancer: results of a national survey of 1984 and 1990. Cancer 1995; 76:1934–47.
4. FIGO Committee on Gynecologic Oncology. Revised FIGO staging for carcinoma of the vulva, cervix, and endometrium. Int J Gynaecol Obstet 2009;105:103–4.
5. Society of Gynecologic Oncology. Clinical practice guidelines: cervical cancer. Oncology 1998;12: 134–8.
6. Morris M, Mitchell MF, Silva EG, et al. Cervical conization as definitive therapy for early invasive squamous carcinoma of the cervix. Gynecol Oncol 1993;51:193–6.
7. Benedet JL, Anderson GH. Stage IA carcinoma of the cervix revisited. Obstet Gynecol 1996;87: 1052–9.
8. Ostos AG. Studies on 200 cases of early squamous cell carcinoma of the cervix. Int J Gynecol Pathol 1993;12:193–207.
9. Wolf JK, Levenback C, Malpica A, et al. Adenocarcinoma in situ of the cervix: significance of cone biopsy margins. Obstet Gynecol 1996;88: 82–6.
10. Poynor EA, Barakat RR, Hoskins WJ. Management and follow-up of patients with adenocarcinoma in situ of the uterine cervix. Gynecol Oncol 1995;57: 158–64.
11. Im DD, Duska LR, Rosenshein NB. Adequacy of conization margins in adenocarcinoma in situ of the cervix as a predictor of residual disease. Gynecol Oncol 1995;59:179–82.
12. Ostor A, Roma R, Quinn M. Microinvasive adenocarcinoma of the cervix: a clinicopathologic study of 77 women. Obstet Gynecol 1997;89:88–93.
13. Spirtos NM, Schlaerth JB, Kimball RE, et al. Laparoscopic radical hysterectomy (tyle III) with aortic and pelvic lymphadenectomy. Am J Obstet Gynecol 1996;174:1763–7 [discussion: 1767–8].

14. Renaud MC, Plante M, Roy M. Combined laparoscopic and vaginal radical surgery in cervical cancer. Gynecol Oncol 2000;79:59–63.
15. Roy M, Plante M, Renaud MC, et al. Vaginal radical hysterectomy versus abdominal radical hysterectomy in the treatment of early stage cervical cancer. Gynecol Oncol 1996;62:336–9.
16. Schneider A, Possover M, Kamprath S, et al. Laparoscopy-assisted radical vaginal hysterectomy modified according to Schauta-Stoeckel. Obstet Gynecol 1996;88:1057–60.
17. Querleu D. Laparoscopically assisted radical vaginal hysterectomy. Gynecol Oncol 1993;51:248–54.
18. Dargent D, Martin X, Sacchetoni A, et al. Laparoscopic vaginal radical trachelectomy: a treatment to preserve the fertility of cervical carcinoma patients. Cancer 2000;88:1877–82.
19. Morrow CP, Curtin JP. Surgery for cervical neoplasia. In: Mitchell J, Hardy J, Birch DJ, editors. Gynecol cancer surgery. New York: Churchhill Livingstone Inc; 1996. p. 451–568.
20. DiSaia PJ. Surgical aspects of cervical carcinoma. Cancer 1981;48:548–59.
21. Piver SM, Rutledge F, Smith JP. Five classes of extended hysterectomy for women with cervical cancer. Obstet Gynecol 1974;44:265–72.
22. Abu-Rustum NR, Sonoda Y, Black D, et al. Fertility sparing radical trachelectomy for cervical carcinoma: technique and review of the literature. Gynecol Oncol 2006;103:807–13.
23. Diaz JP, Sonoda Y, Leitao MM, et al. Oncologic outcome of fertility-sparing radical trachelectomy versus radical hysterectomy for stage IB1 cervical carcinoma. Gynecol Oncol 2008;111:255–60.
24. Peters WA 3rd, Liu PY, Barrett RJ 2nd, et al. Concurrent chemotherapy and pelvic radiation therapy compared with pelvic radiation therapy alone as adjuvant treatment after radical surgery in high-risk early-stage cancer of the cervix. J Clin Oncol 2000;18:1606–13.
25. Sedlis A, Bundy BN, Rotman MZ, et al. A randomized trial of pelvic radiation versus no further treatment in selected patients with stage IB carcinoma of the cervix after radical hysterectomy and pelvic lymphadenectomy: a Gynecologic Oncology Group study. Gynecol Oncol 1999;73:177–83.
26. Sutton GP, Bundy BN, Delgado G, et al. Ovarian metastases in stage IB carcinoma of the cervix: a Gynecologic Oncology Group study. Am J Obstet Gynecol 1992;166:50–3.
27. Hoskins WJ. Prognostic factors for risk of recurrence in stage IB and IIA cervical cancer. Baillieres Clin Obstet Gynaecol 1988;2:817–28.
28. Dargent D, Frobert L, Beau G. V factor (tumor volume) and T factor (FIGO classification) is the assessment of cervix cancer prognosis: the risk of lymph node spread. Gynecol Oncol 1985;22:15–22.

29. Keys HM, Bundy BN, Stehman FB, et al. Cisplatin radiation, and adjuvant hysterectomy compared with radiation and adjuvant hysterectomy for bulky stage IB cervical carcinoma. N Engl J Med 1999; 340:1154–61.

30. Stehman FB, Perez CA, Kurman RJ, Thigpen JT. Uterine cervix. In: Hoskins WJ, Perez CA, Young RC, editors. Principles and practice of gynecologic oncology. 2nd edition. Philadelphia: Lippincott-Raven; 1997. p. 758–858.

31. Morris M, Eifel PJ, Lu J, et al. Pelvic radiation with concurrent chemotherapy compared with pelvic and paraaortic radiation for high-risk cervical cancer. N Engl J Med 1999;340:1137–43.

32. Rose PG, Bundy BN, Watkins EB, et al. Concurrent cisplatin-based radiotherapy and chemotherapy for locally advanced cervical cancer. N Engl J Med 1999;340:1144–53.

33. Whitney CW, Sause W, Bundy BN, et al. Randomized comparison of fluorouracil plus cisplatin versus hydroxyurea as an adjunct to radiation therapy in stage IIB-IVA carcinoma of the cervix with negative paraaortic lymph nodes: a Gynecologic Oncology Group and Southwest Oncology Group study. J Clin Oncol 1999;17:1339–48.

34. Barber HR. Relative prognostic significance of preoperative and operative findings in pelvic exenteration. Surg Clin North Am 1969;49:431–47.

35. Shingleton HM, Soong SJ, Gelder MS, et al. Clinical and histopathologic factors predicting recurrence and survival after pelvic exenteration for cancer of the cervix. Obstet Gynecol 1989;73:1027–34.

36. Curtin JP, Hoskins WJ. Pelvic exenteration for gynecologic cancers. Surg Oncol Clin N Am 1994;3:267–76.

37. Beller U, Sideri M, Maisonneuve P, et al. Carcinoma of the vagina. J Epidemiol Biostat 2001;6:153–74.

38. Kurman RJ, Trimble CL, Shah KV. Human papilloma virus and the pathogenesis of vulvar carcinoma. Curr Opin Obstet Gynecol 1992;4:582–5.

39. Carli P, De Magnis A, Mannine F, et al. Vulvar carcinoma associated with lichen sclerosis: experience at the Florence, Italy vulvar clinic. J Reprod Med 2003;48:313–8.

40. Hietanen SH, Kurvinen K, Syrjanen K, et al. Mutation of tumor suppressor gene p53 is frequently found in vulvar carcinoma cells. Am J Obstet Gynecol 1995; 173:1477–9.

41. Trimble CL, Hildesheim A, Brinton LA, et al. Heterogenous etiology of squamous carcinoma of the vulva. Obstet Gynecol 1996;87:59–64.

42. Beahrs OH, Henson DE, Hutter RV, et al, editors. Manual for staging of cancer. 4th edition. Philadelphia: JB Lippincott; 1992. p. 177–80.

43. Parry-Jones E. Lymphatics of the vulva. J Obstet Gynaecol Br Emp 1963;70:751–5.

44. Iverson T, Aas M. Lymph drainage from the vulva. Gynecol Oncol 1983;16:179–82.

45. Kelley JL III, Burke TW, Tornos C, et al. Minimally invasive vulvar carcinoma: an indication for conservative surgical therapy. Gynecol Oncol 1991;144: 240–5.

46. Farias-Eisner R, Cirisano FD, Grouse D, et al. Conservative and individualized surgery for early squamous carcinoma of the vulva: the treatment of choice for stage I and II (T12-2N0-1M0) disease. Gynecol Oncol 1994;53:55.

47. Figge CD, Gaudenz R. Invasive carcinoma of the vulva. Am J Obstet Gynecol 1974;119:382–7.

48. Rutledge F, Smith JP, Franklin EW. Carcinoma of the vulva. Am J Obstet Gynecol 1970;106:1117–21.

49. DeHulla JA, Hollema H, Lolkema S, et al. Vulvar carcinoma. The price of less radical surgery. Cancer 2002;95:2331.

50. Stehman FB, Bundy BN, Dvoretsky PM, et al. Early stage I carcinoma of the vulva treated with ipsilateral superficial inguinal lymphadenectomy and modified radical hemivulvectomy: a prospective study of the Gynecologic Oncology Group. Obstet Gynecol 1992;79:490–4.

51. Bosquet JG, Magrina JF, Magtibay PM, et al. Patterns of inguinal groin metastases in squamous cell carcinoma of the vulva. Gynecol Oncol 2007;105:742–6.

52. Homesley HD, Bundy BN, Sedlis A, et al. Prognostic factors for groin node metastasis in squamous cell carcinoma of the vulva (a Gynecology Oncology Group study). Gynecol Oncol 1993;49:279.

53. Hampl M, Hantschmann P, Michels W, et al. Validation of the accuracy of the sentinel lymph node procedure in patients with vulvar cancer: results of a multicenter study in Germany. Gynecol Oncol 2008;111:282–8.

54. Parthasarathy A, Cheung MK, Osann K, et al. The benefit of adjuvant radiation therapy in single node positive squamous cell vulvar carcinoma. Gynecol Oncol 2006;103:1095.

55. DeHulla JA, van der Zee AG. Surgery and radiotherapy in vulvar cancer. Crit Rev Oncol Hematol 2006;60:38.

56. Hopkins MP, Reid GC, Morley GW. The surgical management of recurrent squamous cell carcinoma of the vulva. Obstet Gynecol 1990;75:1001–7.

NEOPLASTIC LESIONS OF THE CERVIX

Kay J. Park, MD

KEYWORDS
- Cervical cancer • Neoplastic lesions • HPV • Invasive squamous carcinoma
- Glandular neoplasms

ABSTRACT

This review presents a discussion of the gross and microscopic features, diagnosis, differential diagnosis, and prognosis of neoplastic lesions of the cervix. Biomarkers are discussed for each entity presented – cervical intraepithelial neoplasia, squamous carcinoma, glandular neoplasms, adenocarcinoma in situ, adenosquamous carcinoma, and others.

SQUAMOUS NEOPLASTIC LESIONS OF THE CERVIX

CERVICAL INTRAEPITHELIAL NEOPLASIA AND INVASIVE SQUAMOUS CARCINOMA

Cervical dysplasia is caused by Human Papillomavirus (HPV) infection of low or high oncogenic risk type. Infection by low risk HPV may result in low grade dysplasia/cervical intraepithelial neoplasia (CIN) 1, the majority of which will regress if left untreated. Approximately 30% of low grade lesions persist while only 10% progress to high grade dysplasia within 2 years.[1–3] High grade lesions are precursors to invasive squamous carcinoma with a probability of progression to invasion greater than 12% over 10 to 20 years.[2] Condyloma acuminatum (genital wart) is a benign lesion that is also associated with low risk HPV; most commonly types 6 and 11. High risk HPV infection results in either high grade or low grade dysplasia, with approximately 50% of low grade lesions being associated with high risk HPV.[4,5] The epithelial alterations that define CIN 1, 2 and 3 are well defined with neoplastic basaloid cells involving the lower third, lower third to two-thirds and two-thirds to full thickness of the squamous epithelium, respectively. However, studies have shown that there is great variation in interobserver variability in both identifying lesions and in assigning a grade.[6] Ancillary immunohistochemical stains have been shown to be useful in decreasing the variability.

CERVICAL INTRAEPITHELIAL NEOPLASIA (SPECTRUM OF DYSPLASIA AND CARCINOMA IN-SITU)

Cervical intraepithelial neoplasia is classified on a three-tiered grading system based on the level of immature cellular proliferation of the squamous epithelium, cytologic atypia and mitotic activity: low grade squamous intraepithelial lesions (LSIL)/CIN 1 and high grade squamous intraepithelial lesions (HSIL)/CIN 2 and CIN 3.

Gross Features

Dysplastic lesions are usually within the cervical transformation zone but may also extend into the endocervical canal or mature squamous epithelium. Condylomata can also affect the mature squamous epithelium. Lesions can be visualized at colposcopy and can show a variety of gross appearances. Low grade lesions are typically flat with a smooth surface, except for condyloma acuminatum, which has an exophytic, warty, papillary-like appearance. The application of 3 to 5% acetic acid or Lugol's iodine will highlight the abnormal areas. LSILs can appear white (leukoplakia) even before application of acetic acid and are characterized by indistinct borders. There may be fine mosaicism or punctuation with a regular pattern of vascular changes with equal intercapillary distances. High grade lesions will typically have sharply demarcated edges and lack the geographic or indistinct margins of LSIL. They may have raised, rolled or peeling borders and display

Department of Pathology, Memorial Sloan Kettering Cancer Center, 1275 York Avenue, New York, NY 10065, USA
E-mail address: ParkK@MSKCC.ORG

Surgical Pathology 4 (2011) 17–86
doi:10.1016/j.path.2010.12.006
1875-9181/11/$ – see front matter © 2011 Elsevier Inc. All rights reserved.

a dense, dull acetowhitening due to increased nuclear density and less reflection of incident light. The vascular pattern is more coarse than that seen in LSIL, with punctuation, mosaicism and umbilicated patterns. These areas will appear less white.

Microscopic Features and Diagnosis

Condyloma acuminatum is a low grade lesion with a papillary, warty appearance, both grossly and histologically. The papillae consist of fibrovascular cores lined by atypical cells resembling those seen in LSIL. The lesions commonly display hyperkeratosis, acanthosis, dyskeratosis and parakeratosis. Koilocytosis and bi- or multinucleation are common **Fig. 1**. Condylomata are much more common in the vulva and vagina than in the cervix where flat low grade lesions predominate.

LSIL/CIN 1 is characterized by a proliferation of immature basal/parabasal squamous cells and mitotic figures that extend no higher than the lower

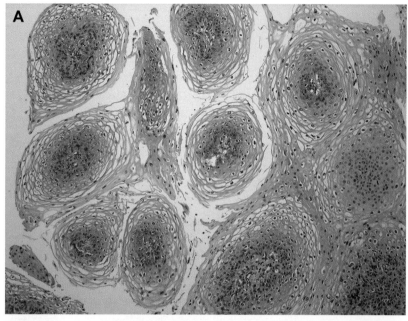

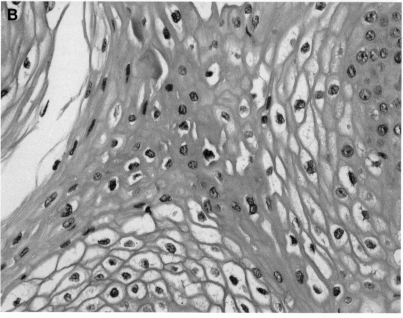

Fig. 1. Condyloma acuminatum.

Fig. 2. CIN 1 (koilocytes).

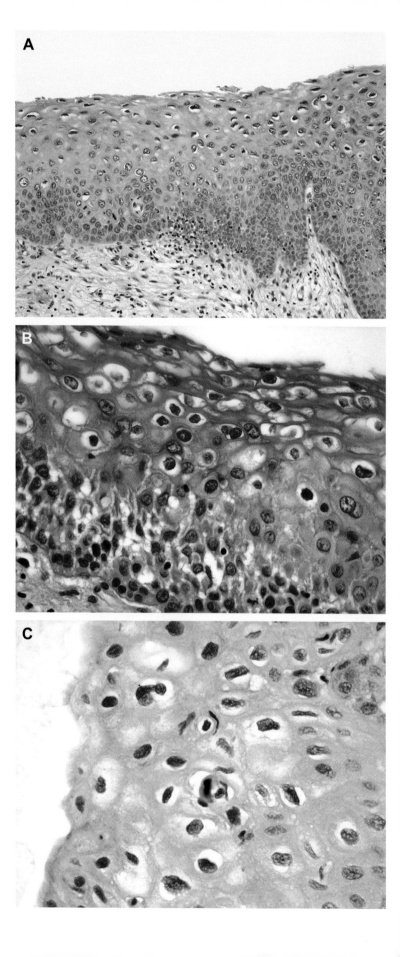

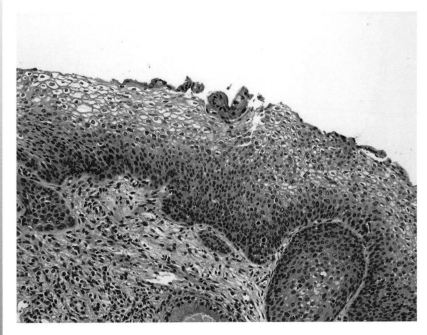

Fig. 3. CIN 2.

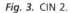

CINI should
not have abnormal or
any mitoses above
lower 1/3

one third of the thickness of the epithelium. The surface cells display nuclear enlargement, irregular nuclear contours, nuclear hyperchromasia and often have a clear cytoplasmic halo surrounding the nuclei (koilocytotic effect) **Fig. 2**. These histologic changes signify a productive viral infection and the nuclei of these lesions are packed with newly formed viral particles that are ready to be shed and infect other cells. CIN 1 lesions should not have any abnormal mitotic figures or mitoses above the lower one-third of the epithelium.

HSIL/CIN 2 is characterized by increased proliferation of immature basal squamous cells that extend above the lower one-third but not beyond two-thirds of the epithelial thickness **Fig. 3**. These lesions can also show some koilocytotic nuclear features which can sometimes make distinguishing CIN 2 and CIN 1 difficult. Studies of cytology

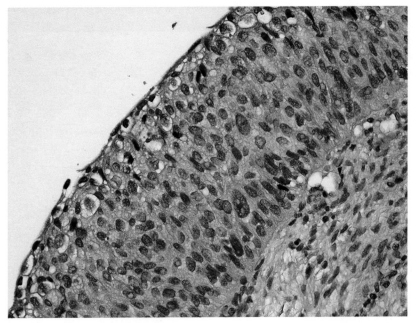

Fig. 4. CIN 3.

Fig. 5. HSIL with multi-nucleation/ and markedly enlarged nuclei.

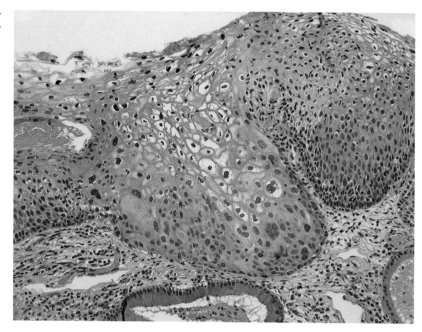

and routine histology sections have shown that the diagnosis of CIN 1 and 2 is not as consistent as normal squamous epithelium or CIN 3.[7]

HSIL/CIN 3 (carcinoma in-situ) is characterized by greater than two-thirds to full thickness involvement of the epithelium by immature basal cells **Fig. 4**. At the molecular level, viral DNA has been integrated into the host DNA and,

therefore, these are no longer productive viral infections. Therefore, the typical nuclear features of low grade lesions may not be present. High grade lesions (CIN 2 and CIN 3) can also be characterized by atypical mitotic figures, markedly enlarged nuclei (greater than 5 times the size of a parabasal cell) and multinucleation with 5 or more nuclei **Fig. 5**.[8]

Fig. 6. Atypical immature metaplasia.

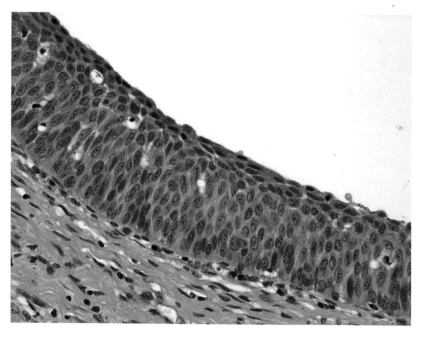

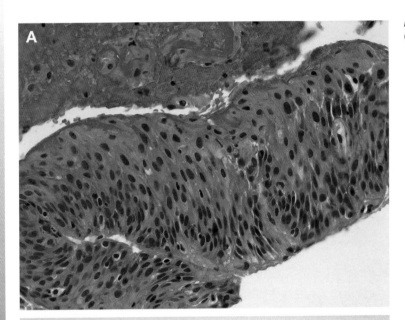

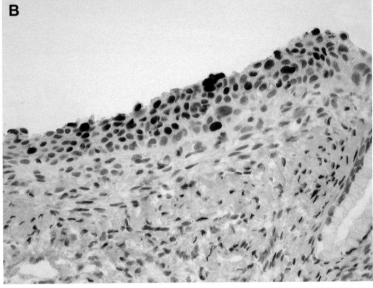

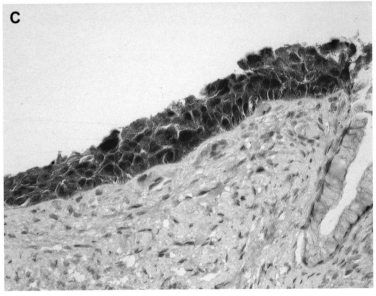

Fig. *7.* Eosinophilic dysplasia (*A*), MIB-1 (*B*), p16 (*C*).

CIN variant lesions

There are some morphologic variants of squamous dysplastic lesions that may pose diagnostic difficulties.

Atypical immature metaplasia

Atypical immature metaplasia (AIM) is an entity that was first described by Crum and colleagues[9] in 1983 and by their description, was a lesion similar to condyloma, ie, a low grade lesion. It is a loosely defined term that has shifted in meaning over the years and now includes lesions that span the spectrum from benign metaplasias to high grade dysplasia. There is lack of a uniform definition and inconsistencies in morphologic criteria that perpetuate this confusion. Studies have shown that AIM can be HPV positive or negative, variably positive with p16 and display a large range of proliferative rates with Mib-1/Ki-67 (see text on biomarkers below).[10–12] HPV and p16 positive AIM

Fig. 8. Benign LSIL mimic (*A, B*).

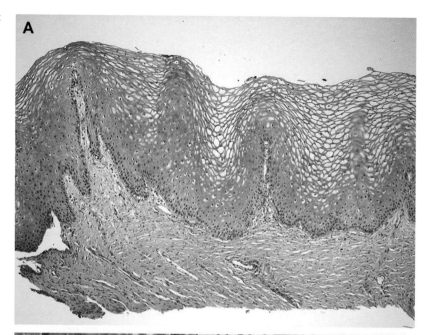

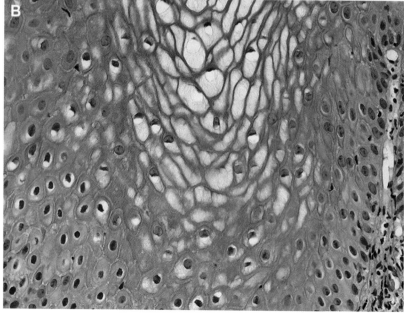

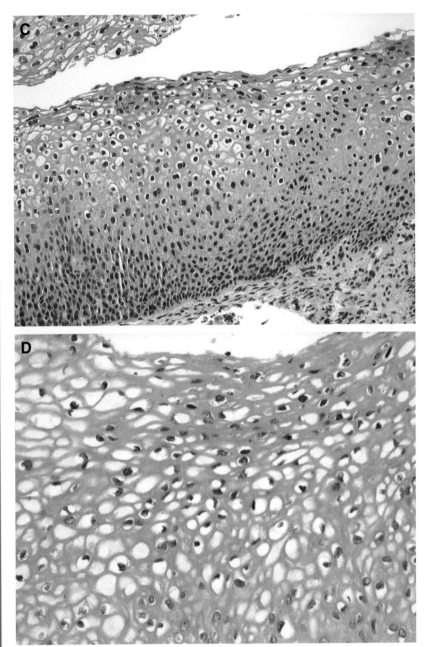

Fig. 8. LSIL (*C, D*).

lesions have been shown to be followed subsequently by bona fide HSIL. HPV and p16 positive AIMs with low Mib-1 labeling might represent early or regressing SILs. Therefore, atypical immature metaplasia represents a spectrum of processes that are difficult for pathologists to recognize by histology alone **Fig. 6**.

Eosinophilic dysplasia (ED)

Another variant described by Ma and colleagues[13] is so-called eosinophilic dysplasia.

This is a descriptive term that has been used for intraepithelial lesions showing both squamous metaplasia and dysplasia. These are considered different from AIM due to the significant amount of cytoplasmic maturation and presence of clearly demonstrable dysplastic features. The histologic features are as follows: nuclei 2- to 3-fold larger than normal basal cells; nuclear to cytoplasmic ratio only mildly to moderately increased due to the presence of moderate to abundant cytoplasm; focal hyperchromasia with slightly coarse chromatin and mildly irregular nuclear contours; variable nucleoli; absence of usual HSIL features such as coarse clumped chromatin and frank nuclear membrane irregularity **Fig. 7**. Mitotic figures may not be present. ED is always adjacent to squamous metaplasia and almost always adjacent to conventional LSIL or HSIL. Intermediate or high risk HPV has been detected in ED, supporting that these are in fact truly dysplastic lesions. Because of the lack of obvious histologic features of dysplasia, ED can be misinterpreted as a benign metaplastic process and there is high interobserver variability in the diagnosis of these lesions.[13] Immunohistochemistry can be very useful in the diagnosis of ED since the majority of the lesions are diffusely and strongly positive for p16 and hyper-proliferative with Mib-1.[13] If the immunostains do not support an HPV associated lesion, a diagnosis of atypical metaplasia is sufficient.

Fig. 9. Squamous atrophy (*A*) versus HSIL (*B*).

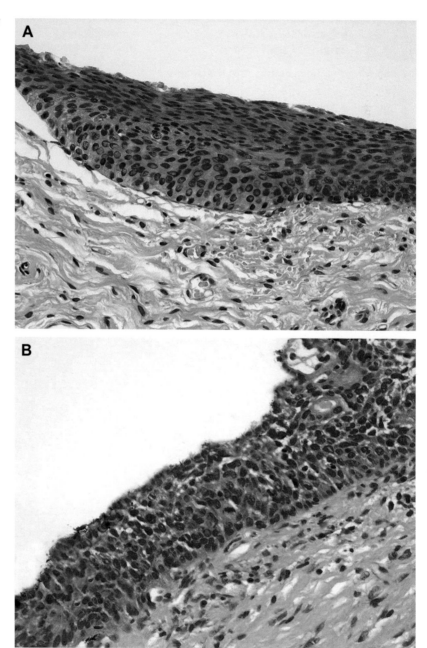

Differential Diagnosis

The differential diagnoses for each lesion are listed in the Differential Diagnosis box for Squamous Neoplastic Lesions of the Cervix that follows. Information regarding the use of immunohistochemistry for differential diagnosis is contained in the subsequent "Biomarkers" section.

Squamous papillomas are benign lesions that usually occur in clusters near the hymenal ring (vulva). Although they may be difficult to differentiate from condylomata grossly, they lack the complex arborizing architecture and koilocytes of condyloma and are not associated with HPV infection.

Mild cytologic changes that occur in normal squamous epithelium can be misinterpreted as LSIL. These include cytoplasmic glycogenation or vacuolization, which can mimic koilocytosis, slight nuclear enlargement due to inflammation, and metaplastic changes. These benign alterations, however, do not have the marked nuclear enlargement, irregular nuclear contours, nuclear hyperchromasia, basal cell proliferation and increased mitotic activity of true low grade lesions **Fig. 8**.

Squamous atrophy can be confused with HSIL due to the loss of cytoplasm which increases the nucleus to cytoplasm ratio and imparts a dark, immature appearance at low power. However, on closer examination, the cells are not enlarged, the nuclei are smooth with regular borders, they do not overlap and there are no mitotic figures **Fig. 9**.

Squamous metaplasia can also mimic both low grade and high grade lesions, depending on the level of cytologic atypia and amount of cytoplasm. Background inflammation can enhance the cytologic atypia and even increase mitotic activity, further obscuring the true nature of the lesion. Again, this benign process does not have the nuclear pleomorphism, loss of cell polarity, nuclear hyperchromasia or clumped chromatin of HSIL and in a reactive setting, may show prominent nucleoli which are not typically seen in squamous dysplasia **Fig. 10**.

ΔΔ Differential Diagnosis
SQUAMOUS NEOPLASTIC LESIONS OF THE CERVIX

- Condyloma acuminatum versus squamous papilloma
- LSIL versus benign squamous mucosa with glycogenization and "pseudokoilocytosis"
- LSIL versus reactive atypia
- LSIL versus atypical or immature squamous metaplasia
- HSIL versus atrophy
- LSIL versus HSIL
- HSIL versus atypical or immature squamous metaplasia
- HSIL versus urothelial carcinoma involving the cervix

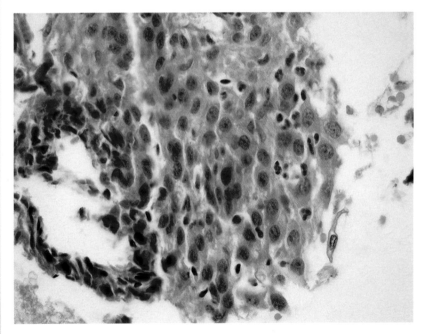

Fig. 10. Reactive atypia with prominent nucleoli and background inflammation.

Urothelial carcinoma from the genitourinary tract, including bladder, ureters and renal pelvis, can extend into the gynecologic tract and involve various sites. It can present as Paget's disease of the vulva or vagina and also extend into the cervix and endometrial cavity, mimicking gynecologic primaries.[14–21] When urothelial carcinoma involves cervical mucosa in a superficial spreading pattern, it can easily mimic a high grade lesion and without the appropriate clinical information, can lead to incorrect diagnosis and treatment **Fig. 11.**

Biomarkers

There are many immunohistochemical studies that can be used to help distinguish between dysplasia and benign mimics. The biomarkers used in HPV associated lesions are based on the proliferative and oncogenic activity of the virus in the host cell.

HPV

The human papillomavirus is a doubled-stranded DNA virus of approximately 8000 base pairs covered by a protein capsid shell composed of

Fig. 11. Urothelial carcinoma involving cervix mimicking CIN.

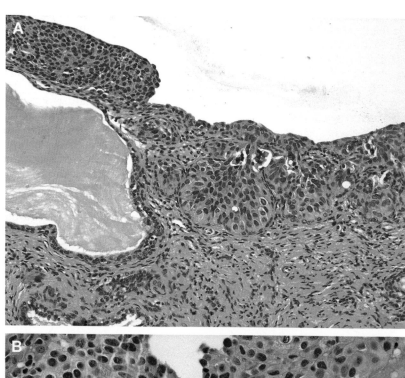

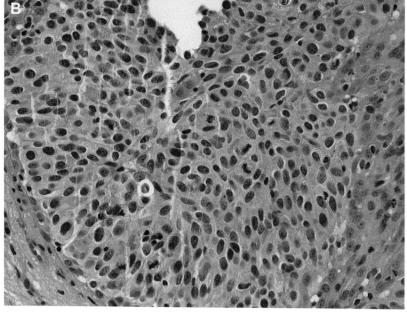

[handwritten margin note: p16 overexpressed when Hr HPV integrates with cell genome. Gives diffuse strong cytoplasmic and or nuclear staining]

two proteins L1 and L2. The genes are divided into early (E1, E2, E4, E5, E6 and E7) and late genes (L1 and L2), encoding transcriptional and structural proteins, respectively. There is also the Long Control Region (LCR), the point of origin of DNA replication and regulation of HPV gene expression. E6 and E7 are the two oncogenic proteins which destroy host cell p53 (E6) and inactivate host cell pRb (E7) **Fig. 12**.

P16INK4a

P16INK4a is a tumor suppressor gene that encodes a protein involved in cell cycle regulation.[22] P16 is a cyclin dependent kinase (CDK) 4 inhibitor and a product of the INK4a gene on chromosome 9 (9p21) which specifically binds to cyclin D-CDK4/6 complexes to control the cell cycle at the G1-S interphase. When p16 binds to CDK, this prevents the phosphorylation of pRb, subsequently preventing cell cycle activation and setting up a negative feedback loop with pRb so that cell proliferation is held in check **Fig. 13**. When high risk HPV DNA integrates into the host cell genome, the viral oncoprotein E7 binds to pRb, rendering it inactive and as a result, the feedback loop is lost and p16 is overexpressed **Fig. 13**. This manifests as diffuse, strong, cytoplasmic and or/nuclear staining in squamous and glandular lesions associated with high risk

HPV infection. It is now well established that p16 is a robust surrogate marker for infection with high risk HPV in high grade CIN lesions.[22–29] P16 expression can be seen in 57% to 87.5% of LSILs and 84% to 100% of HSILs.[22–24,29] P16 overexpression is also a marker of E7 gene activity.

High grade lesions will usually have a strong, diffuse, band-like positivity for p16, either nuclear or cytoplasmic or both. The staining can be full or partial thickness but maintains the strong diffuse pattern in most cases **Fig. 14**. LSILs tend to show partial thickness staining, however, they can also show full thickness, diffuse staining and, therefore, the pattern of staining is not generally used to grade the lesion **Fig. 15**.[29] In some instances, both high and low grade lesions can show only focal strong p16 staining, as can other benign processes like normal squamous epithelium and squamous metaplasia. Therefore, focal p16 staining should not be considered as evidence of a high-risk HPV associated lesion. Furthermore, p16 staining can be seen in non-HPV related lesions of cervical and non-cervical tissues and, therefore, the interpretation of the results is highly dependent on the context.

If the differential diagnosis is between HSIL and urothelial carcinoma, p16 may not necessarily be very helpful since urothelial carcinoma can have diffuse strong staining with the marker.[30,31]

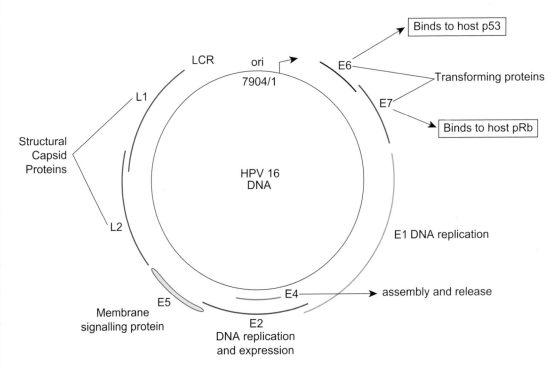

HPV DNA : Double stranded DNA N 8000 base pairs
LCR : Long control region

Fig. 12. HPV DNA.

Fig. 13. (A) Diagram of the role of p16 in normal cell cycle; (B) Diagram of p16 with HPV infection.

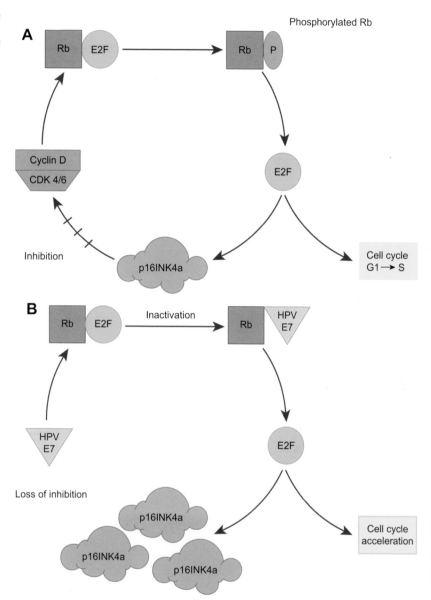

Mib-1/Ki-67

Mib-1 is a monoclonal antibody that targets the Ki-67 antigen, a cellular proliferation marker that is detected during all active phases of the cell cycle (G1, S, G2 and mitosis). In normal and metaplastic squamous epithelium, Mib-1 positivity is confined to the parabasal cell layer.[32] Since HPV associated lesions have an increased rate of cellular proliferation as compared with normal squamous or glandular epithelium, Mib-1 can be used to detect the increased activity and distinguish benign atypia from dysplasia **Fig. 16**.[32] The parabasal cells of squamous mucosa and any inflammatory cells present serve at positive internal controls and should always show positive staining with Mib-1. In squamous intraepithelial lesions, Mib-1 expression is increased in the parabasal cells and extends to the intermediate and superficial layers.[32–34] Typically, a Mib-1 stain is considered abnormal or increased when a cluster of at least two strongly stained epithelial nuclei are present in the upper two thirds of the epithelium.[34–36] High grade lesions tend to have a higher density of Mib-1 positive nuclei than low grade lesions, but the type of HPV does not show any significant differences in staining patterns.[32]

One possible pitfall in the interpretation of Mib-1 immunostaining is the presence of intraepithelial

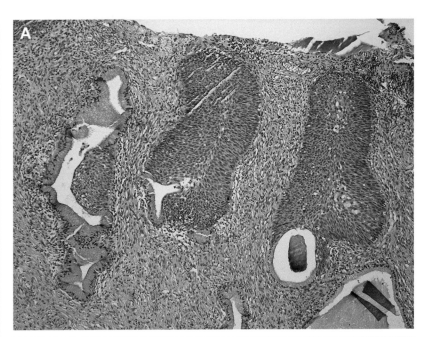

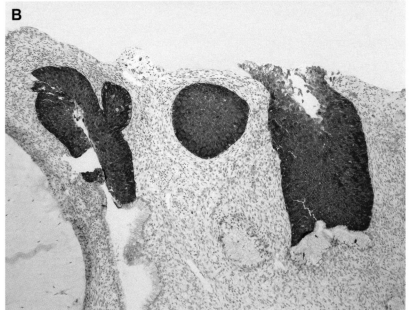

Fig. 14. HSIL (*A*) with strong and diffuse p16 staining (*B*).

inflammatory cells which can be present at all layers of the epithelium and show positive nuclear staining. Also, tangential sectioning through the basal aspect of the squamous mucosa can also mimic diffuse Mib-1 positivity as well as appear immature on histology **Fig. 17**.

ProEx C

ProEx C is a recently developed immunohisto-chemical assay that targets the expression of topoisomerase II-alpha (TOP2A) and minichromo-some maintenance protein-2 (MCM2), two genes that have been shown to be overexpressed in cervical cancers.[37–40] It is a nuclear stain that is positive in squamous dysplasia and has the same pattern as Mib-1 with normal parabasal cells serving as internal positive controls and increased staining in the upper layers with increasing grade of the lesion. Studies have shown that ProEx C is comparable to p16 and Mib-1 in the detection of

Fig. 15. LSIL (*A*) with weak band-like p16 staining (*B*).

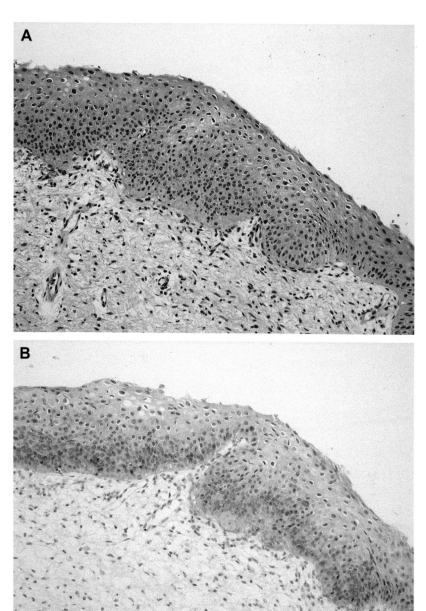

high grade lesions in formalin fixed tissue sections and in distinguishing them from benign mimics.[40–42] One recent study showed that the combination of p16 and ProEx C was more predictive of non-SILs than p16 combined with Mib-1, suggesting that ProEx C may be more effective than Mib-1 for distinguishing reactive epithelial changes from squamous dysplasia **Fig. 18**.[42]

In situ hybridization (ISH)

In situ hybridization is a direct assay that detects individual HPV DNA fragments within infected cells and can be used in formalin fixed paraffin embedded tissue **Fig. 19**. However, this method suffers from low sensitivity, and of all the direct probe methods, it is the least specific for HPV detection (72% for condylomatous lesions and 30% for invasive cancer cells).[43–45] A recent in situ test, the INFORM HPV 3 (Ventana Medical Systems) test was shown to correlate with PCR-based assays, however, the assay detected significantly fewer HPV positive cases among patients with cervical carcinomas than the PCR method.[46] Because of its relatively low sensitivity,

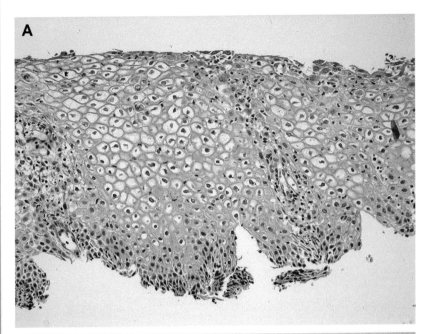

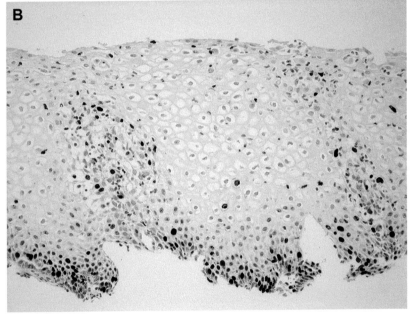

Fig. 16. Benign atypia with inflammation, hematoxylin and eosin (*A*); Mib-1 in benign mucosa (*B*).

especially in the setting of HPV DNA integration into the host genome, this test is less useful for detecting high grade lesions and invasive carcinomas.

Prognosis

Most squamous dysplastic lesions (>90%) spontaneously regress within 2 years in young immunocompetent patients due to the body's cell mediated immune response.[47] However, a small percentage of both low and high grade lesions persist and a smaller percentage still will progress to invasive carcinoma, with the risk of persistence and progression increasing with age. The mean age of women with HSIL is 28 and the mean age of women with invasive carcinoma is 50. The average time to progression is 10 to 20 years, a long in-situ phase of the disease that is amenable to detection through screening.[48]

Fig. 16. Benign atypia with inflammation, Mib-1 in LSIL (*C*); Mib-1 in HSIL (*D*).

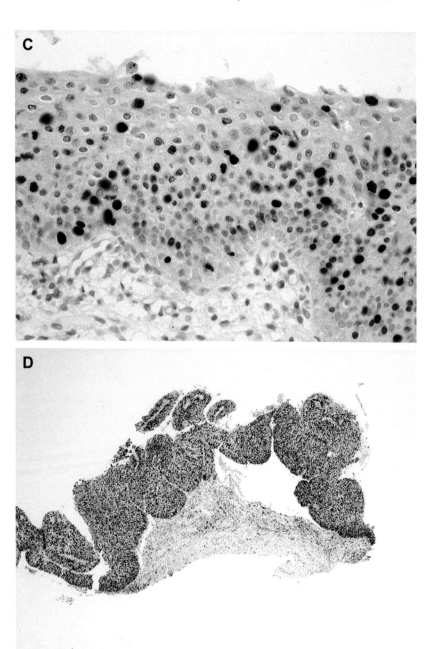

INVASIVE SQUAMOUS CARCINOMA

Cervical carcinoma is the 14th most common malignancy in women in the United States with approximately 12,000 cases diagnosed in the United States each year, accounting for about 4,000 deaths,[49] squamous cell carcinoma (SCC) being by far the most common histologic subtype. Infection with high risk HPV is a necessary but insufficient factor in the pathogenesis of cervical squamous carcinoma and in countries with well established screening programs, the incidence and mortality from cervical cancer has dramatically decreased in recent decades. However, cervical cancer is still the 2nd most common cancer in women worldwide causing over 250,000 deaths yearly.[50] It is now well established that the majority of cervical cancers are etiologically associated with high risk HPV infection and nearly all squamous carcinomas are

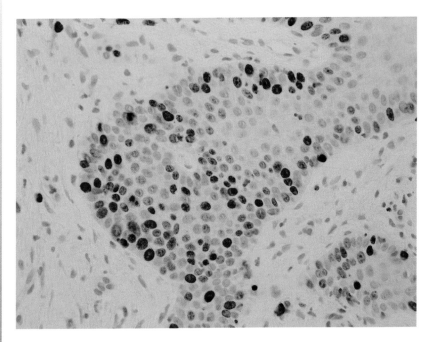

Fig. 17. False Mib-1 through tangential sectioning of basal cell layer.

HPV related[51] with HPV types 16 and 18 accounting for approximately 70% of all cervical cancer.[5] Other high risk types of HPV include, in descending order of frequency, 45, 31, 33, 52, 58 and 35.[5] Other epidemiologic risk factors associated with cervical cancer including smoking, multiple sexual partners, early age at first intercourse, obesity and use of oral contraceptives (the last two in particular for adenocarcinoma).

Gross Features

Cervical squamous carcinomas can be exophytic, warty and papillary or grow in an endophytic pattern which enlarges the cervix without a visible lesion. In populations lacking screening for early detection, circumferential, bulky and deeply invasive lesions are common. Large lesions have a tendency to grow radially and invade the parametrium and/or longitudinally to involve the vagina.

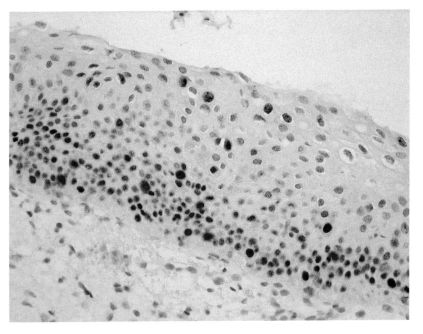

Fig. 18. ProEx C staining in LSIL.

Fig. 19. In situ hybridization in LSIL (*A*) and HSIL (*B*).

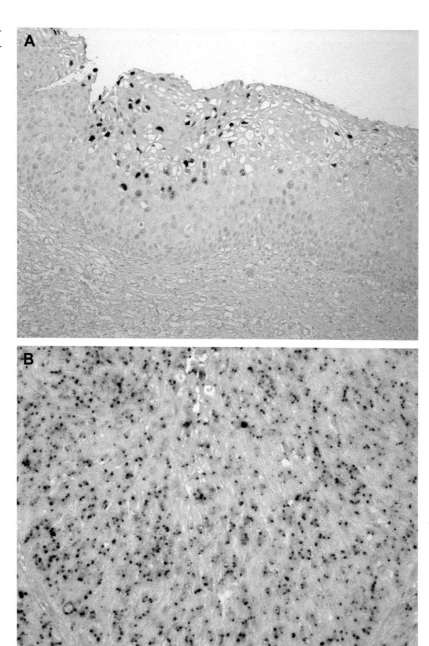

Microscopic Features and Diagnosis

The World Health Organization classifies squamous carcinomas of the cervix into the following subtypes: keratinizing, non-keratinizing, basaloid, warty, verrucous, papillary, lymphoepithelioma-like and squamotransitional.[52] Tumors that invade up to 3 mm and up to 7 mm in horizontal extent are considered early invasive (or microinvasive) carcinomas **Fig. 20**.

Keratinizing SCC is characterized by keratin pearls composed of circular whorls of squamous cells with central nests of keratin. Also present are intercellular bridges, keratohyaline granules and cytoplasmic keratinization. Nuclei are typically large and hyperchromatic with coarse chromatin, and mitotic figures are infrequent except at the periphery of the tumor in less well differentiated areas. Necrosis can be present. The tumor invades in irregular nests and sheets often with an associated desmoplastic or inflammatory stromal reaction. This subtype is usually considered to be well differentiated.

Measuring depth of invasion in early stage squamous carcinoma

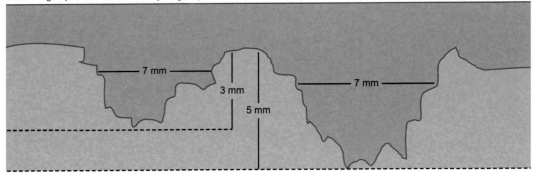

Fig. 20. Diagram for measuring invasive SCC.

Non-keratinizing SCC is composed of recognizable squamous cells that may have individual cell keratinization and intercellular bridges without keratin pearls. There may be more cellular pleomorphism and increased mitotic figures than in well differentiated SCC.

Basaloid SCC is composed of immature, cytoplasm depleted, blue cells with a high nuclear to cytoplasmic ratio resembling HSIL **Fig. 21**. This imparts a poorly differentiated appearance to the tumor. There can be some keratinization of the cells but frank keratin pearl formation is rare.

Warty SCC, also known as condylomatous SCC, has an exophytic, papillary gross appearance. On histology, the cells have a prominent koilocytotic appearance. Most cervical carcinomas have a mixed histology of both basaloid and warty appearance **Fig. 22**.

Verrucous carcinoma is a rare subtype of squamous carcinoma that grossly resembles a giant condyloma. It is histologically highly differentiated with an undulating, hyperkeratotic surface and a broad pushing invasive front, rather than being irregular and infiltrative. The cells have abundant eosinophilic cytoplasm with at most minimal atypia and little mitotic activity. Unlike condylomas, these tumors have broad papillae, lack fibrovascular cores and do not have koilocytosis. It is important to extensively sample tumors that appear verrucous since any severe atypia or infiltrative invasion pattern takes the tumor out of the verrucous category. This has important clinical

Fig. 21. Basaloid SCC.

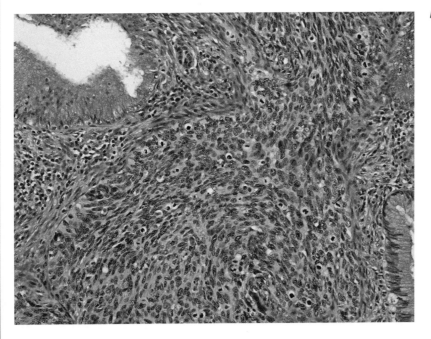

Fig. 22. Warty SCC.

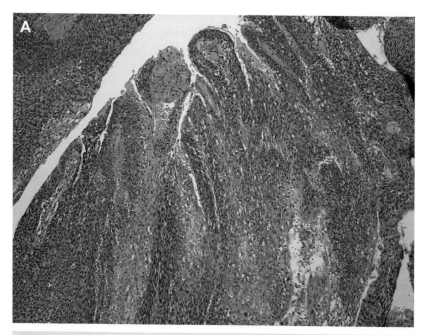

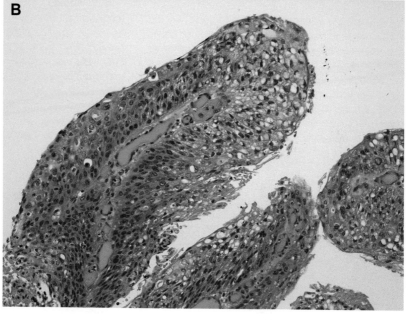

implications since verrucous carcinomas are known to locally recur but have limited potential for distant metastases and may be treated more conservatively that conventional SCC. The association of this tumor to infection with HPV is not definitive, although there are isolated case reports and small series that have shown the presence of HPV in these tumors.[53–55]

Papillary SCC is a tumor in which thin or broad papillae are lined by immature basaloid cells resembling HSIL that lack significant koilocytotic change (which is more characteristic of a warty carcinoma). Superficial biopsies may not show the invasive component, therefore, it is important for the entire lesion to be excised and the epithelial stromal junction evaluated to exclude stromal invasion. These tumors are typically associated with HPV type 16.[56]

Lymphoepithelioma-like carcinoma (LEC) of the cervix is another rare variant that is histologically similar to the nasopharyngeal counterpart. It consists of poorly defined islands of large undifferentiated cells with abundant cytoplasm and uniform, vesicular nuclei with prominent nucleoli. The cell borders are indistinct. Cells grow in syncytial sheets that are intimately associated with a prominent lymphoplasmacytic infiltrate and occasional eosinophils **Fig. 23**. Cytokeratins will highlight the tumors cells while the inflammatory cells are largely composed of T-lymphocytes. It is postulated that the intense chronic inflammation signifies cell-mediated immunity and some evidence suggests that these tumors having a favorable prognosis. LEC is more prevalent in Asia than in Western countries and has been shown to be associated with the Epstein-Barr virus (EBV) in Taiwan and Japan[57] but not in the United States.[58]

Squamotransitional carcinomas of the cervix resemble urothelial carcinoma of the urinary tract. They have a papillary architecture and can be indistinguishable from either urothelial carcinoma or papillary SCC. HPV 16 has been detected in these tumors with an immunohistochemical profile similar to cervical SCC (CK7 positive, CK20 negative).[59–62]

Another rare variant that is not included in the WHO classification of squamous carcinomas is the spindle cell variant of SCC or sarcomatoid carcinoma. This was first described in 1983 and can occur in the lower genital tract, including vulva, vagina and cervix.[63] The morphology of these tumors is similar to counterparts in other organ sites, like the upper respiratory and digestive tracts and skin. These tumors have areas of

> ## △△ **Differential Diagnosis**
> ### INVASIVE SQUAMOUS CARCINOMA
>
> - HSIL versus early invasive SCC
> - SCC versus endometrial endometrioid adenocarcinoma with squamous differentiation
> - SCC versus epithelioid trophoblastic tumor (ETT)
> - SCC versus urothelial carcinoma
> - SCC with spindle cell features versus sarcoma versus MMMT

spindled or sarcomatoid morphology growing in fascicles resembling fibrosarcoma or leiomyosarcoma with markedly atypical, pleomorphic spindle cells and may show other areas of conventional squamous carcinoma merging with the spindle cells.[64] Areas of heterologous differentiation (chondorsarcoma or osteosarcoma) are not seen, however, multinucleated giants cells may be present.[63–66] Lack of overt squamous differentiation may necessitate staining with an epithelial immunohistochemical marker such as cytokeratin to establish squamous origin but it is important to note that these can also co-express vimentin and smooth muscle actin.[64] These tumors are highly aggressive with a poor prognosis.[63,64]

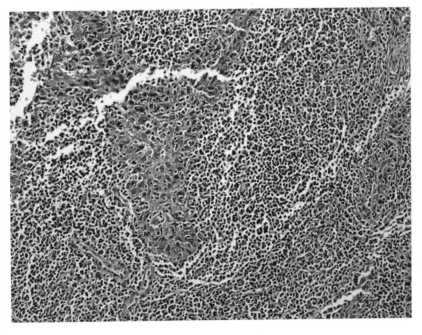

Fig. 23. Lymphoepithelioma like carcinoma of cervix.

Fig. 24. Extensive involvement of endocervical glands by HSIL sometimes raises concern for invasive carcinoma.

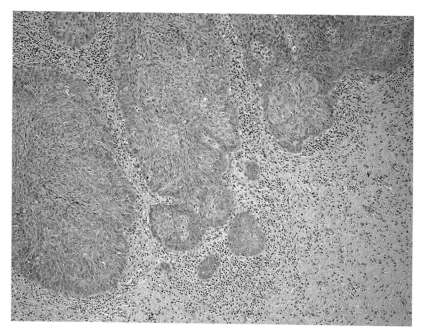

Recognizing stromal invasion arising from HSIL can be difficult, especially in a setting of exuberant inflammation, entrapped squamous cells in a biopsy site, endocervical gland involvement by HSIL and poorly oriented specimens **Fig. 24**. Histologic features strongly supporting invasion include stromal desmoplasia, irregular or scalloped margins, and abundant, paradoxically mature eosinophilic cytoplasm **Fig. 25**. Immunohistochemical staining with cytokeratins and basement membrane stains (collagen IV or laminin) may highlight areas of early invasion that may otherwise be difficult to detect on H&E alone.[67]

The differential diagnosis for SCC of the cervix depends on the predominant morphology of the tumor. For conventional keratinizing and non-

Fig. 25. Microinvasive SCC (desmoplasia, paradoxic maturation, irregular scalloped margins).

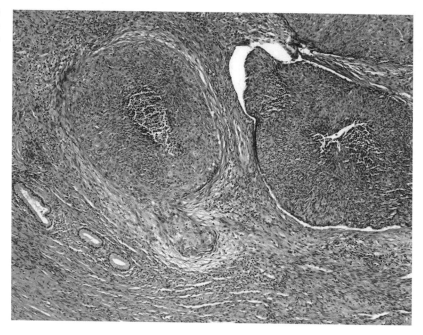

keratinizing SCC, the main differential is an endometrial endometrioid adenocarcinoma with squamous differentiation extending into the cervix. Endometrioid adenocarcinomas can have an exuberant squamous component that obscures the glandular portions of the tumor, however, the main bulk of the tumor should be within the endometrial cavity and one should look for focal areas of glandular differentiation. Since endometrial adenocarcinomas are not associated with high risk HPV infection, a p16 stain should not show the characteristic diffuse strong staining pattern that is seen in true cervical squamous carcinomas, although a considerable degree of staining may be seen.

Another unusual lesion that mimics keratinizing and non-keratinizing SCC of the cervix is epithelioid trophoblastic tumor (ETT). ETT is a gestational trophoblastic tumor of intermediate trophoblastic cells that can occur in the lower uterine segment and endocervical canal and mimic a squamous neoplasm.[68] It is composed of mononucleate epithelioid cells that are small and uniform with clear or eosinophilic cytoplasm and occasional pleomorphic cells. The tumor can grow along the cervical epithelium and secrete eosinophilic hyaline-like material resembling keratin, mimicking a keratinizing SCC of the cervix. However, the clinical, morphologic and immunohistochemical profile will help to distinguish between the two. ETT expresses trophoblastic proteins like hPL (human placental lactogen), hCG (human chorionic gonadotropin) and PLAP (placental alkaline phosphatase), as well as inhibin-alpha and Mel-CAM (CD146) a cell adhesion molecule.[68] Clinically, patients with ETT will have elevated serum hCG levels and may have a history of hydatidiform mole or choriocarcinoma.[68] Unlike SCC, these tumors lack p16 overexpression.

Primary urothelial carcinoma involving the lower genital tract can mimic a papillary or squamotransitional SCC. Urothelial carcinoma can grow in a pagetoid pattern into the vulva, vagina and cervix, as well as invade the underlying stroma in infiltrative or papillary patterns. CK7 and CK20 may be helpful if the CK20 is positive since cervical SCC is generally not positive for this marker.

The primary differential diagnoses for spindle cell variant of SCC are sarcoma and malignant mixed Müllerian tumor (MMMT/carcinosarcoma). Sarcomas should not have any overt epithelial differentiation. MMMTs have very distinct separation between the malignant epithelial and sarcomatous components as opposed to the merging of the two areas in sarcomatoid carcinoma. **Table 1** provides a summary of useful immunohistochemical

Table 1
Useful immunohistochemical stains in the differential diagnosis of squamous cell carcinoma

	SCC	EMC-SM	UC	ETT	MMMT
AE1/AE3	+	+	+	+	+/-
CK7	+	+	+	-	+/-
CK20	-	-	+/-	-	-
P16	+++	+/-	+/-	-	+/-
HPL	-	-	-	+	-
INH	-	-	-	+	-
HCG	-	-	-	+	-
Mel-Cam	-	-	-	+	-

Abbreviations: EMC-SM, endometrioid adenocarcinoma with squamous metaplasia; ETT, epithelioid trophoblastic tumor; MMMT, malignant mixed Müllerian tumor/carcinosarcoma; SCC, squamous cell carcinoma; UC, urothelial carcinoma; +, focal positive staining; ++, moderate positive staining; +++, diffuse positive staining; -, negative staining; +/-, can be positive or negative.

markers in the differential diagnosis of squamous cell carcinoma.

Staging and Prognosis

Cervical cancer is staged clinically rather than surgically because of the prevalence of the disease in under-developed nations where medical and technological advances are limited. Most gynecologists use the FIGO (International Federation of Gynecology and Obstetrics) staging system which was recently revised in 2009.[69] Staging is based on the size of the tumor, depth of stromal invasion and extension beyond the uterus (**Table 2**). Stage I tumors are confined to the cervix and any extension into the uterine corpus is disregarded. IA tumors have a horizontal extent no greater than 7 mm with stage IA1 tumors having stromal invasion no greater than 3 mm and IA2 tumors having stromal invasion between 3 and 5 mm. Depth of invasion is measured from the nearest basement membrane from which the tumor appears to originate. All clinically visible tumors are considered stage IB, regardless of size or depth of invasion.

There is a clear difference in survival depending on stage of disease with near 99% 5 year survival for stage IA1 to 65% for IIB and 43% for IIIB.[70] Among treated patients, the 5-year survival for stage I is 90 to 95%, stage II 50 to 70%, stage III 30% and stage IV less than 20%.[71] Independent prognostic factors include depth of invasion, size of tumor, lymphovascular invasion, lymph node status and parametrial invasion.[72–77]

The standard treatment for patients with stage IA1 disease without lymphovascular invasion is

Table 2
Carcinoma of the cervix uteri

Stage I	The carcinoma is strictly confined to the cervix (extension to the corpus would be disregarded)
IA	Invasive carcinoma which can be diagnosed only by microscopy, with deepest invasion ≤5 mm and largest extension ≥7 mm
IA1	Measured stromal invasion of ≤3.0 mm in depth and extension of ≤7.0 mm
IA2	Measured stromal invasion of >3.0 mm and not >5.0 mm with an extension of not >7.0 mm
IB	Clinically visible lesions limited to the cervix uteri or pre-clinical cancers greater than stage IA[a]
IB1	Clinically visible lesion ≤4.0 cm in greatest dimension
IB2	Clinically visible lesion >4.0 cm in greatest dimension
Stage II	Cervical carcinoma invades beyond the uterus, but not to the pelvic wall or to the lower third of the vagina
IIA	Without parametrial invasion
IIA1	Clinically visible lesion ≤4.0 cm in greatest dimension
IIA2	Clinically visible lesion >4 cm in greatest dimension
IIB	With obvious parametrial invasion
Stage III	The tumor extends to the pelvic wall and/or involves lower third of the vagina and/or causes hydronephrosis or non-functioning kidney[b]
IIIA	Tumor involves lower third of the vagina, with no extension to the pelvic wall
IIIB	Extension to the pelvic wall and/or hydronephrosis or non-functioning kidney
Stage IV	The carcinoma has extended beyond the true pelvis or has involved (biopsy proven) the mucosa of the bladder or rectum. A bullous edema, as such, does not permit a case to be allotted to Stage IV
IVA	Spread of the growth to adjacent organs
IVB	Spread to distant organs

[a] All macroscopically visible lesions—even with superficial invasion—are allotted to stage IB carcinomas. Invasion is limited to a measured stromal invasion with a maximal depth of 5.00 mm and a horizontal extension of not >7.00 mm. Depth of invasion should not be >5.00 mm taken from the base of the epithelium of the original tissue—superficial or glandular. The depth of invasion should always be reported in mm, even in those cases with "early (minimal) stromal invasion" (~1 mm). The involvement of vascular/lymphatic spaces should not change the stage allotment.
[b] On rectal examination, there is no cancer-free space between the tumor and the pelvic wall. All cases with hydronephrosis or non-functioning kidney are included, unless they are known to be due to another cause.

simple hysterectomy or a cone excision with negative margins. The risk of lymph node metastases is minimal and, therefore, a lymph node dissection is not warranted. The presence of lymphovascular invasion does not change the stage of the disease, however, it may affect patient management since it has been shown to be an adverse prognostic factor in early stage cervical cancer.[78] Higher stage tumors require a more radical treatment, either radical hysterectomy or trachelectomy (cervicectomy) with lymph node dissections for IA2 to IB1 tumors. Patients with stage IB2 tumors and beyond typically go straight to chemoradiation without surgical intervention. It is unclear whether hysterectomy is necessary after primary chemoradiation.

GLANDULAR NEOPLASMS OF THE CERVIX

ADENOCARCINOMA IN SITU OF THE CERVIX

Adenocarcinoma in situ (AIS) of the cervix, a recognized precursor lesion of invasive adenocarcinoma, was first described in 1953 by Friedell and McKay.[79] AIS occurs in the cervical transformation zone and can extend far into the endocervical canal, as well as show multifocal distribution.[80,81] Evidence supporting AIS as a precursor lesion includes:

1. AIS is diagnosed in a population 10 to 20 years younger than those with invasive adenocarcinoma, with a mean age of about 35 years.[82–88]

2. AIS is frequently found adjacent to invasive adenocarcinoma.[84,88]
3. Similar HPV types are found in both in situ and invasive adenocarcinomas[88]
4. Cases of untreated AIS preceding invasive disease have been identified.[84,88–91]

Detection of glandular lesions has traditionally been more difficult than detecting squamous lesions for a variety of reasons. Glandular lesions are less common so the recognition of abnormal glandular cells on a Pap is more difficult. Because the lesion may only involve glands that are below the epithelial surface or occur high up in the endocervical canal away from the transformation zone, it may not be clinically visualized colposcopically or adequately sampled. Similar to squamous intraepithelial lesions of the cervix, glandular lesions are also associated with high risk HPV infection,[92,93] and AIS can be found co-existing with HSIL.

Gross Features

Adenocarcinoma in situ is typically not visible grossly at colposcopic evaluation and the application of acetowhite solution may not elicit the same kind of vascular changes as in squamous lesions.

Microscopic Features and Diagnosis

AIS is characterized by preserved architecture of normal endocervical glands with alterations in the surface and invaginating glandular epithelium. The cells show nuclear enlargement, coarse chromatin, small or inconspicuous nucleoli, increased mitotic and apoptotic activity and cellular overlapping with nuclear pseudostratification. The mitotic figures are easily identified, usually located on the luminal side of the cells. Apoptotic bodies are also readily visible, often in the same glands with mitoses. The nuclei maintain their columnar shape but are enlarged and darker compared with normal endocervical glands. The pseudostratification should reach the level of the luminal surface, even if only focally, which is an important feature in distinguishing other benign mimics. There are morphologic variants of endocervical AIS which have traditionally been called "endometrioid," endocervical and intestinal types. Endocervical type was always described as resembling normal endocervical glands with retention of some cytoplasm and mucin, while the endometrioid type was said to resemble proliferative or hyperplastic endometrium with mucin depletion. However, this separation has no biologic or clinical relevance and the term "endometrioid" is misleading. Both endometrioid and endocervical types have the same nuclear morphology, mitotic and apoptotic activity and immunohistochemically stain like HPV associated endocervical neoplasia rather than endometrial endometrioid adenocarcinoma (see biomarkers section below). Intestinal type AIS displays apical intracytoplasmic mucin with goblet cells. There can be a mixture of the various morphologies within a single tumor and all are associated with high risk HPV infection.

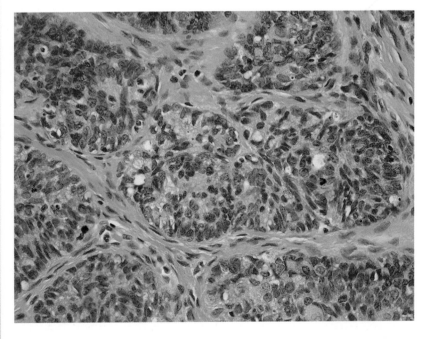

Fig. 26. Stratified mucin-producing intraepithelial lesion (SMILE).

Fig. 27. (*A–C*) Adenocarcinoma in situ.

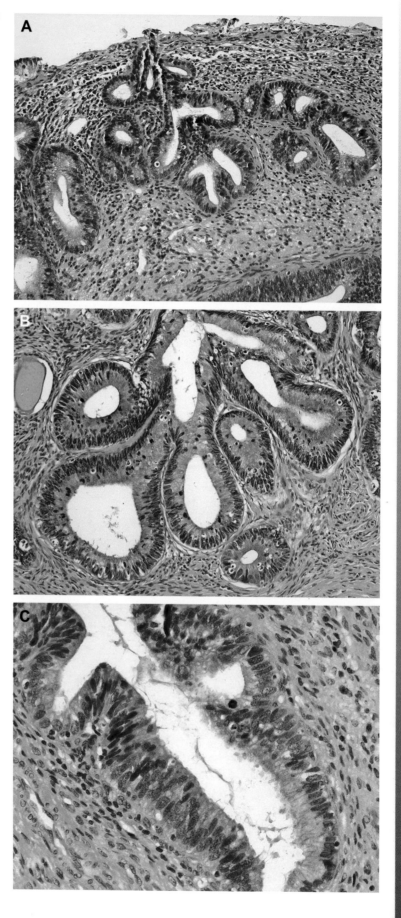

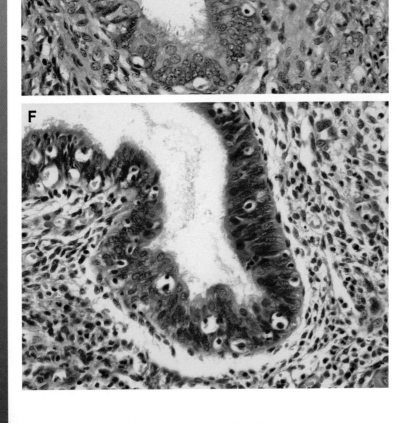

Fig. 27. Reactive glandular atypia with inflammation (*D*); tubal metaplasia (*E, F*).

AIS variant

Stratified mucin-producing intraepithelial lesion (SMILE) is an HPV associated intraepithelial columnar cell neoplasm that is thought to arise from the reserve cells of the cervical transformation zone **Fig. 26**.[94] The morphologic appearance of these lesions is between a squamous and glandular lesion, composed of immature stratified cells that, while similar to SIL, display intracytoplasmic mucin or cytoplasmic vacuoles that separate the cells in the mid to lower layers of the epithelium. However, unlike conventional AIS, overt gland formation is not seen. The most consistent feature of SMILE is the spacing of nuclei by mucin which can be highlighted with a mucicarmine stain. These lesions are often found adjacent to HSIL, AIS, adenocarcinoma, squamous carcinoma and adenosquamous carcinoma. Although the natural history of these lesions has not been fully elucidated, it is reported that they may recur in the form of either SIL or AIS. It is recommended in the reporting of these lesions that the term "SMILE" not be used, but rather AIS or adenosquamous carcinoma in situ since many gynecologists will not be familiar with the terminology.

Differential Diagnosis

There are some benign glandular lesions that can mimic endocervical AIS and it is important to be able to recognize these and differentiate them from true precancerous lesions **Fig. 27**.

Tubal/tuboendometrioid metaplasia (TM/TEM) is a benign metaplastic process that can affect glandular cells along the entire Müllerian tract. Tubal metaplasia resembles cells of the normal fallopian tube containing secretory cells, intercalated/peg cells and ciliated cells. There should be no apoptotic bodies and either no or rare mitotic figures present. If ciliated cells are readily identified, the distinction from AIS is not difficult. Tuboendometrioid

metaplasia is diagnosed when the cells lose distinctive tubal features (ciliated and secretory cells) and take on a more endometrioid appearance, resembling the elongated, pseudostratified appearance of proliferative-type endometrium. These cells have a slightly increased nuclear to cytoplasmic ratio and are mucin depleted, which can mimic AIS. However, they tend not to show the architectural complexity, nuclear hyperchromasia, pleomorphism or irregularity of cervical adenocarcinoma in situ, nor do they have the increased apoptotic and mitotic activity. Tubal and tuboendometrioid metaplasia can involve the upper endocervix/lower uterine segment, as well as deep endocervical glands with dilated irregular gland formation and stromal reaction around the glands; this latter feature in particular may erroneously suggest a diagnosis of invasive adenocarcinoma.[95]

Immunostains can be helpful since tuboendometrioid metaplasia should be positive for ER, PR and vimentin with low Mib-1, while the opposite applies to AIS. P16 should show diffuse strong staining in AIS, while TEM will be either negative or focal with p16.[96]

Reactive glandular atypia is cytologic atypia of benign endocervical glands caused by or associated with a variety of processes which include inflammation, infection, papillary endocervicitis and radiation changes. In reactive changes, the nuclei are typically enlarged, have prominent nucleoli but lack nuclear hyperchromasia, and mitotic/apoptotic activity is absent or minimal as is pseudostratification. Papillary endocervicitis features exaggerated papillary projections with a dense acute and/or chronic inflammatory infiltrate.[97] Radiation causes cellular enlargement with retention of the nuclear to cytoplasmic ratio. The cytoplasm can show vacuolization and eosinophilia. The nuclei can appear round and vesicular with prominent nucleoli and can also have a smudged hyperchromatic appearance.[98] Reactive glandular cells should have low Mib-1 proliferation rates and negative or only focal p16 staining, unlike endocervical AIS.

In curettage specimens, fragments of proliferative endometrium in the endocervical sample may mimic AIS since proliferative glands are pseudostratified with dark nuclei and mitotic figures. The absence of apoptoses and presence of endometrial stroma should be helpful in identifying endometrium. Endometriosis in the cervix can also pose diagnostic problems, especially if deeply placed with an infiltrative appearance, but the presence of stroma and hemorrhage around the glands should be diagnostic. Also, endometrial tissue is positive for ER, PR and vimentin, and

△△ **Differential Diagnosis**
GLANDULAR NEOPLASMS
OF THE CERVIX

- Tubal/tuboendometrioid metaplasia
- Reactive glandular atypia
- Proliferative endometrium and endometriosis
- So-called "glandular dysplasia"
- Other proliferating glandular lesions and hyperplasias

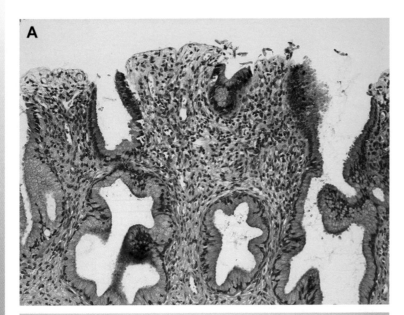

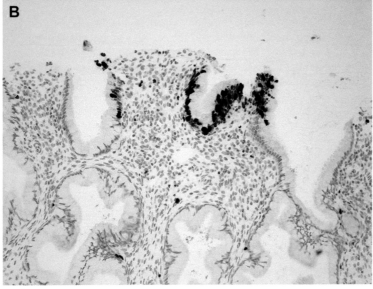

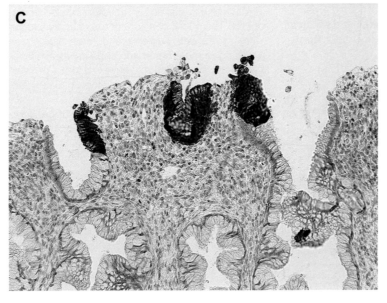

Fig. 28. Biomarkers in AIS (*A*), Mib-1 (*B*), p16 (*C*).

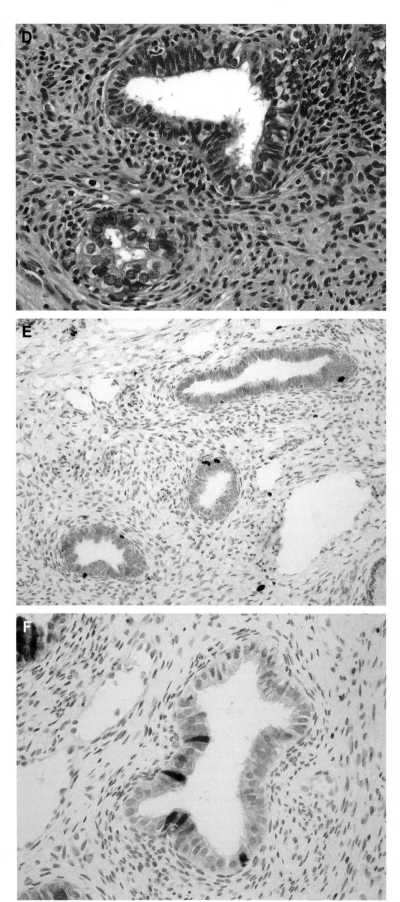

Fig. 28. Biomarkers in tubal metasplasia (*D*), Mib-1 (*E*), p16 (*F*).

negative or focally positive for p16 and CEA (monoclonal), which can be used in difficult cases.

So called "glandular dysplasia" is an ill-defined entity that describes atypical glandular lesions that display a "lesser degree of abnormality" than adenocarcinoma in situ.[99–101] The diagnostic criteria remain largely subjective, it is not reproducible and the clinical significance of this entity is still unknown. Therefore, this terminology should not be used for clinical purposes.[88]

There are other proliferative glandular lesions of the cervix that are less diagnostically difficult but are mentioned here for completeness. These include tunnel clusters, microglandular hyperplasia (MGH), mesonephric hyperplasia, lobular endocervical glandular hyperplasia, ectopic prostatic tissue and Arias-Stella change.

Biomarkers

Useful biomarkers in the diagnosis of AIS are similar to ones used in squamous dysplasia **Fig. 28**. If the differential diagnosis is between AIS and a benign glandular lesion (eg, reactive atypia or microglandular hyperplasia), the most useful stains are Mib-1/Ki-67, p16 and ProEx C since AIS will show diffuse strong staining with all 3 markers. Each marker individually may show variations within AIS and benign mimics, however, used in combination, the three stains are very helpful in making the distinction.[96,102–109] TEM and endometriosis are usually negative or focally positive for p16 with Mib-1 generally staining less than 10% of the nuclei, whereas AIS will show diffuse strong p16 staining and Mib-1 labeling greater than 10%.[96] ProEx C will also have a much higher distribution of staining in AIS versus TEM, endometriosis or reactive endocervical cells.[110] Other useful markers include ER/PR and vimentin, which are generally negative in AIS but positive in tuboendometrioid metaplasia, proliferative endometrium and endometriosis. Another immunostain that shows preferential staining in these lesions, but not in AIS is Bcl-2, which has a diffuse cytoplasmic staining pattern in TEM and endometriosis.[96,111] The mechanism for this staining is not known. **Table 3** provides a summary of useful immunohistochemical markers in the differential diagnosis of non-invasive glandular lesions.

Intestinal type AIS/adenocarcinoma may be confused with a tumor of intestinal origin. Unlike colorectal adenocarcinomas, cervical AIS intestinal type should be diffusely and strongly positive for CK7. However, CK20 and CDX-2, hindgut markers usually positive in intestinal tumors, may show positive staining in intestinal type AIS,

Table 3
Useful immunohistochemical markers in the differential diagnosis of non-invasive glandular lesions

	AIS	TEM	EM	RGA	MGH
Mib-1	>10%	<10%	<10%		<10%
P16	+++	+/-	+/-	+/-	+/-
ProEx C	>67%	<33%	<67%	<67%	<10%
ER/PR	-	+++	+++	-	+/-
Bcl-2	-	+++	+++		
Vimentin	-	+++	+++		

Abbreviations: AIS, adenocarcinoma in situ; EM, endometriosis; MGH, microglandular hyperplasia; RGA, reactive glandular atypia; TEM, tuboendometrioid metaplasia; +++, diffusely positive staining; -, negative staining; +/-, can be positive or negative.

sometimes diffusely.[112,113] Therefore, the results should be interpreted carefully in conjunction with p16.

Prognosis and Treatment

The most important factors in the management of adenocarcinoma in situ are complete excision and exclusion of invasion. Although most AIS lesions start at the transformation zone, they may not be visualized on colposcopy, although they may extend into the endocervical canal by as much as 2 cm.[80,114–116] Therefore, a LEEP (loop electrosurgical excision procedure) cone excision is insufficient for most cases and either a cold knife cone with negative margins or simple hysterectomy (depending on patient's age) is more appropriate. AIS can also involve multiple quadrants and be multicentric (separated by more than 2 mm of normal mucosa) so that a negative cone margin may not necessarily predict complete excision, although the rate of residual disease is higher in cases with positive margins.[80–82,89,117–120]

INVASIVE ENDOCERVICAL ADENOCARCINOMA OF USUAL (HPV-ASSOCIATED) TYPE

Invasive adenocarcinoma comprises approximately 20 to 25% of all cervical cancer cases with the incidence increasing in recent years, especially relative to squamous carcinoma and cervical cancer overall.[121–125] Compared to squamous carcinomas, a larger percentage of cervical adenocarcinomas is etiologically unrelated to infection by high risk HPV,[126] although these latter tumors, discussed in detail in subsequent sections of this review, are still very uncommon. In general, the detection of adenocarcinoma may be more problematic than squamous carcinoma due to its location higher in the endocervical canal resulting in sampling error, as well as less well defined criteria for detection in cytologic specimens. There are numerous histologic types of cervical adenocarcinoma that have different etiologic origins and prognostic implications, although these are much rarer than the usual type of endocervical adenocarcinoma.

Gross Features

Endocervical adenocarcinoma can have either an exophytic or endophytic gross appearance. Exophytic tumors can be papillary and polypoid and may not necessarily show stromal invasion. Endophytic tumors can invade deep into the cervical wall without evidence of a surface lesion, but these will circumferentially enlarge the cervix which results in a "barrel cervix." Like invasive squamous carcinomas, large lesions have

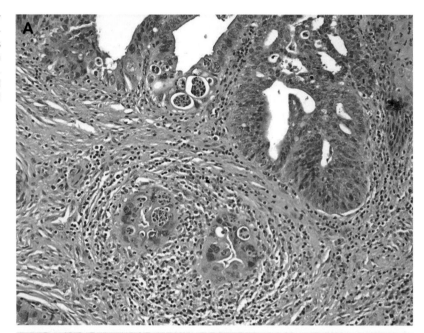

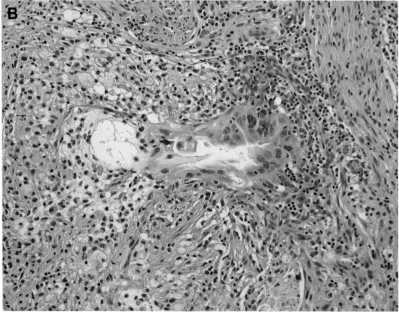

Fig. 29. Patterns of early invasion in adenocarcinoma; (*A*) Detached glands with abundant cytoplasm showing stromal response. (*B*) Irregular fragmented glands with stromal desmoplasia.

a tendency to grow radially and invade the para-metrium, and/or longitudinally to involve the vagina.

Microscopic Features and Diagnosis

The two unequivocal signs of invasion in cervical adenocarcinoma include:

1. Histologically malignant irregular, fragmented glands or single cells that are within the cervical stroma
2. Desmoplastic stromal reaction around the malignant glands.[88]

It is important to note that the glands and single cells must exhibit a cytologically malignant appearance since there are other benign processes that can cause gland fragmentation and stromal reactions. Obvious deeply invasive adenocarcinomas do not usually pose diagnostic problems, especially in excision specimens like cone biopsies or hysterectomies. However, the presence of invasion can be difficult to detect in small biopsies and cases with early invasion ("microinvasive" or "early invasive" adenocarcinoma," defined as stromal invasion less than or equal to 3 mm) **Fig. 29**. Other less definitive histologic features suggestive of invasion are architecturally complex, branching, irregular or small glands growing confluently, cribriform growth without intervening stroma within a single gland profile, and the presence of malignant appearing glands below the deepest normal gland.[88] This last feature becomes problematic because although normal cervical glands should be confined to the inner third of the cervix and no deeper than 1 cm, benign glands in various patterns can be found deep within the stroma, eg, Nabothian cysts, tunnel cluster, endocervical hyperplasia, deep endocervical glands and mesonephric ducts remnants.[88,127] In about 20% of cases, it is impossible to distinguish AIS from early invasive adenocarcinoma.[128]

Measuring depth of invasion

Since early cervical cancer is staged based on the size of the tumor and depth of stromal invasion, it can be particularly difficult to assign a stage in cases of adenocarcinoma where there is no obvious mucosal-stromal junction as in squamous epithelium. Normal endocervical glands can be complex with secondary branching and deep invaginations into the cervical wall.[129] Therefore, invasion may not necessarily originate from the surface glandular epithelium - it can arise from any gland profile regardless of its location. According to the World Health Organization (WHO)

Classification of Tumors, both the depth of invasion and the width of the invasive component must be measured. In practice, tumor thickness rather than "depth of invasion" is reported.[52] Invasion thickness is measured from the surface rather than the point of origin, the latter being difficult to establish in some cases **Fig. 30**. The use of the term "microinvasive adenocarcinoma" is discouraged since it implies a negligible risk of lymph node metastasis in a setting where the method of measuring invasion is inconsistent.[52,88]

Villoglandular adenocarcinoma

This is a well differentiated morphologic variant of endocervical adenocarcinoma that grows with a frond-like pattern resembling villous adenoma of the colon. The epithelium is tall columnar, usually well to moderately differentiated with scattered mitoses. It is important to distinguish this tumor from usual endocervical adenocarcinoma because of its reported favorable prognosis with 5 year survival between 57 to 77%, as compared with 30% for all adenocarcinomas.[130–132] The patients tend to be approximately a decade younger than for usual endocervical adenocarcinoma.[133,134] These tumors are traditionally treated more conservatively (cone biopsy instead of hysterectomy) if there is no more than superficial invasion because they have been reported to rarely metastasize to lymph nodes or spread beyond the uterus.[135–138] However, there are conflicting data regarding the prognosis of this disease, partly due to the fact

Uterine cervix cross section

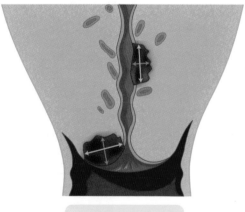

⟵⟶ Horizontal spread

⟵⟶ Depth of invasion

Measuring depth of
invasion and horizontal extent of tumor

Fig. 30. Diagram showing how to measure thickness and horizontal spread of invasive adenocarcinoma.

that there has been a lack of reproducibility in making the diagnosis.[139–141] HPV types 16 and 18 are the most common HPVs associated with this tumor.[142–144]

Gross Features

The tumor has been described as polypoid or papillary, resembling condyloma acuminatum. It can be white, friable, fungating or nodular with papillary excrescences and cervical erosion.[134]

Microscopic Features and Diagnosis

The papillary component can be of variable thickness, although the papillae are usually thin and only occasionally short and broad. The papillae have central cores composed of spindle cells and acute and chronic inflammatory cells. The stromal invasive component is usually absent or only superficial, although rare cases of deep invasion have been reported.[134] The invasive component infiltrates the stroma with elongated branching glands separated by fibromatous stroma similar to that in the papillary cores, with occasional desmoplasia or myxoid change at the advancing front.[134] The cells lining the papillae are typically stratified and relatively mucin-depleted although occasional mucin, including goblet cells, can be seen. Small papillae can be seen budding from larger papillae, but not to the degree typically seen in serous carcinomas. The tumor can be associated with in situ squamous or adenocarcinoma.

The cytology of the cells should show mild to moderate atypia at most, so as to appear almost benign, a distinguishing characteristic that separates villoglandular adenocarcinoma from usual type endocervical adenocarcinoma with papillary architecture. The tumor can be difficult to detect on cytology due to the mild atypia.[145]

Differential Diagnosis

The most common differential diagnoses for invasive endocervical adenocarcinomas are well differentiated endometrioid endometrial adenocarcinoma and cervical adenocarcinoma in situ. If the tumor metastasizes to the ovaries, then the differential is between a primary ovarian neoplasm and metastasis from the cervix, endometrium or other site.

Endometrial endometrioid adenocarcinoma typically has a complex cribriform growth pattern with enlarged, round, vesicular nuclei with occasionally prominent nucleoli and some mitotic figures. In contrast, endocervical adenocarcinoma has more columnar and pseudostratified nuclei that are hyperchromatic with occasional nucleoli

△△ Differential Diagnosis
INVASIVE ENDOCERVICAL ADENOCARCINOMA OF USUAL TYPE

- Well differentiated endometrioid endometrial adenocarcinoma versus cervical adenocarcinoma
- AIS versus invasive cervical adenocarcinoma
- Usual endocervical adenocarcinoma versus villoglandular adenocarcinoma
- Villoglandular adenocarcinoma versus benign papillary lesions (Müllerian papilloma, papillary adenofibroma, papillary endocervicitis, endocervical polyp)
- Villoglandular adenocarcinoma versus other malignancies (endocervical adenosarcoma, minimal deviation adenocarcinoma, metastatic endometrial adenocarcinoma)
- Primary ovarian mucinous/endometrioid neoplasm versus metastatic cervical adenocarcinoma

and numerous luminal mitoses and apoptotic bodies. The difficulties in distinguishing the two tumors can arise from either endometrial adenocarcinoma extending into the cervix or endocervical adenocarcinoma invading up into the lower uterine segment and endometrium/myometrium.

Usual endocervical adenocarcinoma can have papillary growth with focal areas of villoglandular pattern. However, the diagnosis of villoglandular adenocarcinoma should be reserved for tumors that are exclusively or predominantly composed of the villoglandular pattern with at most moderate cytologic atypia. The diagnosis of villoglandular adenocarcinoma is based primarily on the exophytic, non-invasive component since the invasive portion often loses its papillary configuration and an elongated, branching glandular pattern predominates.[130,134] Definitive diagnosis of villoglandular adenocarcinoma should not be made in curettage or biopsy specimens since this might result in inappropriately conservative surgical management of a conventional adenocarcinoma that had villoglandular features that were present only focally.[146]

Differentiating AIS from invasive adenocarcinoma is covered above in the previous section.

Metastatic endocervical adenocarcinoma to the ovaries can present synchronously or metachronously with the primary tumor (and can sometimes precede the development of a clinically apparent cervical adenocarcinoma) and can resemble

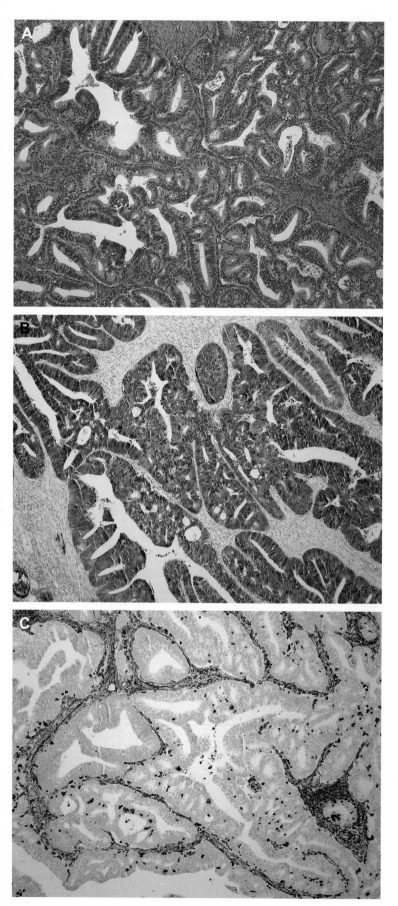

Fig. 31. Biomarkers in endocervical versus endometrial endometrioid adenocarcinoma [(*A*) cervix H&E, (*B*) p16, (*C*) vimentin].

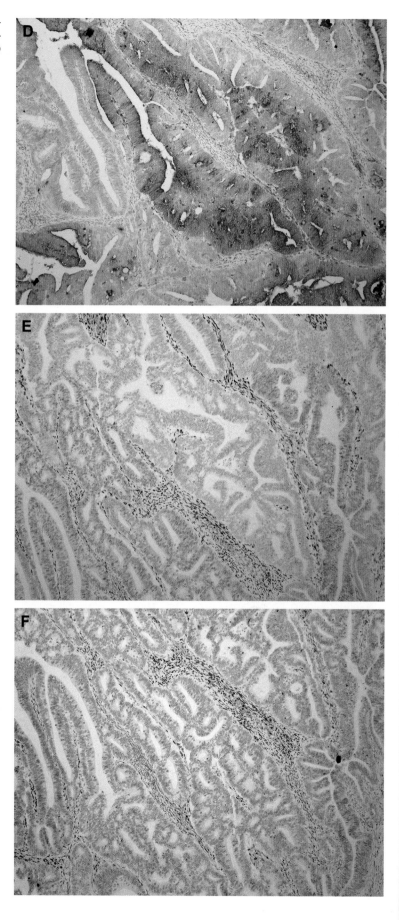

Fig. 31. Biomarkers in endocervical versus endometrial endometrioid adenocarcinoma [(*D*) CEA, (*E*) ER, (*F*) PR].

ovarian mucinous or endometrioid borderline tumors or well differentiated adenocarcinomas. It has also been reported that extensive cervical adenocarcinoma in situ without evidence of obvious stromal invasion can metastasize to the ovaries.[147] Although metastatic endocervical adenocarcinoma can usually be diagnosed readily using a variety of morphologic and clinical indices (bilateral ovarian involvement, ovarian surface involvement, nodular growth pattern, known primary tumor), cases with unilateral involvement and expansile growth lacking destructive stromal invasion can be particularly challenging. The metastases can grow in papillary, villoglandular or confluent glandular patterns, mimicking primary ovarian borderline tumors and carcinomas. Metastatic endocervical adenocarcinoma nuclei are typically enlarged, elongated, and hyperchromatic, and somewhat more atypical than those seen in well differentiated endometrioid adenocarcinomas, with numerous luminal mitoses and apoptotic bodies.[148] They also can show hybrid mucinous and endometrioid features, which is a useful clue to the presence of metastatic endocervical adenocarcinoma.[148]

Biomarkers

Various immunohistochemical markers can be helpful in distinguishing endocervical from endometrial endometrioid adenocarcinoma. Endocervical tumors are typically positive for p16, CEA(m) and negative for ER, PR and vimentin **Fig. 31**, while the opposite is true for endometrial endometrioid adenocarcinoma, although there may be some overlap of staining patterns.[149,150] Endometrial endometrioid adenocarcinomas may show some p16 staining, but it is usually not in the diffuse strong pattern that is typically seen in endocervical adenocarcinomas. Cervical adenocarcinomas may show ER or PR nuclear positivity, but it is generally only focal or weak, unlike the usual diffuse strong pattern seen in well differentiated endometrial endometrioid adenocarcinomas.

To differentiate metastatic endocervical adenocarcinoma from primary ovarian mucinous or endometrioid neoplasm, p16, ER and PR can be very useful.[148] Metastatic endocervical adenocarcinoma should be diffusely p16 positive, hormone receptor negative (or only focally positive) and display HPV positivity by in situ hybridization (although this test can be less sensitive than p16 immunohistochemistry).[147] **Table 4** summarizes the immunohistochemical stains that can help differentiate endocervical from well differentiated endometrioid endometrial adenocarcinoma.

Table 4
Immunohistochemical stains to help differentiate between endocervical and endometrial endometrioid adenocarcinoma

	Endocervical ACA	WD Endometrial Endometrioid ACA
p16	+++	+/-
CEA (monoclonal)	+++	+/-
ER	+/-	+++
PR	+/-	+++
Vimentin	+/-	+++

Abbreviations: WD, well differentiated; +++, diffusely positive staining; -, negative staining; +/-, can be focally positive or negative.

Prognosis

The prognosis for cervical carcinoma is dependent on clinical stage and lymph node status with overall survival steadily decreasing with increase in stage. Most studies looking at cervical cancer have focused on squamous cell carcinoma since adenocarcinoma comprises a small subset of cervical cancer overall. Therefore, information on the natural history and optimal management of adenocarcinoma of the cervix is limited. In a review article from Gien and colleagues[151] in 2010 looking at pooled literature on cervical adenocarcinoma, it is reported that there are epidemiologic, as well as prognostic differences between squamous and adenocarcinomas. Although some studies have shown no differences in survival between these two histologic subtypes, the majority have shown that adenocarcinoma carries a worse prognosis with 10%–20% differences in 5-year overall survival rates.[151] Comparing stage for stage, patients with adenocarcinoma have a significantly lower survival rate than those with squamous carcinoma. One study demonstrated that 5-year overall survival rates for adenocarcinoma decreased with increasing FIGO stage (stage I: 80%; stage II: 37%; stage III less than 11%).[152]

Tumor size has also been shown to be prognostically significant in larger tumors (>4 cm) with differences seen between squamous and glandular histology. In one study, the overall survival for squamous carcinomas greater than 4 cm was 73% compared with only 59% for adenocarcinoma ($P<.1$) reflecting the greater risk of developing distant metastases in patients with adenocarcinomas (25%) compared with those with squamous carcinoma (14%).[153] For patients with tumor size greater than 4 cm and progressively advanced disease, concurrent chemoradiation is the primary treatment. There appears to be no survival difference between squamous and adenocarcinomas less than 2 cm with no lymphovascular invasion treated by radical surgery.[151]

Lymph node status is also prognostically important. Not only has the incidence of lymph node metastasis been reported to be higher in adenocarcinomas, but the survival significantly decreases in patients with lymph node metastases and is worse in patients with adenocarcinoma than squamous carcinoma.[154–157]

ADENOSQUAMOUS CARCINOMA

Adenosquamous carcinoma of the cervix is a mixture of both squamous and glandular components, also associated with high risk HPV infection. Most studies on adenosquamous carcinoma combine it with adenocarcinoma, however, when they are separately analyzed, they show a worse overall survival rate in greater than stage 1 disease.[158]

ADENOCARCINOMA VARIANTS AND NEUROENDOCRINE CARCINOMA

Although the majority of cervical adenocarcinomas are of the usual (ie, HPV-associated endocervical) type, there are other rare variants that are morphologically, etiologically and prognostically different. As such, they pose a different spectrum of diagnostic issues. With the exception of glassy cell, adenoid basal and adenoid cystic carcinoma, the following tumors are either not etiologically associated with HPV infection or have an uncertain association.

- "Endometrioid" adenocarcinoma
- Minimal deviation/adenoma malignum/gastric type adenocarcinoma
- Mesonephric carcinoma
- Clear cell carcinoma
- Serous carcinoma
- Glassy cell carcinoma
- Adenoid cystic carcinoma
- Adenoid basal epithelioma/carcinoma.

"ENDOMETRIOID" ADENOCARCINOMA OF THE CERVIX

Similar to the endometrioid variant of endocervical AIS, invasive endometrioid adenocarcinoma of the

cervix is a misleading term that describes what is essentially usual type endocervical adenocarcinoma with mucin depletion. True endometrioid adenocarcinoma probably does rarely occur in the cervix in the setting of endometriosis, in which case, the tumor will look and stain like an endometrial endometrioid adenocarcinoma (ER/PR/vimentin positive, p16/CEA negative).

MINIMAL DEVIATION (ADENOMA MALIGNUM)/GASTRIC TYPE ADENOCARCINOMA

Minimal deviation adenocarcinoma (MDA) is a malignant, histologically highly differentiated mucinous cervical adenocarcinoma in which the majority of the epithelial cells resemble benign endocervical glands with abundant apical mucin, although a minor component of less well differentiated tumor is usually present Fig. 32.[159,160] It may be difficult to differentiate from benign processes, especially in small biopsies, because of the deceptively bland appearance of tumor cells. Patients with Peutz-Jeghers syndrome (PJS) tend to develop minimal deviation adenocarcinomas, although sporadic cases also occur. Approximately 10% of patients with MDA have PJS.[159,161]

Gastric type adenocarcinoma of the cervix is a recently described mucinous adenocarcinoma of the cervix defined as having voluminous clear or eosinophilic cytoplasm containing gastric type mucin, with distinct cell borders and moderate to severe cytologic atypia Fig. 33. It is postulated that MDA is a well differentiated form of gastric type adenocarcinoma, since gastric type mucin is also characteristic of MDA.[162–164]

Minimal deviation adenocarcinoma comprises approximately 1 to 3% of uterine cervical adenocarcinomas, however, the true incidence is difficult to determine accurately since it is such a rare tumor and diagnostic criteria vary among studies.[165,166] It is well accepted now that these tumors, unlike the usual type of endocervical adenocarcinoma, are not etiologically related to infection by high risk HPV.[167–170] Instead of typical adenocarcinoma in situ, lobular endocervical glandular hyperplasia (LEGH) is thought to be a precursor lesion to MDA.[168,171–173] LEGH is characterized by glands growing in a lobular architecture, with small to moderate, sized round glands often surrounding cystically dilated glands Fig. 34. Unlike MDA, these lesions retain a lobular contour and branching glands and associated stromal desmoplasia is not seen. They have a gastric phenotype (like MDA) and are often found adjacent to MDA.

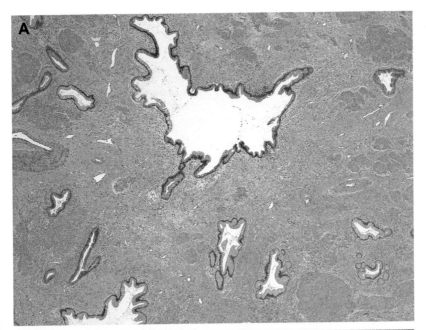

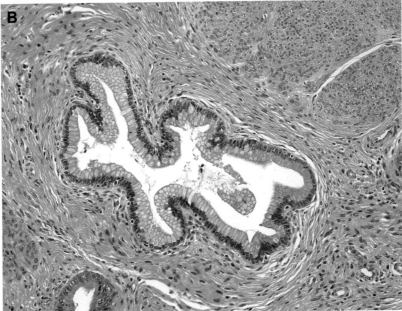

Fig. 32. Minimal deviation adenocarcinoma. (*A*) Large, irregular, "claw-like" glands deep within cervical stroma. (*B*) Glands lined by bland cells with abundant apical mucin.

Gross Features

The cervix is typically indurated, enlarged or "barrel-shaped" but can also be grossly unremarkable. The mucosal surface can be hemorrhagic, friable or mucoid and cut sections can show tan, white firm tumors as well as mucin-filled cysts. These tumors tend to arise high up in the endocervical canal, not at the transformation zone, and they occasionally involve the lower uterine segment.

Microscopic Features and Diagnosis

The glands of minimal deviation adenocarcinoma are typically enlarged, dilated, irregularly shaped and are lined by predominantly bland mucinous epithelium. The nuclei tend to be basally located with abundant apical mucin and nucleoli are generally inconspicuous. However, there is almost always a focus with higher grade cytologic atypia and a less well differentiated appearance, which

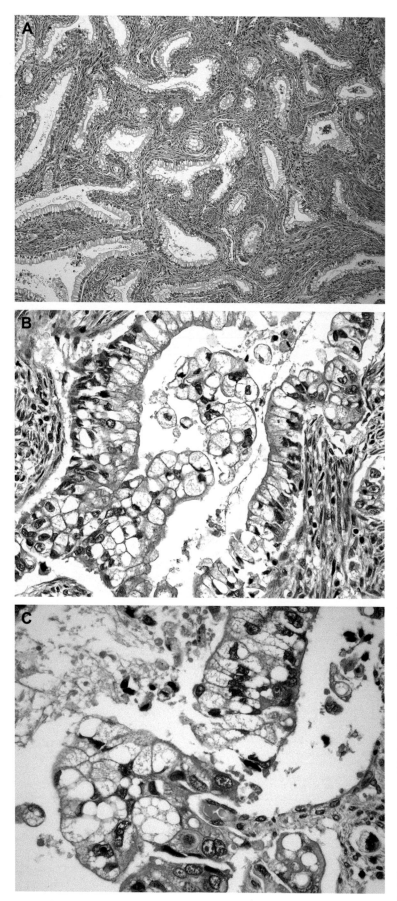

Fig. 33. Gastric type adenocarcinoma. (*A*) Deep stromal invasion by irregular glands. (*B* and *C*) Glands lined by cells with voluminous clear cytoplasm with distinct cell borders and moderate to severe nuclear atypia.

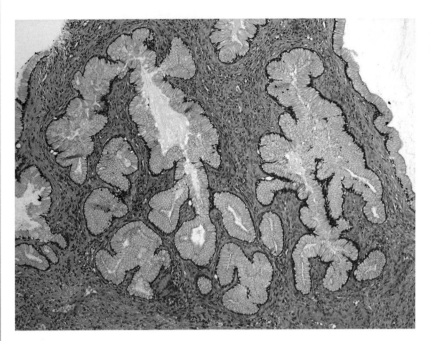

Fig. 34. Lobular endocervical glandular hyperplasia (LEGH).

is the most helpful in distinguishing this lesion from other benign processes. The glands can be closely packed or widely spaced apart and usually invade deep into the cervical wall. Although this is a feature that helps in the recognition of an invasive neoplasm, it can only be appreciated in large cone biopsies or hysterectomy, not biopsies or curettings. There may or may not be desmoplastic stromal changes at the invasive front and vascular or perineural invasion may be seen.

Gastric type adenocarcinoma is less well differentiated than minimal deviation adenocarcinoma and can have mildly to severely atypical nuclei. The cytoplasm is usually abundant and ranges from optically clear to eosinophilic, with very distinct cell borders sometimes resembling plant cells. These features have to be present in greater than 10% of the total area of the tumor. The majority of these tumors have well formed glands, however, papillary or cribriform growth can be seen. The nuclei are ovoid and irregular, tend to be vesicular and can have prominent eosinophilic nucleoli. There can be mucin extravasation into the stroma due to gland disruption.

Differential Diagnosis

The differential diagnosis for minimal deviation adenocarcinoma includes many benign cervical lesions, including deeply placed Nabothian cysts, lobular endocervical glandular hyperplasia (LEGH), diffuse laminar endocervical hyperplasia, tunnel clusters, endocervicosis, adenomyosis of endocervical type, microglandular hyperplasia, mesonephric remnants and hyperplasia, and intestinal or pyloric gland metaplasia. Other malignancies in the differential diagnosis are metastatic gastric adenocarcinoma, invasive endometrioid adenocarcinoma of endometrium with cervical involvement, and usual type endocervical adenocarcinoma. Because of the emphasis on the deceptively bland nature of tumor cells in MDA, there is a tendency to overcall benign glandular lesions as carcinoma. Therefore, the diagnosis of minimal deviation adenocarcinoma should only be made in the presence of obvious features of malignancy – focal desmoplasia/stromal loosening, deep stromal invasion, clearly malignant cytology, less well differentiated areas, vascular or perineural invasion.[159]

Biomarkers

Minimal deviation and gastric type adenocarcinoma have similar immunohistochemical staining patterns. CEA stains in a cytoplasmic pattern, more often in the less well differentiated areas, unlike benign endocervical glands, which tend to have either luminal or no staining. Microglandular hyperplasia is also negative for CEA, and therefore, this stain may be used to differentiate benign lesions from MDA. However, MDA can have very focal CEA staining that can be misleading in small biopsies.[159,174] Other useful stains in differentiating benign endocervical glands from MDA are ER, PR, CA125 and gastric mucin.[175] Normal endocervical glands are ER, PR and CA125 positive,

Fig. 35. Gastric-type differentiation (HIK1083 immunostain) in endocervical adenocarcinoma.

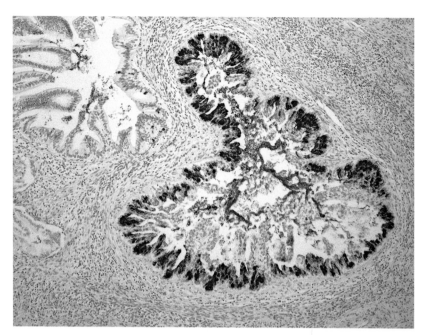

and negative for gastric mucin, while the opposite is generally true for MDA.

HIK1083 is a gastric type mucin immunohistochemical marker that is consistently positive in minimal deviation and gastric type adenocarcinomas **Fig. 35**.[162–164] This antibody is directed to alpha 1,4-GlcNAc-capped O-glycans expressed in gastric gland mucin and reacts to gastric cancer cells, as well as to normal, metaplastic and cancer cells of the pancreas and bile duct.[176,177] HIK1083 also stains lobular endocervical glandular hyperplasia, further supporting the idea that LEGH, MDA and gastric type adenocarcinoma of the cervix are all related.

Since MDA and gastric type adenocarcinomas are not related to HPV infection, they do not show the expected diffuse strong p16 positivity of usual type endocervical adenocarcinoma. The stain is usually negative or if present, is only weak and focal.[172] Therefore, it cannot be used to differentiate MDA from benign lesions.

Prognosis

Historically, minimal deviation adenocarcinomas were reported to have a worse prognosis than usual type endocervical adenocarcinoma. However, there are conflicting data in the literature with some studies showing worse outcome for MDA and others showing no difference.[159,162,165,178,179] The results may be due to overdiagnosis of benign lesions as MDA, falsely improving outcome, lack of early recognition of MDA resulting in delayed treatment resulting in worse outcome, and high diagnostic interobserver variability. In the one study looking at gastric type adenocarcinomas, these tumors had a worse outcome compared with non-gastric type endocervical adenocarcinoma.[162]

MESONEPHRIC ADENOCARCINOMA

Mesonephric adenocarcinoma is an adenocarcinoma of the cervix that is derived from mesonephric (Wolffian) duct remnants in the lateral cervical wall. These remnants can be seen in up to 22% of adults and 40% of newborns and children,[180,181] but the tumor is rare with only a few dozen cases reported in the literature. Patient age ranges from 34 to 73 years with a mean age of 52 at presentation.[182] Although studies are limited, mesonephric adenocarcinoma is likely not associated with high risk HPV infection.[126,170]

Gross Features

The tumor can be exophytic or endophytic, nodular, polypoid or friable, usually involves the lateral cervical wall and can extend into the vagina, protrude into the endocervical canal and into the lower uterine segment or endometrium. The endophytic tumors can diffusely enlarge the cervix without forming a grossly discernible mass and sometimes no grossly visible abnormality is present.

Microscopic Features

The tumor arises from deep lateral wall meso-nephric remnants, can extend to and involve the cervical mucosal surface and often shows entire thickness involvement of the cervical wall. There are five morphologic patterns that are usually inter-mixed within the same tumor: tubular, ductal, solid, retiform and sex-cord-like.[183] A malignant spindle cell component may also be present, in which case the tumor would be designated malignant mixed mesonephric tumor (MMMT).

The tubular pattern most closely resembles native mesonephric remnants and is characterized by back-to-back, small round, uniform tubules lined by cuboidal to flattened cells. Some lumens contain dense eosinophilic hyaline secretions like those seen in normal mesonephric remnants.[183]

The ductal pattern resembles endometrioid adenocarcinomas with glands that vary in size and shape and may contain intraglandular papillae lined by one to several layers of columnar cells **Fig. 36**.

The retiform pattern is characterized by elon-gated slit-like branching tubules which can contain intraluminal papillae with hyalinized fibrous cores. They can also form sieve-like patterns with cysts. The cells can vary from columnar to cuboidal to flattened and eosinophilic colloid-like material may be present in cyst spaces.[183]

The sex-cord-like pattern consists of cells growing in cords and trabeculae reminiscent of sex-cord tumors of the ovary.

The mixed tumor variant has a malignant sarco-matous component that is typically homologous, resembling endometrial stromal or nonspecific sarcoma, although heterologous elements like bone or cartilage may be present.

Cytologically, the nuclei show mild to moderate atypia, and may have prominent nucleoli. Mitotic figures are not difficult to identify, especially in the ductal pattern. The tumors can be infiltrative or pushing at the invasive front and a desmoplastic stromal response may or may not be present. Benign mesonephric remnants or hyperplasia may be seen adjacent to and confluent with the tumor.

Differential Diagnosis

The differential diagnosis includes benign lesions like mesonephric hyperplasia, as well as other malignant tumors like endometrial endometrioid adenocarcinoma and usual type endocervical adenocarcinoma.

Mesonephric hyperplasia resembles the tubular variant of mesonephric adenocarcinoma, espe-cially when the hyperplasia is in a diffuse pattern. Hyperplasia can be infiltrative, deep in the cervical stroma without a desmoplastic response. Features that would support a diagnosis of carci-noma are the presence of other carcinoma growth patterns, lymphovascular invasion, nuclear atypia, mitotic activity exceeding 1 per 10 HPFs and necrotic luminal debris. Clinically, patients with carcinomas tend to be symptomatic while hyper-plasia is always an incidental finding.[182,184] Prolif-eration marker Mib-1/Ki-67 may also be helpful since adenocarcinoma has an average

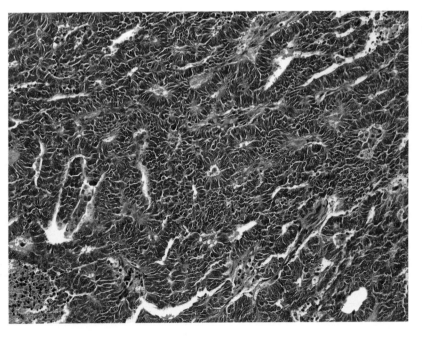

Fig. **36.** Mesonephric adeno-carcinoma (ductal pattern).

proliferation index of 15% versus only 1 to 2% in hyperplasia.[182]

Endometrioid endometrial adenocarcinomas can invade into the cervical mucosa and stroma and be mistaken for a primary cervical cancer. Conversely, primary mesonephric adenocarcinoma of the cervix can be mistaken as extension from an endometrial primary. The presence of adjacent mesonephric remnants, absence of squamous metaplasia, and the presence of other mesonephric adenocarcinoma patterns are useful in making the correct diagnosis. Immunohistochemistry is also useful.

Biomarkers

Mesonephric remnants and adenocarcinoma are usually diffusely and strongly positive for pancytokeratin, Cam 5.2, CK7, EMA and vimentin, with other positive markers including calretinin (88%), inhibin (30%, focal) and androgen receptor (33%).[182,185] CD10 has also been described to be a consistently positive marker for mesonephric adenocarcinoma, but it is usually focal and found in the ductal type.[186] Since mesonephric glands are derived from Wolffian ducts, they do not stain with the usual Müllerian type immunohistochemical markers ER and PR, and in conjunction with calretinin and inhibin, may be helpful in distinguishing endometrial endometrioid adenocarcinoma from mesonephric adenocarcinoma.[186] CEA(m) and CK20 are consistently negative markers.

Prognosis

Due to the rarity of the tumor, little is known regarding optimal therapy or prognosis. In a review article looking at all published reported cases, local recurrence and distant metastasis were commonly found, including to bone, lung, pleura, abdomen and liver.[187] Median and mean times to recurrence were 2.1 and 3.6 years, respectively, and most patients with recurrence died within 1 year, despite therapy. Also of note, many of the metastatic mesonephric adenocarcinomas occurred in the setting of MMMT.[187]

CLEAR CELL CARCINOMA

Clear cell carcinoma is an invasive adenocarcinoma of the cervix composed mainly of clear or hobnail cells arranged in tubulocystic, papillary and/or solid architectural patterns. This histologic subtype of adenocarcinoma is not limited to the cervix, but may occur in other gynecologic organs like ovary and endometrium. However, clear cell carcinoma of the cervix and vagina has a specific clinical association with in utero exposure to diethylstilbestrol (DES), a synthetic non-steroid estrogenic hormone prescribed to pregnant women as a preventative measure against abortion in the 1960s and 1970s. It is estimated that 1 to 4 million women in the U.S. have used DES during pregnancy and the estimated chance of developing clear cell carcinoma is 1 in 1000 for DES-exposed women.[188,189] Despite the association with DES in younger patients, clear cell carcinoma of the cervix and vagina appear to have bimodal peak distribution with the two peaks occurring at mean ages of 26 and 71.[190] Possible non-DES etiologic causes are as yet unknown. Although there are conflicting data from small series and isolated case reports, based on larger studies, HPV likely does not play an etiologic role.[126,170,191–196]

Gross Features

The tumor is usually located in the endocervical canal, not necessarily in the transformation zone, and can have an exophytic or endophytic appearance. Because of its location, it may not be visible on colposcopic examination.

Microscopic Features

Clear cell carcinomas that arise in any of the Müllerian organs are histologically identical. There are three histologic growth patterns, tubulocystic (most common), papillary and solid (least common) and these can occur in mixed patterns **Fig. 37**. The cells can range from flat to hobnail with mild to severe nuclear atypia. The tubulocystic pattern tends to have the flat, mildly atypical cells with minimal cytoplasm. The cytoplasm can be eosinophilic or optically clear due to glycogenization. Mitoses are infrequent. The cells may also have intracytoplasmic or luminal mucin and in rare cases, there is an abundance of cytoplasmic vacuoles which can show a targetoid appearance due to central condensation of eosinophilic secretions.[197] The papillary pattern may be complex and may contain dense eosinophilic hyaline cores, a very helpful feature in making the diagnosis.[197]

Differential Diagnosis

The differential diagnosis includes other cervical adenocarcinoma variants, metastatic clear cell carcinoma from other sites, as well as benign processes such as Arias-Stella reaction, adenosis and microglandular hyperplasia. Endometrioid adenocarcinoma with clear cell/secretory change can have sub- or supranuclear vacuoles in columnar cells. They do not usually have the tubulocystic or papillary configuration, the stromal hyaline deposition, or cuboidal cell shape of clear

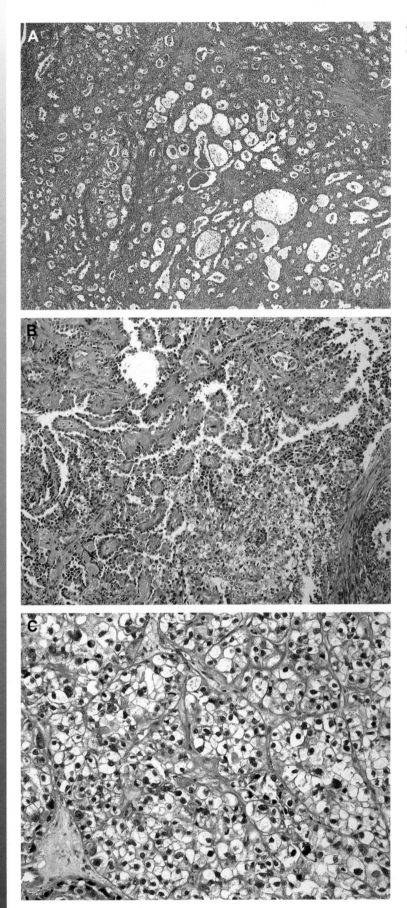

Fig. 37. Clear cell carcinoma [(*A*) tubulocystic, (*B*) papillary, (*C*) solid)].

cell carcinomas. Endometrioid tumors are typically well differentiated and express diffuse ER/PR positivity, unlike most clear cell carcinomas, which tend to be negative for hormonal markers. The gastric type of endocervical adenocarcinoma is another variant that can mimic clear cell carcinoma. These tumors are defined as having voluminous clear to eosinophilic cytoplasm with distinct cell borders and gastric type mucin (see section above). These tumors will stain with gastric type mucins MUC6 and HIK1083.[162,163] PAS and PAS-D special stains should also differentially stain the glycogen of clear cell carcinomas (PAS-D sensitive) and the mucin of gastric type endocervical adenocarcinoma (PAS-D resistant). Clear cell carcinomas from other gynecologic sites are identical to those arising in the cervix, therefore, direct extension or metastasis must be excluded by clinical history and examination of the other sites.

Benign processes such as Arias-Stella reaction, adenosis and microglandular hyperplasia will lack the distinct histologic characteristics of clear cell carcinoma. Adenosis and hyperplasia do not have the cytologic atypia of clear cell and Arias-Stella is usually mitotically inactive.

Biomarkers

Not much is known specifically about cervical clear cell carcinomas. However, ovarian and endometrial clear cell carcinomas have been more extensively studied and demonstrate consistent staining for CK7, CA125 and 34βE12, Leu-M1, vimentin, BCL-2 and CEA with variable staining for ER and PR.[198–201] Nuclear staining for hepatocyte nuclear factor-1β (HNF-1β) has also been found Fig. 38.[202,203] This is a transcription factor normally expressed in liver, kidney and pancreas and thought to be associated with glucose homeostasis. The extent to which cervical clear cell carcinoma stains for this marker is unknown. A recent case report of a cervical clear cell carcinoma in a pregnant patient showed positive staining for pankeratin, Cam 5.2, CK7, CK8, CK18, CK19, EMA, CA125 and p53, although the extent of p53 positivity was not mentioned.[204] Immunohistochemical overexpression of p53 in cervical clear cell carcinomas has been reported sporadically, however, no corresponding gene mutation has been found.[205]

Prognosis

The most important prognostic indicator in clear cell cervical carcinoma is stage, with 3-year overall survival of 91% for stage I/II versus 22% for stage III/IV.[206] Other factors that predict for worse outcome include no surgical resection, metastasis at the time of diagnosis, lymph node metastasis and solid histologic growth.[207,208] The tubulocystic variant appears to have a better prognosis, whereas the effects of tumor size and grade are controversial, with some studies showing an association with unfavorable outcome and others not.[206,208–210] Ovarian preservation does not seem to have any prognostic

Fig. 38. HNF1-β expression in clear cell carcinoma of the cervix.

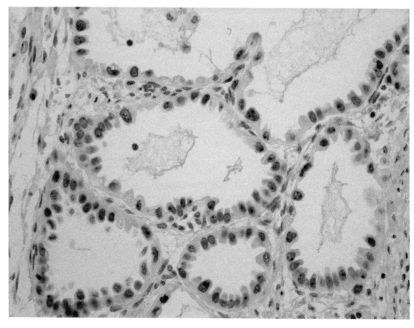

significance.[206,211] In early stage disease, the presence of positive lymph nodes has a negative impact on 5-year progression free survival (31% versus 92%) and overall survival (80% versus 100%) in one multi-institutional retrospective review. In early stage patients without lymph node involvement, adjuvant radiation therapy did not impact progression free or overall survival.[206] The median time to recurrence in this study was 12 months, however, there are reports of recurrences occurring 8 to 20 years after primary treatment.[211]

SEROUS CARCINOMA

Serous carcinoma of the cervix is an extremely rare entity and extension from an endometrial or extra-uterine site should always be excluded. In the largest case series of cervical serous carcinomas (17 cases), 3.4% of the invasive cervical adenocarcinomas were of pure or mixed serous type.[212] Ages ranged from 26 to 70 years with a biphasic distribution.[212,213]

Gross Features

Usually based in the endocervical canal, the tumor can be polypoid, exophytic, show ulceration or induration.

Microscopic Features

The tumor histologically resembles other serous carcinomas of the gynecologic tract. It grows in complex papillae with cellular budding and psammoma bodies **Fig. 39**.[52] There can be non-papillary areas of the tumor that show a more glandular growth pattern with elongated, slit-like spaces, like serous carcinomas from other Müllerian sites. More solid or confluent areas can be seen. The cells usually show marked pleomorphism with prominent nucleoli. There can be occasional bizarre multinucleated giant cells, some of which contain abundant eosinophilic cytoplasm. Mitotic figures (MF) are numerous with most tumors showing greater than 30 MF per 10 high power fields.

Differential Diagnosis

The main differential diagnosis is serous carcinoma originating from the endometrium or other extrauterine sites like the ovary or fallopian tube. Since endometrial/ovarian/tubal/peritoneal serous carcinomas are much more common than cervical serous carcinomas, secondary cervical involvement must be excluded before an unequivocal diagnosis can be rendered. In young patients, it is particularly important to carefully exclude both drop metastasis from an adnexal serous carcinoma (possibly related to BRCA-1 mutation) or endocervical adenocarcinoma associated with HPV infection.

Well differentiated villoglandular adenocarcinoma of the cervix is a tumor with a papillary growth pattern that can be mistaken for serous carcinoma. However, the cytologic atypia is no more than mildly atypical in these tumors and they should not display the pleomorphism, budding or mitotic activity of serous carcinoma. The distinction of these tumors is important since the villoglandular variant has an excellent prognosis.

Clear cell carcinomas with a predominantly papillary growth pattern can appear histologically similar to serous carcinoma. However, they should have some of the more characteristic features such as hyaline stromal deposition, hobnail cells and should be less mitotically active than serous carcinomas.

Most tumors thought to be cervical serous carcinomas most likely represent usual type endocervical adenocarcinoma with a papillary growth pattern or drop metastasis from an endometrial or extrauterine serous carcinoma. This is supported by the conflicting data regarding HPV association and p53 overexpression, as discussed in the following section.[126,170,214–216] True cervical serous carcinoma is, therefore, an extremely rare tumor.

Biomarkers

Serous carcinomas are positive for keratins (AE1/AE3, EMA), B72.3 and CA125, negative for vimentin and have high proliferation rates with Mib-1.[213,217] Unlike serous carcinomas from other sites, they can be positive for CEA (most of these presumably representing high grade, papillary endocervical adenocarcinomas of usual type), although not as consistently as mucinous tumors.[213,218] Unlike usual type endocervical adenocarcinoma, but like endometrioid adenocarcinoma, these can be ER/PR positive, and WT1 is usually negative (although focal positivity may be present).[213] One reported case with an in situ serous component was diffusely positive with p53 but negative for p16 in both the invasive and in situ components.[216] In general, p53 has been found to be positive from 6 to 90% of cases, typically present in advanced stage cases with staining patterns ranging from focal weak to diffuse.[213,219–223] Since there is not consistent overexpression of p53 in cervical serous carcinomas, this suggests either difficulties with consistent and accurate diagnosis, or that there are other genetic factors involved in the pathogenesis of these tumors.

Fig. 39. Serous carcinoma. (*A*) Complex papillae with slit-like spaces. (*B*) Papillary buds and cells with severe nuclear atypia and abundant mitotic figures.

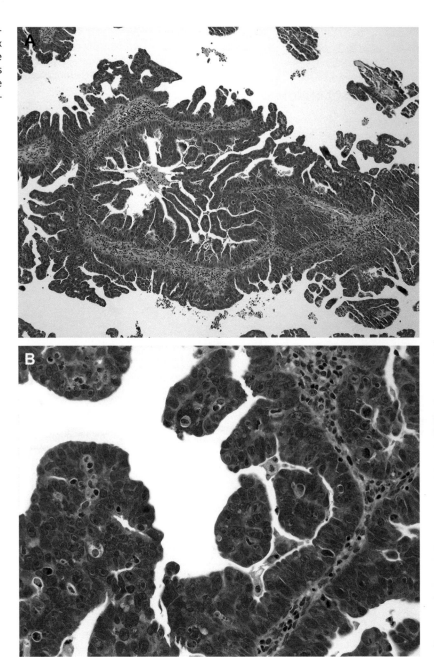

Prognosis

Due to the rarity of serous carcinomas and the likelihood that many are etiologically related to endocervical adenocarcinoma of the usual type, it is difficult to draw definitive conclusions regarding the biologic behavior of these tumors. The tumors are aggressive and rapidly fatal in advanced stages, however, patients with stage I disease appear to have similar outcomes as patients with the usual type of endocervical adenocarcinoma.[212,218,224,225] The limited number of cases reported, the fact that they presented at different stages and were treated differently complicate the accurate analysis of prognosis.[213] Paraneoplastic cerebellar degeneration, a debilitating neurodegenerative disease and a rare complication of cancer, has been reported to occur in the setting of serous carcinomas, including two cases of cervical serous carcinomas.[226]

GLASSY CELL CARCINOMA

Glassy cell carcinoma of the cervix is a rare tumor originally described by Glucksmann and Cherry in 1956 and thought to be a poorly differentiated variant of adenosquamous carcinoma.[227] It typically occurs in young women, grows rapidly and develops distant metastases.

Gross Features

These tumors can be exophytic, fungating, ulcerating, barrel-shaped and necrotic.

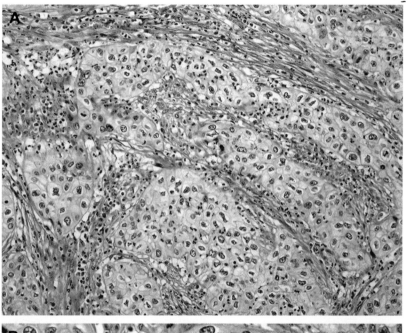

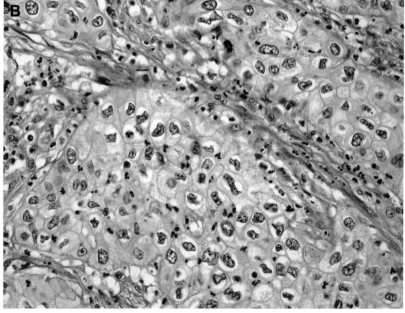

Fig. 40. Glassy cell carcinoma. (*A*) Conspicuous neutrophilic and eosinophilic tumor infiltration. (*B*) Tumor cells with abundant amphophilic cytoplasm and plant cell-like cell borders

Microscopic Features

The tumor is composed of cells with abundant ground-glass or amphophilic cytoplasm, sometimes with a fine cytoplasmic granularity, distinct cell borders and high grade nuclei with prominent nucleoli **Fig. 40**.[227,228] Cells are generally polygonal, but spindle forms can be seen, as well as bizarre multinucleated giant cells. Mitoses are numerous and the tumor is often associated with a prominent inflammatory infiltrate composed of plasma cells, lymphocytes and eosinophils that are present in between tumor nests and at the tumor-stromal junction. Associated in situ squamous carcinoma has also been reported.[229] It is thought that glassy cell carcinoma arises from pluripotential reserve cells that have the ability to differentiate into squamous or glandular type cells. Ultrastructural studies have shown that these tumors have characteristics of both squamous and glandular cells, along with abundant polyribosomes and rough endoplasmic reticulum that likely account for the glassy appearance.[229,230] Glassy cell carcinoma can also occasionally coexist with usual adenocarcinoma showing a gradual transition between the two components.[231]

Differential Diagnosis

Tumors in the differential include non-keratinizing squamous cell carcinoma, especially with cytoplasmic glycogenization, and clear cell carcinoma. These tumors, however, usually do not have the characteristic exuberant inflammatory infiltrate nor the prominent nucleoli of glassy cell carcinoma.

Benign lesions can also be in the differential, including decidualized cells, especially in pregnant women, as well as reactive changes that can occur due to inflammation or healing.

How about implantation site nodules

Biomarkers

Many of the markers that have been studied in glassy cell carcinoma support the dual squamous-glandular phenotype of this tumor. Both high molecular weight (positive in squamous cells) and low molecular weight (positive in glandular cells) cytokeratins are positive.[232] Glassy cell carcinoma also sporadically expresses intracytoplasmic mucin, as demonstrated by Alcian blue and MUC2 positivity, but also shows strong membranous staining with MUC1, a membrane bound mucin core protein expressed on squamous cells.[232] ER and PR are usually negative with only a few cases having been reported as expressing these markers.[233] HPV 18 has been detected in these tumors, which is consistent with the finding that HPV 18 is most commonly associated with glandular tumors of the cervix.[232,234,235] There has been no evidence of loss of heterozygosity at the p53 gene or p53 overexpression by immunohistochemistry.[232] Her2/neu overexpression has been detected in up to 45% of glassy cell carcinomas, but the significance and the relation to actual gene amplification in these cases is unknown.[233]

Prognosis

This tumor has traditionally been thought to be an aggressive form of cervical cancer and was initially thought to be more common in pregnant women and resistant to surgical and radiation therapy.[228,230,231,236–240] Since the tumor is so rare, there are no specific data on best treatment. Both adjuvant and neoadjuvant chemotherapy have been used to treat this tumor.[241–245]

ADENOID BASAL EPITHELIOMA/CARCINOMA

Adenoid basal epithelioma is an HPV-positive, clinically indolent neoplasm with basaloid features that is associated with typical squamous dysplasia and is usually an incidental finding in cervices sampled for other reasons. This tumor has also been called adenoid basal carcinoma, but because of its predominantly benign clinical behavior, it has been suggested that the term "epithelioma" be used rather than "carcinoma." It is rare, representing less than 1% of all cervical carcinomas and typically affects non-white postmenopausal women.[246,247] It is also thought to represent a precursor lesion to other frankly malignant tumors ranging from squamous to glandular to neuroendocrine carcinomas.[248]

Gross Features

Adenoid basal epitheliomas do not form obvious gross lesions. They are usually incidental findings, most commonly detected in cervices removed for dysplasias or other unrelated reasons.

Microscopic Features

This tumor is composed of small discrete epithelial nests that are round to oval and often have a lobule-like arrangement. The cells are uniform, small, cuboidal, oval or spindled and generally have bland nuclei without conspicuous nucleoli. Basaloid cells are often palisaded at the periphery of the nests **Fig. 41**. There is usually a glandular component in which the cuboidal or basaloid cells surround a distinct lumen.[249] The glands can vary from minor to encompassing the entire tumor. They may form cribriform structures with eosinophilic luminal secretions, which

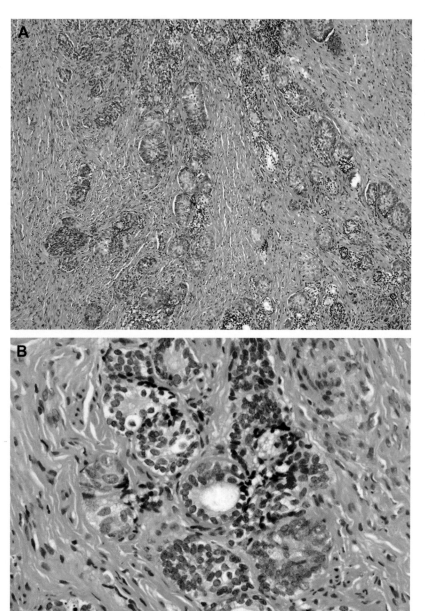

Fig. 41. Adenoid basal epithelioma. (*A*) Small discrete epithelial nests with no obvious stromal response. (*B*) Glandular and basaloid phenotype with uniform bland appearing cells.

can mimic adenoid cystic carcinoma. Necrosis is not seen and mitotic activity can range from 0 to 9 per 10 high power fields.[250] Squamous metaplasia can be seen in the central portions of the nests, which when expanded, can mimic squamous carcinoma. The nests can be located deep in the cervical wall and may or may not be connected to the overlying epithelium and in 90% of cases, adenoid basal epithelioma is associated with a concurrent high grade dysplastic lesion.[250] Although desmoplastic stromal response is uncommon, there can be loosening and edematous changes in the stroma.

Similar to high grade squamous intraepithelial lesions, adenoid basal epitheliomas are believed to be benign precursors to invasive malignancies and the term adenoid basal "carcinoma" should be reserved for those cases in which there is an associated invasive carcinoma with obvious malignant cytologic features (increased cytologic atypia, mitotic activity with abnormal mitotic figures *and* deeply infiltrative growth of these malignant components).[248] Squamous carcinoma, adenoid cystic carcinoma and small cell neuroendocrine carcinoma have all been described in association with adenoid basal tumors.[248] This divergent morphologic potential suggests that adenoid basal tumors may arise from the putative cervical reserve cell.

Differential Diagnosis

Adenoid cystic carcinoma, basaloid squamous carcinoma, mucoepidermoid carcinoma and adenosquamous carcinoma are all in the differential diagnosis of adenoid basal epithelioma. Morphologically, the main differential is adenoid cystic carcinoma, but this tumor is typically a large visible mass with nodules, prominent cribriforming, sieve-like pattern, hyaline cylinders or thick circumferential bands of hyaline basement membrane material, solid sheets, malignant nuclei, comedo-like necrosis or lymphatic invasion.

Biomarkers

Cytokeratins are generally positive in adenoid basal epithelioma, although different portions of the tumor can stain differentially. CK AE1/AE3, Cam 5.2 and 34BE12 are positive while CEA and EMA are positive only in the ductal cells, CK7 is positive in the basaloid and periluminal cells (about half of cases), and p63 is positive in the basaloid component.[249,251–256] Unlike conventional squamous and adenocarcinomas of the cervix, the Mib-1/Ki-67 proliferation index is markedly decreased in the basaloid component when features of HSIL are lacking.[257] But since this is also an HPV-associated neoplasm, p16 has a diffusely strong staining pattern.[248,258]

Prognosis

Completely excised adenoid basal epitheliomas with clear margins do not recur or metastasize. If the lesion extends to margins, then there is the possibility that an associated invasive carcinoma exists beyond that margin. Therefore, the recommendation is to treat these like in situ squamous lesions. When adenoid basal epitheliomas are associated with other malignancies, the overall prognosis is mostly dependent on the stage, grade and other clinicopathologic parameters of the associated malignancy.[247]

ADENOID CYSTIC CARCINOMA

Adenoid cystic carcinoma of the cervix resembles that of salivary gland origin and is an extremely rare variant. It is known to be associated with high risk HPV infection, most commonly HPV type 16.[259,260] The origin of the tumor is thought to be cervical reserve cells rather than true myoepithelial cells.[259,261,262] However, ultrastructurally, cervical adenoid cystic carcinoma shows similar findings to the salivary gland counterpart, including pseudocysts, intercellular spaces, basal laminin and true glandular lumens.[261,263]

Gross Features

These tumors usually form an obvious cervical mass, are grossly exophytic or endophytic and can vary greatly in size.

Microscopic Features

Histologically, these tumors are similar to adenoid cystic carcinomas of the salivary gland **Fig. 42**. There are two morphologic patterns, the usual type and the solid variant. The tumor can grow in nests of cells with focal cribriforming, sheets, trabeculae and cords.[249] Hyaline basement membrane-like material that stains with collagen type IV and laminin is often deposited within glandular lumen.[261,264] There is usually at least focal palisading of nuclei at the periphery of tumor nests. Cytologically, in contrast to adenoid basal epithelioma, the main differential diagnosis, the cells are slightly larger and more pleomorphic with high mitotic counts; there can be necrosis, which may be extensive.[146] However, small foci of squamous differentiation and nests similar to adenoid basal epithelioma can also be present, which can cause diagnostic confusion. The stromal response may be myxoid, fibroblastic or hyaline and adenoid cystic carcinoma has been reported to be the epithelial component of malignant mixed Müllerian tumors (MMMT) of the cervix.[251,260,265–269]

The solid variant is a histologically distinct variant lacking the characteristic cribriform pattern of conventional adenoid cystic carcinoma. The tumor cells are undifferentiated or basaloid, growing in cords, nests, trabeculae and nodules with possible squamous differentiation and necrosis.[270] They produce PAS-positive basement membrane like material that in some areas compresses the tumor cells - this feature can help distinguish these from basaloid squamous carcinomas. These tumors are also negative for neurosecretory granules and myoepithelial cells.[270] Occasional large vesicular nuclei with

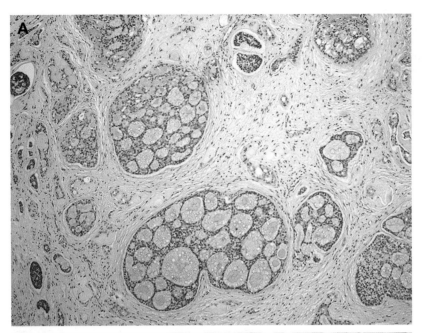

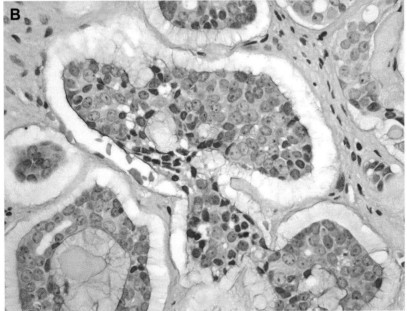

Fig. 42. Adenoid cystic carcinoma. (*A*) Cribriform glands with hyaline basement membrane-like luminal secretions. (*B*) Tumor cells with moderate to severe cytologic atypia.

prominent nucleoli have been described, especially in those tumors with solid growth or necrosis.

Differential Diagnosis

Other poorly differentiated carcinomas enter the differential diagnosis, including squamous, glandular and neuroendocrine tumors. However, the most commonly mistaken entity with adenoid cystic carcinoma is adenoid basal epithelioma/carcinoma. Adenoid basal epithelioma is a well differentiated, usually indolent neoplasm that is incidentally discovered in the cervix and often associated with an overlying squamous dysplasia (see previous section). This is in contrast to adenoid cystic carcinoma which usually presents with a large clinically visible mass. It is important to make the distinctions between these two tumors since they have entirely different clinical outcomes. There has been a reported case of a mixed adenoid cystic and adenoid basal carcinoma with morphologic transition between the two components, suggesting that these tumors are etiologically related and that one may possibly arise from the other.[251]

Biomarkers

The majority of cervical adenoid cystic carcinomas have been shown to be positive for cytokeratin MNF116 and Cam 5.2.[251] CK7 is positive in about 50% of cases while EMA and CEA stain the luminal membranes of glands only.[251] S100 protein has been shown to be both positive and negative, the significance of which is unknown.[249,251]

Prognosis

Most patients are over the age of 60 with a high proportion of black women, although occasional cases occurring in women less than 40 have been reported.[271] The majority of women present with postmenopausal bleeding and an obvious mass on clinical examination. Both local and distant recurrences occur in early and late stage disease with lung being the most common site of distant metastasis.[272–274] The abdominal cavity

and brain can also be involved.[272] The prognosis for high stage disease is poor.

NEUROENDOCRINE TUMORS

Neuroendocrine tumors of the cervix are rare and can occur alone or in the setting of invasive or in situ cervical squamous or adenocarcinoma, which may be a minor or major component **Fig. 43**.[275] It is postulated that endocrine cell hyperplasia in normal cervical glands may be a precursor to these tumors.[276] A variety of peptides and hormones are present, such as calcitonin, gastrin, serotonin, substance P, vasoactive intestinal peptide, pancreatic polypeptide, somatostatin and adrenocorticotrophic hormone, however, their clinical significance is limited.[277–285] Since the morphologic features of endocrine tumors in the cervix are comparable to those in the lung, the terminology from pulmonary neuroendocrine tumor classification has been adopted to also describe cervical neuroendocrine tumors.[275]

Classification of Cervical Neuroendocrine Tumors

- Typical (Classical) Carcinoid Tumor
- Atypical Carcinoid Tumor
- Large Cell Neuroendocrine Tumor
- Small Cell Carcinoma.

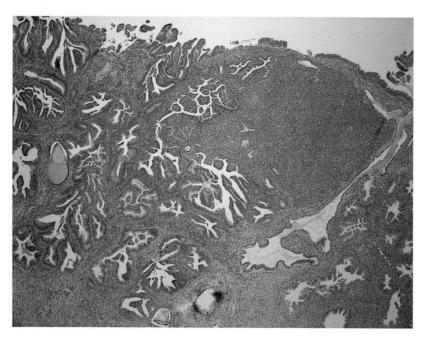

Fig. 43. Endocervical adenocarcinoma with neuroendocrine tumor.

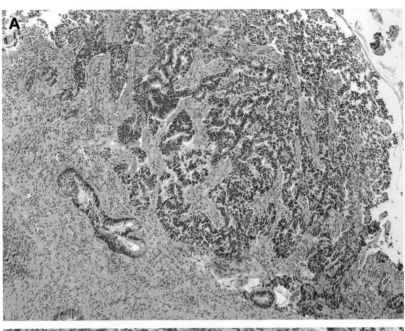

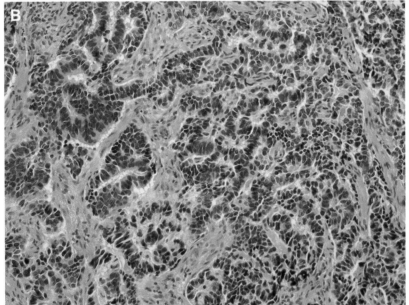

Fig. 44. Cervical carcinoid (*A, B*).

Typical (Classical) Carcinoid Tumor

These tumors display trabecular, nodular or cord-like architectural patterns and rosette-like structures are common. The cells are small, round, uniform with finely granular chromatin and inconspicuous nucleoli (**Fig. 44**). Mitoses are rare and greater than 70% show positive reaction to neuroendocrine markers (chromogranin, synaptophysin, neuron specific enolase). However, these tumors should be easily recognized on light microscopy.

Fig. 44. Cervical carcinoid. Chromogranin (*C*), synaptophysin (*D*).

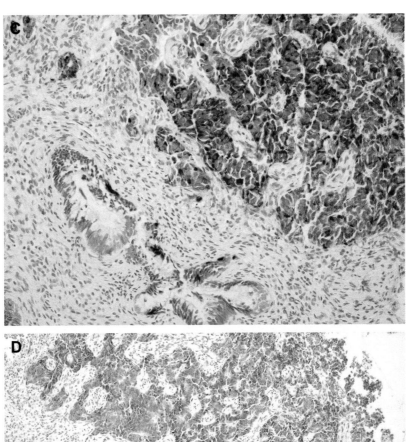

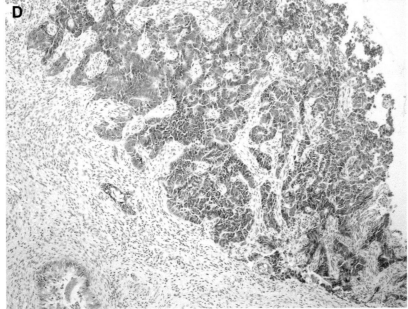

ATYPICAL CARCINOID TUMOR

In contrast to typical carcinoids, atypical carcinoids are hypercellular with cytologic atypia, increased mitoses (5–10 per 10 high power fields) and foci of necrosis.[275] The growth pattern is the same as typical carcinoid with similar staining patterns.

LARGE CELL NEUROENDOCRINE TUMOR

This is a poorly differentiated, high grade malignant tumor morphologically and biologically closer to small cell carcinoma than to typical carcinoid.[275] The growth pattern is organoid, trabecular or cord-like with prominent peripheral palisading and variable necrosis. The cells are large with abundant cytoplasm, vesicular nuclei and prominent nucleoli and mitotic figures are numerous (greater than 10 per 10 HPF) (**Fig. 45**). Since poorly differentiated carcinomas of the cervix may have a neuroendocrine appearance, large cell neuroendocrine carcinoma of the cervix must be confirmed by stains or electron microscopy.[275]

Small Cell Carcinoma

Similar to small cell carcinoma of the lung, these cells are small, fusiform with scant cytoplasm and hyperchromatic nuclei with finely granular chromatin and absent or inconspicuous nucleoli. Numerous mitotic figures and extensive necrosis are characteristic. The tumors cells may grow in sheets, nests, trabeculae or cords and peripheral

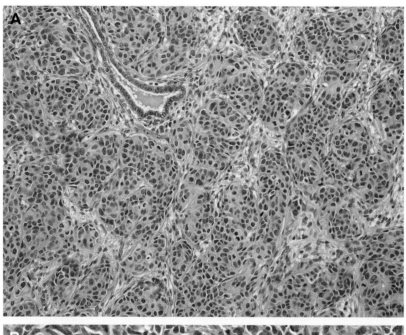

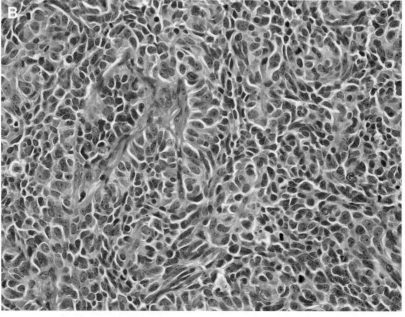

Fig. 45. Large cell neuro-endocrine carcinoma. (*A*) Organoid growth of cells with, (*B*) abundant cyto-plasm, vesicular nuclei and prominent nucleoli.

palisading and prominent perivascular growth are common **Fig. 46**. Staining for neuroendocrine markers is not necessary for the diagnosis since approximately 60% do not react with chromogranin or synaptophysin and about one-third do not express neuron specific enolase.[275] A small percentage of cervical small cell carcinomas express TTF-1 staining, similar to other extrapulmonary small cell carcinomas.[286–288]

Neuroendocrine tumors of the cervix are etiologically related to infection by high risk HPV, most commonly HPV 16 and 18.[282,289–296] Clinically, atypical carcinoids, large cell neuroendocrine and small cell carcinomas are all biologically aggressive with poor 5-year survival.[283,293,297,298] Due to the rarity of these tumors, optimal treatment options are not standardized, however, studies have shown that stage (limited versus metastatic)

Fig. 46. Small cell carcinoma. (*A*) Sheets and nests of tumor cells with, (*B*) hyperchromatic nuclei with finely granular chromatin and inconspicuous nucleoli.

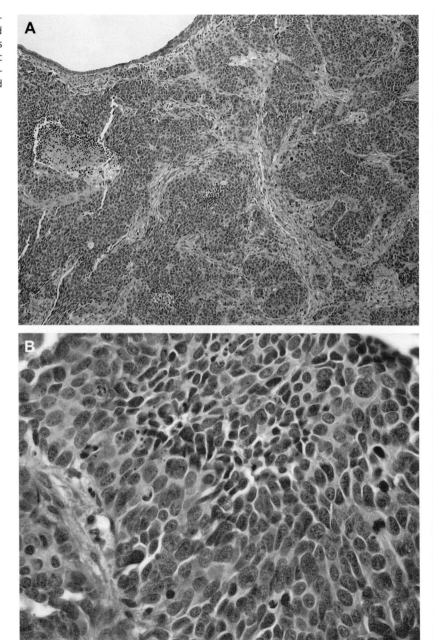

and initial treatment with chemotherapy have the most prognostic impact in small cell carcinomas.[298]

REFERENCES

1. Nasiell K, Roger V, Nasiell M. Behavior of mild cervical dysplasia during long-term follow-up. Obstet Gynecol 1986;67(5):665–9.
2. Ostor AG. Natural history of cervical intraepithelial neoplasia: a critical review. Int J Gynecol Pathol 1993;12(2):186–92.
3. Schlecht N, Platt RW, Duarte-Franco E, et al. Human papillomavirus infection and time to progression and regression of cervical intraepithelial neoplasia. J Natl Cancer Inst 2003;95(17):1336–43.
4. Clifford GM, Rana RK, Franceschi S, et al. Human papillomavirus genotype distribution in low-grade cervical lesions: comparison by geographic region and with cervical cancer. Cancer Epidemiol Biomarkers Prev 2005;14(5):1157–64.
5. Munoz N, Bosch FX, de Sanjosé S, et al. Epidemiologic classification of human papillomavirus types associated with cervical cancer. N Engl J Med 2003;348(6):518–27.
6. Dalla Palma P, Giorgi Rossi P, Collina G, et al. The reproducibility of CIN diagnoses among different pathologists: data from histology reviews from a multicenter randomized study. Am J Clin Pathol 2009;132(1):125–32.
7. Schiffman M, Solomon D. Findings to date from the ASCUS-LSIL Triage Study (ALTS). Arch Pathol Lab Med 2003;127(8):946–9.
8. Park K, Ellenson LH, Pirog EC. Low-grade squamous intraepithelial lesions of the cervix with marked cytological atypia-clinical follow-up and human papillomavirus genotyping. Int J Gynecol Pathol 2007;26(4):457–62.
9. Crum CP, Egawa K, Fu YS, et al. Atypical immature metaplasia (AIM). A subset of human papilloma virus infection of the cervix. Cancer 1983;51(12):2214–9.
10. Duggan MA, Akbari M, Magliocco AM. Atypical immature cervical metaplasia: immunoprofiling and longitudinal outcome. Hum Pathol 2006;37(11):1473–81.
11. Geng L, Connolly DC, Isacson C, et al. Atypical immature metaplasia (AIM) of the cervix: is it related to high-grade squamous intraepithelial lesion (HSIL)? Hum Pathol 1999;30(3):345–51.
12. Iaconis L, Hyjek E, Ellenson LH, et al. p16 and Ki-67 immunostaining in atypical immature squamous metaplasia of the uterine cervix: correlation with human papillomavirus detection. Arch Pathol Lab Med 2007;131(9):1343–9.
13. Ma L, Fisk JM, Zhang RR, et al. Eosinophilic dysplasia of the cervix: a newly recognized variant of cervical squamous intraepithelial neoplasia. Am J Surg Pathol 2004;28(11):1474–84.
14. Mondaini N, Giubilei G, Raspollini MR, et al. Recurrence of vaginal implantation of transitional cell carcinoma of the urinary tract. Gynecol Oncol 2005;97(2):669–70.
15. Brown HM, Wilkinson EJ. Cytology of secondary vulvar Paget's disease of urothelial origin: a case report. Acta Cytol 2005;49(1):71–4.
16. Yazgan C, Erden A, Yagci O, et al. Clitoral metastasis from transitional cell carcinoma of the renal pelvis: CT and MRI findings. Int Urol Nephrol 2004;36(3):331–3.
17. Wilkinson EJ, Brown HM. Vulvar Paget disease of urothelial origin: a report of three cases and a proposed classification of vulvar Paget disease. Hum Pathol 2002;33(5):549–54.
18. Kumar R, Kumar S, Hemal AK. Vaginal and omental metastasis from superficial bladder cancer. Urol Int 2001;67(1):117–8.
19. Lerner LB, Andrews SJ, Gonzalez JL, et al. Vulvar metastases secondary to transitional cell carcinoma of the bladder. A case report. J Reprod Med 1999;44(8):729–32.
20. Bulbul MA, Kaspar H, Nasr R, et al. Urothelial carcinoma of the vagina six years following cystectomy for invasive cancer. A case report. Eur J Gynaecol Oncol 1999;20(3):233–4.
21. Arnould L, Chalabreysse L, Belichard C, et al. Genital carcinoma secondary to pagetoid spread from a pagetoid urothelial carcinoma in-situ. Histopathology 1998;32(6):575–7.
22. Klaes R, Friedrich T, Spitkovsky D, et al. Overexpression of p16(INK4A) as a specific marker for dysplastic and neoplastic epithelial cells of the cervix uteri. Int J Cancer 2001;92(2):276–84.
23. Agoff SN, Lin P, Morihara J, et al. p16(INK4a) expression correlates with degree of cervical neoplasia: a comparison with Ki-67 expression and detection of high-risk HPV types. Mod Pathol 2003;16(7):665–73.
24. Keating JT, Cviko A, Riethdorf S, et al. Ki-67, cyclin E, and p16INK4 are complimentary surrogate biomarkers for human papilloma virus-related cervical neoplasia. Am J Surg Pathol 2001;25(7):884–91.
25. Lorenzato M, Caudroy S, Bronner C, et al. Cell cycle and/or proliferation markers: what is the best method to discriminate cervical high-grade lesions? Hum Pathol 2005;36(10):1101–7.
26. Murphy N, Ring M, Heffron CC, et al. p16INK4A, CDC6, and MCM5: predictive biomarkers in cervical preinvasive neoplasia and cervical cancer. J Clin Pathol 2005;58(5):525–34.
27. Sano T, Oyama T, Kashiwabara K, et al. Expression status of p16 protein is associated with human papillomavirus oncogenic potential in cervical and genital lesions. Am J Pathol 1998;153(6):1741–8.

28. Wang SS, Trunk M, Schiffman M, et al. Validation of p16INK4a as a marker of oncogenic human papillomavirus infection in cervical biopsies from a population-based cohort in Costa Rica. Cancer Epidemiol Biomarkers Prev 2004;13(8): 1355–60.

29. Kong CS, Balzer BL, Troxell ML, et al. p16INK4A immunohistochemistry is superior to HPV in situ hybridization for the detection of high-risk HPV in atypical squamous metaplasia. Am J Surg Pathol 2007;31(1):33–43.

30. Yin M, Bastacky S, Parwani AV, et al. p16ink4 immunoreactivity is a reliable marker for urothelial carcinoma in situ. Hum Pathol 2008;39(4):527–35.

31. Raspollini MR, Nesi G, Baroni G, et al. p16(INK4a) expression in urinary bladder carcinoma. Arch Ital Urol Androl 2006;78(3):97–100.

32. al-Saleh W, Delvenne P, Greimers R, et al. Assessment of Ki-67 antigen immunostaining in squamous intraepithelial lesions of the uterine cervix. Correlation with the histologic grade and human papillomavirus type. Am J Clin Pathol 1995;104(2): 154–60.

33. Mittal K, Demopoulos RI, Tata M. A comparison of proliferative activity and atypical mitoses in cervical condylomas with various HPV types. Int J Gynecol Pathol 1998;17(1):24–8.

34. Pirog EC, Baergen RN, Soslow RA, et al. Diagnostic accuracy of cervical low-grade squamous intraepithelial lesions is improved with MIB-1 immunostaining. Am J Surg Pathol 2002;26(1):70–5.

35. Isacson C, Kessis TD, Hedrick L, et al. Both cell proliferation and apoptosis increase with lesion grade in cervical neoplasia but do not correlate with human papillomavirus type. Cancer Res 1996;56(4):669–74.

36. Pirog EC, Chen YT, Isacson C. MIB-1 immunostaining is a beneficial adjunct test for accurate diagnosis of vulvar condyloma acuminatum. Am J Surg Pathol 2000;24(10):1393–9.

37. Chen Y, Miller C, Mosher R, et al. Identification of cervical cancer markers by cDNA and tissue microarrays. Cancer Res 2003;63(8):1927–35.

38. Santin AD, Zhan F, Bignotti E, et al. Gene expression profiles of primary HPV16- and HPV18-infected early stage cervical cancers and normal cervical epithelium: identification of novel candidate molecular markers for cervical cancer diagnosis and therapy. Virology 2005;331(2):269–91.

39. Shroyer KR, Homer P, Heinz D, et al. Validation of a novel immunocytochemical assay for topoisomerase II-alpha and minichromosome maintenance protein 2 expression in cervical cytology. Cancer 2006;108(5):324–30.

40. Shi J, Liu H, Wilkerson M, et al. Evaluation of p16INK4a, minichromosome maintenance protein 2, DNA topoisomerase IIalpha, ProEX C, and p16INK4a/ProEX C in cervical squamous intraepithelial lesions. Hum Pathol 2007;38(9):1335–44.

41. Badr RE, Walts AE, Chung F, et al. BD ProEx C: a sensitive and specific marker of HPV-associated squamous lesions of the cervix. Am J Surg Pathol 2008;32(6):899–906.

42. Pinto AP, Schlecht NF, Woo TY, et al. Biomarker (ProEx C, p16(INK4A), and MiB-1) distinction of high-grade squamous intraepithelial lesion from its mimics. Mod Pathol 2008;21(9):1067–74.

43. Sambrook J, Russell D, editors. Molecular cloning: a laboratory manual. 3rd edition. Cold Spring Harbor (NY): Cold Spring Harbor Laboratory Press; 2001.

44. Caussy D, Orr W, Daya AD, et al. Evaluation of methods for detecting human papillomavirus deoxyribonucleotide sequences in clinical specimens. J Clin Microbiol 1988;26(2):236–43.

45. Ausubel F, editor. Short protocols in molecular biology: a compendium of methods from current protocols in molecular biology. 4th edition. New York: Wiley; 1999.

46. Guo M, Gong Y, Deavers M, et al. Evaluation of a commercialized in situ hybridization assay for detecting human papillomavirus DNA in tissue specimens from patients with cervical intraepithelial neoplasia and cervical carcinoma. J Clin Microbiol 2008;46(1):274–80.

47. Ho GY, Bierman R, Beardsley L, et al. Natural history of cervicovaginal papillomavirus infection in young women. N Engl J Med 1998;338(7):423–8.

48. Baseman JG, Koutsky LA. The epidemiology of human papillomavirus infections. J Clin Virol 2005; 32(Suppl 1):S16–24.

49. U.S. Cancer Statistics Working Group. United States Cancer Statistics:2004 incidence and mortality. Atlanta (GA): Department of Health and Human Services and the National Cancer Institute; 2007.

50. Ferlay J. Globocan 2002: cancer incidence, mortality and prevalence worldwide. in IARC Cancer Base No. 5, version 2.0. Lyon (France): IARC Press; 2004.

51. Bosch FX, Lorincz A, Muñoz N, et al. The causal relation between human papillomavirus and cervical cancer. J Clin Pathol 2002;55(4):244–65.

52. Tavassoli FA, Devilee P, editors. Pathology & genetics tumors of the breast and female genital organs. World Health Organization Classification of Tumors. Lyon (France): Oxford University Press; 2000. p. 260.

53. Okagaki T, Clark BA, Zachow KR, et al. Presence of human papillomavirus in verrucous carcinoma (Ackerman) of the vagina. Immunocytochemical, ultrastructural, and DNA hybridization studies. Arch Pathol Lab Med 1984;108(7):567–70.

54. Nishikawa T, Kobayashi H, Shindoh M, et al. A case of verrucous carcinoma associated with human

papillomavirus type 16 DNA. J Dermatol 1993; 20(8):483–8.

55. Yorganci A, Serinsoz E, Ensari A, et al. A case report of multicentric verrucous carcinoma of the female genital tract. Gynecol Oncol 2003;90(2):478–81.

56. Brinck U, Jakob C, Bau O, et al. Papillary squamous cell carcinoma of the uterine cervix: report of three cases and a review of its classification. Int J Gynecol Pathol 2000;19(3):231–5.

57. Tseng CJ, Pao CC, Tseng LH, et al. Lymphoepithelioma-like carcinoma of the uterine cervix: association with Epstein-Barr virus and human papillomavirus. Cancer 1997;80(1):91–7.

58. Weinberg E, Hoisington S, Eastman AY, et al. Uterine cervical lymphoepithelial-like carcinoma. Absence of Epstein-Barr virus genomes. Am J Clin Pathol 1993;99(2):195–9.

59. Lininger RA, Wistuba I, Gazdar A, et al. Human papillomavirus type 16 is detected in transitional cell carcinomas and squamotransitional cell carcinomas of the cervix and endometrium. Cancer 1998;83(3):521–7.

60. Maitra A, Wistuba II, Gibbons D, et al. Allelic losses at chromosome 3p are seen in human papilloma virus 16 associated transitional cell carcinoma of the cervix. Gynecol Oncol 1999;74(3):361–8.

61. Albores-Saavedra J, Young RH. Transitional cell neoplasms (carcinomas and inverted papillomas) of the uterine cervix. A report of five cases. Am J Surg Pathol 1995;19(10):1138–45.

62. Ortega-Gonzalez P, Chanona-Vilchis J, Dominguez-Malagon H. Transitional cell carcinoma of the uterine cervix. A report of six cases with clinical, histologic and cytologic findings. Acta Cytol 2002; 46(3):585–90.

63. Steeper TA, Piscioli F, Rosai J. Squamous cell carcinoma with sarcoma-like stroma of the female genital tract. Clinicopathologic study of four cases. Cancer 1983;52(5):890–8.

64. Brown J, Broaddus R, Koeller M, et al. Sarcomatoid carcinoma of the cervix. Gynecol Oncol 2003; 90(1):23–8.

65. Pang LC. Sarcomatoid squamous cell carcinoma of the uterine cervix with osteoclast-like giant cells: report of two cases. Int J Gynecol Pathol 1998;17(2):174–7.

66. Rodrigues L, Santana I, Cunha T, et al. Sarcomatoid squamous cell carcinoma of the uterine cervix: case report. Eur J Gynaecol Oncol 2000;21(3):287–9.

67. Rush D, Hyjek E, Baergen RN, et al. Detection of microinvasion in vulvar and cervical intraepithelial neoplasia using double immunostaining for cytokeratin and basement membrane components. Arch Pathol Lab Med 2005;129(6):747–53.

68. Shih IM, Kurman RJ. Epithelioid trophoblastic tumor: a neoplasm distinct from choriocarcinoma and placental site trophoblastic tumor simulating carcinoma. Am J Surg Pathol 1998;22(11):1393–403.

69. Pecorelli S, Zigliani L, Odicino F. Revised FIGO staging for carcinoma of the cervix. Int J Gynaecol Obstet 2009;105(2):107–8.

70. Rock JA, Jones HW, editors. TeLinde's operative gynecology. 10th edition. Philadelphia: Lippincott Williams & Wilkins; 2008.

71. Benedet JL, Bender H, Jones H 3rd, et al. FIGO staging classifications and clinical practice guidelines in the management of gynecologic cancers. FIGO Committee on Gynecologic Oncology. Int J Gynaecol Obstet 2000;70(2):209–62.

72. Zaino RJ, Ward S, Delgado G, et al. Histopathologic predictors of the behavior of surgically treated stage IB squamous cell carcinoma of the cervix. A Gynecologic Oncology Group study. Cancer 1992;69(7):1750–8.

73. Roman LD, Felix JC, Muderspach LI, et al. Influence of quantity of lymph-vascular space invasion on the risk of nodal metastases in women with early-stage squamous cancer of the cervix. Gynecol Oncol 1998;68(3):220–5.

74. Comerci G, Bolger BS, Flannelly G, et al. Prognostic factors in surgically treated stage IB-IIB carcinoma of the cervix with negative lymph nodes. Int J Gynecol Cancer 1998;8(1):23–6.

75. Kristensen GB, Abeler VM, Risberg B, et al. Tumor size, depth of invasion, and grading of the invasive tumor front are the main prognostic factors in early squamous cell cervical carcinoma. Gynecol Oncol 1999;74(2):245–51.

76. Takeda N, Sakuragi N, Takeda M, et al. Multivariate analysis of histopathologic prognostic factors for invasive cervical cancer treated with radical hysterectomy and systematic retroperitoneal lymphadenectomy. Acta Obstet Gynecol Scand 2002; 81(12):1144–51.

77. Pickel H, Haas J, Lahousen M. Prognostic factors in cervical cancer. Eur J Obstet Gynecol Reprod Biol 1997;71(2):209–13.

78. Delgado G, Bundy B, Zaino R, et al. Prospective surgical-pathological study of disease-free interval in patients with stage IB squamous cell carcinoma of the cervix: a Gynecologic Oncology Group study. Gynecol Oncol 1990;38(3):352–7.

79. Friedell GH, McKay DG. Adenocarcinoma in situ of the endocervix. Cancer 1953;6(5):887–97.

80. Bertrand M, Lickrish GM, Colgan TJ. The anatomic distribution of cervical adenocarcinoma in situ: implications for treatment. Am J Obstet Gynecol 1987;157(1):21–5.

81. Shin CH, Schorge JO, Lee KR, et al. Conservative management of adenocarcinoma in situ of the cervix. Gynecol Oncol 2000;79(1):6–10.

82. Ostor AG, Duncan A, Quinn M, et al. Adenocarcinoma in situ of the uterine cervix: an experience with 100 cases. Gynecol Oncol 2000;79(2): 207–10.

83. Denehy TR, Gregori CA, Breen JL. Endocervical curettage, cone margins, and residual adenocarcinoma in situ of the cervix. Obstet Gynecol 1997; 90(1):1–6.

84. Boon ME, Baak JP, Kurver PJ, et al. Adenocarcinoma in situ of the cervix: an underdiagnosed lesion. Cancer 1981;48(3):768–73.

85. Gloor E, Ruzicka J. Morphology of adenocarcinoma in situ of the uterine cervix: a study of 14 cases. Cancer 1982;49(2):294–302.

86. Bousfield L, Pacey F, Young Q, et al. Expanded cytologic criteria for the diagnosis of adenocarcinoma in situ of the cervix and related lesions. Acta Cytol 1980;24(4):283–96.

87. Azodi M, Chambers SK, Rutherford TJ, et al. Adenocarcinoma in situ of the cervix: management and outcome. Gynecol Oncol 1999;73(3):348–53.

88. Zaino RJ. Symposium part I: adenocarcinoma in situ, glandular dysplasia, and early invasive adenocarcinoma of the uterine cervix. Int J Gynecol Pathol 2002;21(4):314–26.

89. Poynor EA, Barakat RR, Hoskins WJ. Management and follow-up of patients with adenocarcinoma in situ of the uterine cervix. Gynecol Oncol 1995; 57(2):158–64.

90. Kennedy AW, elTabbakh GH, Biscotti CV, et al. Invasive adenocarcinoma of the cervix following LLETZ (large loop excision of the transformation zone) for adenocarcinoma in situ. Gynecol Oncol 1995;58(2):274–7.

91. Kashimura M, Shinohara M, Oikawa K, et al. An adenocarcinoma in situ of the uterine cervix that developed into invasive adenocarcinoma after 5 years. Gynecol Oncol 1990;36(1):128–33.

92. Tase T, Okagaki T, Clark BA, et al. Human papillomavirus DNA in adenocarcinoma in situ, microinvasive adenocarcinoma of the uterine cervix, and coexisting cervical squamous intraepithelial neoplasia. Int J Gynecol Pathol 1989; 8(1):8–17.

93. Farnsworth A, Laverty C, Stoler MH. Human papillomavirus messenger RNA expression in adenocarcinoma in situ of the uterine cervix. Int J Gynecol Pathol 1989;8(4):321–30.

94. Park JJ, Sun D, Quade BJ, et al. Stratified mucin-producing intraepithelial lesions of the cervix: adenosquamous or columnar cell neoplasia? Am J Surg Pathol 2000;24(10):1414–9.

95. Oliva E, Clement PB, Young RH. Tubal and tuboendometrioid metaplasia of the uterine cervix. Unemphasized features that may cause problems in differential diagnosis: a report of 25 cases. Am J Clin Pathol 1995;103(5):618–23.

96. Cameron RI, Maxwell P, Jenkins D, et al. Immunohistochemical staining with MIB1, bcl2 and p16 assists in the distinction of cervical glandular intraepithelial neoplasia from tubo-endometrial

metaplasia, endometriosis and microglandular hyperplasia. Histopathology 2002;41(4):313–21.

97. Young RH, Clement PB. Pseudoneoplastic glandular lesions of the uterine cervix. Semin Diagn Pathol 1991;8(4):234–49.

98. Lesack D, Wahab I, Gilks CB. Radiation-induced atypia of endocervical epithelium: a histological, immunohistochemical and cytometric study. Int J Gynecol Pathol 1996;15(3):242–7.

99. Jaworski RC. Endocervical glandular dysplasia, adenocarcinoma in situ, and early invasive (microinvasive) adenocarcinoma of the uterine cervix. Semin Diagn Pathol 1990;7(3):190–204.

100. Brown LJ, Wells M. Cervical glandular atypia associated with squamous intraepithelial neoplasia: a premalignant lesion? J Clin Pathol 1986;39(1): 22–8.

101. Casper GR, Ostor AG, Quinn MA. A clinicopathologic study of glandular dysplasia of the cervix. Gynecol Oncol 1997;64(1):166–70.

102. Marjoniemi VM. Immunohistochemistry in gynaecological pathology: a review. Pathology 2004;36(2): 109–19.

103. Pirog EC, Isacson C, Szabolcs MJ, et al. Proliferative activity of benign and neoplastic endocervical epithelium and correlation with HPV DNA detection. Int J Gynecol Pathol 2002;21(1):22–6.

104. Riethdorf L, Riethdorf S, Lee KR, et al. Human papillomaviruses, expression of p16, and early endocervical glandular neoplasia. Hum Pathol 2002; 33(9):899–904.

105. Negri G, Egarter-Vigl E, Kasal A, et al. p16INK4a is a useful marker for the diagnosis of adenocarcinoma of the cervix uteri and its precursors: an immunohistochemical study with immunocytochemical correlations. Am J Surg Pathol 2003; 27(2):187–93.

106. Pavlakis K, Messini I, Athanassiadou S, et al. Endocervical glandular lesions: a diagnostic approach combining a semi-quantitative scoring method to the expression of CEA, MIB-1 and p16. Gynecol Oncol 2006;103(3):971–6.

107. van Hoeven KH, Ramondetta L, Kovatich AJ, et al. Quantitative image analysis of MIB-1 reactivity in inflammatory, hyperplastic, and neoplastic endocervical lesions. Int J Gynecol Pathol 1997;16(1):15–21.

108. Cina SJ, Richardson MS, Austin RM, et al. Immunohistochemical staining for Ki-67 antigen, carcinoembryonic antigen, and p53 in the differential diagnosis of glandular lesions of the cervix. Mod Pathol 1997;10(3):176–80.

109. McCluggage WG, Maxwell P, McBride HA, et al. Monoclonal antibodies Ki-67 and MIB1 in the distinction of tuboendometrial metaplasia from endocervical adenocarcinoma and adenocarcinoma in situ in formalin-fixed material. Int J Gynecol Pathol 1995;14(3):209–16.

110. Aximu D, Azad A, Ni R, et al. A pilot evaluation of a novel immunohistochemical assay for topoisomerase II-alpha and minichromosome maintenance protein 2 expression (ProEx C) in cervical adenocarcinoma in situ, adenocarcinoma, and benign glandular mimics. Int J Gynecol Pathol 2009;28(2):114–9.

111. McCluggage WG, Maxwell P. bcl-2 and p21 immunostaining of cervical tubo-endometrial metaplasia. Histopathology 2002;40(1):107–8.

112. McCluggage WG, Shah R, Connolly LE, et al. Intestinal-type cervical adenocarcinoma in situ and adenocarcinoma exhibit a partial enteric immunophenotype with consistent expression of CDX2. Int J Gynecol Pathol 2008;27(1):92–100.

113. Park KJ, Bramlage MP, Ellenson LH, et al. Immunoprofile of adenocarcinomas of the endometrium, endocervix, and ovary with mucinous differentiation. Appl Immunohistochem Mol Morphol 2009; 17(1):8–11.

114. Andersen ES, Arffmann E. Adenocarcinoma in situ of the uterine cervix: a clinico-pathologic study of 36 cases. Gynecol Oncol 1989;35(1):1–7.

115. Jaworski RC, Pacey NF, Greenberg ML, et al. The histologic diagnosis of adenocarcinoma in situ and related lesions of the cervix uteri. Adenocarcinoma in situ. Cancer 1988;61(6):1171–81.

116. Tobon H, Dave H. Adenocarcinoma in situ of the cervix. Clinicopathologic observations of 11 cases. Int J Gynecol Pathol 1988;7(2):139–51.

117. Hopkins MP. Adenocarcinoma in situ of the cervix–the margins must be clear. Gynecol Oncol 2000; 79(1):4–5.

118. Im DD, Duska LR, Rosenshein NB. Adequacy of conization margins in adenocarcinoma in situ of the cervix as a predictor of residual disease. Gynecol Oncol 1995;59(2):179–82.

119. Muntz HG, Bell DA, Lage JM, et al. Adenocarcinoma in situ of the uterine cervix. Obstet Gynecol 1992;80(6):935–9.

120. Ostor AG, Pagano R, Davoren RA, et al. Adenocarcinoma in situ of the cervix. Int J Gynecol Pathol 1984;3(2):179–90.

121. Smith HO, Tiffany MF, Qualls CR, et al. The rising incidence of adenocarcinoma relative to squamous cell carcinoma of the uterine cervix in the United States–a 24-year population-based study. Gynecol Oncol 2000;78(2):97–105.

122. Davis JR, Moon LB. Increased incidence of adenocarcinoma of uterine cervix. Obstet Gynecol 1975; 45(1):79–83.

123. Devesa SS. Descriptive epidemiology of cancer of the uterine cervix. Obstet Gynecol 1984;63(5): 605–12.

124. Anton-Culver H, Bloss JD, Bringman D, et al. Comparison of adenocarcinoma and squamous cell carcinoma of the uterine cervix: a population-based epidemiologic study. Am J Obstet Gynecol 1992;166(5):1507–14.

125. Horowitz IR, Jacobson LP, Zucker PK, et al. Epidemiology of adenocarcinoma of the cervix. Gynecol Oncol 1988;31(1):25–31.

126. Pirog EC, Kleter B, Olgac S, et al. Prevalence of human papillomavirus DNA in different histological subtypes of cervical adenocarcinoma. Am J Pathol 2000;157(4):1055–62.

127. Clement PB, Young RH. Deep nabothian cysts of the uterine cervix. A possible source of confusion with minimal-deviation adenocarcinoma (adenoma malignum). Int J Gynecol Pathol 1989;8(4):340–8.

128. Ostor AG. Early invasive adenocarcinoma of the uterine cervix. Int J Gynecol Pathol 2000;19(1):29–38.

129. Fluhmann CF. Focal hyperplasis (tunnel clusters) of the cervix uteri. Obstet Gynecol 1961;17:206–14.

130. Abell MR, Gosling JR. Gland cell carcinoma (adenocarcinoma) of the uterine cervix. Am J Obstet Gynecol 1962;83:729–55.

131. Fu YS, Reagan JW, Hsiu JG, et al. Adenocarcinoma and mixed carcinoma of the uterine cervix. I.A. clinicopathologic study. Cancer 1982;49(12):2560–70.

132. Rombaut RP, Charles D, Murphy A. Adenocarcinoma of the cervix. A clinicopathologic study of 47 cases. Cancer 1966;19(7):891–900.

133. Jones MW, Silverberg SG, Kurman RJ. Well-differentiated villoglandular adenocarcinoma of the uterine cervix: a clinicopathological study of 24 cases. Int J Gynecol Pathol 1993;12(1):1–7.

134. Young RH, Scully RE. Villoglandular papillary adenocarcinoma of the uterine cervix. A clinicopathologic analysis of 13 cases. Cancer 1989; 63(9):1773–9.

135. Bouman A, Oosterhuis GJ, Naudin ten Cate L, et al. Villoglandular papillary adenocarcinoma of the cervix. Beware of a wolf in sheep's clothing. Eur J Obstet Gynecol Reprod Biol 1999;87(2):183–9.

136. Garcea A, Nunns D, Ireland D, et al. A case of villoglandular papillary adenocarcinoma of the cervix with lymph node metastasis. BJOG 2003;110(6): 627–9.

137. Khunamornpong S, Maleemonkol S, Siriaunkgul S, et al. Well-Differentiated villoglandular adenocarcinoma of the uterine cervix: a report of 15 cases including two with lymph node metastasis. J Med Assoc Thai 2001;84(6):882–8.

138. Utsugi K, Shimizu Y, Akiyama F, et al. Villoglandular papillary adenocarcinoma of the uterine cervix with bulky lymph node metastases. Eur J Obstet Gynecol Reprod Biol 2002;105(2):186–8.

139. Heatley MK. Villoglandular adenocarcinoma of the uterine cervix-a systematic review of the literature. Histopathology 2007;51(2):268–9.

140. Korach J, Machtinger R, Perri T, et al. Villoglandular papillary adenocarcinoma of the uterine cervix: a

diagnostic challenge. Acta Obstet Gynecol Scand 2009;88(3):355–8.

141. Macdonald RD, Kirwan J, Hayat K, et al. Villoglandular adenocarcinoma of the cervix: clarity is needed on the histological definition for this difficult diagnosis. Gynecol Oncol 2006;100(1):192–4.

142. An HJ, Kim KR, Kim IS, et al. Prevalence of human papillomavirus DNA in various histological subtypes of cervical adenocarcinoma: a population-based study. Mod Pathol 2005;18(4):528–34.

143. Matthews-Greer J, Dominguez-Malagon H, Herrera GA, et al. Human papillomavirus typing of rare cervical carcinomas. Arch Pathol Lab Med 2004;128(5):553–6.

144. Yamazawa K, Matsui H, Seki K, et al. Human papillomavirus-positive well-differentiated villoglandular adenocarcinoma of the uterine cervix: a case report and review of the literature. Gynecol Oncol 2000;77(3):473–7.

145. Chang WC, Matisic JP, Zhou C, et al. Cytologic features of villoglandular adenocarcinoma of the uterine cervix: comparison with typical endocervical adenocarcinoma with a villoglandular component and papillary serous carcinoma. Cancer 1999;87(1):5–11.

146. Young RH, Clement PB. Endocervical adenocarcinoma and its variants: their morphology and differential diagnosis. Histopathology 2002;41(3):185–207.

147. Ronnett BM, Yemelyanova AV, Vang R, et al. Endocervical adenocarcinomas with ovarian metastases: analysis of 29 cases with emphasis on minimally invasive cervical tumors and the ability of the metastases to simulate primary ovarian neoplasms. Am J Surg Pathol 2008;32(12):1835–53.

148. Elishaev E, Gilks CB, Miller D, et al. Synchronous and metachronous endocervical and ovarian neoplasms: evidence supporting interpretation of the ovarian neoplasms as metastatic endocervical adenocarcinomas simulating primary ovarian surface epithelial neoplasms. Am J Surg Pathol 2005;29(3):281–94.

149. McCluggage WG, Sumathi VP, McBride HA, et al. A panel of immunohistochemical stains, including carcinoembryonic antigen, vimentin, and estrogen receptor, aids the distinction between primary endometrial and endocervical adenocarcinomas. Int J Gynecol Pathol 2002;21(1):11–5.

150. Yemelyanova A, Vang R, Seidman JD, et al. Endocervical adenocarcinomas with prominent endometrial or endomyometrial involvement simulating primary endometrial carcinomas: utility of HPV DNA detection and immunohistochemical expression of p16 and hormone receptors to confirm the cervical origin of the corpus tumor. Am J Surg Pathol 2009;33(6):914–24.

151. Gien LT, Beauchemin MC, Thomas G. Adenocarcinoma: a unique cervical cancer. Gynecol Oncol 2010;116(1):140–6.

152. Baalbergen A, Ewing-Graham PC, Hop WC, et al. Prognostic factors in adenocarcinoma of the uterine cervix. Gynecol Oncol 2004;92(1):262–7.

153. Eifel PJ, Burke TW, Morris M, et al. Adenocarcinoma as an independent risk factor for disease recurrence in patients with stage IB cervical carcinoma. Gynecol Oncol 1995;59(1):38–44.

154. Irie T, Kigawa J, Minagawa Y, et al. Prognosis and clinicopathological characteristics of Ib-IIb adenocarcinoma of the uterine cervix in patients who have had radical hysterectomy. Eur J Surg Oncol 2000;26(5):464–7.

155. Berek JS, Hacker NF, Fu YS, et al. Adenocarcinoma of the uterine cervix: histologic variables associated with lymph node metastasis and survival. Obstet Gynecol 1985;65(1):46–52.

156. Shingleton HM, Bell MC, Fremgen A, et al. Is there really a difference in survival of women with squamous cell carcinoma, adenocarcinoma, and adenosquamous cell carcinoma of the cervix? Cancer 1995;76(Suppl 10):1948–55.

157. Nakanishi T, Ishikawa H, Suzuki Y, et al. A comparison of prognoses of pathologic stage Ib adenocarcinoma and squamous cell carcinoma of the uterine cervix. Gynecol Oncol 2000;79(2):289–93.

158. Farley JH, Hickey KW, Carlson JW, et al. Adenosquamous histology predicts a poor outcome for patients with advanced-stage, but not early-stage, cervical carcinoma. Cancer 2003;97(9):2196–202.

159. Gilks CB, Young RH, Aguirre P, et al. Adenoma malignum (minimal deviation adenocarcinoma) of the uterine cervix. A clinicopathological and immunohistochemical analysis of 26 cases. Am J Surg Pathol 1989;13(9):717–29.

160. McKelvey JL, Goodlin RR. Adenoma malignum of the cervix; a cancer of deceptively innocent histological pattern. Cancer 1963;16(5):549–57.

161. Young RH, Welch WR, Dickersin GR, et al. Ovarian sex cord tumor with annular tubules: review of 74 cases including 27 with Peutz-Jeghers syndrome and four with adenoma malignum of the cervix. Cancer 1982;50(7):1384–402.

162. Kojima A, Mikami Y, Sudo T, et al. Gastric morphology and immunophenotype predict poor outcome in mucinous adenocarcinoma of the uterine cervix. Am J Surg Pathol 2007;31(5):664–72.

163. Ishii K, Hidaka E, Katsuyama T, et al. Ultrastructural features of adenoma malignum of the uterine cervix: demonstration of gastric phenotypes. Ultrastruct Pathol 1999;23(6):375–81.

164. Ishii K, Hosaka N, Toki T, et al. A new view of the so-called adenoma malignum of the uterine cervix. Virchows Arch 1998;432:315–22.

165. Kaminski PF, Norris HJ. Minimal deviation carcinoma (adenoma malignum) of the cervix. Int J Gynecol Pathol 1983;2(2):141–52.

166. Scully RE, Bonfiglio TA, editors. Histological typing of female genital tract tumours. Berlin: Springer; 1994.

167. Hashi A, Xu JY, Kondo T, et al. p16INK4a overexpression independent of human papillomavirus infection in lobular endocervical glandular hyperplasia. Int J Gynecol Pathol 2006;25(2):187–94.

168. Nara M, Hashi A, Murata S, et al. Lobular endocervical glandular hyperplasia as a presumed precursor of cervical adenocarcinoma independent of human papillomavirus infection. Gynecol Oncol 2007;106(2):289–98.

169. Xu JY, Hashi A, Kondo T, et al. Absence of human papillomavirus infection in minimal deviation adenocarcinoma and lobular endocervical glandular hyperplasia. Int J Gynecol Pathol 2005; 24(3):296–302.

170. Park KJ, Kiyokawa T, Soslow RA, et al. Unusual endocervical adenocarcinomas: an immunohistochemical analysis with molecular detection of human papillomavirus. Am J Surg Pathol 2011, in press.

171. Kawauchi S, Kusuda T, Liu XP, et al. Is lobular endocervical glandular hyperplasia a cancerous precursor of minimal deviation adenocarcinoma? a comparative molecular-genetic and immunohistochemical study. Am J Surg Pathol 2008;32(12): 1807–15.

172. Mikami Y, Kiyokawa T, Hata S, et al. Gastrointestinal immunophenotype in adenocarcinomas of the uterine cervix and related glandular lesions: a possible link between lobular endocervical glandular hyperplasia/pyloric gland metaplasia and 'adenoma malignum'. Mod Pathol 2004;17(8):962–72.

173. Nucci MR, Clement PB, Young RH. Lobular endocervical glandular hyperplasia, not otherwise specified: a clinicopathologic analysis of thirteen cases of a distinctive pseudoneoplastic lesion and comparison with fourteen cases of adenoma malignum. Am J Surg Pathol 1999;23(8):886–91.

174. Steeper TA, Wick MR. Minimal deviation adenocarcinoma of the uterine cervix ("adenoma malignum"). An immunohistochemical comparison with microglandular endocervical hyperplasia and conventional endocervical adenocarcinoma. Cancer 1986;58(5):1131–8.

175. Toki T, Shiozawa T, Hosaka N, et al. Minimal deviation adenocarcinoma of the uterine cervix has abnormal expression of sex steroid receptors, CA125, and gastric mucin. Int J Gynecol Pathol 1997;16(2):111–6.

176. Nakamura N, Ota H, Katsuyama T, et al. Histochemical reactivity of normal, metaplastic, and neoplastic tissues to alpha-linked N-acetylglucosamine residue-specific monoclonal antibody HIK1083. J Histochem Cytochem 1998;46(7):793–801.

177. Nakajima K, Ota H, Zhang MX, et al. Expression of gastric gland mucous cell-type mucin in normal and neoplastic human tissues. J Histochem Cytochem 2003;51(12):1689–98.

178. Kaku T, Enjoji M. Extremely well-differentiated adenocarcinoma ("adenoma malignum") of the cervix. Int J Gynecol Pathol 1983;2(1):28–41.

179. Silverberg SG, Hurt WG. Minimal deviation adenocarcinoma ("adenoma malignum") of the cervix: a reappraisal. Am J Obstet Gynecol 1975;121(7):971–5.

180. Huffman JW. Mesonephric remnants in the cervix. Am J Obstet Gynecol 1948;56(1):23–40.

181. Sneeden VD. Mesonephric lesions of the cervix; a practical means of demonstration and a suggestion of incidence. Cancer 1958;11(2):334–6.

182. Silver SA, Devouassoux-Shisheboran M, Mezzetti TP, et al. Mesonephric adenocarcinomas of the uterine cervix: a study of 11 cases with immunohistochemical findings. Am J Surg Pathol 2001;25(3):379–87.

183. Clement PB, Young RH, Keh P, et al. Malignant mesonephric neoplasms of the uterine cervix. A report of eight cases, including four with a malignant spindle cell component. Am J Surg Pathol 1995;19(10):1158–71.

184. Seidman JD, Tavassoli FA. Mesonephric hyperplasia of the uterine cervix: a clinicopathologic study of 51 cases. Int J Gynecol Pathol 1995; 14(4):293–9.

185. Fukunaga M, Takahashi H, Yasuda M. Mesonephric adenocarcinoma of the uterine cervix: a case report with immunohistochemical and ultrastructural studies. Pathol Res Pract 2008;204(9):671–6.

186. Ordi J, Romagosa C, Tavassoli FA, et al. CD10 expression in epithelial tissues and tumors of the gynecologic tract: a useful marker in the diagnosis of mesonephric, trophoblastic, and clear cell tumors. Am J Surg Pathol 2003;27(2):178–86.

187. Yap OW, Hendrickson MR, Teng NN, et al. Mesonephric adenocarcinoma of the cervix: a case report and review of the literature. Gynecol Oncol 2006;103(3):1155–8.

188. Melnick S, Cole P, Anderson D, et al. Rates and risks of diethylstilbestrol-related clear-cell adenocarcinoma of the vagina and cervix. An update. N Engl J Med 1987;316(9):514–6.

189. Nordqvist SR. Perspective: DES exposure in utero. What are the effects? In: Ballon SC, editor, In: Gynecologic Oncology: controversies in cancer treatment, vol. 113. Boston: Hall G.K. Medical Publishers; 1981.

190. Hanselaar A, van Loosbroek M, Schuurbiers O, et al. Clear cell adenocarcinoma of the vagina

and cervix. An update of the central Netherlands registry showing twin age incidence peaks. Cancer 1997;79(11):2229–36.

191. Nofech-Mozes S, Khalifa MM, Ismiil N, et al. Detection of HPV-DNA by a PCR-based method in formalin-fixed, paraffin-embedded tissue from rare endocervical carcinoma types. Appl Immunohistochem Mol Morphol 2010;18(1):80–5.

192. Liebrich C, Brummer O, Von Wasielewski R, et al. Primary cervical cancer truly negative for high-risk human papillomavirus is a rare but distinct entity that can affect virgins and young adolescents. Eur J Gynaecol Oncol 2009;30(1):45–8.

193. Hadzisejdc I, Krasević M, Haller H, et al. Distribution of human papillomavirus types in different histological subtypes of cervical adenocarcinoma. Coll Antropol 2007;31(Suppl 2):97–102.

194. Goto K, Takeuchi Y, Yakihara A, et al. Synchronous invasive squamous cell carcinoma and clear cell adenocarcinoma of the uterine cervix: a different human papillomavirus status. Gynecol Oncol 2005;97(3):976–9.

195. Stewart J 3rd, Bevans-Wilkins K, Ye C, et al. Clear-cell endocervical adenocarcinoma in a 19-year-old woman. Diagn Cytopathol 2006;34(12):839–42.

196. Waggoner SE, Anderson SM, Van Eyck S, et al. Human papillomavirus detection and p53 expression in clear-cell adenocarcinoma of the vagina and cervix. Obstet Gynecol 1994;84(3):404–8.

197. Matias-Guiu X, Lerma E, Prat J. Clear cell tumors of the female genital tract. Semin Diagn Pathol 1997; 14(4):233–9.

198. Vang R, Whitaker BP, Farhood AI, et al. Immunohistochemical analysis of clear cell carcinoma of the gynecologic tract. Int J Gynecol Pathol 2001; 20(3):252–9.

199. Murta EF, Nomelini RS, Ferreira FA, et al. Ovarian clear cell carcinoma associated with endometriosis: a case report with immunohistochemical study. Eur J Gynaecol Oncol 2007;28(5):403–5.

200. Nolan LP, Heatley MK. The value of immunocytochemistry in distinguishing between clear cell carcinoma of the kidney and ovary. Int J Gynecol Pathol 2001;20(2):155–9.

201. Howell NR, Zheng W, Cheng L, et al. Carcinomas of ovary and lung with clear cell features: can immunohistochemistry help in differential diagnosis? Int J Gynecol Pathol 2007;26(2):134–40.

202. Kato N, Sasou S, Motoyama T. Expression of hepatocyte nuclear factor-1beta (HNF-1beta) in clear cell tumors and endometriosis of the ovary. Mod Pathol 2006;19(1):83–9.

203. Yamamoto S, Tsuda H, Aida S, et al. Immunohistochemical detection of hepatocyte nuclear factor 1beta in ovarian and endometrial clear-cell adenocarcinomas and nonneoplastic endometrium. Hum Pathol 2007;38(7):1074–80.

204. Terada T. Clear cell adenocarcinoma of the uterine cervix in a young pregnant woman: a case report with immunohistochemical study. Med Oncol 2010. [Online].

205. Waggoner SE, Anderson SM, Luce MC, et al. p53 protein expression and gene analysis in clear cell adenocarcinoma of the vagina and cervix. Gynecol Oncol 1996;60(3):339–44.

206. Thomas MB, Wright JD, Leiser AL, et al. Clear cell carcinoma of the cervix: a multi-institutional review in the post-DES era. Gynecol Oncol 2008;109(3): 335–9.

207. McNall RY, Nowicki PD, Miller B, et al. Adenocarcinoma of the cervix and vagina in pediatric patients. Pediatr Blood Cancer 2004;43(3):289–94.

208. Hanselaar AG, Van Leusen ND, De Wilde PC, et al. Clear cell adenocarcinoma of the vagina and cervix. A report of the central netherlands registry with emphasis on early detection and prognosis. Cancer 1991;67(7):1971–8.

209. Scully RE, Robboy SJ, Welch WR. Pathology and pathogenesis of diethylstilbestrol-related disorders of the female genital tract. In: Herbst AL, editor. Intrauterine exposure to diethylstilbestrol in the human. Chicago: The American College of Obstetricians and Gynecologists; 1978. p. 8–22.

210. Grisaru D, Covens A, Chapman B, et al. Does histology influence prognosis in patients with early-stage cervical carcinoma? Cancer 2001; 92(12):2999–3004.

211. Herbst AL. Behavior of estrogen-associated female genital tract cancer and its relation to neoplasia following intrauterine exposure to diethylstilbestrol (DES). Gynecol Oncol 2000;76(2):147–56.

212. Zhou C, Gilks CB, Hayes M, et al. Papillary serous carcinoma of the uterine cervix: a clinicopathologic study of 17 cases. Am J Surg Pathol 1998;22(1): 113–20.

213. Nofech-Mozes S, Rasty G, Ismiil N, et al. Immunohistochemical characterization of endocervical papillary serous carcinoma. Int J Gynecol Cancer 2006;16(Suppl 1):286–92.

214. Duggan MA, McGregor SE, Benoit JL, et al. The human papillomavirus status of invasive cervical adenocarcinoma: a clinicopathological and outcome analysis. Hum Pathol 1995;26(3):319–25.

215. Milde-Langosch K, Schreiber C, Becker G, et al. Human papillomavirus detection in cervical adenocarcinoma by polymerase chain reaction. Hum Pathol 1993;24(6):590–4.

216. Nofech-Mozes S, Khalifa MA. Endocervical adenocarcinoma in situ, serous type. Int J Gynecol Pathol 2009;28(2):140–1.

217. Batistatou A, Zolota V, Tzoracoleftherakis E, et al. Papillary serous adenocarcinoma of the endocervix: a rare neoplasm. Immunohistochemical profile. Int J Gynecol Cancer 2000;10(4):336–9.

218. Gilks CB, Clement PB. Papillary serous adenocarcinoma of the uterine cervix: a report of three cases. Mod Pathol 1992;5(4):426–31.

219. Holm R, Skomedal H, Helland A, et al. Immunohistochemical analysis of p53 protein overexpression in normal, premalignant, and malignant tissues of the cervix uteri. J Pathol 1993;169(1):21–6.

220. Inoue M, Fujita M, Enomoto T, et al. Immunohistochemical analysis of p53 in gynecologic tumors. Am J Clin Pathol 1994;102(5):665–70.

221. McHugh M, Bose S, Palazzo J. p53 expression in endocervical and endometrial adenocarcinomas. Int J Surg Pathol 1995;2(4):269–74.

222. Moll UM, Chalas E, Auguste M, et al. Uterine papillary serous carcinoma evolves via a p53-driven pathway. Hum Pathol 1996;27(12):1295–300.

223. Tashiro H, Isacson C, Levine R, et al. p53 gene mutations are common in uterine serous carcinoma and occur early in their pathogenesis. Am J Pathol 1997;150(1):177–85.

224. Costa MJ, McIlnay KR, Trelford J. Cervical carcinoma with glandular differentiation: histological evaluation predicts disease recurrence in clinical stage I or II patients. Hum Pathol 1995;26(8):829–37.

225. Singh N, Arif S. Histopathologic parameters of prognosis in cervical cancer–a review. Int J Gynecol Cancer 2004;14(5):741–50.

226. Power DG, McVey GP, Delaney DW, et al. Papillary serous carcinomas of the uterine cervix and paraneoplastic cerebellar degeneration: a report of two cases. Acta Oncol 2008;47(8):1590–3.

227. Glucksmann A, Cherry CP. Incidence, histology, and response to radiation of mixed carcinomas (adenoacanthomas) of the uterine cervix. Cancer 1956;9(5):971–9.

228. Littman P, Clement PB, Henriksen B, et al. Glassy cell carcinoma of the cervix. Cancer 1976;37(5):2238–46.

229. Ulbright TM, Gersell DJ. Glassy cell carcinoma of the uterine cervix. A light and electron microscopic study of five cases. Cancer 1983;51(12):2255–63.

230. Costa MJ, Kenny MB, Hewan-Lowe K, et al. Glassy cell features in adenosquamous carcinoma of the uterine cervix. Histologic, ultrastructural, immunohistochemical, and clinical findings. Am J Clin Pathol 1991;96(4):520–8.

231. Maier RC, Norris HJ. Glassy cell carcinoma of the cervix. Obstet Gynecol 1982;60(2):219–24.

232. Kato N, Katayama Y, Kaimori M, et al. Glassy cell carcinoma of the uterine cervix: histochemical, immunohistochemical, and molecular genetic observations. Int J Gynecol Pathol 2002;21(2):134–40.

233. Kuroda H, Toyozumi Y, Masuda T, et al. Glassy cell carcinoma of the cervix: cytologic features and expression of estrogen receptor, progesterone receptor and Her2/neu protein. Acta Cytol 2006;50(4):418–22.

234. Kenny MB, Unger ER, Chenggis ML, et al. In situ hybridization for human papillomavirus DNA in uterine adenosquamous carcinoma with glassy cell features ("glassy cell carcinoma"). Am J Clin Pathol 1992;98(2):180–7.

235. Smotkin D, Berek JS, Fu YS, et al. Human papillomavirus deoxyribonucleic acid in adenocarcinoma and adenosquamous carcinoma of the uterine cervix. Obstet Gynecol 1986;68(2):241–4.

236. Cherry CP, Glucksmann A. Histology of carcinomas of the uterine cervix and survival rates in pregnant and nonpregnant patients. Surg Gynecol Obstet 1961;113:763–76.

237. Glucksmann A. Relationships between hormonal changes in pregnancy and the development of mixed carcinoma of the uterine cervix. Cancer 1957;10(4):831–7.

238. Pak HY, Yokota SB, Paladugu RR, et al. Glassy cell carcinoma of the cervix. Cytologic and clinicopathologic analysis. Cancer 1983;52(2):307–12.

239. Seltzer V, Sall S, Castadot MJ, et al. Glassy cell cervical carcinoma. Gynecol Oncol 1979;8(2):141–51.

240. Tamimi HK, Ek M, Hesla J, et al. Glassy cell carcinoma of the cervix redefined. Obstet Gynecol 1988;71(6 Pt 1):837–41.

241. Matsuura Y, Murakami N, Nagashio E, et al. Glassy cell carcinoma of the uterine cervix: combination chemotherapy with paclitaxel and carboplatin in recurrent tumor. J Obstet Gynaecol Res 2001;27(3):129–32.

242. Nagai T, Okubo T, Sakaguchi R, et al. Glassy cell carcinoma of the uterine cervix responsive to neoadjuvant intraarterial chemotherapy. Int J Clin Oncol 2008;13(6):541–4.

243. Nasu K, Takai N, Narahara H. Multimodal treatment for glassy cell carcinoma of the uterine cervix. J Obstet Gynaecol Res 2009;35(3):584–7.

244. Seamon LG, Downey GO, Harrison CR, et al. Neoadjuvant chemotherapy followed by post-partum chemoradiotherapy and chemoconsolidation for stage IIIB glassy cell cervical carcinoma during pregnancy. Gynecol Oncol 2009;114(3):540–1.

245. Takekuma M, Hirashima Y, Takahashi N, et al. A case of glassy cell carcinoma of the uterine cervix that responded to neoadjuvant chemotherapy with paclitaxel and carboplatin. Anticancer Drugs 2006;17(6):715–8.

246. Hart WR. Symposium part II: special types of adenocarcinoma of the uterine cervix. Int J Gynecol Pathol 2002;21(4):327–46.

247. Russell MJ, Fadare O. Adenoid basal lesions of the uterine cervix: evolving terminology and clinicopathological concepts. Diagn Pathol 2006;1:18.

248. Parwani AV, Smith Sehdev AE, Kurman RJ, et al. Cervical adenoid basal tumors comprised of adenoid basal epithelioma associated with various types of invasive carcinoma: clinicopathologic features, human papillomavirus DNA detection, and P16 expression. Hum Pathol 2005;36(1): 82–90.

249. Ferry JA, Scully RE. "Adenoid cystic" carcinoma and adenoid basal carcinoma of the uterine cervix. A study of 28 cases. Am J Surg Pathol 1988;12(2): 134–44.

250. Brainard JA, Hart WR. Adenoid basal epitheliomas of the uterine cervix: a reevaluation of distinctive cervical basaloid lesions currently classified as adenoid basal carcinoma and adenoid basal hyperplasia. Am J Surg Pathol 1998;22(8):965–75.

251. Grayson W, Taylor LF, Cooper K. Adenoid cystic and adenoid basal carcinoma of the uterine cervix: comparative morphologic, mucin, and immunohistochemical profile of two rare neoplasms of putative 'reserve cell' origin. Am J Surg Pathol 1999; 23(4):448–58.

252. Hiroi M, Fukunaga T, Miyazaki E, et al. Adenoid basal carcinoma of the uterine cervix: a case report with ultrastructural findings. Med Electron Microsc 2000;33(4):241–5.

253. Lin Z, Liu M, Li Z, et al. DeltaNp63 protein expression in uterine cervical and endometrial cancers. J Cancer Res Clin Oncol 2006;132(12):811–6.

254. Senzaki H, Osaki T, Uemura Y, et al. Adenoid basal carcinoma of the uterine cervix: immunohistochemical study and literature review. Jpn J Clin Oncol 1997;27(6):437–41.

255. Teramoto N, Nishimura R, Saeki T, et al. Adenoid basal carcinoma of the uterine cervix: report of two cases with reference to adenosquamous carcinoma. Pathol Int 2005;55(7):445–52.

256. Yoshida T, Fujiwara K, Shimizu M, et al. Adenoid basal carcinoma of the cervix uteri: a case report. Pathol Int 1997;47(11):775–7.

257. Cviko A, Briem B, Granter SR, et al. Adenoid basal carcinomas of the cervix: a unique morphological evolution with cell cycle correlates. Hum Pathol 2000;31(6):740–4.

258. Zamecnik M, Skrivanek A. Adenoid basal epithelioma of the uterine cervix in 21-year-old patient. Report of a case with histologic and immunohistochemical study. Cesk Patol 2005;41(4):157–62.

259. Daponte A, Grayson W, Moisuc D, et al. Adenoid cystic carcinoma stage Ib1 treated with radical surgery displaying human papilloma virus 33 (HPV 33): immunoelectron microscopy and review. Gynecol Oncol 2003;90(3):673–6.

260. Grayson W, Taylor L, Cooper K. Detection of integrated high risk human papillomavirus in adenoid cystic carcinoma of the uterine cervix. J Clin Pathol 1996;49(10):805–9.

261. Mazur MT, Battifora HA. Adenoid cystic carcinoma of the uterine cervix: ultrastructure, immunofluorescence, and criteria for diagnosis. Am J Clin Pathol 1982;77(4):494–500.

262. Vuong PN, Neveux Y, Schoonaert MF, et al. Adenoid cystic (cylindromatous) carcinoma associated with squamous cell carcinoma of the cervix uteri: cytologic presentation of a case with histologic and ultrastructural correlations. Acta Cytol 1996;40(2):289–94.

263. Lawrence JB, Mazur MT. Adenoid cystic carcinoma: a comparative pathologic study of tumors in salivary gland, breast, lung, and cervix. Hum Pathol 1982;13(10):916–24.

264. Morimura Y, Honda T, Hoshi K, et al. A case of uterine cervical adenoid cystic carcinoma: immunohistochemical study for basement membrane material. Obstet Gynecol 1995;85(5 Pt 2):903–5.

265. Clement PB, Zubovits JT, Young RH, et al. Malignant mullerian mixed tumors of the uterine cervix: a report of nine cases of a neoplasm with morphology often different from its counterpart in the corpus. Int J Gynecol Pathol 1998;17(3):211–22.

266. Grayson W, Taylor LF, Cooper K. Adenoid basal carcinoma of the uterine cervix: detection of integrated human papillomavirus in a rare tumor of putative "reserve cell" origin. Int J Gynecol Pathol 1997;16(4):307–12.

267. Grayson W, Taylor LF, Cooper K. Carcinosarcoma of the uterine cervix: a report of eight cases with immunohistochemical analysis and evaluation of human papillomavirus status. Am J Surg Pathol 2001;25(3):338–47.

268. Mathoulin-Portier MP, Penault-Llorca F, Labit-Bouvier C, et al. Malignant mullerian mixed tumor of the uterine cervix with adenoid cystic component. Int J Gynecol Pathol 1998;17(1):91–2.

269. Takeshima Y, Amatya VJ, Nakayori F, et al. Co-existent carcinosarcoma and adenoid basal carcinoma of the uterine cervix and correlation with human papillomavirus infection. Int J Gynecol Pathol 2002;21(2):186–90.

270. Albores-Saavedra J, Manivel C, Mora A, et al. The solid variant of adenoid cystic carcinoma of the cervix. Int J Gynecol Pathol 1992;11(1):2–10.

271. King LA, Talledo OE, Gallup DG, et al. Adenoid cystic carcinoma of the cervix in women under age 40. Gynecol Oncol 1989;32(1):26–30.

272. Dixit S, Singhal S, Vyas R, et al. Adenoid cystic carcinoma of the cervix. J Postgrad Med 1993; 39(4):211–5.

273. Musa AG, Hughes RR, Coleman SA. Adenoid cystic carcinoma of the cervix: a report of 17 cases. Gynecol Oncol 1985;22(2):167–73.

274. van Dinh T, Woodruff JD. Adenoid cystic and adenoid basal carcinomas of the cervix. Obstet Gynecol 1985;65(5):705–9.

275. Albores-Saavedra J, Gersell D, Gilks CB, et al. Terminology of endocrine tumors of the uterine cervix: results of a workshop sponsored by the College of American Pathologists and the National Cancer Institute. Arch Pathol Lab Med 1997; 121(1):34–9.
276. Chan JK, Tsui WM, Tung SY, et al. Endocrine cell hyperplasia of the uterine cervix. A precursor of neuroendocrine carcinoma of the cervix? Am J Clin Pathol 1989;92(6):825–30.
277. Abeler VM, Holm R, Nesland JM, et al. Small cell carcinoma of the cervix. A clinicopathologic study of 26 patients. Cancer 1994;73(3):672–7.
278. Seckl MJ, Mulholland PJ, Bishop AE, et al. Hypoglycemia due to an insulin-secreting small-cell carcinoma of the cervix. N Engl J Med 1999; 341(10):733–6.
279. Ulich TR, Liao SY, Layfield L, et al. Endocrine and tumor differentiation markers in poorly differentiated small-cell carcinoids of the cervix and vagina. Arch Pathol Lab Med 1986;110(11):1054–7.
280. Akiba Y, Mikami M, Komuro Y, et al. [A case of neuroendocrine carcinoma of uterine cervix with the elevated plasma level of serotonin]. Nippon Sanka Fujinka Gakkai Zasshi 1996;48(10): 897–900 [in Japanese].
281. Gilks CB, Young RH, Gersell DJ, et al. Large cell neuroendocrine [corrected] carcinoma of the uterine cervix: a clinicopathologic study of 12 cases. Am J Surg Pathol 1997;21(8):905–14.
282. Ishida GM, Kato N, Hayasaka T, et al. Small cell neuroendocrine carcinomas of the uterine cervix: a histological, immunohistochemical, and molecular genetic study. Int J Gynecol Pathol 2004; 23(4):366–72.
283. Soga J, Osaka M, Yakuwa Y. Gut-endocrinomas (carcinoids and related endocrine variants) of the uterine cervix: an analysis of 205 reported cases. J Exp Clin Cancer Res 2001;20(3):327–34.
284. Stewart CJ, Taggart CR, Brett F, et al. Mesonephric adenocarcinoma of the uterine cervix with focal endocrine cell differentiation. Int J Gynecol Pathol 1993;12(3):264–9.
285. Toki T, Katayama Y, Motoyama T. Small-cell neuroendocrine carcinoma of the uterine cervix associated with micro-invasive squamous cell carcinoma and adenocarcinoma in situ. Pathol Int 1996;46(7): 520–5.
286. Agoff SN, Lamps LW, Philip AT, et al. Thyroid transcription factor-1 is expressed in extrapulmonary small cell carcinomas but not in other extrapulmonary neuroendocrine tumors. Mod Pathol 2000; 13(3):238–42.
287. Carlson JW, Nucci MR, Brodsky J, et al. Biomarker-assisted diagnosis of ovarian, cervical and pulmonary small cell carcinomas: the role of TTF-1, WT-1 and HPV analysis. Histopathology 2007;51(3): 305–12.
288. Ordonez NG. Value of thyroid transcription factor-1 immunostaining in distinguishing small cell lung carcinomas from other small cell carcinomas. Am J Surg Pathol 2000;24(9):1217–23.
289. Stoler MH, Mills SE, Gersell DJ, et al. Small-cell neuroendocrine carcinoma of the cervix. A human papillomavirus type 18-associated cancer. Am J Surg Pathol 1991;15(1):28–32.
290. Mannion C, Park WS, Man YG, et al. Endocrine tumors of the cervix: morphologic assessment, expression of human papillomavirus, and evaluation for loss of heterozygosity on 1p,3p, 11q, and 17p. Cancer 1998;83(7):1391–400.
291. Yun K, Cho NP, Glassford GN. Large cell neuroendocrine carcinoma of the uterine cervix: a report of a case with coexisting cervical intraepithelial neoplasia and human papillomavirus 16. Pathology 1999;31(2):158–61.
292. Grayson W, Rhemtula HA, Taylor LF, et al. Detection of human papillomavirus in large cell neuroendocrine carcinoma of the uterine cervix: a study of 12 cases. J Clin Pathol 2002;55(2):108–14.
293. Wang KL, Yang YC, Wang TY, et al. Neuroendocrine carcinoma of the uterine cervix: a clinicopathologic retrospective study of 31 cases with prognostic implications. J Chemother 2006;18(2): 209–16.
294. Alphandery C, Dagrada G, Frattini M, et al. Neuroendocrine small cell carcinoma of the cervix associated with endocervical adenocarcinoma: a case report. Acta Cytol 2007;51(4):589–93.
295. Powell JL, McKinney CD. Large cell neuroendocrine tumor of the cervix and human papillomavirus 16: a case report. J Low Genit Tract Dis 2008;12(3): 242–4.
296. Wistuba II, Thomas B, Behrens C, et al. Molecular abnormalities associated with endocrine tumors of the uterine cervix. Gynecol Oncol 1999;72(1): 3–9.
297. Sato Y, Shimamoto T, Amada S, et al. Large cell neuroendocrine carcinoma of the uterine cervix: a clinicopathological study of six cases. Int J Gynecol Pathol 2003;22(3):226–30.
298. Zivanovic O, Leitao MM Jr, Park KJ, et al. Small cell neuroendocrine carcinoma of the cervix: analysis of outcome, recurrence pattern and the impact of platinum-based combination chemotherapy. Gynecol Oncol 2009;112(3):590–3.

PATHOLOGY OF VULVAR NEOPLASMS

Edyta C. Pirog, MD

KEYWORDS

- Vulvar intraepithelial neoplasia • Vulvar carcinoma • Keratinizing squamous cell carcinoma
- Warty carcinoma • Basaloid carcinoma • Verrucous carcinoma • Papillary hidradenoma
- Paget disease • Bartholin gland carcinoma

ABSTRACT

Carcinoma of the vulva is an uncommon malignant neoplasm (approximately one-fifth as frequent as cervical cancer) and represents 4% of all genital cancers in women. Approximately two-thirds of cases occur in women older than 60 years, and squamous cell carcinoma is the most common histologic type. Several different subtypes of squamous cell carcinoma have been described in the vulva; however, in terms of etiology, pathogenesis, and histologic features, most carcinomas belong to one of two categories: keratinizing squamous cell carcinomas associated with chronic inflammatory skin disorders, and basaloid or warty carcinomas related to infection with high oncogenic risk human papillomaviruses. Glandular neoplasms of the vulva arise from the vulvar apocrine sweat glands (papillary hidradenoma and Paget disease) or the Bartholin gland and their cause is not known.

SQUAMOUS NEOPLASTIC LESIONS OF THE VULVA

VULVAR INTRAEPITHELIAL NEOPLASIA (DYSPLASIA, CARCINOMA IN SITU)

Invasive basaloid and warty carcinomas develop from an in situ lesion called usual vulvar intraepithelial neoplasia (uVIN). This form of VIN includes lesions formerly designated as classic VIN or Bowen disease. Invasive keratinizing squamous cell carcinomas (SCCs) develop from a precursor lesion termed differentiated vulvar intraepithelial neoplasia (dVIN), also known as VIN simplex.

According to European and United States epidemiologic data, the incidence of uVIN and dVIN has increased in the recent decades, whereas the incidence of vulvar SCC has remained stable.[1–3]

In 1986 the International Society for the Study of Vulvovaginal Disease (ISSVD) established a 3-tier classification of VIN (VIN 1, 2, and 3) modeled on classification of cervical intraepithelial neoplasia. A separate category of dVIN has been established as a histologic entity equivalent to VIN 3.[4,5] Since that time, clinical studies of the natural history of VIN have shown that VIN 1 does not progress to cancer. This finding was supported by additional evidence from human papillomavirus (HPV) genotyping studies showing that most cases of VIN 1 are caused by low oncogenic risk HPVs.[6,7] In view of these findings, ISSVD revised the VIN classification in 2004[4,5] and excluded VIN 1 from diagnostic categories of vulvar neoplasia, with a recommendation that cases formerly classified as VIN 1 should be diagnosed as HPV-related changes. VIN 2 and VIN 3 were combined into 1 category termed uVIN. The current terminology of vulvar neoplasia includes the following entities:

1. VIN, usual type
   - VIN, basaloid type
   - VIN, warty type
   - VIN, mixed (warty/basaloid) type
2. VIN, differentiated type.

Some cases of VIN, such as pagetoid VIN, cannot be classified into either of these categories, and cases like these may be diagnosed as VIN, unclassified type.

Department of Pathology, Weill Medical College of Cornell University, 525 East 68th Street, ST-1041, New York, NY 10065, USA
E-mail address: ecpirog@med.cornell.edu

Surgical Pathology 4 (2011) 87–111
doi:10.1016/j.path.2010.03.001

Overall, uVIN is seen more often in vulvar biopsies than dVIN. A recent audit of 164 consecutive vulvar biopsies diagnosed as VIN reported a diagnosis of uVIN in 82% of cases and dVIN in 18% of cases.[8]

USUAL VULVAR INTRAEPITHELIAL NEOPLASIA (CLASSIC VIN)

uVIN most commonly occurs in women 40 to 49 years old. The risk factors are the same as those associated with cervical neoplasia and are related to acquisition of HPV infection (eg, young age at first intercourse, multiple sexual partners, male partner with multiple sexual partners, and immunosuppression).[1,8] Cigarette smoking is an additional independent risk factor. The incidence of uVIN has been increasing significantly in recent decades, especially among young women.[3]

GROSS FEATURES

uVIN presents as a raised plaque, papule or verruciform growth involving vulvar skin or mucosal surfaces. The lesions on the skin tend to be pigmented or white hyperkeratotic, whereas the mucosal lesions are most commonly reddish. Most lesions are multifocal, involving labia and perineum; in addition, 10% to 30% of patients with VIN also have vaginal or cervical HPV-related lesions.

MICROSCOPIC FEATURES AND DIAGNOSIS

Nuclear atypia, decreased maturation of squamous cells, and increased mitotic activity are key features of uVIN. These histologic changes are caused by deregulation of the cell cycle by high oncogenic risk HPVs. The HPV type most commonly detected in uVIN is HPV 16, and other high-risk HPV types, such as HPV 18 or 33, are detected less frequently.[9] While HPV-related changes or VIN 1 represent a productive viral infection with high rates of viral replication and no significant effect on the cell cycle, development

of uVIN (VIN 2–3) is a sign of a progressive alteration of the cell cycle by HPV resulting in increased cellular proliferation, decreased or arrested epithelial maturation, and lower rates of viral replication. Derangement of the cell cycle in uVIN may become irreversible and lead to a fully transformed malignant phenotype.

The diagnosis of uVIN is based on identification of nuclear atypia and decreased cellular maturation.[10] The dysplastic cells typically show high nuclear/cytoplasmic (N/C) ratio, nuclear enlargement, pleomorphism, hyperchromasia with coarse, stippled chromatin and multinucleation. In addition, there is an upward expansion of the basal immature cell layer beyond the lower one-third of the epithelial thickness. Depending on the degree of keratinocyte maturation, uVIN lesions may show koilocytic atypia (viral cytopathic effect related to accumulation of viral particles in the nuclei of the superficial keratinocytes). In lesions with arrested keratinocyte differentiation the koilocytic atypia may be only minimal. The mitotic figures may extend to the superficial layers of the epithelium and atypical mitotic figures may be present. Apoptotic bodies (single-cell necrosis) are common. Hyperkeratosis and parakeratosis may be present on the epithelial surface and account for a white gross appearance. Increased pigmentation of the keratinocytes and presence of dermal melanophages contribute to pigmented appearance of VIN.[10]

Two histologic variants of uVIN have been described:

1. Warty VIN shows acanthosis with a slightly raised papillary surface and prominent koilocytosis. The nuclei show marked enlargement, pleomorphism, and multinucleation (**Fig. 1**). The cytoplasm is densely eosinophilic owing to abundant intracytoplasmic keratin.
2. Basaloid VIN typically presents as a flat lesion composed of small, uniform cells with minimal or no maturation, high N/C ratio, and minimal koilocytic changes (**Fig. 2**). The cytoplasm is scant and purple.

Some VIN cases show warty and basaloid (mixed) features. Cases of uVIN with mucinous differentiation have recently been described; this HPV-positive subtype of basaloid VIN may mimic Paget disease of the vulva.[11]

With immunohistochemistry, uVIN overexpresses p16 in a diffuse, bandlike pattern and shows high levels of proliferation with Ki-67 marker. Ki-67 shows a characteristic pattern of staining in uVIN in which positive cells are seen extending from the normal parabasal location into the upper two-thirds of the epithelial thickness.

Key Features
USUAL VULVAR INTRAEPITHELIAL
NEOPLASIA

- Nuclear atypia
- Decreased maturation of the squamous cells
- Increased mitotic activity
- Diffuse, bandlike p16 overexpression
- Ki-67 positive cells present in the upper two-thirds of the epithelial thickness

Fig. 1. Warty VIN (magnification ×400).

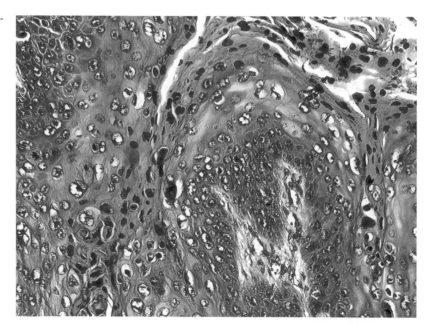

DIFFERENTIAL DIAGNOSIS

The differential diagnosis of uVIN includes epithelial regeneration with reactive atypia, Paget disease, pagetoid urothelial intraepithelial neoplasia, pagetoid spread of rectal carcinoma, and superficial spreading malignant melanoma. In equivocal cases, immunohistochemical staining may be necessary for accurate diagnosis. uVIN shows strong, diffuse, bandlike positivity with p16 immunostain in contrast to regeneration/repair in which p16 stain is negative.[12] Although p16 was shown to be a sensitive and specific marker of uVIN, caution should be used when interpreting p16 staining results. Weak blush staining does not correlate with HPV detection and is occasionally seen in benign vulvar epithelium. Only strong, diffuse nuclear and cytoplasmic staining should be considered a positive result.[12]

Fig. 2. Basaloid VIN (×400).

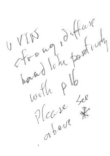

uVIN strong, diffuse bandlike positivity with p16 Please see ★ above

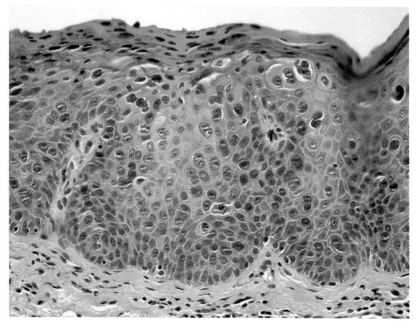

Primary vulvar Paget disease shows positivity for CK7 and carcinoembryonic antigen (CEA); pagetoid spread of urothelial carcinoma shows positivity for CK7 and CK20; rectal carcinoma is positive for CK20[11] (see later discussion on Paget disease), whereas vulvar melanoma is positive for S-100, HMB-45, and melan-A; all of these stains are negative in uVIN.[11]

In cases of VIN equivocal for invasion, double immunostaining for cytokeratin and collagen IV may be useful to confirm migration of invasive keratinocytes through breaks in the basement membrane into the underlying dermis (**Fig. 3**).

PROGNOSIS

Spontaneous regression of VIN lesions has been reported, usually in younger women.[13] The risk of progression to invasive carcinoma is higher in women more than 45 years of age or in women with immunosuppression. VIN in patients who are HIV positive does not seem to improve with retroviral treatment. In a 2-year follow-up of women who were HIV positive and receiving antiviral therapy, 65% of patients required re-excision and 10% of patients developed invasive cancer.[14] Because uVIN is readily identified during vulvar colposcopic examination and most of the patients are treated with excisional biopsies before the

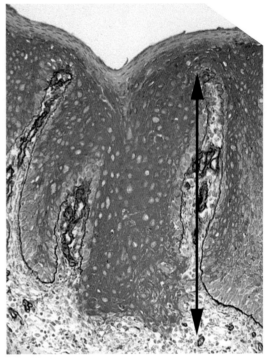

Fig. 3. Superficially invasive carcinoma. Loss of collagen IV staining at the base indicates invasion through the basement membrane. Arrow illustrates measurement of depth of invasion (×200). *Editor's note: This technique, which produces beautiful images, is useful in educational and investigative settings; however, it is not currently considered a standard practice for diagnostic use.*

disease progression, the rate of invasive cancer associated with uVIN is lower than that associated with dVIN (see later discussion).

DIFFERENTIATED VULVAR INTRAEPITHELIAL NEOPLASIA (dVIN)

dVIN is recognized as an immediate precursor of invasive keratinizing SCCs in the vulva. The average age of patients is reported at 66 to 69 years[8,15]; however, cases of dVIN in patients as young as 20 years have been described.[16] dVIN typically develops in a background of vulvar squamous cell hyperplasia (SCH), a chronic inflammatory condition, or long-lasting lichen sclerosus (LS), a lesion with strong links to autoimmune diseases. Although patients with LS have an average 4.5% cumulative risk of vulvar SCCs,[17] neither LS nor SCH is considered a premalignant lesion. Because dVIN is almost always seen in association with SCH and LS, it is postulated that long-standing epithelial irritation in a nonneoplastic epithelial disorder may contribute to a gradual evolution of the malignant phenotype. dVIN is believed to represent a histologically apparent phase of malignant transformation. The consecutive molecular events in LS, SCH, and dVIN leading to malignant transformation are currently unknown. A report of allelic imbalance in SCH and LS supports the hypothesis that both conditions may pose a risk for neoplasia despite the lack of morphologic evidence of atypia.[18] It has long been hypothesized that mutation of the p53 gene may be an early genetic event leading to neoplastic progression in a nonneoplastic disorder such as LS or SCH or in dVIN. Several research projects have been devoted to this issue. Some studies have confirmed the presence of identical p53 gene mutations in LS

and adjacent SCC, whereas other results were inconclusive.[19–22]

GROSS FEATURES

The gross features of dVIN are not specific and the lesion is usually found in the background of skin changes related to long-standing LS or SCH. The most common clinical appearance is that of a white-gray hyperkeratotic plaque, warty papule or flat reddish area. The lesion may be misinterpreted as eczema.[16] This lack of specific gross features accounts for difficulty in clinical diagnosis and may result in delayed excision. dVIN is only diagnosed in approximately one-quarter of patients before development of invasive SCC.[8]

MICROSCOPIC FEATURES AND DIAGNOSIS

dVIN is characterized by marked atypia of the basal layer of the epithelium with a high degree of epithelial maturation and differentiation in the superficial layers.[10] The epidermis is typically thickened with prominent acanthosis. Reverse maturation can occur, in which keratin pearls develop deep within the rete ridges (Fig. 4). In addition, there may be marked interanastomosis of the rete ridges (Fig. 5). The keratinocytes in the basal layers show abundant eosinophilic cytoplasm, prominent intercellular bridges, and

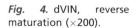

Fig. 4. dVIN, reverse maturation (×200).

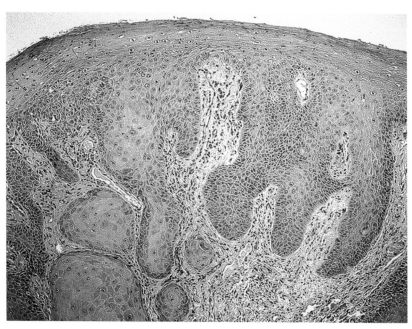

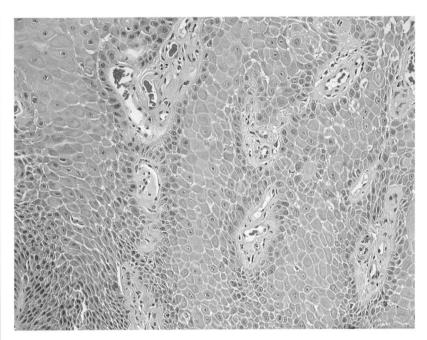

Fig. 5. dVIN with intera-nastomosing of rete ridges (×400).

markedly atypical nuclei with pale vesicular chromatin and prominent cherry-red macronucleoli. Mitotic activity is brisk and atypical mitotic figures may be present (**Fig. 6**). The nuclei in the mid- and superficial epithelial layers may show variable degrees of atypia or no atypia at all. In some cases atypia of the superficial nuclei may be so prominent as to mimic koilocytic atypia of HPV infection (**Fig. 7**). Surface parakeratosis and hyperkeratosis may be marked (**Fig. 8**). Rare subtypes of dVIN

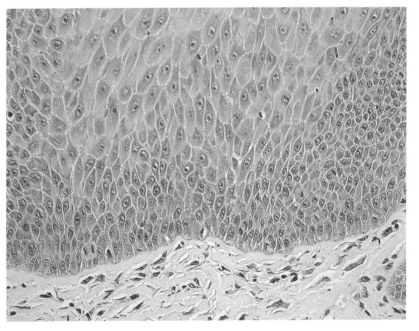

Fig. 6. dVIN, basal cell atypia and brisk mitotic activity (×400).

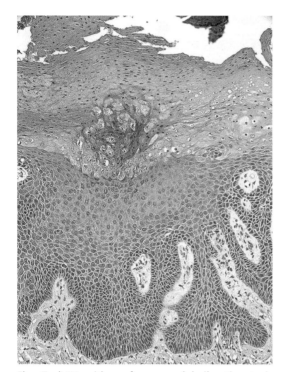

Fig. 7. dVIN with surface pseudokoilocytic atypia (×200). (*Reproduced from* de Koning MNC, Quint WGV, Pirog EC. Prevalence of mucosal and cutaneous human papillomaviruses in different histologic subtypes of vulvar carcinoma. Modern Pathology 2008;21:334; with permission.)

with acantholytic changes (**Fig. 9**) and dVIN with spindle cell features have been reported adjacent to rare variants of acantholytic and spindle cell (sarcomatoid) SCCs.[15] In addition, dVIN with a basaloid pattern mimicking uVIN of the basaloid type has been reported; the lesion is negative for HPV and p16.[23]

It has been suggested that immunopositivity for p53 can serve as an objective marker of dVIN. Positive p53 immunostaining in the basal as well as suprabasal epithelial regions has been shown in up to 80% of cases of dVIN.[24,25] However, some studies have noted that p53 positivity is not specific for dVIN.[26] Positive p53 immunostaining has been found in 25% of biopsies of normal vulvar epithelium and 80% of cases of LS. It has been postulated that, in these cases, p53 immunopositivity may be related to functional overexpression of the protein and not gene alterations.[26] The usefulness of p53 immunostaining in confirmation of the diagnosis of dVIN still requires clarification.

Unlike uVIN, dVIN does not overexpress p16. Proliferative activity assessed with Ki-67 is mostly limited to basal keratinocytes.

DIFFERENTIAL DIAGNOSIS

It may be difficult to distinguish dVIN from background SCH, because the atypia of basal keratinocytes in dVIN shows a gradient of changes rather

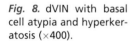

Fig. 8. dVIN with basal cell atypia and hyperkeratosis (×400).

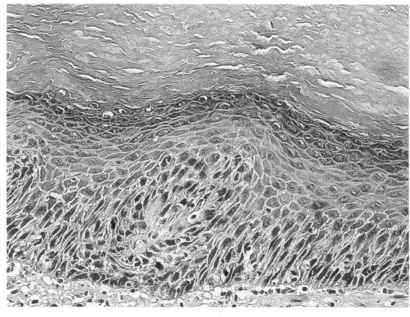

> ⚠️ **Differential Diagnosis**
> **DIFFERENTIATED VULVAR INTRAEPITHELIAL NEOPLASIA**
>
> - Squamous cell hyperplasia
> - Pseudoepitheliomatous hyperplasia
> - Usual vulvar intraepithelial neoplasia

than an abrupt change, and it is therefore subject to individual interpretation. Pseudoepitheliomatous hyperplasia at the edge of the ulcer is another common condition that may mimic dVIN.[27] Cases of dVIN with atypia extending to the superficial layers of the epithelium may be confused with uVIN. Lack of p16 immunostaining in such cases confirms the diagnosis of dVIN.

Verifying the presence of significant basilar nuclear atypia and excluding benign mimics are currently the only ways to confirm a diagnosis of dVIN. p53 immunohistochemical assays are used in some institutions for differential diagnosis, but caution is advised because, as discussed earlier, occasional nonneoplastic lesions may show upregulation of p53 expression in basal keratinocytes. Diffuse immunolabeling above the basal layer suggests a diagnosis of dVIN in the appropriate context.

PROGNOSIS

The progression rate of dVIN to invasive SCC is higher than that of uVIN. de Nieuwenhof and colleagues[2] reported that the overall percentage of patients with dVIN who were subsequently diagnosed with vulvar SCC was 32.8% and the median time of progression to invasion was 22.8 months. The progression rate of uVIN in that study was 5.7% with median time of 41.5 months. In the study of Scurry and colleagues[8] the percentage of patients with dVIN who had prior or concurrent SCC was 73.3%, compared with 27.4% in patients with uVIN. These results were corroborated by another study showing a significant association between the presence of dVIN and the risk of SCC with an odds ratio (OR) of 15.3 compared with 0.5 for patients with uVIN ($P<.0001$).[28]

UNCLASSIFIED VULVAR INTRAEPITHELIAL NEOPLASIA

Rare unclassified variants of VIN include pagetoid VIN. Pagetoid VIN resembles basaloid VIN, but shows pagetoid expansion of the dysplastic cells within the epidermis (**Fig. 10**).[11] Unlike uVIN or dVIN, dysplastic cells in pagetoid VIN are positive for CK7, but, unlike in Paget disease, they are negative for mucin, GCDFP-15, and CEA. Association with HPV is not known. In the few reported cases the patients were in their 20s or 60s.[29]

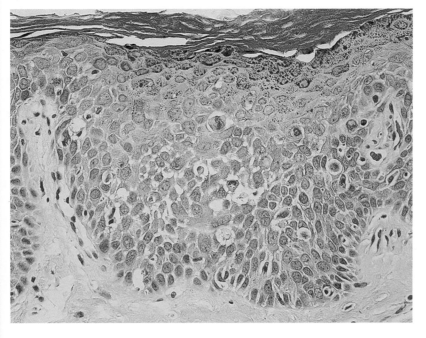

Fig. 9. dVIN with acantholytic changes (×400).

Fig. 10. Pagetoid VIN (×400).

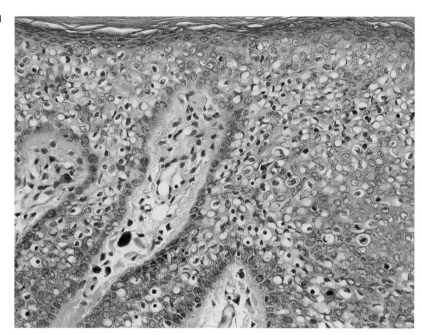

VULVAR CARCINOMA

Several different subtypes of SCC have been described in the vulva. Keratinizing SCCs are the most common type of vulvar cancer and account for approximately 60% of all cases. This type of malignancy is almost invariably associated with chronic inflammatory disorder of the vulvar skin. Basaloid and warty carcinomas are caused by HPV infection and constitute almost 30% of vulvar tumors. Rare verrucous carcinomas account for less than 10% of cases. Keratoacanthoma and basal cell carcinoma may occasionally develop within vulvar skin but, because the histopathologic features of these 2 tumors are the same as in other skin locations, they are not discussed in this review.

Vulvar carcinomas are staged using the International Federation of Gynecology and Obstetrics (FIGO) system combined with the TNM (tumor size, lymph nodes, metastases) system. The staging is based on depth of invasion, overall tumor size, and involvement of other organs (**Table 1**). Depth of invasion is measured from the deepest invasive focus to the tip of the closest dermal papillae (see **Fig. 3**). Tumors consisting of a single lesion measuring less than 2 cm in diameter and with depth of invasion measuring less than 1 mm are designated as superficially invasive SCC (FIGO stage 1A, TNM stage T1a), whereas tumors exceeding these dimensions are referred to as invasive SCC.[30,31] The grading system for vulvar cancer has been developed by the Gynecologic Oncology Group (GOG) and is based on the percentage of undifferentiated cells in the tumor mass. The system has 4 tiers: grade 1, well-differentiated carcinoma (no undifferentiated cells); grade 2, moderately differentiated carcinoma (<50% of undifferentiated cells); grade 3, poorly differentiated carcinoma (>50% of undifferentiated cells), grade 4, undifferentiated carcinoma (entirely composed of undifferentiated cells).

WARTY AND BASALOID CARCINOMA

The peak age for warty and basaloid carcinoma is 55 to 58 years, and thus the patients are, on average, 20 years younger than patients with

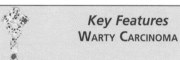

Key Features
WARTY CARCINOMA

- Verrucous architecture
- Large cells with marked cytologic atypia
- Infiltrative growth

Table 1
FIGO 2009 staging of vulvar cancer

Stage	Description
Stage I	Tumor confined to the vulva
IA	Superficially invasive vulvar carcinoma Lesions <2 cm in size confined to the vulva or perineum; invasion <1 mm in depth and no lymph node metastases
IB	Lesions >2 cm in size, confined to the vulva or perineum; or invasion >1 mm in depth and no lymph node metastases
Stage II	Tumor of any size with extension to adjacent perineal structures (one-third lower urethra, one-third lower vagina, anus); no lymph node metastases
Stage III	Tumor of any size with or without extension to perineal structures (one-third lower urethra, one-third lower vagina, anus); with metastases to inguinofemoral lymph nodes
IIIA	With 1 lymph node metastasis (>5 mm), or 1–2 lymph node metastases (<5 mm)
IIIB	With 2 or more lymph node metastases (>5 mm), or 3 or more lymph node metastases (<5 mm)
IIIC	Positive lymph nodes with extracapsular spread
Stage IV	Tumor invades other regional or distant structures
IVA	Tumor invades any of the following: upper urethral or vaginal mucosa, bladder mucosa, rectal mucosa, or fixed to pelvic bone, or fixed to ulcerated inguinofemoral lymph nodes
IVB	Any distant metastasis including pelvic lymph nodes

Modified from Pecorelli S. Revised FIGO staging for carcinoma of the vulva, cervix, and endometrium. Int J Gynaecol Obstet 2009;105(2):103–4; with permission.

keratinizing SCC.[32] Many of the patients have a history of cervical or vaginal dysplasia/carcinoma or immunosuppression. The tumors are related to infection with high oncogenic HPVs and, similar to uVIN, the most common HPV genotype detected in these tumors is HPV 16. Other high-risk HPV types are detected less frequently.[9,32] Based on the results of HPV genotyping, it is expected that current HPV vaccines may prevent almost all basaloid and warty cancer subtypes and therefore reduce the incidence of vulvar cancer by 25% to 35%.[9]

GROSS FEATURES

The gross appearance of warty carcinoma is that of a heavily keratinized verrucous or papillary lesion that may resemble condyloma. Basaloid carcinoma may appear as an indurated dermal mass or an irregular exophytic growth.

MICROSCOPIC FEATURES AND DIAGNOSIS

On histologic examination, warty carcinoma is characterized by exophytic papillary architecture (**Fig. 11**). The fibrovascular cores are covered with layers of large, eosinophilic and markedly keratinized cells.[33] A thick, spiked layer of parakeratosis may be present on the surface. The nuclei show prominent enlargement, pleomorphism, hyperchromasia, multinucleation, and sometimes also koilocytic changes. Cells with giant multiple nuclei are present. The nuclear contours are irregular, angulated and wrinkled, with dark, coarse, or clumped chromatin; no nucleoli are evident. The mitotic activity is sparse. The base of the tumor shows diffuse stromal infiltration with small, irregularly shaped nests and single tumor cells.[33]

Basaloid carcinoma (**Fig. 12**) is characterized by large ovoid nests and elongated bands and cords of small, tightly packed cells resembling immature squamous cells from the basal layer of the epidermis.[33] The cells are uniform, with scant cytoplasm and high N/C ratio. The nuclei are uniform, oval with dark, coarse, stippled chromatin and no nucleoli. The cytoplasm appears bluish

---

Key Features
BASALOID CARCINOMA

- Small basaloid cells with high N/C ratio
- High mitotic activity
- Infiltrative growth

Fig. 11. Warty carcinoma of vulva (×100). (*Reproduced from* de Koning MNC, Quint WGV, Pirog EC. Prevalence of mucosal and cutaneous human papillomaviruses in different histologic subtypes of vulvar carcinoma. Modern Pathology 2008; 21:334; with permission.)

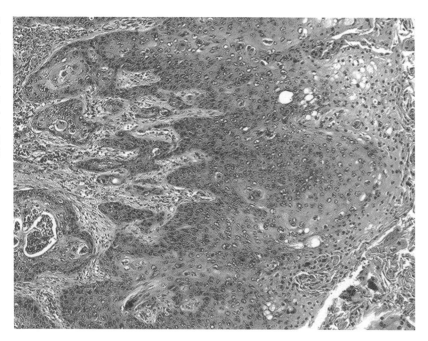

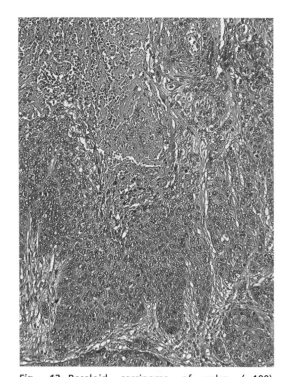

Fig. 12. Basaloid carcinoma of vulva (×100). (*Reproduced from* de Koning MNC, Quint WGV, Pirog EC. Prevalence of mucosal and cutaneous human papillomaviruses in different histologic subtypes of vulvar carcinoma. Modern Pathology 2008;21:334; with permission.)

purple without evidence of maturation or keratin production. However, occasionally small keratin pearls may be encountered. The mitotic activity is brisk. The tumor nests may show apoptosis as well as larger foci of central necrosis. Some basaloid carcinomas may show exophytic papillary architecture in addition to infiltrative growth. P16 is overexpressed in most cases.

DIFFERENTIAL DIAGNOSIS

The gross and low-power appearance of warty carcinoma may be similar to condyloma or verrucous carcinoma. Warty carcinoma can be differentiated from condyloma based on the presence of stromal invasion, and from verrucous carcinoma based on the presence of nuclear atypia and infiltrating tumor growth at the tumor base. Basaloid carcinoma should be differentiated from basal cell carcinoma. The latter tumor shows characteristic peripheral palisading and does not arise within a background of VIN.

Warty and basaloid carcinomas may have features that overlap with keratinizing SCC. Keratin pearls are identified in more than half of basaloid and warty carcinomas. In addition, pseudokoilocytic atypia is identified in almost half of HPV-negative keratinizing carcinomas.[32,34] Correlation between the overall tumor morphology, adjacent in situ lesion, and nuclear chromatin distribution are necessary for accurate diagnosis. Keratinizing tumors exhibit pale, vesicular chromatin and a prominent nucleolus, whereas basaloid/warty tumors show dark, coarse, granular chromatin and inconspicuous nucleoli. In addition, p16 immunostaining may be used as an objective adjunct test to confirm the diagnosis of warty and basaloid carcinoma in equivocal cases.[32,34] A comparison of differentiating clinicopathologic features in keratinizing and basaloid/warty carcinomas is shown in **Table 2**.

PROGNOSIS

The most important risk factors for tumor recurrences and metastases are depth of invasion, tumor size, involvement of lymphatic vessels, and margin clearance. The overall recurrence rate for vulvar cancer is approximately 20% to 25%, with half of patients having multiple recurrences. The recurrences occur most commonly in the vulvar region.

Once the tumor has spread to lymph nodes, the survival is related to the number of lymph nodes involved, the size of metastases (smaller/larger than 5 mm) and extracapsular extension. The FIGO staging system has recently been revised to reflect these prognostic factors (see **Table 1**).[30,31]

Pitfalls
WARTY AND BASALOID CARCINOMA

! Warty and basaloid carcinomas may have overlapping features with keratinizing SCC. Correlation between the overall tumor morphology, adjacent in situ lesion (ie, uVIN vs dVIN) and nuclear chromatin distribution are necessary for accurate diagnosis:

Keratinizing carcinoma:

  ! Nuclei with pale, vesicular chromatin and prominent nucleolus

Basaloid and warty carcinoma:

  ! Nuclei with dark, coarse, granular chromatin and inconspicuous nucleoli

! Accurate diagnosis is important because the overall risk for recurrence is higher in keratinizing carcinoma.

The initial metastatic spread involves inguinal, pelvic, iliac, and periaortic lymph nodes and is followed by involvement of distant organs. These general observations pertain to basaloid, warty, and keratinizing SCCs. The overall 5-year survival of patients is 86%,[1] and ranges from 98% for patients with stage I disease to 31% for patients

Table 2
Comparison of clinicopathologic features of vulvar carcinomas

	Keratinizing Squamous Cell Carcinoma	Warty and Basaloid Carcinoma
Percentage of all vulvar carcinomas	60	30
Average age of patients (y)	75	55
Risk factors	Nonneoplastic epithelial disorder: LS or SCH	HPV infection, immunosuppression
Molecular pathogenetic events	p53 gene mutation	HPV-related malignant transformation with inactivation of p53 and retinoblastoma proteins
Precursor lesion	dVIN	uVIN
Frequency of progression of in situ lesion to invasive cancer (%)	32.8	5.7
Average progression time from in situ lesion to invasion (mo)	22.8	41.5
OR for tumor recurrence	4.3	1.35
Immunohistochemical marker	p53	p16

with stage IV tumors. As is discussed later, survival and recurrence rates for uVIN-associated tumors are superior to those of dVIN-associated tumors.

Examining 1 or 2 sentinel inguinal nodes is a novel way to detect whether the tumor has metastasized in early-stage vulvar cancer.[35] Sentinel node dissection results in fewer adverse side effects compared with the standard approach of groin dissection; however, extensive experience is necessary to ensure that the false-negative rate is negligible.

KERATINIZING SQUAMOUS CELL CARCINOMA (SCC)

The average age of patients with keratinizing squamous cell carcinoma (SCC) is 75 years.[32] Most patients have a long-standing history of a nonneoplastic epithelial disorder of the vulva.

GROSS FEATURES

Superficially invasive SCCs associated with LS, SCH, and dVIN may present as an ulcer, papule, macule, or hyperkeratotic plaque in a background of vulvar inflammation. The often-subtle emergence of an invasive lesion may be misinterpreted for long periods as dermatitis or leukoplakia. Advanced invasive carcinoma presents as an indurated cutaneous mass, frequently with ulceration or as an irregular, keratinized exophytic growth.

MICROSCOPIC FEATURES AND DIAGNOSIS

Keratinizing SCCs are composed of invasive nests and cords of malignant squamous epithelium with prominent central keratin whorls with an onion skin appearance. The tumor cells are large with abundant eosinophilic cytoplasm, large, round to oval nuclei with pale, vesicular chromatin and a single prominent nucleolus. The nuclear atypia may range from minimal to marked. In rare cases, the nuclei may show significant variation of sizes and shapes and multinucleolation, mimicking koilocytic atypia. The invasive nests spread radially within the dermis and may undermine normal skin (**Fig. 13**). Some well-differentiated keratinizing carcinomas show exophytic, papillary architecture rather than infiltrative growth. Although the most keratinizing SCCs are well-differentiated tumors, approximately 10% to 20% of tumors are moderately or poorly differentiated with little or no keratin production. Such tumors are typically composed of small angulated cords of markedly atypical cells with variable amounts of eosinophilic cytoplasm. Poorly differentiated tumors may form solid

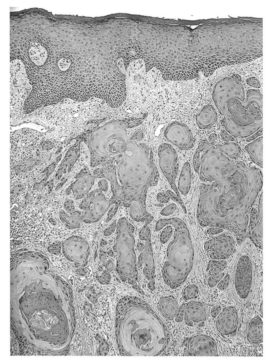

Fig. 13. Keratinizing SCC of the vulva (×100). (*Reproduced from* de Koning MNC, Quint WGV, Pirog EC. Prevalence of mucosal and cutaneous human papillomaviruses in different histologic subtypes of vulvar carcinoma. Modern Pathology 2008;21:334; with permission.)

masses of confluent epithelial growth. Acantholytic SCC and spindle cell SCC are less differentiated variants of keratinizing SCC. Approximately two-thirds to three-quarters of keratinizing SCCs show significant levels of p53 expression using immunohistochemistry.[36]

DIFFERENTIAL DIAGNOSIS

Superficially invasive SCC has to be differentiated from pseudoepitheliomatous hyperplasia and entrapped benign epithelial nests in a previous biopsy site. Pseudoepitheliomatous hyperplasia is a reactive/regenerative change typically present on the edge of an ulcer. It may also be seen as a regenerative response in the areas of epithelial injury in LS.[27] In cases equivocal for invasion, double immunostaining for cytokeratin and collagen IV may be useful to confirm the diagnosis. Invasive keratinizing SCC has to be differentiated from other types of SCC (basaloid, warty, and verrucous) as well as from keratoacanthoma. The latter lesion shows characteristic, well-circumscribed, craterlike growth with a central keratin plug. Superficial biopsy of this lesion may be mistaken for keratinizing SCC.

PROGNOSIS

The OR for a recurrence is higher for tumors arising from dVIN and nonneoplastic epithelial disorder (4.3 with 95% confidence interval [CI] 0.84, 21.92) than from uVIN (1.35 with 95% CI 0.20, 9.01).[28] The disease-specific survival for patients with SCC arising from dVIN has been reported to be significantly worse compared with patients with SCC arising from uVIN (ie, HPV-associated tumors).[37] Whether these differences are specific to tumor type remains to be determined. Most studies have not accounted for the tendency of dVIN-associated squamous carcinoma to present at high stage and in significantly older populations. It has been shown that HPV-related oropharyngeal carcinomas have a significantly better prognosis than HPV-negative tumors, which prove to be relatively resistant to chemotherapy and radiation.[38] It remains to be determined whether survival in different subtypes of vulvar cancer parallels the pattern observed in oropharyngeal carcinomas.

VERRUCOUS CARCINOMA

The tumor most commonly develops in the seventh and eighth decades. Some of the lesions have been described to arise in association with vulvar condylomata and others as developing de novo and growing rapidly to a large size. Formerly, there was long-standing controversy about relationship, or lack thereof, to giant condyloma of Buschke-Lowenstein. Given the overlapping histologic features, it is now believed that giant condyloma of Buschke-Lowenstein and verrucous carcinoma are part of the spectrum of the same process, and because the term giant condyloma of Buschke-Lowenstein is confusing, it is no longer recommended. The association between verrucous carcinoma and HPV is still uncertain. There are rare reports of detection of low oncogenic risk HPVs, such as HPV 6 or 11, in this type of tumor[32]; however, in larger series of vulvar and penile verrucous carcinomas, no HPV DNA has been detected.[39,40] The tumor has been also reported in immunosuppressed patients.[41] Given the architectural appearance, it is tempting to speculate that verrucous carcinoma could evolve from a nonexcised, irritated condyloma in which low oncogenic risk HPVs initiate the growth process, and subsequent chronic epithelial irritation contributes to gradual malignant transformation. However, a strong argument against the connection between condyloma and verrucous carcinoma is that patients with condylomata are, on average, 40 years younger than patients with verrucous carcinoma (25–35 years old vs 65–75 years old). It is also possible that verrucous carcinoma is a well-differentiated variant of the conventional keratinizing SCC, because tumors with mixed verrucous and keratinizng features are sometimes seen.

GROSS FEATURES

Verrucous carcinomas are warty or papillary, cauliflowerlike masses resembling condyloma acuminatum. The tumor most commonly develops on the mucosal surface of the labia but may also arise within the labial skin.

MICROSCOPIC FEATURES AND DIAGNOSIS

Verrucous carcinoma (**Fig. 14**) is composed of papillary fronds of mature keratinocytes with abundant eosinophilic cytoplasm and pale, uniform, vesicular nuclei with small nucleoli. No nuclear atypia or koilocytic atypia is present (**Fig. 15**). The tumor surface shows a thick layer of parakeratosis and hyperkeratosis. The base of the tumor is composed of well-demarcated

Key Features
VERRUCOUS CARCINOMA

- Verrucous architecture
- No cytologic atypia
- Bulbous rete ridges

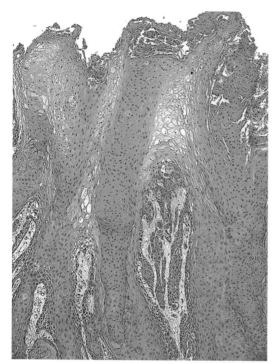

Fig. 14. Verrucous carcinoma of vulva (×100). (*Reproduced from* de Koning MNC, Quint WGV, Pirog EC. Prevalence of mucosal and cutaneous human papillomaviruses in different histologic subtypes of vulvar carcinoma. Modern Pathology 2008;21:334; with permission.)

and circumscribed rete with rounded, bulbous shape, consistent with pushing, expansive tumor growth. Immunostaining for basement membrane component shows thick, continuous basement membrane at the pushing tumor front (**Fig. 16**A).[42] The tumor does not infiltrate the dermis or penetrate the vascular channels as seen in conventional SCC (see **Fig. 16**B).

DIFFERENTIAL DIAGNOSIS

Verrucous carcinoma is differentiated from condyloma based on lack of koilocytic atypia; from warty

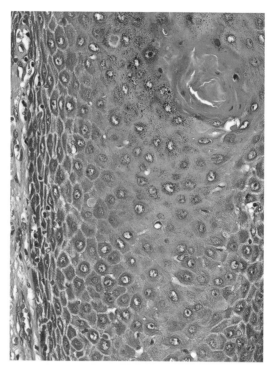

Fig. 15. Verrucous carcinoma of vulva, high-power magnification (×400).

carcinoma based on lack of cytologic atypia and lack of infiltrative growth; and from keratinizing SCC with papillary architecture based on lack of infiltrative growth. Keratinized tumors with verrucous architecture and infiltrative tumor nests at the tumor base should be classified as keratinizing SCC.

PROGNOSIS

The tumor shows indolent local growth with occasional recurrences. If not excised, the expansive, pushing tumor base may erode into the underlying

Differential Diagnosis
Verrucous Carcinoma

- Condyloma
- Warty carcinoma
- Keratinizing squamous cell carcinoma

Pitfall
Verrucous Carcinoma

! Keratinized carcinoma with verrucous architecture and infiltrative growth at the tumor base should be classified as keratinizing SCC and not verrucous carcinoma, because such a lesion has the potential for lymphvascular metastatic spread.

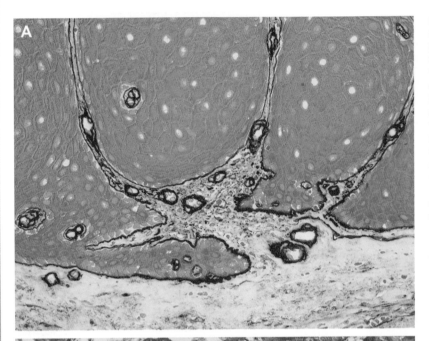

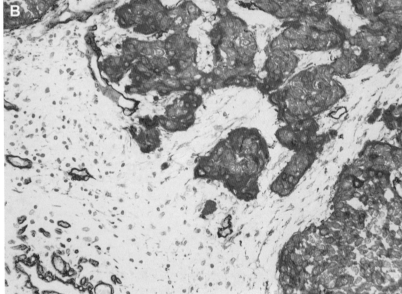

Fig. 16. (*A*) Verrucous carcinoma of vulva, pushing tumor front; double immunostaining for cytokeratin and collagen IV (×400). (*B*) Keratinizing carcinoma of vulva, infiltrative tumor front; double immunostaining for cytokeratin and collagen IV (×400). (*Reproduced from* Rush D, Hyjek E, Baergen RN, et al. Detection of microinvasion in vulvar and cervical intraepithelial neoplasia using double immunostaining for cytokeratin and basement membrane components. Arch Pathol Lab Med 2005;129:747, copyright 2005, College of American Pathologists; with permission.) *Editor's note: This technique, which produces beautiful images, is useful in educational and investigative settings; however, it is not currently considered a standard practice for diagnostic use.*

structures such as the pubic bone. Treatment is with wide local excision. Verrucous carcinoma does not invade the lymphatic channels, and therefore lymph node dissection is not required. Radiotherapy is contraindicated because it may induce anaplastic transformation of the tumor. Sometimes the recurrence may take the form of typical keratinizing SCC with infiltrating tumor growth and metastases.

CONDYLOMA ACUMINATUM

Condylomata acuminata (CONAs) are benign lesions with a distinct warty appearance that involve vulvar skin or mucosal surfaces. CONA are caused by low oncogenic risk HPVs, principally types 6 and 11, and only occasionally are due to high oncogenic risk HPVs.[43] CONA can occur at any age but they are most common in the third decade.

> **Key Features**
> CONDYLOMA ACUMINATUM
>
> - Verrucous architecture
> - Koilocytic atypia
> - Ki-67 staining extending into the upper two-thirds of the epithelial thickness

> **Differential Diagnosis**
> CONDYLOMA ACUMINATUM
>
> - Fibroepithelial polyp
> - Squamous papilloma
> - Seborrheic keratosis
> - Verrucous carcinoma
> - Warty carcinoma

GROSS FEATURES

CONA present as hyperkeratotic cauliflowerlike, warty or papillary lesions. They may be solitary, but more frequently, they are multiple and multi-focal, involving vulvar and perianal regions as well as vaginal mucosa.

MICROSCOPIC FEATURES AND DIAGNOSIS

On histologic examination, they consist of branching papillary cores of stroma covered by thickened squamous epithelium with viral cytopathic effect. Condylomata represent productive viral infection in which HPV replicates and completes its life cycle in mature superficial squamous epithelium causing distinct cytologic changes (koilocytic atypia) characterized by nuclear enlargement, hyperchromasia, coarseness of the chromatin, variations of nuclear sizes and shapes, and cytoplasmic perinuclear halo indicating a disruption of the cytoskeleton before release of the virus into the environment (**Fig. 17**). The degree of viral cytopathic changes depends on the age of the lesion; koilocytic atypia may be prominent at early stages but diminishes in regressing infection. In rare condylomata that are caused by high oncogenic risk HPVs, a high-grade dysplasia may develop within the epithelial lining resulting in the appearance of uVIN. CONAs show variable degrees of surface keratinization with parakeratosis and dense hyperkeratosis.

Ki-67 staining in CONA shows a characteristic pattern of positive cells extending from the normal parabasal location into the upper two-thirds of the epithelial thickness (**Fig. 18**). P16 is negative in CONAs, except for the rare lesions with high-grade dysplasia.

DIFFERENTIAL DIAGNOSIS

Condylomata acuminatum must be differentiated from fibroepithelial polyp, squamous papilloma, and seborrheic keratosis on the benign end of

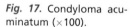

Fig. 17. Condyloma acuminatum (×100).

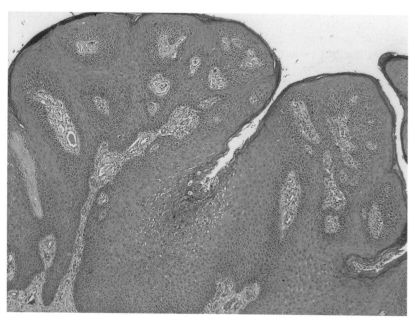

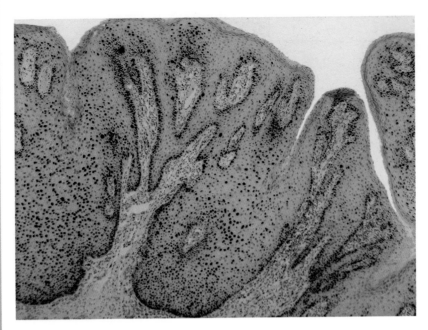

Fig. 18. Ki-67 immunostaining in condyloma acuminatum showing expansion of the positive cells from the normal parabasal location to the superficial layers of the epithelium.

the spectrum, and from verrucous and warty carcinomas on the malignant end of the spectrum. Fibroepithelial polyps (skin tags) lack dense surface hyperkeratosis or parakeratosis, or koilocytic atypia; however, skin adnexal structures are frequently seen within their fibrovascular cores. Squamous papillomas are nonkeratinized, slender papillary growths of unknown cause and lacking koilocytic atypia. In contrast to CONA, fibroepithelial polyps and squamous papillomas show only parabasal staining with Ki-67 marker.[43] Seborrheic keratosis is characteristic for its keratin horn configurations. Ki-67 is usually negative; however, the interpretation may be difficult because of tangential sectioning of the expanded parabasal layer. In contrast to verrucous and warty carcinomas, CONAs show neither a pushing tumor front nor infiltrative invasion.

PROGNOSIS

CONA do not progress to carcinoma and are not considered to be premalignant lesions. They are treated with excision or ablative methods. Recurrences are common in immunocompromised patients.

GLANDULAR NEOPLASTIC LESIONS OF THE VULVA

Like the breast, the vulva contains modified apocrine sweat glands, and tumors with counterparts in the breast may develop in the vulva, namely papillary hidradenoma and extramammary Paget disease. In addition, rare cases of fibroadenoma, ductal carcinoma in situ, and invasive mammary carcinoma arising from apocrine glands, or vulvar ectopic breast tissue have been reported.[44] Invasive adenocarcinomas of the colorectal type, including colloid carcinoma, associated with villous adenoma of the vulva, may also rarely occur.[45]

PAPILLARY HIDRADENOMA

Papillary hidradenoma is identical in appearance to intraductal papillomas of the breast.

GROSS FEATURES

Papillary hidradenoma presents as a firm, sharply circumscribed nodule, most commonly on the labia majora or interlabial folds. It has tendency to ulcerate and, therefore, clinically may be confused with carcinoma.

MICROSCOPIC FEATURES AND DIAGNOSIS

On histologic examination the lesion consists of a well-circumscribed tumor with papillary projections covered by 2 layers of cells: the columnar, secretory cells and the underlying layer of flattened myoepithelial cells. These myoepithelial elements are characteristic of sweat glands and sweat gland tumors (**Fig. 19**). The secretory cells may show apocrine change with voluminous eosinophilic cytoplasm.

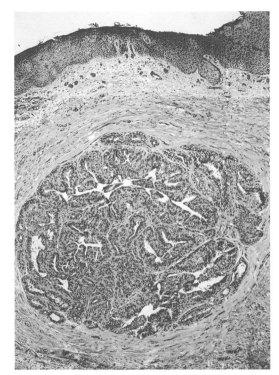

Fig. 19. Papillary hidradenoma (×100). (*Reproduced from* Kumar V, Abbas AK, Fausto N, et al. Robbins and Cotran pathologic basis of disease. 8th edition. Philadelphia (PA): Saunders; 2009. p. 1015, copyright by Elsevier, 2009; with permission.)

DIFFERENTIAL DIAGNOSIS

Hidradenoma has such a distinctive appearance that it rarely creates a diagnostic difficulty.

PROGNOSIS

The tumor is benign and does not recur when completely excised. Rare cases of ductal carcinoma in situ or invasive mammary carcinoma arising within hidradenoma have been reported.[44]

EXTRAMAMMARY PAGET DISEASE

Extramammary Paget disease is a rare lesion of the vulvar skin and the perianal region. The average age of the patients is 65 to 70 years. In contrast to Paget disease of the nipple, in which almost all patients show an underlying ductal breast carcinoma, vulvar lesions are most frequently confined to the epidermis of the skin and adjacent hair follicles and sweat glands. No environmental or genetic risk factors have been identified.

Ultrastructurally, Paget cells display apocrine, eccrine, and keratinocyte differentiation, and

Key Features
PAGET DISEASE

- Large tumor cells lying singly or in clusters within the epidermis and appendages
- Finely granular, pale, eosinophilic cytoplasm
- Large vesicular nuclei with prominent nucleoli
- CK7, CEA, and GCDFP-15 immunopositivity

presumably arise from primitive germinal cells of the mammarylike gland ducts of the vulvar skin.[46,47]

GROSS FEATURES

Paget disease presents as a pruritic, red, crusted, sharply demarcated, maplike area, usually occurring on the labia majora. It may be accompanied by a palpable submucosal thickening or nodule.

MICROSCOPIC FEATURES AND DIAGNOSIS

Histologically, Paget disease is an intraepithelial proliferation of malignant glandular cells (**Fig. 20**), and therefore may be considered as an adenocarcinoma in situ. The diagnostic feature of this lesion is the presence of large tumor cells lying singly or in small clusters within the epidermis and its appendages. These cells are distinguished by a clear separation (halo) from the surrounding epithelial cells (**Fig. 21**) and a finely granular, pale, eosinophilic cytoplasm containing mucopolysaccharide that stains with periodic acid-Schiff, alcian blue and mucicarmine stains.[48] The nuclei are large and vesiculated, with prominent nucleoli. Dermal invasion develops in approximately 12% of patients (**Fig. 22**).[49] The exact

Differential Diagnosis
PAGETOID LESIONS OF THE VULVA

- Primary vulvar Paget: MUCIN+, CK7+, CEA+, GCDFP-15+
- Pagetoid VIN: MUCIN−, CK7+
- Pagetoid urothelial intraepithelial neoplasia: CK7+, CK20+, UP-III+
- Pagetoid spread of rectal carcinoma: CK20+, CK7−, GCDFP-15
- Malignant melanoma in situ: S-100+, HMB-45+

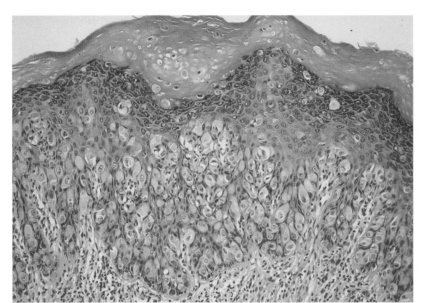

Fig. 20. Paget disease of vulva (×200).

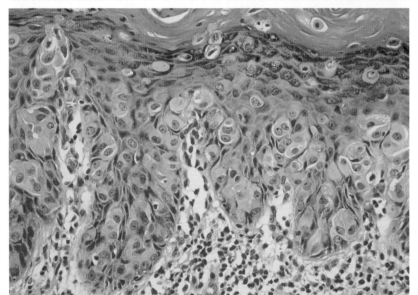

Fig. 21. Paget disease of vulva, high-power magnification (×400) hematoxylin and eosin.

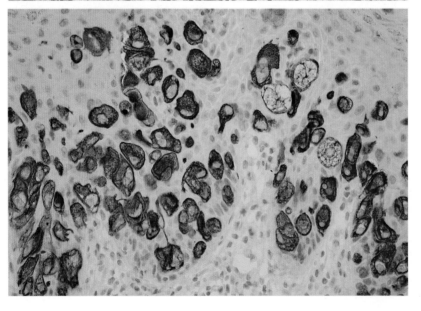

Fig. 22. Paget disease of vulva (×400), cytokeratin 7 immunostaining.

Fig. 23. Invasive Paget disease (×200).

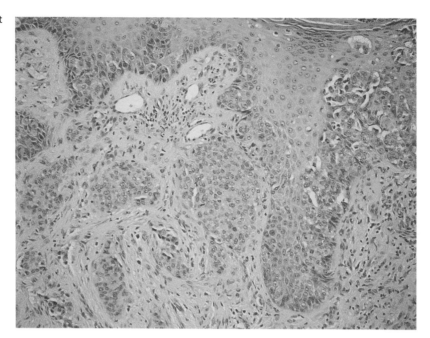

measurement of depth of invasion is important because invasion deeper than 1 mm is associated with a significant risk of lymph node metastases.[50,51] In cases with marked inflammation at the epidermal-stromal interface, immunostains (such as CK7) highlighting Paget cells in the stroma may be helpful in assessing the invasion. Vulvar Paget disease shows immunohistochemical positivity for CK7 (**Fig. 23**), CEA, and gross cystic disease fluid protein 15 (GCDFP-15).

DIFFERENTIAL DIAGNOSIS

Vulvar Paget disease has to be differentiated from pagetoid VIN, pagetoid urothelial intraepithelial neoplasia, pagetoid spread of rectal carcinoma,

Fig. 24. Pagetoid urothelial intraepithelial neoplasia (×400).

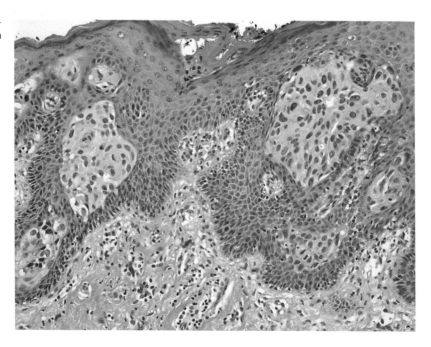

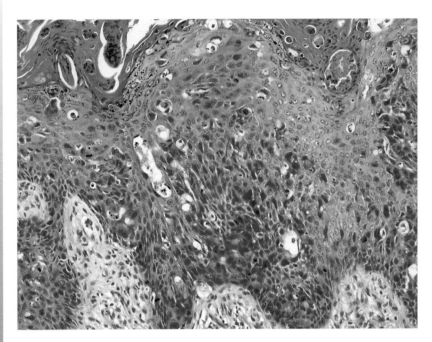

Fig. 25. Pagetoid spread of rectal carcinoma (×400). The rectal primary is a combined adenocarcinoma and small cell carcinoma. Both components colonize the epithelium in an excision from the perianal region.

and superficial spreading malignant melanoma. Special stains may be necessary to confirm the diagnosis. Pagetoid VIN shows positivity for CK7, similar to vulvar Paget disease, but is negative for mucin stains, GCDFP-15, or CEA.[11] Paget disease of urothelial origin (**Fig. 24**) typically shows positivity for CK 7, CK 20, and uroplakin-III (UP-III), but is not immunoreactive with GCDFP-15 or CEA.[52] Rectal carcinoma with pagetoid spread to vulva (**Fig. 25**) shows positivity for CK 20 and is negative for CK7 and GCDFP-15 staining.[53] It is currently not considered the standard of care to perform CK7 and CK 20 immunostains on all vulvar biopsies of Paget disease, but a history of urothelial or rectal carcinoma should encourage immunohistochemical evaluation. Vulvar melanoma shows positivity for S-100, HMB-45, and melan-A immunomarkers,[54] whereas all of these markers are negative in Paget disease.

PROGNOSIS

Paget disease is treated with wide local excision and shows a high recurrence rate.[50] Typically, Paget cells spread beyond the confines of the grossly visible lesion, and therefore they frequently extend far beyond the margins of surgical excision. Mapping biopsies to determine the extent of Paget disease before planning excision are discouraged. Intraepidermal Paget disease may persist for many years, even decades, without invasion or metastases. Once significant invasion develops, the prognosis is poor. Invasive carcinomas tend to be staged like other primary vulvar carcinomas.

BARTHOLIN GLAND CARCINOMAS

Bartholin gland carcinomas are rare tumors of the vulva. Several different histologic types of Bartholin gland carcinomas were described, of which the most common are adenocarcinoma (40%), SCC (40%), adenoid cystic carcinoma (15%), transitional cell carcinoma (<5%), and adenosquamous carcinoma (<5%). For the tumor to be classified as Bartholin gland carcinoma it has to arise at site of the Bartholin gland and a metastasis or direct extension from another site has to be ruled out. The average age of the patients is 50 years.

GROSS FEATURES

Bartholin gland carcinomas present as enlargement or a palpable submucosal mass of the labia majora.

MICROSCOPIC FEATURES AND DIAGNOSIS

Histologically, Bartholin gland adenocarcinomas that arise from the mucinous acini are of mucinous or nonspecific type. The tumor cells are positive for CEA. SCCs, transitional cell carcinomas, and adenosquamous carcinomas develop from the

Fig. 26. Adenoid cystic carcinoma of the vulva (×200). (*Courtesy of* Kay Park, MD.)

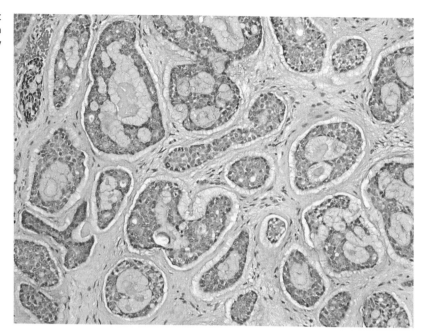

epithelium of the Bartholin duct. Adenoid cystic carcinomas (**Fig. 26**) are similar to those occurring in salivary glands and are positive for CK stain and S-100, a myoepithelial cell marker.[55]

DIFFERENTIAL DIAGNOSIS

Bartholin gland carcinomas have to be differentiated from tumors arising from epidermis, skin appendages, and metastases.

PROGNOSIS

Bartholin gland carcinomas spread to the regional inguinal lymph nodes. The overall 5-year survival in patients without lymph node metastases is 50%, and 18% with positive lymph nodes. Approximately 20% of patients present with lymph node metastases. The prognosis is best for adenoid cystic carcinoma, and least favorable for adenosquamous carcinoma.[55]

Pitfall
PAGET DISEASE

! Invasive Paget disease may be overlooked in cases with marked inflammation at the epidermal-stromal interface. In such cases, immunostaining for CK7 may be used to highlight Paget cells in the stroma.

REFERENCES

1. Saraiya M, Watson M, Wu X, et al. Incidence of in situ and invasive vulvar cancer in the US, 1998–2003. Cancer 2008;113(Suppl 10):2865–72.
2. van de Nieuwenhof HP, Massuger LF, van der Avoort IA, et al. Vulvar squamous cell carcinoma development after diagnosis of VIN increases with age. Eur J Cancer 2009;45(5):851–6.
3. Joura EA, Lösch A, Haider-Angeler MG, et al. Trends in vulvar neoplasia. Increasing incidence of vulvar intraepithelial neoplasia and squamous cell carcinoma of the vulva in young women. J Reprod Med 2000;45(8):613–5.
4. Sideri M, Jones RW, Wilkinson EJ, et al. Squamous vulvar intraepithelial neoplasia: 2004 modified terminology, ISSVD Vulvar Oncology Subcommittee. J Reprod Med 2005;50(11):807–10.
5. Heller DS. Report of a new ISSVD classification of VIN. J Low Genit Tract Dis 2007;11(1):46–7.
6. Logani S, Lu D, Quint WG, et al. Low-grade vulvar and vaginal intraepithelial neoplasia: correlation of histologic features with human papillomavirus DNA detection and MIB-1 immunostaining. Mod Pathol 2003;16(8):735–41.
7. Srodon M, Stoler MH, Baber GB, et al. The distribution of low and high-risk HPV types in vulvar and vaginal intraepithelial neoplasia (VIN and VaIN). Am J Surg Pathol 2006;30(12):1513–8.
8. Scurry J, Campion M, Scurry B, et al. Pathologic audit of 164 consecutive cases of vulvar intraepithelial neoplasia. Int J Gynecol Pathol 2006;25(2):176–81.

9. De Vuyst H, Clifford GM, Nascimento MC, et al. Prevalence and type distribution of human papillomavirus in carcinoma and intraepithelial neoplasia of the vulva, vagina and anus: a meta-analysis. Int J Cancer 2009;124(7):1626–36.

10. Hart WR. Vulvar intraepithelial neoplasia: historical aspects and current status. Int J Gynecol Pathol 2001;20(1):16–30.

11. McCluggage WG, Jamison J, Boyde A, et al. Vulval intraepithelial neoplasia with mucinous differentiation: report of 2 cases of a hitherto undescribed phenomenon. Am J Surg Pathol 2009; 33(6):945–9.

12. Rufforny I, Wilkinson EJ, Liu C, et al. Human papillomavirus infection and p16(INK4a) protein expression in vulvar intraepithelial neoplasia and invasive squamous cell carcinoma. J Low Genit Tract Dis 2005;9(2):108–13.

13. Jones RW, Rowan DM, Stewart AW. Vulvar intraepithelial neoplasia: aspects of the natural history and outcome in 405 women. Obstet Gynecol 2005; 106(6):1319–26.

14. Dedes KJ, Beneder C, Samartzis N, et al. Outcome of treated anogenital intraepithelial neoplasia among human immunodeficiency virus-infected women. J Reprod Med 2008;53(12):947–51.

15. Mulvany NJ, Allen DG. Differentiated intraepithelial neoplasia of the vulva. Int J Gynecol Pathol 2008; 27(1):125–35.

16. Kruse AJ, Bottenberg MJ, Tosserams J, et al. The absence of high-risk HPV combined with specific p53 and p16INK4a expression patterns points to the HPV-independent pathway as the causative agent for vulvar squamous cell carcinoma and its precursor simplex VIN in a young patient. Int J Gynecol Pathol 2008;27(4):591–5.

17. Carlson JA, Ambros R, Malfetano J, et al. Vulvar lichen sclerosus and squamous cell carcinoma: a cohort, case control, and investigational study with historical perspective; implications for chronic inflammation and sclerosis in the development of neoplasia. Hum Pathol 1998;29(9): 932–48.

18. Pinto AP, Lin MC, Sheets EE, et al. Allelic imbalance in lichen sclerosus, hyperplasia, and intraepithelial neoplasia of the vulva. Gynecol Oncol 2000;77(1): 171–6.

19. Kim YT, Thomas NF, Kessis TD, et al. p53 mutations and clonality in vulvar carcinomas and squamous hyperplasias: evidence suggesting that squamous hyperplasias do not serve as direct precursors of human papillomavirus-negative vulvar carcinomas. Hum Pathol 1996;27(4):389–95.

20. Rolfe KJ, MacLean AB, Crow JC, et al. TP53 mutations in vulval lichen sclerosus adjacent to squamous cell carcinoma of the vulva. Br J Cancer 2003;89(12):2249–53.

21. Lee YY, Wilczynski SP, Chumakov A, et al. Carcinoma of the vulva: HPV and p53 mutations. Oncogene 1994;9:1655–9.

22. Ngan HY, Cheung AN, Liu SS, et al. Abnormal expression or mutation of TP53 and HPV in vulvar cancer. Eur J Cancer 1999;35:481–4.

23. Ordi J, Alejo M, Fusté V, et al. HPV-negative vulvar intraepithelial neoplasia (VIN) with basaloid histologic pattern: an unrecognized variant of simplex (differentiated) VIN. Am J Surg Pathol 2009;33(11):1659–65.

24. Yang B, Hart WR. Vulvar intraepithelial neoplasia of the simplex (differentiated) type: a clinicopathologic study including analysis of HPV and p53 expression. Am J Surg Pathol 2000;24(3):429–41.

25. Santos M, Montagut C, Mellado B, et al. Immunohistochemical staining for p16 and p53 in premalignant and malignant epithelial lesions of the vulva. Int J Gynecol Pathol 2004;23(3):206–14.

26. Liegl B, Regauer S. p53 immunostaining in lichen sclerosus is related to ischaemic stress and is not a marker of differentiated vulvar intraepithelial neoplasia (d-VIN). Histopathology 2006;48(3): 268–74.

27. Lee ES, Allen D, Scurry J. Pseudoepitheliomatous hyperplasia in lichen sclerosus of the vulva. Int J Gynecol Pathol 2003;22(1):57–62.

28. Eva LJ, Ganesan R, Chan KK, et al. Differentiated-type vulval intraepithelial neoplasia has a high-risk association with vulval squamous cell carcinoma. Int J Gynecol Cancer 2009;19(4):741–4.

29. Raju RR, Goldblum JR, Hart WR. Pagetoid squamous cell carcinoma in situ (pagetoid Bowen's disease) of the external genitalia. Int J Gynecol Pathol 2003;22(2):127–35.

30. Hacker NF. Revised FIGO staging for carcinoma of the vulva. Int J Gynaecol Obstet 2009;105(2):105–6.

31. Pecorelli S. Revised FIGO staging for carcinoma of the vulva, cervix, and endometrium. Int J Gynaecol Obstet 2009;105(2):103–4.

32. de Koning MN, Quint WG, Pirog EC. Prevalence of mucosal and cutaneous human papillomaviruses in different histologic subtypes of vulvar carcinoma. Mod Pathol 2008;21:334–44.

33. Kurman RJ, Toki T, Schiffman MH. Basaloid and warty carcinomas of the vulva. Distinctive types of squamous cell carcinoma frequently associated with human papillomaviruses. Am J Surg Pathol 1993;17(2):133–45.

34. Santos M, Landolfi S, Olivella A, et al. p16 overexpression identifies HPV-positive vulvar squamous cell carcinomas. Am J Surg Pathol 2006;30(11): 1347–56.

35. Hampl M, Hantschmann P, Michels W, et al. Validation of the accuracy of the sentinel lymph node procedure in patients with vulvar cancer: results of a multicenter study in Germany. Gynecol Oncol 2008;111(2):282–8.

36. Hoevenaars BM, van der Avoort IA, de Wilde PC, et al. A panel of p16(INK4A), MIB1 and p53 proteins can distinguish between the 2 pathways leading to vulvar squamous cell carcinoma. Int J Cancer 2008;123(12):2767–73.

37. van de Nieuwenhof HP, van Kempen LC, de Hullu JA, et al. The etiologic role of HPV in vulvar squamous cell carcinoma fine tuned. Cancer Epidemiol Biomarkers Prev 2009;18(7):2061–667.

38. Vu HL, Sikora AG, Fu S, et al. HPV-induced oropharyngeal cancer, immune response and response to therapy. Cancer Lett 2010;288(2):149–55.

39. Nascimento AF, Granter SR, Cviko A, et al. Vulvar acanthosis with altered differentiation: a precursor to verrucous carcinoma? Am J Surg Pathol 2004; 28(5):638–43.

40. Gualco M, Bonin S, Foglia G, et al. Morphologic and biologic studies on ten cases of verrucous carcinoma of the vulva supporting the theory of a discrete clinico-pathologic entity. Int J Gynecol Cancer 2003; 13(3):317–24.

41. Massad LS, Ahuja J, Bitterman P. Verrucous carcinoma of the vulva in a patient infected with the human immunodeficiency virus. Gynecol Oncol 1999;73(2):315–8.

42. Rush D, Hyjek E, Baergen RN. Detection of microinvasion in vulvar and cervical intraepithelial neoplasia using double immunostaining for cytokeratin and basement membrane components. Arch Pathol Lab Med 2005;129(6):747–53.

43. Pirog EC, Chen YT, Isacson C. MIB-1 immunostaining is a beneficial adjunct test for accurate diagnosis of vulvar condyloma acuminatum. Am J Surg Pathol 2000;24(10):1393–9.

44. Vazmitel M, Spagnolo DV, Nemcova J, et al. Hidradenoma papilliferum with a ductal carcinoma in situ component: case report and review of the literature. Am J Dermatopathol 2008;30(4): 392–4.

45. Dubé V, Lickrish GM, MacNeill KN, et al. Villoglandular adenocarcinoma in situ of intestinal type of the hymen: de novo origin from squamous mucosa? J Low Genit Tract Dis 2006;10(3):156–60.

46. Belousova IE, Kazakov DV, Michal M, et al. Vulvar Toker cells: the long-awaited missing link: a proposal for an origin-based histogenetic classification of extramammary Paget's disease. Am J Dermatopathol 2006;28:84–5.

47. Willman JH, Golitz LE, Fitzpatrick JE. Vulvar clear cells of Toker: precursors of extramammary Paget's disease. Am J Dermatopathol 2005;27:185–7.

48. Preti M, Micheletti L, Massobrio M, et al. Vulvar Paget's disease: one century after first reported. J Low Genit Tract Dis 2003;7(2):122–35.

49. Fanning J, Lambert HC, Hale TM, et al. Paget's disease of the vulva: prevalence of associated vulvar adenocarcinoma, invasive Paget's disease, and recurrence after surgical excision. Am J Obstet Gynecol 1999;180(1 Pt 1):24–7.

50. Crawford D, Nimmo M, Clement PB, et al. Prognostic factors in Paget's disease of the vulva: a study of 21 cases. Int J Gynecol Pathol 1999;18(4):351–9.

51. Shaco-Levy R, Bean SM, Vollmer RT, et al. Paget disease of the vulva: a histologic study of 56 cases correlating pathologic features and disease course. Int J Gynecol Pathol 2010;29(1):69–78.

52. Wilkinson EJ, Brown HM. Vulvar Paget's disease of urothelial origin: a report of three cases and a proposed classification of vulvar Paget's disease. Hum Pathol 2002;33(5):549–54.

53. Goldblum JR, Hart WR. Perianal Paget's disease: a histologic and immunohistochemical study of 11 cases with and without associated rectal adenocarcinoma. Am J Surg Pathol 1998;22:170–9.

54. Glasgow BJ, Wen DR, Al-Jitawi S, et al. Antibody to S-100 protein aids the separation of pagetoid melanoma from mammary and extramammary Paget's disease. J Cutan Pathol 1987;14(4):223–6.

55. Yang SY, Lee JW, Kim WS, et al. Adenoid cystic carcinoma of the Bartholin's gland: report of two cases and review of the literature. Gynecol Oncol 2006;100(2):422–5.

CLINICAL APPROACH TO DIAGNOSIS AND MANAGEMENT OF ENDOMETRIAL HYPERPLASIA AND CARCINOMA

Mario M. Leitao Jr, MD*, Richard R. Barakat, MD

KEYWORDS

- Uterus • Endometrium • Hyperplasia • Complex atypical hyperplasia
- Endometrial carcinoma • Cancer treatment • Sentinel lymph node

ABSTRACT

This article focuses on the most important neoplastic epithelial lesions of the uterus, endometrial hyperplasia and carcinoma. The primary management of hyperplastic lesions and carcinoma is often surgical but nonsurgical options are possible for both, depending on specific patients and tumor characteristics. Many controversies still exist regarding the optimal medical and surgical treatments of hyperplasias and carcinomas of the endometrium. There is a need to more accurately select patients for lymph node sampling or dissection. The role of adjuvant therapies for endometrial carcinomas is still under investigation. This review covers current understanding in the diagnosis and clinical management of endometrial hyperplasias and carcinomas.

ENDOMETRIAL HYPERPLASIA

OVERVIEW

The classification of hyperplasias recognized by the International Society of Gynecologic Pathologists is based on the fact that certain endometrial hyperplasias will more readily progress than others to carcinoma.[1] The four lesions are differentiated based on architectural complexity and the presence of cytologic atypia[2]; they are:

- Simple hyperplasia
- Complex hyperplasia
  - Simple hyperplasia with atypia
  - Complex hyperplasia with atypia

It is often difficult to distinguish complex atypical hyperplasia from well-differentiated carcinoma as discussed in the following article entitled, Complex atypical hyperplasia and differentiated endometrioid adenocarcinoma, but it is important to distinguish complex atypical hyperplasia from myoinvasive well-differentiated carcinoma[3] at hysterectomy. Distinguishing complex atypical hyperplasia and carcinoma at endometrial biopsy or dilation and curettage is significantly more challenging.

Atypical Hyperplasia

Atypical hyperplasia is considered a precursor to endometrial carcinoma. Kurman and colleagues[2] retrospectively reviewed 170 patients with any degree of endometrial hyperplasia untreated for at least 1 year. The risk of progression to carcinoma was 1% for simple hyperplasia, 3% for complex hyperplasia, 8% for simple atypical hyperplasia, and 29% for complex atypical hyperplasia.

Division of Gynecology, Department of Surgery, Memorial Sloan-Kettering Cancer Center, 1275 York Avenue, New York, NY 10065, USA
* Corresponding author.
E-mail address: leitaom@mskcc.org

Surgical Pathology 4 (2011) 113–130
doi:10.1016/j.path.2010.03.002
1875-9181/11/$ – see front matter © 2011 Elsevier Inc. All rights reserved.

The risk for simple atypical versus complex atypical hyperplasia was not statistically different.

The most important determinant of risk for progression to carcinoma was the presence of cytologic atypia, with only 2% of hyperplasias without atypia versus 23% of atypical hyperplasias progressing to carcinoma. Degrees of atypia, epithelial stratification, and mitotic activity did not predict progression. The time to progression from hyperplasia to carcinoma is long for both, with median times of 9.5 years for non-atypical hyperplasia and 4.1 years for atypical hyperplasia.

13 of 170 patients developed carcinoma and 12 of 13 had stage I disease. All were alive without evidence of disease 4 to 25 years after definitive therapy.

Underlying carcinoma with hyperplasia

There is risk of having an underlying occult carcinoma at the time of a hyperplasia diagnosis. Rates of underlying carcinoma are as high as 43% in patients with atypical hyperplasia.[4–6] The presence of architectural complexity (simple versus complex) in atypical hyperplasia does not confer a greater risk.[5] Simple and complex hyperplasias without cytologic atypia appear to carry a low risk of association with an underlying malignancy. Reported rates in the literature of underlying carcinoma, as reviewed by other investigators, range from 15% to 57%.[5,6] The majority of these "occult" malignancies are early-stage, endometrioid adenocarcinomas with excellent prognoses after treatment.

Gynecologic Oncology Group trial

The Gynecologic Oncology Group (GOG) conducted a large prospective trial in patients with atypical hyperplasias of the endometrium.[7,8] Patients with atypical hyperplasias on a preoperative endometrial biopsy underwent an immediate hysterectomy, and the findings in the uterus were analyzed to determine the rate of underlying carcinoma.[7] There was also an analysis of the inter- and intraobserver reproducibility of an endometrial biopsy diagnosis and correlation with findings in the hysterectomy specimen.[8] A total of 289 cases with a referring diagnosis of atypical endometrial hyperplasia (AEH) on biopsy were analyzed in this prospective series.[7] Table 1 details the findings. The mean age of the cohort was 58 years and the median time from biopsy to hysterectomy was 6 weeks, with a range from 0 to 53 weeks. Carcinoma was diagnosed in the hysterectomy in 123 (43%) for the 289 cases. Of these 123 cases with cancer in the hysterectomy, most (115/123 [94%]) were International Federation of Gynecology and Obstetrics (FIGO) grade 1. Myoinvasion was seen in 18 of 123 (30.6%) cases. The investigators defined "high-risk" cancer cases as those with any myoinvasion or grade 2/3 lesions. High-risk lesions, according to these criteria, were seen in 43 (35%) of 123 cases. Patient age was significantly associated with a high-risk cancer being found in the hysterectomy but not time from biopsy to hysterectomy. However, if "high-risk" was defined as tumors with myoinvasion and grade 2 or 3 or tumors with deep myoinvasion of any grade (cases in which the risk of nodal spread is of concern),[9,10] then only 16 (14%) of the 118 cancer cases would be "high risk" and necessitate treatment beyond simple hysterectomy. Overall, approximately 6% (ie, 14% of 43%) of AEH patients in this trial would have needed either lymphadenectomy or other adjuvant therapy.

The aforementioned 289 cases were subjected to a blinded review by 3 study pathologists and the findings in the hysterectomy were then analyzed based on this study panel review.[7,8]

Diagnosis of atypical endometrial hyperplasia

The difficulty in diagnosing AEH in an endometrial biopsy is clearly demonstrated (Fig. 1). The study

---

Table 1
Characteristics of the concurrent endometrial carcinomas found in women with a referring institution biopsy diagnosis of atypical endometrial hyperplasia (AEH) in GOG 167

FIGO 1988 Stage	Grade 1	Grade 2	Grade 3	Total
IA	77 (63%)	2 (1.6%)	1 (0.8%)	80 (65%)
IB	22 (17.9%)	2 (1.6%)	1 (0.8%)	25 (20%)
IC	13 (10.6%)	0 (0)	0 (0)	13 (10.6%)
No stage	3 (2.4%)	2 (1.6%)	0 (0)	5 (4.1%)
Total	115 (93.5%)	6 (4.9%)	2 (1.6%)	123

Values are N (% of total cancer cases).
From Trimble CL, Kauderer J, Zaino R, et al. Concurrent endometrial carcinoma in women with a biopsy diagnosis of atypical endometrial hyperplasia: a Gynecologic Oncology Group study. Cancer 2006;106:812–19; with permission.

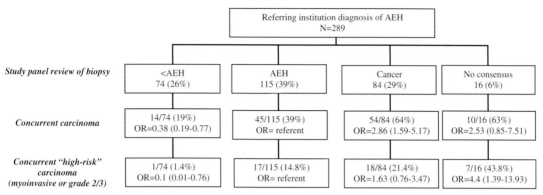

Referring institution diagnosis of AEH N=289			

Study panel review of biopsy	<AEH 74 (26%)	AEH 115 (39%)	Cancer 84 (29%)	No consensus 16 (6%)
Concurrent carcinoma	14/74 (19%) OR=0.38 (0.19-0.77)	45/115 (39%) OR= referent	54/84 (64%) OR=2.86 (1.59-5.17)	10/16 (63%) OR=2.53 (0.85-7.51)
Concurrent "high-risk" carcinoma (myoinvasive or grade 2/3)	1/74 (1.4%) OR=0.1 (0.01-0.76)	17/115 (14.8%) OR= referent	18/84 (21.4%) OR=1.63 (0.76-3.47)	7/16 (43.8%) OR=4.4 (1.39-13.93)

Fig. 1. GOG pathologist study panel review of referring institution biopsy diagnosis of AEH and correlation with the finding of concurrent endometrial carcinoma in GOG 167. (*Data from* Trimble CL, Kauderer J, Zaino R, et al. Concurrent endometrial carcinoma in women with a biopsy diagnosis of atypical endometrial hyperplasia: a Gynecologic Oncology Group study. Cancer 2006;106:812–19.)

panel diagnosis remained as AEH in only 115 (39%) of the 289 cases but the rate of carcinoma was still 39% (45/115) in this group. The odds of carcinoma in the hysterectomy was significantly lower with a study panel diagnosis of less than AEH and significantly higher if the panel felt the biopsy was worse than AEH. The reproducibility of the referring institutions' pathologists' diagnosis of AEH by the study panel of pathologists was poor.[8] However, the level of reproducibility among the subspecialist study panel was also poor.[8] These findings clearly highlight the need for improved reproducibility of the diagnosis of AEH in endometrial biopsies, as it may have important implications in the clinical management of these patients.

Recent work has suggested that AEH may be stratified into subcategories that may be more likely than others to be associated with an underlying carcinoma.[11] The sampling method also seems to have significance because AEH diagnosed in dilatation and curettage specimens may be less strongly associated with carcinoma on follow-up as compared with AEH diagnosed on biopsy alone.[12]

Recently, the authors reviewed 197 consecutive cases of AEH treated at their institution.[13] Fifty-six percent of AEH cases with features "bordering on carcinoma" were associated with an underlying carcinoma in the hysterectomy specimen, compared with 28% of typical AEH cases. The risk of an underlying carcinoma was significantly less if AEH was diagnosed via dilatation and curettage (27%) compared with an office pipelle biopsy (46%).

Endometrial intraepithelial neoplasia

Classification of an entity referred to as endometrial intraepithelial neoplasia (EIN) has been reported to more accurately predict an underlying carcinoma[14,15] as compared to the hyperplasia classification described earlier. In practice, strict application of EIN criteria sometimes result in disordered proliferative endometrium, a physiologic variant of normal in the perimenopausal state, and benign papillary change being categorized as EIN. The EIN classification system is based on a D-score (DS), which takes into account glandular volume, architectural complexity, and nuclear abnormality, and is facilitated with computer software.[14,15] EIN is diagnosed if DS is less than 1. In a large multicenter retrospective review, EIN seemed to be the strongest predictor of a future diagnosis of carcinoma[14]; however, this requires validation by other groups in a prospective fashion before this can be routinely incorporated into general clinical use.

TREATMENT

Endometrial Hyperplasia

The risk of underlying carcinoma is low in patients with endometrial hyperplasias lacking atypia. A conservative approach is preferred, especially if a patient desires fertility preservation. Weight loss alone may reverse the process. If a patient remains relatively asymptomatic, then close observation may be sufficient without any medical or surgical intervention. Hormonal medications, or possibly a progesterone-containing intrauterine device (IUD), may be considered in patients with excessive vaginal bleeding.

If they do not desire a more conservative approach, hysterectomy is a reasonable option in postmenopausal women, or in women who have completed childbearing.

In postmenopausal women and those in whom childbearing is no longer an issue, hysterectomy is the preferred choice of treatment for all atypical hyperplasias. Bilateral salpingo-oophorectomy is not absolutely required, especially in premenopausal women because removal of both ovaries in patients without a known gynecologic malignancy may result in an increased overall morbidity and mortality in women younger than 50 years.[16] Therefore, the risks of bilateral oophorectomy must be weighed against the risk of requiring additional surgery to remove the ovaries if carcinoma is diagnosed at hysterectomy. Lymphadenectomy at the time of surgery for AEH is considered by some surgeons, but this will result in overtreatment and lead to unnecessarily increased surgical risk for the vast majority of patients. A simple hysterectomy with or without removal of the ovaries and without lymphadenectomy seems to be the most appropriate surgical treatment for AEH at this time. Patients need to know that additional surgery or therapy may be required in certain situations where an underlying carcinoma is identified.

In young premenopausal women with AEH who desire future fertility, hysterectomy is not an acceptable option and a conservative approach may be considered. Also, some patients are simply not fit to undergo any surgical procedure. The most commonly used agents for treating AEH are progestational. Conservative management of AEH and endometrial carcinoma, are discussed in greater detail later in this article.

Intraoperative frozen section assessment of atypical hyperplasias

Very few published data address the value of intraoperative frozen section to determine which AEH patients should be offered lymphadenectomy. The most recent report included only 23 relevant cases.[17] The accuracy of frozen section in terms of identifying carcinoma was only 65% in this small series. Data from the authors' institution of 130 AEH cases demonstrated a sensitivity of 42% and specificity of 97%, with an accuracy of 79% for predicting a final pathologic diagnosis of carcinoma.[13] However, in 110 cases where the frozen section demonstrated no cancer, only 1 (0.9%) case had a high-risk carcinoma (myoinvasive and FIGO grade 2/3 or deeply myoinvasive of any grade) on permanent sections. In the 20 cases in which carcinoma was reported at frozen section, 5 (25%) were found to have high-risk carcinoma after final pathologic evaluation of the hysterectomy specimen. Any potential benefit of frozen section assessments must be weighed against the additional costs, additional operative times needed while awaiting the frozen section, and the potential for overtreatment. The value of frozen section will need to be further investigated. The concept of sentinel lymph node identification in the surgical management of these patients is interesting but must still be considered investigational.

ENDOMETRIAL CARCINOMA

OVERVIEW

Endometrial cancer is the most common gynecologic malignancy and the fourth most common malignancy overall in the United States, with approximately 40,000 new cases diagnosed annually.[18] An estimated 136,000 new cases were diagnosed worldwide in 2002.[19] This section focuses on endometrial carcinomas, with the most common histologic subtype by far being endometrioid.[20] In general, all histologic subtypes of endometrial carcinomas are approached in a similar clinical fashion, except for some differences in the treatment of serous and clear cell carcinomas.

Staging of Endometrial Carcinoma

Endometrial carcinomas are surgically staged using a system devised by the FIGO. American Joint Committee on Cancer TNM correlates exist, but the FIGO system is preferred over the TNM system by the majority of physicians who routinely treat patients with gynecologic malignancies. The FIGO system, developed in 1988 (**Table 2**), was recently revised in 2009 (**Table 3**).[21] Major changes from 1988 to 2009 are:

- Collapse of stage IA and IB from the 1988 system into stage IA
- Cervical mucosal involvement and peritoneal cytology results are removed as criteria
- Parametrial and pelvic peritoneal involvement are accounted for in the new system
- The 2009 system subdivides stage IIIC based on whether pelvic or para-aortic nodes are involved.

The 2009 system is now in use worldwide but there exists some controversy about some of the changes. The concordance of this 2009 revised system with outcomes compared with the 1988 system needs to be tested and validated. Clinical decisions should not be altered by this new system and must still rely on other routinely used clinicopathologic features. The stage distribution and 5-year overall survival based on the 1988 staging system are shown in **Fig. 1**.[20] More than 80% of patients will present with disease confined to the uterine fundus and/or cervix, with very good outcomes.

Table 2
1988 FIGO staging system for endometrial carcinoma

Stage	Criteria
IA	Tumor limited to endometrium
IB	Tumor invades ≤50% myometrium
IC	Tumor invades >50% myometrium
IIA	Extension to cervical mucosa
IIB	Extension to cervical stroma
IIIA	Extension to uterine serosa, adnexae, or positive peritoneal cytology
IIIB	Vaginal metastases
IIIC	Metastasis to pelvic and/or para-aortic lymph nodes
IVA	Extension to bladder and/or rectal mucosa
IVB	Distant metastasis including intra-abdominal and/or inguinal lymph nodes

Surgical Management of Endometrial Carcinomas Grossly Confined to Uterus

The standard treatment for patients who present with disease grossly confined to the uterus and who are suitable surgical candidates is to perform a total hysterectomy with bilateral salpingo-oophorectomy. Routine preoperative imaging before hysterectomy is not cost effective, as it is costly and rarely affects management.[22] However, preoperative imaging is reasonable to consider in selected patients who have:

- Grade 3 tumors
- Serous or clear cell carcinomas
- Long-standing unevaluated vaginal bleeding
- Symptoms that might suggest the presence of extrauterine disease.

The greatest controversy in the initial management of patients with endometrial carcinoma grossly confined to the uterus is whether to perform a lymphadenectomy. The potential value of lymphadenectomy is twofold:

1. Most importantly, lymphadenectomy will allow proper staging and affect postoperative therapies.
2. There is a possible "therapeutic" benefit for both node-negative and -positive patients.

A select group of patients probably will not derive any benefit from lymphadenectomy; however, accurately identifying this select group preoperatively has been challenging.

The incidence of nodal metastasis in patients with disease grossly confined to the uterus was established by a prospective trial conducted by the GOG.[23] **Table 4** details the rate of pelvic and para-aortic nodal metastasis seen in this trial. Patients with FIGO grade 1 tumors invading less

Table 3
2009 FIGO staging system for endometrial carcinoma

Stage	Criteria
IA	Tumor limited to endometrium or invades ≤50% myometrium
IB	Tumor invades >50% myometrium
II	Extension to cervical stroma
IIIA	Extension to uterine serosa and/or adnexae
IIIB	Extension to vagina, parametria, and/or pelvic peritoneum
IIIC1	Metastasis to pelvic lymph nodes
IIIC2	Metastasis to para-aortic lymph nodes regardless of pelvic node status
IVA	Extension to bladder and/or rectal mucosa
IVB	Distant metastasis including intra-abdominal and/or inguinal lymph nodes

Table 4
Rate of pelvic and para-aortic nodal metastasis based on final depth of myometrial invasion and final FIGO grade in GOG 33

Depth of Myometrial Invasion	Grade 1 (%)	Grade 2 (%)	Grade 3 (%)
Limited to endometrium	0/0	3/3	0/0
Inner-third myoinvasion	3/1	5/4	9/4
Middle-third myoinvasion	0/5	9/0	4/0
Outer-third myoinvasion	11/6	19/14	34/23

Values are reported as percentage pelvic node metastasis/percentage para-aortic node metastasis.
From Creasman WT, Morrow CP, Bundy BN, et al. Surgical pathologic spread patterns of endometrial cancer: a Gynecologic Oncology Group study. Cancer 1987;60:2035–41; with permission.

than the outer third of the myometrium as well as tumors limited to the endometrium of any grade had the lowest rate of nodal metastasis (5% or less). Patients with invasion into the outer third of the myometrium had the highest risk. Chi and colleagues[24] presented similar data using the 1988 FIGO staging criteria for myometrial invasion (none, <50% myoinvasion, or >50% myoinvasion) in a cohort of patients with endometrioid carcinoma. These data are shown in **Table 5**, are retrospective, and may actually underestimate the rate of nodal positivity as cases were excluded if fewer than 8 pelvic lymph nodes were obtained. In addition, there were small numbers in some of the subgroups, such as there were only 5 cases with FIGO grade 1 and outer half myoinvasion.

A review of the Surveillance Epidemiology and End Results (SEER) database did not find a significant difference in survival among patients with FIGO grade 1 or 2 endometrioid adenocarcinoma confined to the uterus (1988 FIGO stages IA–IC) based on whether or not lymph nodes were removed.[25] Other investigators have reported similar observations regarding the lack of obvious value for lymphadenectomy in select "low-risk" patients.[26,27] However, lymphadenectomy appeared to be beneficial in high-risk stage I and II carcinomas.

"Risk" is defined differently in various publications but can be generalized based on the association between uterine features and nodal metastasis, as described in **Table 6**.[9,10] Serous and clear cell carcinomas are considered high risk regardless of other uterine features. The survival of patients with high-risk stage I and II endometrial cancers is significantly improved if a lymphadenectomy is performed, but this benefit is not seen in patients with low-risk cancers.[25–27] The number of lymph nodes retrieved is associated with outcome, with a pelvic nodal count of more than 11 appearing to be important.[26,27] Although it is debatable, the benefit of lymphadenectomy is likely related to the greater probability of identifying nodal metastases in a group of patients with a high risk of nodal metastasis (ie, it allows accurate stage assignment). The presence of nodal metastasis is strongly associated with clinical outcomes. Para-aortic nodal metastasis results in a significantly worse outcome compared with pelvic only nodal metastasis.[28]

Adjuvant Therapy for Early-Stage Endometrial Carcinoma

Accurate staging of patients with endometrial carcinomas will have tremendous impact on

Table 5
Rate of pelvic nodal metastasis based on final depth of myometrial invasion using FIGO criteria and final FIGO grade

Depth of Myometrial Invasion (FIGO Stage)	Grade 1 (%)	Grade 2 (%)	Grade 3 (%)
Limited to endometrium (IA)	0	4	0
Inner-half myoinvasion (IB)	0	10	7
Outer-half myoinvasion (IC)	0[a]	17	28

[a] There were only 5 cases in this group.
From Chi DS, Barakat RR, Paleyakar MJ, et al. The incidence of pelvic node metastasis by FIGO staging for patients with adequately surgically staged endometrial adenocarcinoma of endometrioid histology. Int J Gynecol Cancer 2008;18: 269–73; with permission.

Table 6
Risk groupings using final FIGO grade and depth of invasion in hysterectomy specimen and based on the risk of nodal metastasis (LR, low-risk; HR, high-risk)

Depth of Myometrial Invasion (DOI)	Grade 1	Grade 2	Grade 3[a]
Limited to endometrium	LR-FIGO	LR-FIGO	LR-FIGO
<50% DOI	LR-FIGO	*HR-FIGO*	*HR-FIGO*
≥50% DOI	*HR-FIGO*	*HR-FIGO*	*HR-FIGO*

[a] Serous/clear cell (pure or mixed) considered as grade 3.

postoperative treatment recommendations and is likely to reduce the use of external pelvic radiotherapy.[29] Observation alone, or possibly intravaginal brachytherapy in select cases, appears to be all that is needed for well-staged FIGO stage I endometrial carcinomas that are nonserous or clear cell.[30–33] The role of adjuvant external beam radiotherapy (RT) in stage I/II endometrial carcinoma has been evaluated in 4 randomized trials.[34–37] The results are summarized in **Table 7**. The studies varied in terms of the specific inclusion criteria as well as comprehensive staging requirements and the use of vaginal brachytherapy. The 3 most recent studies included only what was considered intermediate- or high-risk cases. All 4 studies demonstrated a reduction in local recurrence with the use of adjuvant external pelvic radiotherapy but no impact on survival, either disease-specific or overall.

Subgroups were identified within each of the 4 aforementioned studies that had the greatest risk of recurrence. All of these subgroups were based on the following as prognostic factors:

- Age
- Tumor grade
- Lymph-vascular space invasion (LVSI)
- Myoinvasion

Adjuvant pelvic RT appeared to affect outcome in these higher risk subgroups in the Aalders trial and GOG 99.[34,36] The PORTEC and ASTEC/EN 5 trials did not find a difference in these higher risk groups with the use of radiotherapy.[35,37]

GOG 99 described a "high-intermediate" risk (HIR) group based on age, tumor grade, LVSI, and myoinvasion (**Table 8**).[36] Local control using pelvic RT was greatest in this HIR group, and survival seemed to be different but not statistically significant. The distant recurrence rate was high in this subgroup (10% for RT arm and 19% for no RT arm), suggesting a possible role for systemic therapy. Chemotherapy was compared with radiotherapy alone (pelvic ± para-aortic) in 2 randomized trials that included

very heterogeneous patient populations, all of which were "intermediate-" or "high-risk" cases, stages I to III.[38,39] RT was associated with a decreased local recurrence rate whereas chemotherapy was associated with a decreased distant recurrence rate.[38] Subgroup analysis suggested that chemotherapy may improve outcomes in selected patients, such as those older than 70 years with certain tumor characteristics (ie, grade 3, stage IC–II, and IIIA cytology positive).[39] This benefit was not seen in "low-intermediate" cases and also not in the higher risk group with nodal involvement.[39] This result is contradictory to GOG 122, which demonstrated a significant survival benefit for chemotherapy compared with whole abdominal radiotherapy in stage III and IV endometrial cancers.[40]

It is difficult to know whether any potential benefit from systemic therapy in stage I or II endometrial endometrioid carcinomas derives from treating unknown metastatic disease because the majority of completed trials to date have not required comprehensive and accurate nodal surgical evaluation. There are no trials assessing the role of adjuvant systemic therapy in a cohort of patients with stage I or II endometrial endometrioid carcinomas who have been accurately staged surgically. Retrospective reports of patients with stage I endometrial endometrioid carcinomas that have been accurately staged surgically report 5- and 10-year overall survivals of much greater than 90% regardless of the depth of myoinvasion, grade, or use of adjuvant RT.[30–32]

Serous carcinomas account for a small proportion of endometrial carcinomas and are either underrepresented in all prospective trials or grouped together with endometrioid and clear cell carcinomas. Based on retrospective reports, all patients with uterine serous carcinomas currently are offered adjuvant chemotherapy except for those without any residual disease in the hysterectomy specimens.[41] The GOG is currently conducting a randomized trial in a group of patients considered to be HIR as defined by

Table 7
Randomized trials of adjuvant external pelvic radiotherapy in stage I/II endometrial carcinomas

Series	Included Cases	LND Required	IVRT Used	Local Recurrence Rate		Distant Recurrence Rate		Disease-Specific Survival		Overall Survival	
				No RT	RT	No RT	RT	No RT	RT	No RT	RT
Aalders (1980)[34] No RT arm (N = 277) RT arm (N = 263)	Stage I All grades Any invasion Any histology	No	Yes Required Both arms							5-year 91%	5-year 89%
PORTEC (2000)[35] No RT arm (N = 360) RT arm (N = 354)	IC (grade 1) IB/IC (grade 2) All grade 3 Any histology	No	No	5-year 13.7%[a]	5-year 4.2%[a]	5-year 7%	5-year 7.9%	5-year 94%	5-year 90.8%	5-year 85%	5-year 81%
GOG 99 (2004)[36] No RT arm (N = 202) RT arm (N = 190)	IB/IC IIA (occult) Any grade Excluded serous/clear cell	Yes	No	4-year 7%[a]	4-year 2%[a]	4-year 8%	4-year 5%	4-year 92%	4-year 95%	4-year 86%	4-year 92%
ASTEC/EN.5 (2009)[37,b] No RT arm (N = 453) RT arm (N = 452)	IA/IB (grade 3) IC/II (all grades) Serous (any) Clear cell (any)	No	Yes Optional Both arms	5-year 6.1%[a]	5-year 3.2%[a]			5-year 89.9%	5-year 88.5%	5-year 83.9%	5-year 83.5%

Stage is based on FIGO 1988.
Abbreviations: IVRT, intravaginal brachytherapy; LND, lymph node dissection; RT, external pelvic radiotherapy.
[a] Statistically significant difference.
[b] Cases with pelvic nodal metastasis included.

Table 8
High-intermediate risk (HIR) groupings for stage I endometrial carcinoma described in GOG 99

HIR groupings
1. Age $\geq$ 70 y with 1 risk factor
2. Age $\geq$ 50 y with 2 risk factors
3. Any age with 3 risk factors

Risk factors
Grade 2 or 3, presence of lymph-vascular space invasion (LVSI), outer-third myoinvasion

From Keys HM, Roberts JA, Brunetto VI, et al. A phase III trial of surgery with or without adjunctive external pelvic radiation therapy in intermediate risk endometrial adenocarcinoma: a Gynecologic Oncology Group study. Gynecol Oncol 2004;92:744–51; with permission.

GOG 99 (see **Table 8**), but will also include occult stage IIB as well as serous and clear cell carcinomas. Patients will be randomized to receive either pelvic RT (optional vaginal brachytherapy for stage II patients or stage I serous/clear carcinomas) or vaginal brachytherapy with 3 cycles of chemotherapy.

The rates of pelvic and para-aortic nodal metastasis in all of the reports referenced here are based on final pathologic tumor grades and depth of myoinvasion, and not preoperative tumor grades or intraoperative assessments. However, assessment of the risk of nodal metastasis, and therefore the need for nodal dissection, is often based on the preoperative tumor grade and intraoperative assessment of the depth of myoinvasion. *This is a flawed extrapolation of the data.* Work defining which endometrial carcinoma patients benefit from lymphadenectomy is ongoing.

Preoperative and Intraoperative Assessments in the Surgical Triage of Endometrial Carcinomas

Most surgeons routinely perform nodal dissections at the time of hysterectomy in patients with a preoperative diagnosis of FIGO grade 3, serous, or clear cell carcinomas. Some surgeons routinely perform a lymphadenectomy in all cases of endometrial carcinoma regardless of preoperative grade. However, many make intraoperative assessments as to the need for lymphadenectomy in patients with preoperative grade 1 and 2 endometrioid adenocarcinomas. The preoperative grade is used in conjunction with an intraoperative assessment of myometrial invasion to decide whether to perform a lymphadenectomy. However, preoperative tumor grade based on

endometrial sampling by various methods fails to correlate with final pathologic grade in many studies.[9,42–51] Approximately 20% of patients with a preoperative FIGO grade 1 or 2 carcinoma will be found to have a higher grade on final pathologic assessment.

Frozen section (FSC) assessment of grade was reported to correlate with the final pathologic grade in 95% of cases by Malviya and colleagues,[43] but this finding was not confirmed in another series by Case and colleagues,[50] who reported only a 62% correlation. 61% of cases with a FSC assessment of grade 1 or less were upgraded on final pathologic assessment.

Dilation and curettage under anesthesia (D&C) also appears to result in tumor upgrading less often in carcinoma than does office endometrial sampling.[10] However, performing a D&C after an office biopsy diagnosis of FIGO grade 1 carcinoma is likely not beneficial, if the surgeon's practice is to routinely perform lymphadenectomy regardless of preoperative grade. This procedure would lead to additional exposure to anesthetic risks as well as significant additional costs without benefit. Patients with preoperative tumor FIGO grades of 1 or 2 will be found to have disease beyond the uterine fundus at presentation in approximately 15% of cases.[46–49]

Intraoperative assessment of myometrial invasion is also an inaccurate predictor of the actual depth of myometrial invasion. Frumovitz and colleagues[47] reported that a frozen section diagnosis of "no myometrial invasion" was inaccurate in 72% of cases. Twenty-six percent of cases with a frozen section assessment of "myometrial invasion less than 50%" actually had deeper invasion, cervical invasion, and/or extrauterine disease.

The combination of preoperative grade and intraoperative assessments of myometrial invasion has a low predictive value for final pathologic findings in the hysterectomy specimen.[47] The modeled risk of pelvic and para-aortic lymph node metastasis is also not acceptable in general, with a risk of missing nodal metastases in up to 6% of cases if lymphadenectomy is not performed based on these preoperative and intraoperative assessments.[52]

The authors recently reported a large series of patients (N = 490) treated at their institution with a preoperative diagnosis of FIGO grade 1 endometrioid adenocarcinoma.[9,10,53] Overall, 16% of these cases were found to be of higher grade after final pathologic assessment of the hysterectomy specimen. Using the risk groupings described in **Table 6**, 22% of cases were found to be at high risk for nodal metastasis. Frozen section assessment of myoinvasion was performed in 270 of these cases. High-risk cancers were found in only 4% of cases in which the FSC assessment was negative for carcinoma or myoinvasion. It would seem reasonable to consider avoiding lymphadenectomy in this subgroup of patients. High-risk cancer in patients younger than 55 years with FIGO grade 1 carcinoma associated with atypical hyperplasia was only 2%, regardless of FSC assessment.[53] Based on these findings and reports by other investigators, the authors suggest an algorithm for the operative management of patients diagnosed with endometrial carcinoma and without gross extrauterine disease (**Table 9**).

Specific Management Considerations for Endometrial Carcinoma Involving the Cervix

Patients with obvious involvement of the uterine cervix should undergo a lymphadenectomy regardless of grade. The rates of pelvic and para-aortic nodal metastasis are approximately 36% and 22%, respectively.[54] The 5-year disease-specific survival also appears to be improved in patients with FIGO stage II disease who have undergone a lymphadenectomy (90%) compared with those who have not (82%; $P<.001$).[25]

A radical hysterectomy instead of merely a simple hysterectomy should be considered in patients with obvious cervical involvement. Patients who undergo a radical hysterectomy appear to have an improved survival compared with those who have undergone a simple hysterectomy.[54–57] Radical hysterectomy was associated with an improved outcome regardless of RT use, and postoperative RT may be avoided in select cases of stage II endometrial carcinomas treated with radical hysterectomy. The role of parametrectomy after a simple hysterectomy with occult cervical invasion has not been evaluated, and is not routinely offered at the authors' institution.

Role of Lymphadenectomy in Stage III or IV Endometrial Carcinomas

Lymphadenectomy in patients with stage III and IV endometrial carcinoma has been reported to be associated with an improved outcome.[24,58–60] A SEER database review reported a 5-year disease-specific survival of 74% for patients who underwent a lymphadenectomy compared with 63% for those who had not.[25] Similar outcomes in terms of both recurrence rates and survival have been reported by other investigators.[58–60] These reports are limited by their retrospective nature and the lack of uniform use of adjuvant chemotherapy in patients with nodal metastasis. The value of lymphadenectomy in patients with known stage III or IV endometrial carcinoma, beyond the value of accurate staging in patients without gross extrauterine disease, needs to be tested in a randomized fashion before being routinely performed. Randomized trials in clinically early-stage endometrial carcinomas (ie, occult high stage carcinoma) failed to demonstrate a survival advantage for lymphadenectomy,[61,62] although lymphadenectomy statistically improved surgical staging. The GOG is currently comparing chemotherapy alone with combined chemoradiation in patients with stage III and IV optimally resected patients.

Morbidity of Lymphadenectomy

The morbidity of lymphadenectomy is a concern to many surgeons, but the published data are limited. Various studies have reported conflicting data as to whether there is an increased rate of complications with lymphadenectomy at the time of hysterectomy.[63–68] These data are hard to interpret, as most of the reports do not describe the extent of lymphadenectomy. Franchi

Table 9
Suggested algorithm for the intraoperative decision to perform lymphadenectomy at the time of hysterectomy

Situation	Lymphadenectomy
Frozen section assessment of DOI not planned	
Preop grade 1 *not* in a background of AEH	YES
Preop grade 1 in background of AEH, age ≥ 55 y	YES
Preop grade 1 in background of AEH, age <55 y	NO
Frozen section assessment of DOI planned	
Preop grade 1, *no* cancer identified or *no* myoinvasion	NO
Preop grade 1, *any* myoinvasion	YES
ANY preop grade 2 or higher—*frozen section limited*	YES

Abbreviations: AEH, atypical endometrial hyperplasia; DOI, depth of myoinvasion.

and colleagues[69] reported an overall perioperative complication rate of 46% if 14 or more pelvic lymph nodes were removed compared with 22% with fewer than 14 nodes. The complication rate was 17% if pelvic node dissection was not omitted.

It is now becoming increasingly apparent that symptomatic lower extremity lymphedema may be a consequence of lymphadenectomy for endometrial cancer. Abu-Rustum and colleagues[70] reported a 3.4% rate of symptomatic lower extremity lymphedema in cases in which 10 or more nodes were retrieved. No lymphedema was reported in the patients in whom a lymphadenectomy had not been performed or in whom a lymphadenectomy was performed but less than 10 nodes were retrieved. The rate was 5% in the group of patients with 10 or more nodes retrieved followed by adjuvant RT. These rates are likely underestimated due to the retrospective nature of the report, which relied entirely on medical chart review. A prospective evaluation of the true incidence of lower extremity lymphedema after lymphadenectomy is needed.

Sentinel Lymph Node Mapping Concept in Endometrial Carcinomas

The value of accurately identifying nodal metastasis in patients at highest risk, while attempting to minimize the morbidity of lymphadenectomy in all patients, can be mitigated slightly by the suggested algorithm in **Table 9**. However, a significant number of patients must still have a comprehensive lymphadenectomy to accurately identify nodal metastasis. The concept of sentinel lymph node (SLN) identification may possibly lessen the risks of full lymphadenectomy in many more cases. The technique and its feasibility have been described.[71,72] An SLN can be identified in 85% of cases with only cervical injections of blue dye without preoperative lymphoscintigraphy. The accuracy of SLN mapping will need to be determined in a large prospective cohort that undergoes SLN identification in all cases followed by an immediate pelvic and para-aortic lymphadenectomy before it can safely replace full lymphadenectomy. However, if the accuracy and safety of SLN mapping in endometrial cancer can be prospectively confirmed, then a significant proportion of patients will be spared the morbidity of extensive lymphadenectomy. The clinical significance of isolated tumor cells and micrometastases identified on enhanced pathologic evaluation of the SLNs is unknown, and will also need to be determined.

TREATMENT

Surgical Approach

The standard surgical approach in patients with endometrial carcinoma has been a laparotomy. Multiple retrospective series have described the feasibility, lower complication rates, shorter postoperative hospitalizations, and oncologic soundness of a minimally invasive approach using laparoscopy for many gynecologic cancers, including endometrial carcinomas. The results of GOG LAP2, the only large randomized trial comparing laparotomy and laparoscopy in endometrial cancer, were recently published.[73,74] GOG LAP2 confirmed the improved perioperative outcomes, shorter lengths of hospitalizations, and improved quality of life with a laparoscopic approach compared with laparotomy. Laparoscopy, if technically possible, should be considered the standard approach in these patients. Further follow-up of this study will determine the long-term oncologic outcomes. Surgery in obese patients is challenging, but laparoscopy should still be considered in these patients. In morbidly obese patients in whom a minimally invasive approach is not possible, a panniculectomy may be considered to improve surgical outcomes.[75]

Management Considerations in Grossly Metastatic Endometrial Carcinomas

The management of patients with gross extra-uterine disease is controversial. Surgical tumor cytoreduction is routinely performed in patients with metastatic ovarian carcinoma. The role of surgical cytoreduction in endometrial carcinoma is not well defined. The possible benefit of surgical cytoreduction was suggested in 1994.[76] The median overall survival in this study was 19 months for patients with stage IV disease who underwent surgery and were left with no gross "bulky" residual disease compared with 8 months for patients with stage IV disease who were deemed inoperable. The exact amount of residual disease was not better quantified.

The possible benefit of surgical cytoreduction was subsequently reported by other investigators in relatively small heterogeneous retrospective series of patients who all underwent surgery during which the residual tumor amount was quantified (**Table 10**).[77–81] Optimal cytoreduction was defined differently in each series, but median overall survival was consistently greater in patients in whom an optimal surgical cytoreduction was achieved. These series were retrospective and, therefore, limited by selection bias. In addition, all histologies were included in most, and the value

Table 10
Surgical cytoreduction for advanced-stage (FIGO stage III and IV) endometrial carcinoma

Study	FIGO Stage	Optimal Definition (cm)	Optimal (N)	Suboptimal (N)	Median Overall Survival (Months)		P value
					Optimal	Suboptimal	
Chi et al (1997)[77]	IV	≤ 2	24	21	31	12	<.01[c]
Bristow et al (2000)[78]	IVB	≤ 1	36	29	34	11	.0001[c]
Ayhan et al (2002)[79]	IVB	≤ 1	22	15	25	10	<.001[c]
Lambrou, et al (2004)[80]	III/IV	≤ 2	42	16	18	7	.001[c]
Van Wijk et al (2006)[81]	III/IV	No gross	50	17[a]	66%[b]	41%[b]	<.01

[a] Includes 5 patients who did not undergo surgery.
[b] 5-year overall survival.
[c] Retained significance on multivariate analysis. Van Wijk did not report.

of surgical cytoreduction may possibly differ based on histology (serous vs nonserous).

It is reasonable to consider an attempt at surgical cytoreduction if patients are able to undergo surgery and it is felt that all disease can be resected without significant morbidity. Chemotherapy is always considered in patients with grossly metastatic disease, regardless of whether surgery is performed. The standard most active regimen has been combination doxorubicin and cisplatin (AP regimen) as determined by GOG 122.[40] The addition of paclitaxel to AP (TAP regimen) showed a possible benefit in patients with measurable disease, but not in those without measurable disease in GOG 184.[82] GOG 209 has recently completed accrual and will determine whether a much less toxic regimen, carboplatin and paclitaxel, can replace the standard TAP regimen. The use of radiation along with chemotherapy, in various sequence schedules, is also considered, but the benefit over chemotherapy alone in stage III or IV endometrial carcinoma has not been proven. A current GOG study, comparing chemotherapy alone with concurrent chemoradiation in this cohort of patients, will help to better define an optimal regimen.

Fertility-Preserving Options for Patients with Endometrial Atypical Hyperplasia or Carcinomas

The standard treatment for AEHs and endometrial carcinomas is total hysterectomy, bilateral salpingo-oophorectomy, and possibly lymphadenectomy followed by tailored adjuvant therapy in some. In a very select group of young women who desire preservation of fertility, a conservative approach may be considered. The only endometrial carcinomas that are suitable for conservative management are well-differentiated (FIGO grade 1) endometrioid adenocarcinomas confined to the endometrium without evidence of myoinvasion.

Pretreatment evaluation of patients with AEH or carcinoma considering conservative therapy includes:

- Detailed history and physical examination to look for signs and symptoms of advanced metastatic disease
- Dilatation and curettage (D&C) under anesthesia
- Radiologic imaging, preferably contrast-enhanced magnetic resonance imaging (MRI)
- MRI to detect myoinvasion is reasonable if there is any suspicion for carcinoma.

All of these evaluations may underestimate the extent of disease but, in combination, should provide an adequate evaluation in patients that will be followed closely. There is a concern of coexisting ovarian malignancies in young women with endometrial cancer. Walsh and colleagues[83] noted that 25% of women aged 45 years or younger who were diagnosed with an endometrial cancer were found to have coexisting ovarian malignancies. The risk was only approximately 5% if the ovaries were grossly normal. Therefore, it is reasonable to consider a diagnostic laparoscopy to rule out adnexal or intraperitoneal disease before initiating conservative therapies. **Fig. 2** details a suggested algorithm for the conservative management of AEH or endometrial carcinoma.

Patients must be made aware of the limitations of the available data and the potential risks they may be incurring, as deaths after conservative therapy have been reported.[84,85] Strict adherence to therapy and close follow-up is of utmost importance.

Conservative management of atypical hyperplasia and early-stage endometrial carcinoma has mainly involved the use of progestins with the occasional use of other agents. Various regimens have been used to conservatively treat atypical

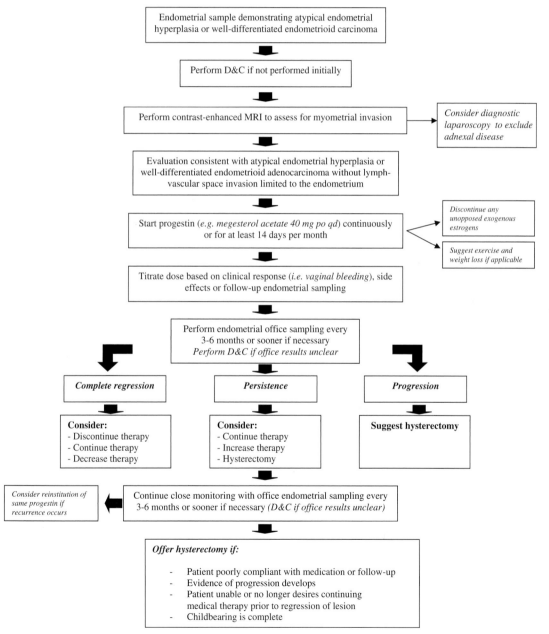

Fig. 2. Suggested algorithm for conservative treatment of atypical endometrial hyperplasias and well-differentiated early-stage endometrioid adenocarcinoma.

hyperplasia and well-differentiated early-stage carcinoma, with megesterol acetate (Megace) and medroxyprogesterone acetate (Provera) being the most extensively studied.[86–88] Complete response rates of 82% for AEH and 55% for carcinomas can be expected.[88] The majority of those who experience a complete response will be expected to do so within 16 weeks of initiating therapy.[88]

Therapy may be discontinued for those who demonstrate complete regression with maintained close follow-up, and it may be reinitiated if a recurrence develops. Attempts at childbearing should be encouraged as soon as possible. Ovulation induction appears safe.[4,88–90] Hysterectomy should be offered to any patient who has evidence of progression, declines further medical therapy without regression of their disease or poor compliance, or once childbearing is complete or no longer desired.

Collaborative Approach to Pathologic Diagnosis and Clinical Treatment

It is obvious that the clinical decisions in the treatment of patients with endometrial hyperplasias and carcinomas are highly reliant on pathologic diagnoses with multiple key pathologic factors that are highly relevant:

- First is the importance of determining which patients undergoing biopsy or curettage have neoplasms that might be myoinvasive. An example is the distinction between AEH and adenocarcinoma.
- Second, pathologists should make every effort to accurately report the histologic subtype of carcinoma, when present, and assign an unambiguous grade.
- Other important pathologic features must be provided: The depth of myoinvasion should be reported in millimeters and the thickness of the myometrium in that area should also be reported. The presence, or absence, of LVSI should be clearly noted.
- Last, the distinction between synchronous and metastatic carcinomas must be made.

All of these goals can be accomplished in the vast majority of cases in clinical practice, although it is acknowledged that there are many ambiguities in diagnostic and staging criteria that do not address every patient's unique situation.[91] The value of an open dialog between pathologists and clinicians taking care of these patients cannot be overemphasized.

A summary of the pitfalls of clinical management of endometrial hyperplasias and carcinomas follows.

Pitfalls
CLINICAL MANAGEMENT OF ENDOMETRIAL HYPERPLASIAS AND CARCINOMAS

! A significant proportion of patients with AEH actually have an underlying carcinoma, and these patients should be informed of this risk as well as the risk of possibly requiring additional surgery or treatments.

! Preoperative and intraoperative assessments of tumor FIGO grade or depth of myometrial invasion are not entirely accurate, and a higher grade and/or more myoinvasive lesion may be found after final pathologic assessment of the hysterectomy specimen.

! Incomplete pathologic evaluations will have significant impact on the clinical management of these patients.

! Pelvic and para-aortic lymphadenectomy is still considered standard for patients diagnosed with endometrial carcinomas of any grade, but this is being constantly reevaluated.

! There is a group of patients with endometrial carcinoma in whom a lymphadenectomy is unnecessary, but the ability to accurately identify this group is not optimal.

! Patients must be informed that additional surgical procedures and/or treatments may be required if only a hysterectomy is performed for a known diagnosis of endometrial carcinoma.

! The role of adjuvant radiation and chemotherapy in patients stage I or II endometrial carcinoma remains to be determined, but to date there are no randomized data to support the role of adjuvant therapies in patients who have been comprehensively staged.

! The appropriate therapy in stage III and IV endometrial carcinoma is under continuous investigation and the optimal strategy has yet to be determined.

! Fertility preservation may be possible in a select group of patients with endometrial carcinomas, but great care must be taken and there is risk associated with this approach.

REFERENCES

1. Barakat RR, Grigsby PW, Sabbatini P, et al. Corpus: epithelial tumors. In: Hoskins WJ, Perez CA, Young RC, editors. Principles and practice of gynecologic oncology. 3rd edition. Philadelphia: Lippincott-Raven; 2000. p. 919–59.

2. Kurman RJ, Kaminski PF, Norris HJ. The behavior of endometrial hyperplasia: a long-term study of "untreated" hyperplasia in 170 patients. Cancer 1985;56:403–12.

3. Kurman RJ, Norris HJ. Evaluation of criteria for distinguishing atypical endometrial hyperplasia from well-differentiated carcinoma. Cancer 1982;49:2547–59.

4. Randall TC, Kurman RJ. Progestin treatment of atypical hyperplasia and well-differentiated carcinoma of the endometrium in women under age 40. Obstet Gynecol 1997;90 :434–40.

5. Hunter JE, Tritz DE, Howell MG, et al. The prognostic and therapeutic implications of cytologic atypia in patients with endometrial hyperplasia. Gynecol Oncol 1994;55:66–71.

6. Janicek MF, Rosenshein NB. Invasive endometrial cancer in uteri resected for atypical endometrial hyperplasia. Gynecol Oncol 1994;52:373–8.

7. Trimble CL, Kauderer J, Zaino R, et al. Concurrent endometrial carcinoma in women with a biopsy diagnosis of atypical endometrial hyperplasia: a Gynecologic Oncology Group Study. Cancer 2006;106:812–9.

8. Zaino RJ, Kauderer J, Trimble CL, et al. Reproducibility of the diagnosis of atypical endometrial hyperplasia: a Gynecologic Oncology Group study. Cancer 2006;106:804–11.

9. Leitao MM Jr, Kehoe S, Barakat RR, et al. Accuracy of preoperative endometrial sampling diagnosis of FIGO grade 1 endometrial adenocarcinoma. Gynecol Oncol 2008;111:244–8.

10. Leitao MM Jr, Kehoe S, Barakat RR, et al. Comparison of D&C and office endometrial biopsy accuracy in patients with FIGO grade 1 endometrial adenocarcinoma. Gynecol Oncol 2009;113:105–8.

11. Miller C, Bidus MA, Pulcini JP, et al. The ability of endometrial biopsies with atypical complex hyperplasia to guide surgical management. Am J Obstet Gynecol 2008;199:69.e1–4.

12. Suh-Burgmann E, Hung Y, Armstrong MA. Complex atypical hyperplasia: the risk of unrecognized adenocarcinoma and value of preoperative dilation and curettage. Obstet Gynecol 2009;114:523–9.

13. Leitao MM Jr, Han G, Lee LX, et al. Complex atypical hyperplasia of the uterus: characteristics and prediction of underlying carcinoma risk. Am J Obstet Gynecol 2010;203:349.e1–6.

14. Baak JP, Mutter GL, Robboy S, et al. The molecular genetics and morphometry-based endometrial intraepithelial neoplasia classification system predicts disease progression in endometrial hyperplasia more accurately than the 1994 World Health Organization classification system. Cancer 2005;103:2304–12.

15. Hecht JL, Ince TA, Baak JP, et al. Prediction of endometrial carcinoma by subjective endometrial intraepithelial neoplasia diagnosis. Mod Pathol 2005;18:324–30.

16. Parker WH, Broder MS, Chang E, et al. Ovarian conservation at the time of hysterectomy and long-term health outcomes in the Nurses' Health Study. Obstet Gynecol 2009;113:1027–37.

17. Indermaur MD, Shoup B, Tebes S, et al. The accuracy of frozen pathology at time of hysterectomy in patients with complex atypical hyperplasia on preoperative biopsy. Am J Obstet Gynecol 2007;196:e40–2.

18. Jemal A, Siegel R, Ward E, et al. Cancer statistics, 2009. CA Cancer J Clin 2009;59:225–49.

19. Parkin DM, Bray F,. Ferlay J, et al. Global cancer statistics, 2002. CA Cancer J Clin 2005;55:74–108.

20. Creasman WT, Odicino F, Maisonneuve P, et al. Carcinoma of the corpus uteri. Int J Gynaecol Obstet 2006;95:S105–44.

21. Mutch DG. Meeting report: The new FIGO staging system for cancers of the vulva, cervix, endometrium and sarcomas. Gynecol Oncol 2009;115:325–8.

22. Bansal N, Herzog TJ, Brunner-Brown A, et al. The utility and cost effectiveness of preoperative computed tomography for patients with uterine malignancies. Gynecol Oncol 2008;111:208–12.

23. Creasman WT, Morrow CP, Bundy BN, et al. Surgical pathologic spread patterns of endometrial cancer: a Gynecologic Oncology Group study. Cancer 1987;60:2035–41.

24. Chi DS, Barakat RR, Paleyakar MJ, et al. The incidence of pelvic node metastasis by FIGO staging for patients with adequately surgically staged endometrial adenocarcinoma of endometrioid histology. Int J Gynecol Cancer 2008;18:269–73.

25. Chan JK, Wu H, Cheung MK, et al. The outcomes of 27,063 women with unstaged endometrioid uterine cancer. Gynecol Oncol 2007;106:282–8.

26. Cragun JM, Havrilesky LJ, Calingaert B, et al. Retrospective analysis of selective lymphadenectomy in apparent early-stage endometrial cancer. J Clin Oncol 2005;23:3668–75.

27. Lutman CV, Havrilesky LJ, Cragun JM, et al. Pelvic lymph node count is an important prognostic variable for FIGO stage I and II endometrial carcinoma with high-risk histology. Gynecol Oncol 2006;102:92–7.

28. Morrow CP, Bundy BN, Kurman RJ, et al. Relationship between surgical-pathological risk factors and outcome in clinical stage I and II carcinoma of the endometrium: a Gynecologic Oncology Group study. Gynecol Oncol 1991;40:55–65.

29. Barakat RR, Lev G, Hummer AJ, et al. Twelve-year experience in the management of endometrial cancer: a change in surgical and postoperative radiation approaches. Gynecol Oncol 2007;105:150–6.

30. Ayhan A, Taskiran C, Celik C, et al. Is there a survival benefit to adjuvant radiotherapy in high-risk surgical

stage I endometrial cancer? Gynecol Oncol 2002; 86:259–63.

31. Straughn JM Jr, Huh WK, Kelly FJ, et al. Conservative management of stage I endometrial carcinoma after surgical staging. Gynecol Oncol 2002;84:194–200.

32. Straughn JM Jr, Huh WK, Orr JW Jr, et al. Stage IC adenocarcinoma of the endometrium: survival comparisons of surgically staged patients with and without adjuvant radiation therapy. Gynecol Oncol 2003;89:295–300.

33. Lukka H, Chambers A, Fyles A, et al. Adjuvant radiotherapy in women with stage I endometrial cancer: a systematic review. Gynecol Oncol 2006;102:361–8.

34. Aalders J, Abeler V, Kolstad P, et al. Postoperative external irradiation and prognostic parameters in stage I endometrial carcinoma: clinical and histopathologic study of 540 patients. Obstet Gynecol 1980;56:419–27.

35. Creutzberg CL, van Putten WLJ, Koper PCM, et al. Surgery and postoperative radiotherapy versus surgery alone for patients with stage-1 endometrial carcinoma: multicentre randomized trial. Lancet 2000;355:1404–11.

36. Keys HM, Roberts JA, Brunetto VL, et al. A phase III trial of surgery with or without adjunctive external pelvic radiation therapy in intermediate risk endometrial adenocarcinoma: a Gynecologic Oncology Group study. Gynecol Oncol 2004;92:744–51.

37. ASTEC/EN5 Study Group, Blake P, Swart AM, et al. Adjuvant external beam radiotherapy in the treatment of endometrial cancer (MRC ASTEC and NCIC CTG EN.5 randomised trials): pooled trial results, systematic review, and meta-analysis. Lancet 2009;373:137–46.

38. Maggi R, Lissoni A, Spina F, et al. Adjuvant chemotherapy vs radiotherapy in high-risk endometrial carcinoma: results of a randomized trial. Br J Cancer 2006;95:266–71.

39. Susumu N, Sagae S, Udagawa Y, et al. Randomized phase III trial of pelvic radiotherapy versus cisplatin-based combined chemotherapy in patients with intermediate- and high-risk endometrial cancer: a Japanese Gynecologic Oncology Group study. Gynecol Oncol 2008;108:226–33.

40. Randall ME, Filiaci VL, Muss H, et al. Randomized phase III trial of whole-abdominal irradiation versus doxorubicin and cisplatin chemotherapy in advanced endometrial carcinoma: a Gynecologic Oncology Group study. J Clin Oncol 2006;24:36–44.

41. Fader AN, Drake RD, O'Malley DM, et al. Platinum/taxane-based chemotherapy with or without radiation therapy favorably impacts survival outcomes in stage I uterine papillary serous carcinoma. Cancer 2009;115:2119–27.

42. Daniel AG, Peters WA 3rd. Accuracy of office and operating room curettage in the grading of endometrial carcinoma. Obstet Gynecol 1988;71:612–4.

43. Malviya VK, Deppe G, Malone JM Jr, et al. Reliability of frozen section examination in identifying poor prognostic indicators in stage I endometrial adenocarcinoma. Gynecol Oncol 1989;34:299–304.

44. Stovall TG, Photopulos GJ, Potson WM, et al. Pipelle endometrial sampling in patients with known endometrial carcinoma. Obstet Gynecol 1991;77: 954–6.

45. Larson DM, Johnson KK, Broste SK, et al. Comparison of D&C and office endometrial biopsy in predicting final histopathologic grade in endometrial cancer. Obstet Gynecol 1995;86:38–42.

46. Obermair A, Geramou M, Gucer F, et al. Endometrial cancer: accuracy of the finding of a well differentiated tumor at dilatation and curettage compared to the findings at subsequent hysterectomy. Int J Gynecol Cancer 1999;9:383–6.

47. Frumovitz M, Singh DK, Meyer L, et al. Predictors of final histology in patients with endometrial cancer. Gynecol Oncol 2004;95:463–8.

48. Eltabbakh GH, Shamonki J, Mount SL. Surgical stage, final grade, and survival of women with endometrial carcinoma whose preoperative endometrial biopsy shows well-differentiated tumors. Gynecol Oncol 2005;99:309–12.

49. Ben-Schachar I, Pavelka J, Cohn DE, et al. Surgical staging for patients presenting with grade 1 endometrial carcinoma. Obstet Gynecol 2005;105: 487–93.

50. Case AS, Rocconi RP, Straughn JM Jr, et al. A prospective blinded evaluation of the accuracy of frozen section for the surgical management of endometrial cancer. Obstet Gynecol 2006;108:1375–9.

51. Traen K, Holund B, Mogensen O. Accuracy of preoperative tumor grade and intraoperative gross examination of myometrial invasion in patients with endometrial cancer. Acta Obstet Gynecol Scand 2007;86:739–41.

52. Frumovitz M, Slomovitz BM, Singh DK, et al. Frozen section analyses as predictors of lymphatic spread in patients with early-stage uterine cancer. J Am Coll Surg 2004;199:388–93.

53. Leitao MM Jr, Kehoe S, Barakat RR, et al. Endometrial sampling diagnosis of FIGO grade 1 endometrial adenocarcinoma in a background of complex atypical hyperplasia (CAH) and final hysterectomy pathology. Am J Obstet Gynecol 2010;202:278. e1–6.

54. Mariani A, Webb MJ, Keeney GL, et al. Role of wide/radical hysterectomy and pelvic node dissection in endometrial cancer with cervical involvement. Gynecol Oncol 2001;83:72–80.

55. Cohn DE, Woeste EM, Cacchio S, et al. Clinical and pathologic correlates in surgical stage II endometrial carcinoma. Obstet Gynecol 2007;109:1062–7.

56. Cornelison TL, Trimble EL, Kosary CL. SEER data, corpus uteri cancer: treatment trends versus survival

for FIGO stage II, 1988–1994. Gynecol Oncol 1999; 74:350–5.

57. Sartori E, Gadducci A, Landoni F, et al. Clinical behavior of 203 stage II endometrial cancer cases: the impact of primary surgical approach and of adjuvant radiation therapy. Int J Gynecol Cancer 2001;11:430–7.

58. Denschlag D, Tan L, Patel S, et al. Stage III endometrial cancer: preoperative predictability, prognostic factors, and treatment outcomes. Am J Obstet Gynecol 2007;196:546.e1–7.

59. Fujimoto T, Nanjyo H, Nakamura A, et al. Para-aortic lymphadenectomy may improve disease-related survival in patients with multipositive pelvic lymph node stage IIIC endometrial cancer. Gynecol Oncol 2007;107:253–9.

60. Mariani A, Dowdy SC, Cliby WA, et al. Efficacy of systematic lymphadenectomy and adjuvant radiotherapy in node-positive endometrial cancer patients. Gynecol Oncol 2006;101:200–8.

61. Panici PB, Basile S, Maneschi F, et al. Systematic pelvic lymphadenectomy vs no lymphadenectomy in early-stage endometrial carcinoma: randomized clinical trial. J Natl Cancer Inst 2008;100: 1707–16.

62. ASTEC study group. Efficacy of systematic pelvic lymphadenectomy in endometrial cancer (MRC ASTEC trial): a randomized study. Lancet 2009; 373:125–36.

63. Moore DH, Fowler WC Jr, Walton LA, et al. Morbidity of lymph node sampling in cancers of the uterine corpus and cervix. Obstet Gynecol 1989;74:180–4.

64. Arduino S, Leo L, Febo G, et al. Complications of pelvic and para-aortic lymphadenectomy in patients with endometrial cancer. Eur J Gynaecol Oncol 1997;18:208–10.

65. Homesley HD, Kadar N, Barrett RJ, et al. Selective pelvic and periaortic lymphadenectomy does not increase morbidity in surgical staging of endometrial carcinoma. Am J Obstet Gynecol 1992;167: 1225–30.

66. Giannice R, Susini T, Ferrandina G, et al. Systematic pelvic and aortic lymphadenectomy in elderly gynecologic oncologic patients. Cancer 2001;92: 2562–8.

67. Berclaz G, Hanggi W, Kratzer-Berger A, et al. Lymphadenectomy in high risk endometrial carcinoma stage I and II: no more morbidity and no need for external radiation. Int J Gynecol Cancer 1999;9: 322–8.

68. Larson DM, Johnson K, Olson KA. Pelvic and para-aortic lymphadenectomy for surgical staging of endometrial cancer: morbidity and mortality. Obstet Gynecol 1992;79:998–1001.

69. Franchi M, Ghezzi F, Riva C, et al. Postoperative complications after pelvic lymphadenectomy for the surgical staging of endometrial cancer. J Surg Oncol 2001;78:232–40.

70. Abu-Rustum NR, Alektiar K, Iasonos A, et al. The incidence of symptomatic lower-extremity lymphedema following treatment of uterine corpus malignancies: a 12-year experience at Memorial Sloan-Kettering Cancer Center. Gynecol Oncol 2006;103:714–8.

71. Abu-Rustum NR, Khoury-Collado F, Gemignani ML. Techniques of sentinel lymph node identification for early-stage cervical and uterine cancer. Gynecol Oncol 2008;111:S44–50.

72. Abu-Rustum NR, Khoury-Collado F, Pandit-Taskar N, et al. Sentinel lymph node mapping for grade 1 endometrial cancer: is it the answer to the surgical staging dilemma? Gynecol Oncol 2009;113:163–9.

73. Walker JL, Piedmonte MR, Spirtos NM, et al. Laparoscopy compared with laparotomy for comprehensive surgical staging of uterine cancer; Gynecologic Oncology Group Study LAP2. J Clin Oncol 2009;27:5331–6.

74. Kornblith AB, Huang HQ, Walker JL, et al. Quality of life of patients with endometrial cancer undergoing laparoscopic International Federation of Gynecology and Obstetrics staging compared with laparotomy: a Gynecologic Oncology Group Study. J Clin Oncol 2009;27:5337–42.

75. Eisenhauer EL, Wypych KA, Mehrara BJ, et al. Comparing surgical outcomes in obese women undergoing laparotomy, laparoscopy, or laparotomy with panniculectomy for the staging of uterine malignancy. Ann Surg Oncol 2007;14:2384–91.

76. Goff BA, Goodman A, Muntz HG, et al. Surgical stage IV endometrial carcinoma: a study of 47 cases. Gynecol Oncol 1994;52:237–40.

77. Chi DS, Welshinger M, Venkatraman ES, et al. The role of surgical cytoreduction in stage IV endometrial carcinoma. Gynecol Oncol 1997;67:56–60.

78. Bristow RE, Zerbe MJ, Rosenshein NB, et al. Stage IVB endometrial carcinoma: the role of cytoreductive surgery and determinants of survival. Gynecol Oncol 2000;78:85–91.

79. Ayhan A, Taskiran C, Celik C, et al. The influence of cytoreductive surgery on survival and morbidity in stage IVB endometrial cancer. Int J Gynecol Cancer 2002;12:448–53.

80. Lambrou NC, Gomez-Marin O, Mirhashemi R, et al. Optimal surgical cytoreduction in patients with stage III and stage IV endometrial carcinoma: a study of morbidity and survival. Gynecol Oncol 2004;93: 653–8.

81. Van Wijk FH, Huikeshoven FJ, Abdulkadir L, et al. Stage III and IV endometrial cancer: a 20-year review of patients. Int J Gynecol Cancer 2006;16:1648–55.

82. Homesley HD, Filiaci V, Gibbons SK, et al. A randomized phase III trial in advanced endometrial

carcinoma of surgery and volume directed radiation followed by cisplatin and doxorubicin with or without paclitaxel: a Gynecologic Oncology Group study. Gynecol Oncol 2009;112:543–52.

83. Walsh C, Holschneider C, Hoang Y, et al. Coexisting ovarian malignancy in young women with endometrial cancer. Obstet Gynecol 2005;106: 693–9.

84. Ota T, Yoshida M, Kimura M, et al. Clinicopathologic study of uterine endometrial carcinoma in young women aged 40 years and younger. Int J Gynecol Cancer 2005;15:657–62.

85. Ferrandina G, Zannoni GF, Gallota V, et al. Progression of conservatively treated endometrial carcinoma after full term pregnancy: a case report. Gynecol Oncol 2005;99:215–7.

86. Ramirez PT, Frumovitz M, Bodurka DC, et al. Hormonal therapy for the management of grade 1 endometrial adenocarcinoma: a literature review. Gynecol Oncol 2004;94:133–8.

87. Chiva L, Lapuente F, Gonzalez-Cortijo L, et al. Sparing fertility in young patients with endometrial cancer. Gynecol Oncol 2008;111:S101–4.

88. Ushijima K, Yahata H, Yoshikawa H, et al. Multicenter phase II study of fertility-sparing treatment with medroxyprogesterone acetate for endometrial carcinoma and atypical hyperplasia in young women. J Clin Oncol 2007;25:2798–803.

89. Bokhman JV, Chepick OF, Volkova AT, et al. Can primary endometrial carcinoma stage I be cured without surgery and radiation therapy? Gynecol Oncol 1985;20:139–55.

90. Lowe MP, Cooper BC, Sood AK, et al. Implementation of assisted reproductive technologies following conservative management of FIGO grade 1 endometrial adenocarcinoma and/or complex hyperplasia with atypia. Gynecol Oncol 2003;91:569–72.

91. Zaino RJ. FIGO staging of endometrial adenocarcinoma: a critical review and proposal. Int J Gynecol Pathol 2009;28:1–9.

SELECTED TOPICS IN THE MOLECULAR PATHOLOGY OF ENDOMETRIAL CARCINOMA

Bojana Djordjevic, MD[a], Russell R. Broaddus, MD, PhD[b],*

KEYWORDS

- Endometrial cancer • Estrogen • PTEN • Microsatellite instability
- Epithelial-to-mesenchymal transition

ABSTRACT

In the developed world, endometrial carcinoma is the most common malignant tumor of the female gynecologic tract. Numerous epidemiologic studies indicate that exposure to unopposed estrogen is a significant risk factor for developing endometrial cancer, particularly endometrioid-type endometrial carcinoma; however, a number of other molecular pathways and mechanisms are also important in endometrial cancer. In this review, the authors highlight some of the more interesting molecular pathways in endometrial cancer, such as the PTEN/PI3K/AKT pathway, microsatellite instability, and molecular mediators of epithelial-to-mesenchymal transition.

OVERVIEW

Endometrial cancer is a complex disease that has a number of distinguishing factors that makes it unique compared with other cancers:

1. It is heterogeneous in that different histotypes are readily identifiable by routine pathologic examination.
2. Hormones, particularly estrogen, play an important role in its pathogenesis.
3. A large number of women are at-risk for this malignancy.

Endometrial cancer is heterogeneous in that different histotypes are readily identifiable by routine pathologic examination. These histotypes are broadly divided into endometrioid carcinoma and non-endometrioid carcinoma.

The non-endometrioid tumors include uterine serous carcinoma, malignant mixed mullerian tumor, and clear cell carcinoma. Traditionally, the non-endometrioid tumors tend to be more clinically aggressive as they are associated with advanced stage at diagnosis and overall poor prognosis. Using both pathologic and clinical features, Bokhman[1] in 1983 recognized that endometrial carcinomas could be classified into two broad categories. The Type I tumors (approximately 65%) were well-to-moderately differentiated adenocarcinomas that had minimal myometrial invasion, were responsive to progestin therapy, and had an excellent prognosis. The Type II tumors (approximately 35%) were poorly differentiated adenocarcinomas with deep myometrial invasion and metastasis to lymph nodes and were associated with a worse prognosis. The Bokhman model is certainly informative in that it recognizes that endometrial cancer is a heterogeneous disease. However, this model is overly

This work was supported by NIH 1P50CA098258-01 (SPORE in Uterine Cancer).
[a] Department of Pathology and Laboratory Medicine, University of Ottawa, Ottawa, Ontario, Canada
[b] Department of Pathology, University of Texas M.D. Anderson Cancer Center, Box 85, 1515 Holcombe Boulevard, Houston, TX 77030, USA
* Corresponding author.
E-mail address: rbroaddus@mdanderson.org

Surgical Pathology 4 (2011) 131–147
doi:10.1016/j.path.2010.12.001

simplistic. Not all low grade endometrioid carcinomas are indolent, as some of these tumors are associated with deep myometrial invasion and/or recurrence after surgery. Furthermore, a subset of grade 3 endometrioid adenocarcinoma is known to have minimal myometrial invasion and small risk of recurrence after surgery.

A second distinguishing feature of endometrial cancer is that hormones, particularly estrogen, play an important role in its pathogenesis. This is discussed in subsequent sections of this review.

A third distinguishing feature of endometrial cancer is that there is a large number of at-risk women for this malignancy. Important and common risk factors include obesity and exposure to tamoxifen for the treatment/prevention of breast cancer. In addition, women with the familial cancer syndrome Lynch syndrome are at significant risk for developing endometrial cancer. It is important to point out here that, in contrast to other common malignancies, the incidence of endometrial cancer is actually rising in the United States.[2]

Because endometrial cancer is a heterogeneous disease, its molecular pathogenesis will necessarily be complex. This review provides selected topics of special importance that have been chosen to allow for the better understanding of the complexity of the molecular pathogenesis of endometrial cancer.

ESTROGEN

Estrogen acts by binding to its receptors (primarily ERα) in the nucleus. This in turn induces a conformational change of the receptor and allows its dimerization and interaction with co-factor molecules. The estrogen receptors are bound to the hormone response element of target genes. Activation of the receptor allows transcriptional regulation of the target genes, which mediate the effects of estrogen.[3] Alternatively, estrogen receptors can bind to other transcription factors such as AP1, SP1 or nuclear factor κB.[4] Overall, estrogen has a proliferative effect in the endometrium. Excessive estrogen stimulation is thought to lead to an accumulation of genetic and epigenetic changes that histologically manifest themselves as endometrial hyperplasia and low grade endometrioid adenocarcinoma.[5]

HYPERESTROGENISM

The hyperestrogenic state can result from a variety of causes. Pathologic examples include polycystic ovary disease, ovarian stromal hyperplasia and hyperthecosis, and estrogen producing tumors, such as the granulosa cell tumor of the ovary. All of these conditions can occur in association with endometrial hyperplasia and carcinoma. From the iatrogenic standpoint, the relationship of estrogen replacement therapy (particularly the earlier versions with higher doses of estrogen and no progestin component) and increased incidence of endometrial carcinoma is well-known. More modern versions of hormone replacement therapy, with lower doses of estrogen and with the addition of progestin, however, are not associated with increased risk of development of endometrial cancer.[6]

Obesity has been linked by strong epidemiologic evidence to increased risk of endometrial carcinoma. While an average woman has a 3% lifetime risk of endometrial carcinoma, obese women have a 9 to 10% lifetime risk of endometrial carcinoma. In addition, obese women account for a higher proportion of both post-menopausal and premenopausal endometrial cancer patients.[7–9] Initially, hyperestrogenism was considered to be the main mechanism by which obesity was linked to increased risk of endometrial cancer, due to the increased conversion of adrenal and ovarian androgens to estrogen in adipose tissues by the enzyme aromatase.[10] However, the obese state is complex metabolically; the contribution of other abnormalities associated with obesity, such as insulin resistance and adipokine production, to the development of endometrial cancer is unknown at this time.

If endometrial cancer, particularly low grade endometrioid carcinoma, was chiefly due to relative hyperestrogenism, then one would expect that these types of tumors would globally over-express genes known to be induced by estrogen. Interestingly, many estrogen-regulated genes (including progesterone receptor, IGF-1 and cyclin D1), are not significantly upregulated in endometrial complex hyperplasia with atypia, the precursor to endometrioid carcinoma, or in grade 1 endometrioid carcinoma.[11] Other estrogen-induced genes, such as EIG121, are highly over-expressed in endometrioid-type endometrial carcinoma, particularly the lower grade tumors.[12,13] Therefore, instead of a global increase in estrogen-induced genes, endometrioid carcinoma is instead associated with a selective increase in expression of such genes.

The endometrium from women taking estrogen-based hormone replacement therapy exhibits an increase in the expression of both pro-proliferative factors (IGF-I and IGF-IR) and growth inhibitory factors (RALDH2, sFRP1 and sFRP4).[12,14] Such an induction of inhibitors of endometrial proliferation contributes to the fact that modern estrogen-based hormone replacement therapy does not induce endometrial hyperplasia or carcinoma.

Fig. 1. Balanced effects of unopposed estrogen treatment on the normal endometrium. Estrogen treatment induces endometrial pro-proliferative and growth inhibitory factors that together act to induce controlled endometrial proliferation. An imbalance of these factors likely contributes to the molecular pathogenesis of low-grade endometrioid-type endometrial carcinomas.

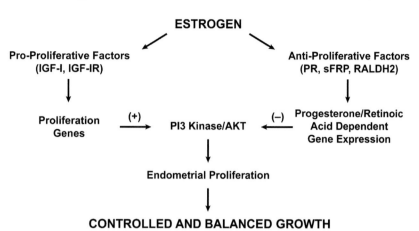

Estrogen's Action in the Endometrium – A Balance

However, endometrioid-type endometrial carcinoma is primarily associated with upregulation of the pro-proliferative factors, without the accompanying induction of growth inhibitory factors. Therefore, the development of endometrioid carcinoma is associated with a disruption of the balance between proliferative and anti-proliferative signaling (**Fig. 1**).[12] One factor that may tip the scales in favor of the proliferative signals is insulin resistance, but this remains to be proven.

TAMOXIFEN

Tamoxifen is widely used for its anti-estrogenic effects in breast tissue for the treatment of estrogen receptor positive breast carcinoma or for the prevention of breast cancer. Tamoxifen paradoxically acts as an estrogen receptor agonist in the uterus. Consequently, tamoxifen use in postmenopausal women is associated with increased rate of large endometrial polyps[15] and endometrial carcinoma.[16] Furthermore, incipient endometrial carcinomas are known to arise more frequently in endometrial polyps of patients on tamoxifen therapy compared with healthy postmenopausal controls.[17] Although breast cancer and endometrial cancer share many of the same risk factors, long term use of tamoxifen results in an additional relative risk of endometrial cancer of 1.3 to over 7, which appears to be related to duration of tamoxifen exposure.[18]

In addition to endometrioid carcinomas arising in women on tamoxifen therapy,[19,20] several studies[21–25] have reported endometrial carcinomas of the non-endometrioid type (serous, clear cell, malignant mixed mullerian tumor) in patients on tamoxifen therapy. These latter studies contradict the initial thinking that tamoxifen's effects in the uterus are due to its action as an estrogen receptor agonist. The explanation for this discrepancy may come from recent genomic studies which have demonstrated that tamoxifen in the endometrium regulates the transcription of a number of genes, only a small subset of which are also regulated by estrogen.[26,27] Therefore, the effect of tamoxifen on the endometrium is not entirely due to stimulation of the estrogen receptor.

PTEN/PI3K/AKT PATHWAY

Because of the general lack of success of conventional chemotherapy or hormone-based therapy for the treatment of advanced or recurrent endometrial carcinoma, efforts have been made to attempt targeted therapy. Much of this attention has been devoted to the PTEN/PI3K/AKT pathway due to a relatively high frequency of molecular anomalies of its components in endometrial cancer. Specifically, compounds that inhibit PI3K as well as both PI3K and mTOR (a downstream target of the pathway) are currently being developed.[28]

PTEN

PTEN (phosphatase and tensin homolog) is a tumor suppressor gene located at chromosome 10q23.[29,30] PTEN plays a key role in the PTEN-PI3K-AKT pathway. While PI3K (phosphatidylinositol -3- kinase) converts the lipid second messenger phosphatidylinositol (4,5) biphosphate into phosphatidylinositol (3,4,5) triphosphate, PTEN drives this reaction in the opposite direction, dephosphorylating phosphatidylinositol (3,4,5) triphosphate into phosphatidylinositol (4,5) bi-phosphate. The net effect of phosphatidylinositol (3,4,5) triphosphate is the activation of protein kinase B (or AKT) by phosphorylation. Loss of PTEN is highly correlated with activation of AKT in vivo.[31,32] A key downstream target of AKT is the mTOR complex 1, whose activation eventually results in inhibition of apoptosis and cell cycle arrest. In the absence of functional PTEN, there-fore, this process occurs unchecked.

PTEN also regulates cell survival pathways such as the mitogen-activated protein kinase pathway, independent of its activities in the PI3K -AKT pathway.[33]

INCIDENCE OF PTEN LOSS IN ENDOMETRIAL CARCINOMA

Sporadic PTEN loss is detected in 34%–55% of endometrial cancers.[34,35] PTEN mutations occur frequently in complex atypical hyperplasia, sug-gesting that they are an early event in endometrial carcinogenesis.[36] By histotype, PTEN mutations occur most frequently in endometrioid-type endo-metrial carcinomas. In their examined cohort of endometrial carcinomas, Tashiro and colleagues[37] found PTEN mutations in 50% of the endometrioid subtype and no PTEN mutations in the serous subtype. Similarly, Risinger and colleagues[38] iden-tified PTEN mutations in 37% of endometrioid tumors and in only 5% of serous/clear cell endo-metrial carcinomas.

The types of PTEN mutations in endometrial carcinomas are highly variable, ranging from frameshifts, splice-site mutations and point muta-tions (missense and nonsense).[34,39,40] In terms of location, mutations occur throughout the coding region. Such mutational heterogeneity makes PTEN mutational analysis difficult for clinical purposes. However, two groups have noted a particular mutation predilection for stretches of adenosine mononucleotide repeats, suggesting that such regions make the PTEN gene vulnerable to mutations in the setting of microsatellite instability.[34,39] PTEN mutations in endometrial carcinoma are typically hemizygous, affecting one allele. However, Mutter and colleagues[36] have shown that the number of endometrial tumors with PTEN protein loss as detected by immunohistochemistry significantly exceeds the number of tumors with detected mutations, and therefore immunohistochemistry may be a better method of detecting functional loss of PTEN in endometrial tumors (**Fig. 2**). Similar observations have been made with PTEN in hematologic malignancies[41] and breast carcinomas.[42] It is possible that epigenetic mechanisms, such as promoter methylation, or increased protein degra-dation in the hemizygous state are responsible for this discrepancy.[36] PTEN promoter methylation has been observed in approximately 19% of endo-metrial cancers.[43,44]

PROGNOSTIC SIGNIFICANCE OF PTEN

The prognostic significance of PTEN loss in endometrial carcinoma is uncertain, owing to contradicting data in the literature. Some investigators[38] reported that PTEN mutations in endometrial carcinoma are associated with early stage disease and increased survival. In particular, PTEN mutations outside exons 5, 6, and 7 have been identified as independent predictors of increased survival.[40] In contrast, others[45] showed that advanced stage endometrial carcinomas had lower PTEN expression by quantitative PCR compared with their early stage counterparts, and that immunohistochemical loss of PTEN protein expression was associated with metastatic disease.[46] Furthermore, PTEN positive staining by immunohistochemistry has been shown to be an independent prognostic indicator of favorable survival in patients with advanced endometrial cancer.[32,47,48] In this patient group, a combination of positive PTEN expression and negative phosphorylated-AKT (the activated form of AKT) expression by immunohistochemistry was a predictor of increased survival.[48] In terms of the significance of epigenetic mechanisms of PTEN silencing, PTEN promoter methylation has been associated with advanced stage endometrial carcinoma.[43]

PI3K AND PIK3CA MUTATIONS IN ENDOMETRIAL CARCINOMA

The PIK3CA gene is located on chromosome 3q26.3 and encodes the catalytic subunit, p110α, of PI3K. Constitutive phosphorylation of AKT has been ascribed to elevated PIK3CA catalytic activity in vitro in the setting of PIK3CA mutations.[49] PIK3CA mutations occur in 36%[50] to 39%[51] of endometrial carcinomas. Unlike PTEN mutations, PIK3CA mutations are uncommon in complex atypical hyperplasia,[51] suggesting that they do not represent an early event in endometrial carcinogenesis. However, PIK3CA mutations have been found to co-exist with PTEN mutations in up to 27% of endometrial carcinomas.[51] Unlike PTEN mutations, which are highly variable in type and location, PIK3CA acti-vating mutations are predominantly missense and occur in the kinase (exon 20) and helical

Fig. 2. PTEN immunohistochemistry in endometrial carcinoma. (*A*) Representative example of positive PTEN immunohistochemistry. Note that the entire tumor is strongly positive for cytoplasmic PTEN expression. (*B*) Representative example of negative PTEN immunohistochemistry. Note the importance of positive staining of internal positive control cells (normal blood vessels, normal myometrium, normal endometrium).

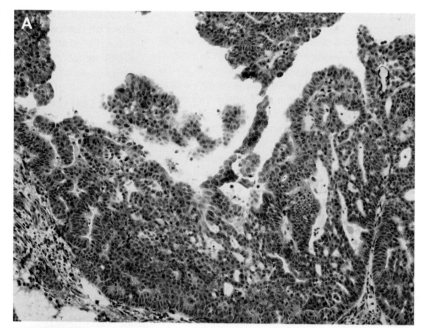

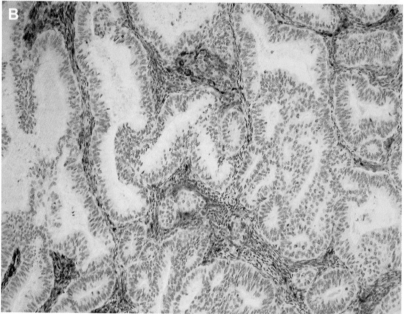

domain (exon 9).[52,53] In addition, some investigators have noted an amplification of the 3q26.32 region[54,55] of *PIK3CA* in endometrial carcinomas. It has been suggested that *PIK3CA* mutations, especially those in exon 20, represent a marker of myometrial invasion and higher grade in endometrioid carcinomas.[52,55] Furthermore, the amplification of the 3q26.3 region has been linked to poor outcome.[54]

In terms of the histologic subtype of endometrial carcinoma, *PIK3CA* mutations, both in exon 9

and in exon 20, have been identified in 28% of endometrioid tumors.[52] For non-endometrioid endometrial carcinomas, several studies have shown a preponderance of exon 20 mutations in the non-endometrioid carcinomas and mixed endometrioid/non-endometrioid carcinomas.[55–57] Recent studies have identified mutations in the *PI3K* regulatory subunit, p85α, in glioblastomas that relieve the inhibitory effect of p85α on p110α. It is not known whether such mutations are also present in endometrial carcinoma.[58]

IGF-I RECEPTOR

Estrogen induces increases in insulin growth factor –I (IGF-I) expression, resulting in activation of the IGF-I receptor (IGF-IR). Although IGF-I is an estrogen-induced gene, and estrogen exposure has been linked to the development of endometrial cancer, increased tissue IGF-I is not a characteristic feature of endometrial hyperplasia or carcinoma.[11] Rather, a large percentage of cases of endometrial complex hyperplasia with atypia and endometrioid-type endometrial carcinoma are associated with increased IGF-IR.[11] Interestingly, this upregulation of IGF-IR is associated with the phosphorylation of AKT, implying activation of the PTEN/PI3K/AKT pathway,[11] and thereby promoting cell survival through inhibition of downstream apoptotic pathways.[59,60] The mechanisms by which estrogen receptor and the PTEN/PI3K/AKT pathway may cross-talk are not yet known.

KRAS

Recently, pharmacologically useful inhibitors of the PTEN-PI3K-AKT pathway have been identified, and these may be employed in the targeted therapy of cancers with activation of this pathway.[28] There is recent evidence from other cancer systems that the presence of KRAS mutation confers resistance to targeting of the PTEN-PI3K-AKT pathway.[61–63] Therefore, a discussion of KRAS mutations in endometrial cancer is relevant in this context.

KRAS is an oncogene located at 12p12.1 that encodes a protein member of the small GTPase superfamily. The key role of RAS in the RAS/RAF/MAP kinase pathway is the recruitment of RAF to the plasma membrane. This process eventually leads to the translocation of MAP kinase to the nucleus where it promotes transcription of genes involved in cell proliferation.[64] KRAS can also bind to and upregulate PIK3CA, thus promoting cell proliferation and survival.[65] KRAS activating mutations occur almost exclusively in codon 12 as single point mutations.[66–69] The incidence of KRAS mutations in endometrial carcinoma is 14 to 36%.[66,67,69,70] KRAS mutation likely occurs early in endometrial carcinogenesis, as mutation has been identified in foci of atypical complex hyperplasia in specimens with endometrial carcinoma.[66,69,70] The prognostic significance of KRAS mutations in endometrial carcinomas is somewhat controversial. Some investigators claim that KRAS mutation confers a good prognosis,[69] while others observed an association of KRAS mutation and metastasis.[71] Another group suggested that KRAS mutations have an adverse effect on outcome in postmenopausal patients.[72] In some studies, however, no relationship between KRAS mutation status and prognostic outcome could be established.[68,70,73]

MICROSATELLITE INSTABILITY

Defects in DNA mismatch repair are characterized by high levels of microsatellite instability (MSI-high) as measured in endometrial tumor DNA compared with DNA from normal tissues. MSI-high endometrial cancers arise from molecular abnormalities of the mismatch repair genes. The Hereditary Non-Polyposis Colorectal Cancer Syndrome (HNPCC or Lynch Syndrome) is associated with germline mutations of MLH1, MSH2, MSH6, PMS2, and other less common genes. On the other hand, MSI-high endometrial cancer can also be found in the sporadic setting due to methylation with subsequent transcriptional silencing of the MLH1 gene promoter. MSI-high tumors due to MLH1 methylation have been well-described in the literature and occur in 15%–25% of sporadic endometrial and colon carcinomas.[74–78] Much of what is known regarding MSI-high colon and endometrial carcinoma has been derived from studies of sporadic tumors; the relevance to the Lynch syndrome-associated tumors is not clear.

Editor's Comment: Content relevant to microsatellite instability can also be found in Familial Tumors of the Uterine Corpus by Karuna Garg and Robert Soslow. Factual information discussed there is similar, but it is complimentary as the point of view and organization differ. Details regarding tissue testing to detect microsatellite instability can be found in that article.

CLINICAL AND PATHOLOGIC FEATURES OF MSI-HIGH ENDOMETRIAL CANCER

It has been suggested that endometrial carcinoma is important in women with Lynch syndrome because it can act as a "sentinel cancer," preceding the diagnosis of colorectal cancer in 51% of these women by a median time of 11 years.[79] However, recent work indicates that endometrial cancer itself is an important cancer in these women, frequently requiring adjuvant treatment in addition to surgery. The clinical and pathologic features of endometrial cancers among 3 different patient groups (sporadic MSI-high endometrial cancer, Lynch syndrome-associated MSI-high endometrial cancer, and MS-stable sporadic endometrial cancers in women younger than 50) have been compared.[78] The last group was included, because women with Lynch syndrome-associated endometrial cancer are often younger (mean age 46.8 years in the M.D. Anderson Cancer Center patient cohort). The young women with sporadic endometrial cancer were proven to be negative for *MLH1* and *MSH2* mutations by formal genetic testing. Remarkably, one of the clearest differences between these 3 groups was that the sporadic younger than 50 group (41/42, 97.6%) and the sporadic MLH1 methylation group (25/26, 96.2%) were almost entirely composed of tumors with endometrioid histology. In contrast, the Lynch syndrome group was more heterogeneous, with 43/50 (86%) tumors with endometrioid histotype. Amongst the 3 groups, there were no statistical differences in myometrial invasion, presence of lymphatic/vascular invasion, and stage. Importantly, 22% of Lynch Syndrome endometrial carcinomas were Stage II, III, or IV, implying the need for adjuvant chemotherapy and/or radiation therapy in addition to hysterectomy.

The relationship between the histologic type of endometrial carcinoma and type of mismatch repair protein abnormality has been the subject of recent investigations.

In the general population, non-endometrioid endometrial carcinoma is typically diagnosed in older women with a mean age of 65 to 68 years.[80–84] However, in Lynch syndrome, the mean age of diagnosis of these non-endometrioid tumors is 46.4 years, similar to the mean age of endometrial cancer diagnosis in the Lynch Syndrome group overall (46.8 years). Clear cell carcinoma, uterine serous carcinoma, and malignant mixed mullerian tumors have been identified as non-endometrioid tumors in Lynch syndrome. In their study of 23 Italian women with Lynch syndrome-associated endometrial cancer, Carcangiu and colleagues[85] found an extraordinarily high percentage (43%) of non-endometrioid carcinomas; 50% of these non-endometrioid tumors were clear cell carcinoma. From the published literature, non-endometrioid tumors do not typically constitute such a high percentage of the Lynch syndrome-associated endometrial cancer population. Interestingly, one study found that all of the non-endometrioid tumors arose in women with *MSH2* mutations.[78] In the population-based study of Hampel and colleagues[86] and subsequent follow-up,[87] two Lynch Syndrome-associated non-endometrioid endometrial carcinomas were identified, both in women with *MSH6* mutations. In our subsequent studies, we have identified only one woman with a *MLH1* mutation and a non-endometrioid endometrial carcinoma. Compared to endometrial cancers in the Lynch syndrome and sporadic younger than 50 groups, endometrial cancers in the sporadic MLH1 methylated group had a greater percentage of grade 2 and grade 3 endometrioid tumors.[78] This suggests that there may be a genotype-phenotype relationship in which microsatellite instability due to loss of MLH1, either by methylation of the promoter or due to gene mutation, is almost exclusively associated with higher grade endometrioid tumors, while microsatellite instability due to defects in the MSH2/MSH6 pair can result in a more varied spectrum of endometrial carcinoma histology. More studies including non-endometrioid tumors will be needed to verify this possible genotype-phenotype relationship.

It has been well-established by a number of different studies that patients with MSI-high colorectal cancer have a significantly improved survival compared with patients with MS-stable colorectal cancer.[88,89] Several studies have examined the clinical significance of MSI-high endometrial cancer. In one of the largest studies, Black and colleagues[90] found that 20% (93/473) of endometrial carcinomas were MSI-high. As compared with the MS-stable tumors, MSI-high tumors were predominantly endometrioid (94% vs 77%), had a higher proportion with myometrial invasion, and were of more advanced stage. Overall, the patients with MSI-high tumors had a better disease free survival and disease specific survival. In contrast, another large prospective study of 446 women with endometrial cancer determined that MSI status has no effect on survival.[91] Therefore, for endometrial cancer, the issue of the impact of MSI on survival remains controversial. Specific associations between mechanisms of MSI development (ie, genetic versus epigenetic) and clinical outcome have not been studied rigorously. It is possible that lack of attention to this, specifically, has led to confounding and, perhaps, misleading results.

MICROSCOPIC FEATURES OF MSI-HIGH ENDOMETRIAL CARCINOMA

There is a considerable amount of literature on the presence or absence of distinctive microscopic features in MSI-high colorectal carcinoma. Some of the microscopic features that have been associated with the presence of MSI-high include poor differentiation, mucinous features, signet ring cell differentiation, mixed tumor histology, tumor cells growing in a medullary-type pattern, increased tumor infiltrating lymphocytes, and a Crohn's like inflammatory infiltrate at the tumor periphery.[92] Most of these studies have not distinguished between sporadic MSI-high due to MLH1 methylation versus MSI-high due to germline mutation of a DNA mismatch repair gene. It is therefore unclear if there are microscopic differences between these two MSI-high groups. It must be noted, however, that these distinctive microscopic features may not be present in a substantial subset of colorectal carcinoma. Up to 40% of colorectal carcinomas do not have such distinguishing microscopic characteristics.[92] Therefore, microscopic features alone cannot be used independently of other factors to determine which colorectal cancer patients should be evaluated for Lynch syndrome at present.

Microscopic features of MSI-high endometrial carcinoma have also been studied, but not to the extent of that for MSI-high colorectal carcinoma.[93,94] Again, as is the case for colorectal cancer, the source of the microsatellite instability (MLH1 methylation versus germline mutation of a DNA mismatch repair gene) was not delineated in these studies. One study found that MSI-high endometrial cancers were associated with higher tumor grade, presence of squamous metaplasia, deeper myometrial invasion, presence of lymphatic/vascular invasion, and extra-uterine spread.[93] High numbers of tumor infiltrating lymphocytes and the presence of peritumoral lymphocytes have been associated with MSI-high.[94] At the higher numbers of tumor infiltrating lymphocytes (42 lymphocytes per 10 high power fields), these counts had a sensitivity of 85% in predicting MSI-high status, but a specificity of only 46%. Although the published data for endometrial cancer is more limited, it is our opinion that microscopic features of endometrial cancer are not sufficiently sensitive and specific to be used in the clinical setting as accurate predictors of the presence of high levels of microsatellite instability (**Fig. 3**). Another point of view is presented in Familial Tumors of the Corpus by Karuna Garg and Robert Soslow.

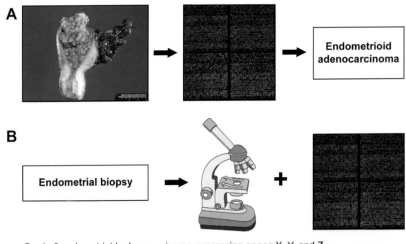

Grade 2 endometrioid adenocarcinoma expressing genes X, Y, and Z, which are predictive of deep myometrial invasion and disease outside the uterus.

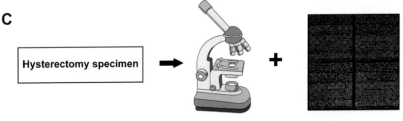

Grade 2 endometrioid adenocarcinoma. Depth of myometrial invasion 6 mm (total myometrial thickness 20 mm). Tumor expresses genes A, B, and C which are predictive of recurrence and are associated with shortened survival.

Fig. 3. Incorporation of genomic data into the clinical and pathologic evaluation of endometrial carcinoma. Current state of the knowledge. (*A*) Researcher's approach: grind up tumor. Answer is provided by genomic analysis. In practicality, such information has limited clinical usefulness, as this distinction can usually be made quickly and with less expense using light microscopic evaluation of H&E stained slides of endometrial tumor. (*B*) and (*C*) Informed pathologist's approach. In (*B*) and (*C*), scenarios are presented in which such molecular data could potentially represent "value added" to the pathology report and aid in planning the surgical hysterectomy approach and type of staging procedure to be performed (*B*) or in choosing which patients might benefit from adjuvant chemotherapy or radiation treatment following hysterectomy (*C*).

MSI-HIGH ENDOMETRIAL CANCER ARISING IN THE LOWER UTERINE SEGMENT

Pathologically, the endometrium comprises two distinct areas, the uterine corpus proper and the lower uterine segment (LUS). Endometrial carcinoma most commonly arises in the mucosa of the corpus, which includes the body and fundus of the uterus. In a large series, only 3.5% of endometrial carcinomas were derived from the LUS.[95] Interestingly, the mean age of the women with LUS tumors was significantly younger (54.2 years) compared with the women with uterine corpus endometrial carcinoma (63.0 years).[95] A relatively high percentage (34.2%) of the LUS carcinomas was MSI-high; 28.6% of the LUS carcinomas were confirmed to be from women with Lynch syndrome.[95] This percentage of Lynch syndrome-associated endometrial cancers is startling when compared with the incidence of Lynch syndrome in the general endometrial cancer patient population (1%–2%)[77,96,97] or in young women (50 years of age or younger) with endometrial cancer (9%–11%).[78,86]

CLINICALLY AGGRESSIVE ENDOMETRIAL CANCER

The previous sections have focused on molecular pathways thought to be more important in the early development of endometrial carcinoma. In the following sections, selected molecular changes in the more clinically aggressive endometrial cancers are discussed. Much of the literature on this topic has focused on identifying molecular changes that distinguish low-grade endometrioid carcinoma (typically good prognosis) from non-endometrioid carcinoma (typically poor prognosis). Molecular changes in recurrent endometrioid carcinomas have not been the subject of as much study, mainly because of the relatively lower numbers of these patients at any one institution.

p53

p53 is a tumor suppressor gene located on chromosome 17p13.1 that regulates a variety of cellular processes, most notably promoting apoptosis, DNA repair, and cell cycle arrest. Although the majority of p53 mutations are concentrated in the core domain (120–292 bp) they can occur throughout the entire genome.[98] Point mutations are the most common. An interesting property of many p53 mutations is their transdominant negative capacity, whereby the altered gene product acts antagonistically to the wild type allele and results in abrogation of

function even in the heterozygous state. Furthermore, some transdominant negative p53 mutants can have gain-of-function effects, which act to enhance tumorigenicity and resistance to therapy.[98] Unlike recessive mutants, the transdominant mutants are not associated with a conformational protein change and they tend to accumulate in the cell.[99] By immunohistochemistry this is detected as a strong positive signal.

p53 mutation is typically associated with uterine serous carcinoma,[100–102] but p53 mutations are not unique to uterine serous carcinomas. In a recent study by Catasus and colleagues,[55] p53 mutations were observed in 54% of non-endometrioid (serous and clear cell) carcinomas, in 50% mixed non-endometrioid and endometrioid carcinomas, in 17% of high grade endometrioid carcinomas and in 2% of endometrioid carcinomas. Similarly, Lax and colleagues[103] reported p53 mutations in 93% of serous carcinomas, compared with 17% in endometrioid endometrial carcinomas. Furthermore, it has been found that a much higher proportion of serous endometrial carcinomas contain dominant negative mutations compared with endometrioid endometrial carcinomas.[104] Several studies have reported a negative association between increased tumor immunohistochemical signal for p53 and survival.[105–107]

GENOMIC STUDIES

Immunohistochemistry for p53 is commonly used clinically to help distinguish endometrioid from non-endometrioid endometrial carcinomas. While sometimes helpful as a diagnostic adjunct, this approach has limitations and requires careful correlation with histology. Several genomic studies have recently employed cDNA microarray technology to identify numerous other genes that can help to discriminate between endometrial cancer histotypes.[108,109] The main advantage of this type of genomic approach is the potential identification of novel genes and pathways not previously examined in endometrial cancer. However, many of the identified genes or ESTs (expressed sequence tags) have no known biologic function or have only been superficially studied. For example, in one microarray study of different histotypes of endometrial cancer, the EST KIAA1324 was identified to be one of the best molecular signatures to distinguish endometrioid from non-endometrioid carcinomas.[108] The function of KIAA1324, however, is entirely unknown so expression was not verified by qRT-PCR in this study. A separate microarray study identified this same EST to be induced 3-fold in the human endometrium by estrogen-based hormone replacement therapy.[13] It was subsequently shown that this EST (termed *Estrogen Induced Gene 121; EIG121*) was significantly upregulated 21-fold in grade 1 endometrioid endometrial carcinomas compared with benign endometrium. Furthermore, *EIG121* expression was significantly suppressed in the non-endometrioid tumors uterine serous carcinoma and uterine malignant mixed mullerian tumor. In fact, the level of *EIG121* mRNA in these non-endometrioid carcinomas was only less than 5% of that of the benign endometrium.[13] Therefore, these separate studies have both identified *EIG121* to be an excellent single gene biomarker to distinguish endometrioid from non-endometrioid endometrial carcinomas. The *EIG121* genes show high sequence conservation among a variety of different species, and their genomic structure, exon/intron boundaries, and exon sizes are nearly identical. This strongly suggests that *EIG121* fulfills some important (albeit currently unknown) biologic function.

EPITHELIAL-TO-MESENCHYMAL TRANSITION

Epithelial-to-mesenchymal transition (EMT) can be thought of as a genetic reprogramming of epithelial tumor cells as they become invasive and metastatic.[110,111] Typically, the genes regulating EMT are also important in regulating the migration of cells during the course of normal embryologic development. EMT is characterized by loss of expression of epithelial markers of differentiation, gain of expression of mesenchymal markers, a more spindled or fibroblastic cell appearance, cellular secretion of proteases and other enzymes that degrade the extracellular matrix, and the acquisition of increased cellular motility.[110,111] In addition to its importance in mediating cancer cell invasion and metastasis, EMT has also been recently implicated in the development of chemotherapy and targeted therapy resistance.[112–114] EMT is regulated by a number of different transcription factors; the expression of these transcription factors is dysregulated in endometrial cancer as will be discussed below.

ZEB1 is a transcription factor linked to EMT. ZEB1 represses the expression of the epithelial marker E-cadherin as well as the expression of other markers of epithelial differentiation. In the normal endometrium, expression of ZEB1 is confined to endometrial stromal cells.[115,116] Interestingly, in grade 1 and grade 2 endometrioid adenocarcinomas, ZEB1 expression is also confined to stromal cells. However, in a subset of grade 3 endometrioid adenocarcinomas, uterine serous carcinoma, and uterine malignant mixed

mullerian tumor, increased ZEB1 expression was detected in the tumor epithelial cells.[115,116] In the MMMT cases, expression was microscopically observed in both the carcinoma and sarcomatous components. Importantly, manipulation of ZEB1 levels in endometrial cancer cell lines via over-expression or sh-RNA mediated knock down resulted in altered endometrial cancer cell in vitro migration.[116] These in vitro findings provide direct evidence for the role of ZEB1 in controlling endometrial cancer cell motility.

SNAIL is a second transcription factor commonly associated with EMT. In the published literature, SNAIL expression has only been examined in endometrioid-type endometrial carcinomas, so comparison to non-endometrioid tumors cannot be made at this time. In one study, approximately 29% of primary endometrioid carcinomas demonstrated positive immunohistochemical expression for SNAIL; expression was not significantly correlated to grade or stage.[117] In metastases of endometrioid carcinoma, SNAIL immunohistochemical expression was detected in approximately 54% of cases.[117] One small study found that SNAIL expression in endometrioid carcinomas was significantly and negatively correlated to expression of E-cadherin,[118] but a second larger study did not observe such a correlation.[117]

TWIST is another transcription factor associated with induction of EMT. In one small study of 70 endometrioid-type endometrial carcinomas, high immunohistochemical expression of TWIST was significantly associated with decreased E-cadherin tumor expression and poor overall survival.[119] However, TWIST expression was not associated with stage or grade. In a Cox proportional hazard analysis, TWIST expression, patient's age, and stage were identified as independent predictive factors of patient survival.[119]

HOXA10 is a transcription factor that controls uterine genesis during embryonic development and functional endometrial differentiation in the adult. In normal endometrial glands, there is strong HOXA10 immunohistochemical expression.[120] With increasing endometrioid tumor grade, there is decreased expression of HOXA10.[120] Grade 3 endometrioid carcinomas and uterine serous carcinomas had little-to-no expression of HOXA10.[120] Enforced expression of HOXA10 in SPEC2 endometrial cancer cells caused these cells to grow in tight aggregates, upregulate E-cadherin expression, and decrease their ability to invade in vitro in Matrigel and in vivo in nude mice.[120] These effects of HOXA10 were likely due to increased expression of HOXA10 inhibiting the expression of the EMT transcription factor SNAIL.[120]

It is clear from the above discussion that a number of EMT-related transcription factors are important in regulating endometrial cancer invasion and metastasis. Other than inducing down-regulation of epithelial markers to decrease cell-cell adhesion, the mechanisms by which these transcription factors act is unknown. Specifically, the cellular effectors of these transcription factors have been poorly described to date. One such cellular effector for endometrial cancer may be S100A4. The *S100* gene family encodes a number of different calcium-binding proteins of uncertain biologic function. Relevant to cancer, a number of different *S100* genes are upregulated in different cancer types; intriguingly, overexpression of *S100* genes is typically associated with advanced, deeply invasive tumors, metastatic tumors, and tumors with a poor prognosis. S100A4 mRNA and protein are selectively overexpressed in grade 3 endometrioid carcinomas and the non-endometrioid carcinomas uterine serous carcinoma and uterine malignant mixed mullerian tumor.[121] Similar to the transcription factor ZEB1, expression of S100A4 is confined to stromal cells in normal endometrium and lower grade endometrioid carcinomas.[121] Knockdown of S100A4 significantly inhibits in vitro endometrial cancer cell migration and invasion.[122]

Understanding the molecular mechanisms of EMT has shed considerable light on the molecular mechanisms of endometrial cancer invasion and metastasis. It is less clear, however, how such knowledge can be exploited clinically. The EMT-related transcription factors and S100A4 are unlikely to represent effective therapeutic targets, because of their widespread expression in normal mesenchymal cells and connective tissue. Calculation of the expression of these genes, however, may prove to be useful in gene panels to help predict endometrial cancer recurrence or advanced endometrial cancer stage; this information would be tremendously useful for clinical decisions regarding the use of adjuvant chemotherapy/radiotherapy following hysterectomy or the extent of surgical staging accompanying hysterectomy.

SUMMARY – GAPS IN OUR CURRENT UNDERSTANDING OF ENDOMETRIAL CANCER

As can be ascertained from the preceding discussion, considerably more is known about molecular events important in early endometrial

Fig. 4. Utility of the paraffin block in the molecular assessment of endometrial carcinoma. From routinely acquired formalin-fixed, paraffin-embedded tissues, a variety of laboratory-based assays can be performed, including immunohistochemistry, in situ hybridization, DNA extraction and PCR-based amplification, and fluorescent in situ hybridization. Transcript (mRNA) quantification via quantitative real-time PCR can also be performed using formalin-fixed, paraffin-embedded tissues, but this technique requires more technical expertise.

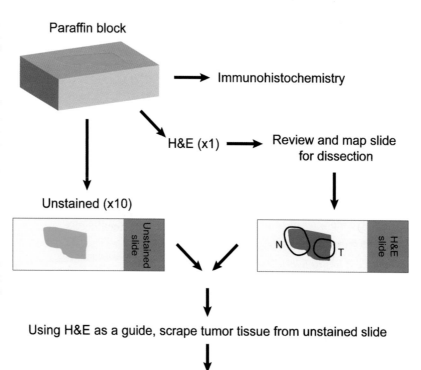

carcinogenesis. Much less is known regarding the molecular mechanisms of endometrial cancer invasion, metastasis, and recurrence. Better understanding of such molecular mechanisms is crucial to make a stronger impact on treatment of advanced endometrial cancer. More detailed study of the current genomic data that is available for endometrial cancer could potentially be fruitful. Significant gaps in our current knowledge include, but are not limited to, the following:

1. Identify the molecular effectors of EMT transcription factors. Can any of these effectors be exploited for targeted therapy?

2. Identify the molecular mechanisms by which estrogen receptor and the PTEN/PI3K/AKT pathway may cross-talk.

3. Identify the factors that make the endometrium particularly susceptible to carcinogenesis via loss of DNA mismatch repair machinery.

4. Understand how microsatellite instability interacts with other molecular mechanisms (such as PTEN loss) to contribute to endometrial cancer development.

5. Better understand the molecular mechanisms by which normal endometrial stromal cells regulate endometrial epithelial biology. Then, determine the fate of normal endometrial

---

Box 1
Laboratory assays useful in pathologic assessments of endometrial cancer

Immunohistochemistry

1. Identify origin in an endocervical or endometrial biopsy with poorly differentiated adenocarcinoma.

    Endometrial origin– ER positive, vimentin positive, CEA negative, p16 negative or patchy positive

    Endocervical origin– ER negative, vimentin negative, CEA positive, p16 diffusely positive

2. Determine if a metastatic adenocarcinoma is of endometrial versus colon origin

    Endometrial – ER positive, vimentin positive, cytokeratin 7 positive, cytokeratin 20 negative, CDX2 negative

    Colon- ER negative, vimentin negative, cytokeratin 7 negative, cytokeratin 20 positive, CDX2 positive

3. Determine if an endometrial carcinoma is endometrioid or non-endometrioid

    Endometrioid – p53 negative or weakly/focally positive

    Non-endometrioid – p53 strongly and diffusely positive

4. Help determine if an endometrial cancer is related to Lynch syndrome

    MLH1, MSH2, MSH6, PMS2

5. Identify therapeutic targets

    ER, PR, HER-2/neu, EGFR, PTEN

PCR-based Amplification of DNA

1. Help determine if an endometrial cancer is related to Lynch syndrome

    Microsatellite instability analysis and MLH1 methylation analysis

2. Identify therapeutic targets

    PIK3CA mutation analysis

3. Possible modifier of response to PI3K Pathway targeted therapy

    KRAS mutation analysis

Fluorescent in situ hybridization

Identify therapeutic targets - HER-2/neu

In situ hybridization

Help to identify origin in an endocervical or endometrial biopsy with poorly differentiated adenocarcinoma

    Endometrial origin – HPV in situ hybridization negative

    Endocervical origin – HPV in situ hybridization positive

stromal cells, which are typically "lost" in the development of complex hyperplasia and endometrioid carcinomas.

6. More fully delineate the roles of other hormones and hormone receptors, particularly progesterone and progesterone receptor, in the molecular pathogenesis of endometrial cancer.

7. Identify molecular alterations that distinguish recurrent endometrioid-type endometrial carcinoma from the primary tumor. This type of study would likely require the resources of a cooperative oncology group or the collaboration of a number of different institutions. The study of recurrences becomes especially important in the era of targeted therapy. Do the recurrent tumors express the same targets as their primary counterparts?

Another significant hurdle in the endometrial cancer field is that clinical translation of laboratory-based, experimental results has been a challenge. For example, numerous publications have reported genetic differences in endometrioid compared with non-endometrioid endometrial carcinomas. However, translation of this knowledge base into clinically useful and relevant pathology laboratory-based assays has yet to occur (**Fig. 4**). Therefore, the laboratory-based assays currently in use for the clinical evaluation of endometrial carcinomas are somewhat limited. Assays in current clinical use are summarized in **Box 1**.

REFERENCES

1. Bokhman JV. Two pathogenetic types of endometrial carcinoma. Gynecol Oncol 1983;15(1):10–7.

2. Jemal A, Siegel R, Ward E, et al. Cancer statistics, 2009. CA Cancer J Clin 2009;59(4):225–49.

3. Glass CK, Rosenfeld MG. The coregulator exchange in transcriptional functions of nuclear receptors. Genes Dev 2000;14(2):121–41.

4. Shang Y. Molecular mechanisms of oestrogen and SERMs in endometrial carcinogenesis. Nat Rev Cancer 2006;6(5):360–8.

5. Kurman RJ, Kaminski PF, Norris HJ. The behavior of endometrial hyperplasia. A long-term study of 'untreated' hyperplasia in 170 patients. Cancer 1985;56(2):403–12.

6. Austin DF, Roe KM. The decreasing incidence of endometrial cancer: public health implications. Am J Public Health 1982;72(1):65–8.

7. Lu KH, Schorge JO, Rodabaugh KJ, et al. Prospective determination of prevalence of Lynch syndrome in young women with endometrial cancer. J Clin Oncol 2007;25(33):5158–64.

8. Schottenfeld D. Epidemiology of endometrial neoplasia. J Cell Biochem 1995;59(Suppl 23):151–9.

9. Soliman PT, Oh JC, Schmeler KM, et al. Risk factors for young premenopausal women with endometrial cancer. Obstet Gynecol 2005;105(3):575–80.

10. Sherman ME. Theories of endometrial carcinogenesis: a multidisciplinary approach. Mod Pathol 2000;13(3):295–308.

11. McCampbell AS, Broaddus RR, Loose DS, et al. Overexpression of the insulin-like growth factor I receptor and activation of the AKT pathway in hyperplastic endometrium. Clin Cancer Res 2006; 12(21):6373–8.

12. Westin SN, Broaddus RR, Deng L, et al. Molecular clustering of endometrial carcinoma based on estrogen-induced gene expression. Cancer Biol Ther 2009;8(22):1–9.

13. Deng L, Broaddus RR, McCampbell A, et al. Identification of a novel estrogen-regulated gene, EIG121, induced by hormone replacement therapy and differentially expressed in type I and type II endometrial cancer. Clin Cancer Res 2005;11(23): 8258–64.

14. Deng L, Shipley GL, Loose-Mitchell DS, et al. Coordinate regulation of the production and signaling of retinoic acid by estrogen in the human endometrium. J Clin Endocrinol Metab 2003;88(5):2157–63.

15. Schlesinger C, Kamoi S, Ascher SM, et al. Endometrial polyps: a comparison study of patients receiving tamoxifen with two control groups. Int J Gynecol Pathol 1998;17(4):302–11.

16. Killackey MA, Hakes TB, Pierce VK. Endometrial adenocarcinoma in breast cancer patients receiving antiestrogens. Cancer Treat Rep 1985; 69(2):237–8.

17. Cohen I, Bernheim J, Azaria R, et al. Malignant endometrial polyps in postmenopausal breast cancer tamoxifen-treated patients. Gynecol Oncol 1999;75(1):136–41.

18. Senkus-Konefka E, Konefka T, Jassem J. The effects of tamoxifen on the female genital tract. Cancer Treat Rev 2004;30(3):291–301.

19. Cohen I, Azaria R, Fishman A, et al. Endometrial cancers in postmenopausal breast cancer patients with tamoxifen treatment. Int J Gynecol Pathol 1999;18(4):304–9.

20. Barakat RR, Wong G, Curtin JP, et al. Tamoxifen use in breast cancer patients who subsequently develop corpus cancer is not associated with a higher incidence of adverse histologic features. Gynecol Oncol 1994;55(2):164–8.

21. Dallenbach-Hellweg G, Schmidt D, Hellberg P, et al. The endometrium in breast cancer patients on tamoxifen. Arch Gynecol Obstet 2000;263(4): 170–7.

22. Deligdisch L, Kalir T, Cohen CJ, et al. Endometrial histopathology in 700 patients treated with tamoxifen for breast cancer. Gynecol Oncol 2000;78(2): 181–6.

23. Magriples U, Naftolin F, Schwartz PE, et al. High-grade endometrial carcinoma in tamoxifen-treated breast cancer patients. J Clin Oncol 1993;11(3):485–90.

24. Bergman L, Beelen ML, Gallee MP, et al. Risk and prognosis of endometrial cancer after tamoxifen for breast cancer. Comprehensive Cancer Centres' ALERT Group. Assessment of Liver and Endometrial cancer Risk following Tamoxifen. Lancet 2000;356(9233):881–7.

25. Silva EG, Tornos CS, Follen-Mitchell M. Malignant neoplasms of the uterine corpus in patients treated for breast carcinoma: the effects of tamoxifen. Int J Gynecol Pathol 1994;13(3):248–58.

26. Wu H, Chen Y, Liang J, et al. Hypomethylation-linked activation of PAX2 mediates tamoxifen-stimulated endometrial carcinogenesis. Nature 2005;438(7070):981–7.

27. Pole JC, Gold LI, Orton T, et al. Gene expression changes induced by estrogen and selective estrogen receptor modulators in primary-cultured human endometrial cells: signals that distinguish the human carcinogen tamoxifen. Toxicology 2005;206(1):91–109.

28. Engelman JA. Targeting PI3K signalling in cancer: opportunities, challenges and limitations. Nat Rev Cancer 2009;9(8):550–62.

29. Steck PA, Pershouse MA, Jasser SA, et al. Identification of a candidate tumour suppressor gene, MMAC1, at chromosome 10q23.3 that is mutated in multiple advanced cancers. Nat Genet 1997;15(4):356–62.

30. Li J, Yen C, Liaw D, et al. PTEN, a putative protein tyrosine phosphatase gene mutated in human brain, breast, and prostate cancer. Science 1997;275(5308):1943–7.

31. Choe G, Horvath S, Cloughesy TF, et al. Analysis of the phosphatidylinositol 3'-kinase signaling pathway in glioblastoma patients in vivo. Cancer Res 2003;63(11):2742–6.

32. Terakawa N, Kanamori Y, Yoshida S. Loss of PTEN expression followed by Akt phosphorylation is a poor prognostic factor for patients with endometrial cancer. Endocr Relat Cancer 2003;10(2):203–8.

33. Eng C. PTEN: one gene, many syndromes. Hum Mutat 2003;22(3):183–98.

34. Kong D, Suzuki A, Zou TT, et al. PTEN1 is frequently mutated in primary endometrial carcinomas. Nat Genet 1997;17(2):143–4.

35. Risinger JI, Hayes AK, Berchuck A, et al. PTEN/MMAC1 mutations in endometrial cancers. Cancer Res 1997;57(21):4736–8.

36. Mutter GL, Lin MC, Fitzgerald JT, et al. Altered PTEN expression as a diagnostic marker for the earliest endometrial precancers. J Natl Cancer Inst 2000;92(11):924–30.

37. Tashiro H, Blazes MS, Wu R, et al. Mutations in PTEN are frequent in endometrial carcinoma but rare in other common gynecological malignancies. Cancer Res 1997;57(18):3935–40.

38. Risinger JI, Hayes K, Maxwell GL, et al. PTEN mutation in endometrial cancers is associated with favorable clinical and pathologic characteristics. Clin Cancer Res 1998;4(12):3005–10.

39. Bussaglia E, del Rio E, Matias-Guiu X, et al. PTEN mutations in endometrial carcinomas: a molecular and clinicopathologic analysis of 38 cases. Hum Pathol 2000;31(3):312–7.

40. Minaguchi T, Yoshikawa H, Oda K, et al. PTEN mutation located only outside exons 5, 6, and 7 is an independent predictor of favorable survival in endometrial carcinomas. Clin Cancer Res 2001;7(9):2636–42.

41. Dahia PL, Aguiar RC, Alberta J, et al. PTEN is inversely correlated with the cell survival factor Akt/PKB and is inactivated via multiple mechanismsin haematological malignancies. Hum Mol Genet 1999;8(2):185–93.

42. Perren A, Weng LP, Boag AH, et al. Immunohistochemical evidence of loss of PTEN expression in primary ductal adenocarcinomas of the breast. Am J Pathol 1999;155(4):1253–60.

43. Salvesen HB, MacDonald N, Ryan A, et al. PTEN methylation is associated with advanced stage and microsatellite instability in endometrial carcinoma. Int J Cancer 2001;91(1):22–6.

44. Macdonald ND, Salvesen HB, Ryan A, et al. Molecular differences between RER+ and RER- sporadic endometrial carcinomas in a large population-based series. Int J Gynecol Cancer 2004;14(5):957–65.

45. Gao Q, Ye F, Xia X, et al. Correlation between PTEN expression and PI3K/Akt signal pathway in endometrial carcinoma. J Huazhong Univ Sci Technolog Med Sci 2009;29(1):59–63.

46. Salvesen HB, Stefansson I, Kalvenes MB, et al. Loss of PTEN expression is associated with metastatic disease in patients with endometrial carcinoma. Cancer 2002;94(8):2185–91.

47. Kanamori Y, Kigawa J, Itamochi H, et al. PTEN expression is associated with prognosis for patients with advanced endometrial carcinoma undergoing postoperative chemotherapy. Int J Cancer 2002;100(6):686–9.

48. Uegaki K, Kanamori Y, Kigawa J, et al. PTEN-positive and phosphorylated-Akt-negative expression is a predictor of survival for patients with advanced endometrial carcinoma. Oncol Rep 2005;14(2):389–92.

49. Kang S, Bader AG, Vogt PK. Phosphatidylinositol 3-kinase mutations identified in human cancer are oncogenic. Proc Natl Acad Sci U S A 2005;102(3):802–7.

50. Oda K, Stokoe D, Taketani Y, et al. High frequency of coexistent mutations of PIK3CA and PTEN genes in endometrial carcinoma. Cancer Res 2005; 65(23):10669–73.

51. Hayes MP, Wang H, Espinal-Witter R, et al. PIK3CA and PTEN mutations in uterine endometrioid carcinoma and complex atypical hyperplasia. Clin Cancer Res 2006;12(20 Pt 1):5932–5.

52. Catasus L, Gallardo A, Cuatrecasas M, et al. PIK3CA mutations in the kinase domain (exon 20) of uterine endometrial adenocarcinomas are associated with adverse prognostic parameters. Mod Pathol 2008;21(2):131–9.

53. Miyake T, Yoshino K, Enomoto T, et al. PIK3CA gene mutations and amplifications in uterine cancers, identified by methods that avoid confounding by PIK3CA pseudogene sequences. Cancer Lett 2008;261(1):120–6.

54. Salvesen HB, Carter SL, Mannelqvist M, et al. Integrated genomic profiling of endometrial carcinoma associates aggressive tumors with indicators of PI3 kinase activation. Proc Natl Acad Sci U S A 2009; 106(12):4834–9.

55. Catasus L, Gallardo A, Cuatrecasas M, et al. Concomitant PI3K-AKT and p53 alterations in endometrial carcinomas are associated with poor prognosis. Mod Pathol 2009;22(4):522–9.

56. Catasus L, D'Angelo E, Pons C, et al. Expression profiling of 22 genes involved in the PI3K-AKT pathway identifies two subgroups of high-grade endometrial carcinomas with different molecular alterations. Mod Pathol 2010;23(5):694–702.

57. Hayes MP, Douglas W, Ellenson LH. Molecular alterations of EGFR and PIK3CA in uterine serous carcinoma. Gynecol Oncol 2009;113(3):370–3.

58. McLendon R, Friedman A, Bigner D, et al. Comprehensive genomic characterization defines human glioblastoma genes and core pathways. Nature 2008;455(7216):1061–8.

59. Rutanen EM. Insulin-like growth factors in endometrial function. Gynecol Endocrinol 1998;12(6): 399–406.

60. Lee YR, Park J, Yu HN, et al. Up-regulation of PI3K/ Akt signaling by 17beta-estradiol through activation of estrogen receptor-alpha, but not estrogen receptor-beta, and stimulates cell growth in breast cancer cells. Biochem Biophys Res Commun 2005; 336(4):1221–6.

61. Engelman JA, Chen L, Tan X, et al. Effective use of PI3K and MEK inhibitors to treat mutant Kras G12D and PIK3CA H1047R murine lung cancers. Nat Med 2008;14(12):1351–6.

62. Ihle NT, Lemos R Jr, Wipf P, et al. Mutations in the phosphatidylinositol-3-kinase pathway predict for antitumor activity of the inhibitor PX-866 whereas oncogenic Ras is a dominant predictor for resistance. Cancer Res 2009;69(1):143–50.

63. Torbett NE, Luna-Moran A, Knight ZA, et al. A chemical screen in diverse breast cancer cell lines reveals genetic enhancers and suppressors of sensitivity to PI3K isoform-selective inhibition. Biochem J 2008;415(1):97–110.

64. Chon HS, Hu W, Kavanagh JJ. Targeted therapies in gynecologic cancers. Curr Cancer Drug Targets 2006;6(4):333–63.

65. Catasus L, Gallardo A, Prat J. Molecular genetics of endometrial carcinoma. Diagn Histopathol 2009;15:554–63.

66. Duggan BD, Felix JC, Muderspach LI, et al. Early mutational activation of the c-Ki-ras oncogene in endometrial carcinoma. Cancer Res 1994;54(6): 1604–7.

67. Enomoto T, Inoue M, Perantoni AO, et al. K-ras activation in premalignant and malignant epithelial lesions of the human uterus. Cancer Res 1991; 51(19):5308–14.

68. Esteller M, Garcia A, Martinez-Palones JM, et al. The clinicopathological significance of K-RAS point mutation and gene amplification in endometrial cancer. Eur J Cancer 1997;33(10):1572–7.

69. Sasaki H, Nishii H, Takahashi H, et al. Mutation of the Ki-ras protooncogene in human endometrial hyperplasia and carcinoma. Cancer Res 1993; 53(8):1906–10.

70. Semczuk A, Berbec H, Kostuch M, et al. K-ras gene point mutations in human endometrial carcinomas: correlation with clinicopathological features and patients' outcome. J Cancer Res Clin Oncol 1998;124(12):695–700.

71. Fujimoto I, Shimizu Y, Hirai Y, et al. Studies on ras oncogene activation in endometrial carcinoma. Gynecol Oncol 1993;48(2):196–202.

72. Ito K, Watanabe K, Nasim S, et al. K-ras point mutations in endometrial carcinoma: effect on outcome is dependent on age of patient. Gynecol Oncol 1996;63(2):238–46.

73. Caduff RF, Johnston CM, Frank TS. Mutations of the Ki-ras oncogene in carcinoma of the endometrium. Am J Pathol 1995;146(1):182–8.

74. Kane MF, Loda M, Gaida GM, et al. Methylation of the hMLH1 promoter correlates with lack of expression of hMLH1 in sporadic colon tumors and mismatch repair-defective human tumor cell lines. Cancer Res 1997;57(5):808–11.

75. Herman JG, Umar A, Polyak K, et al. Incidence and functional consequences of hMLH1 promoter hypermethylation in colorectal carcinoma. Proc Natl Acad Sci U S A 1998;95(12):6870–5.

76. Salvesen HB, MacDonald N, Ryan A, et al. Methylation of hMLH1 in a population-based series of endometrial carcinomas. Clin Cancer Res 2000; 6(9):3607–13.

77. Goodfellow PJ, Buttin BM, Herzog TJ, et al. Prevalence of defective DNA mismatch repair and MSH6

mutation in an unselected series of endometrial cancers. Proc Natl Acad Sci U S A 2003;100(10): 5908–13.

78. Broaddus RR, Lynch HT, Chen LM, et al. Pathologic features of endometrial carcinoma associated with HNPCC: a comparison with sporadic endometrial carcinoma. Cancer 2006;106(1):87–94.

79. Lu KH, Dinh M, Kohlmann W, et al. Gynecologic cancer as a "sentinel cancer" for women with hereditary nonpolyposis colorectal cancer syndrome. Obstet Gynecol 2005;105(3):569–74.

80. Abeler VM, Kjorstad KE. Clear cell carcinoma of the endometrium: a histopathological and clinical study of 97 cases. Gynecol Oncol Mar 1991; 40(3):207–17.

81. Christopherson WM, Alberhasky RC, Connelly PJ. Carcinoma of the endometrium. II. Papillary adenocarcinoma: a clinical pathological study, 46 cases. Am J Clin Pathol 1982;77(5):534–40.

82. Webb GA, Lagios MD. Clear cell carcinoma of the endometrium. Am J Obstet Gynecol 1987;156(6): 1486–91.

83. Doss LL, Llorens AS, Henriquez EM. Carcinosarcoma of the uterus: a 40-year experience from the state of Missouri. Gynecol Oncol 1984;18(1):43–53.

84. Olah KS, Dunn JA, Gee H. Leiomyosarcomas have a poorer prognosis than mixed mesodermal tumours when adjusting for known prognostic factors: the result of a retrospective study of 423 cases of uterine sarcoma. Br J Obstet Gynaecol 1992;99(7):590–4.

85. Carcangiu ML, Radice P, Casalini P, et al. Lynch syndrome-related endometrial carcinomas show a high frequency of nonendometrioid types and of high FIGO grade endometrioid types. Int J Surg Pathol 2010;18(1):21–6.

86. Hampel H, Frankel W, Panescu J, et al. Screening for Lynch syndrome (hereditary nonpolyposis colorectal cancer) among endometrial cancer patients. Cancer Res 2006;66(15):7810–7.

87. Hampel H, Panescu J, Lockman J, et al. Comment on: screening for Lynch syndrome (Hereditary Nonpolyposis Colorectal Cancer) among Endometrial cancer patients. Cancer Res 2007;67(19):9603.

88. Popat S, Hubner R, Houlston RS. Systematic review of microsatellite instability and colorectal cancer prognosis. J Clin Oncol 2005;23(3):609–18.

89. Funaioli C, Pinto C, Mutri V, et al. Does biomolecular characterization of stage II/III colorectal cancer have any prognostic value? Clin Colorectal Cancer 2006;6(1):38–45.

90. Black D, Soslow RA, Levine DA, et al. Clinicopathologic significance of defective DNA mismatch repair in endometrial carcinoma. J Clin Oncol 2006;24(11):1745–53.

91. Zighelboim I, Goodfellow PJ, Gao F, et al. Microsatellite instability and epigenetic inactivation of MLH1 and outcome of patients with endometrial carcinomas of the endometrioid type. J Clin Oncol 2007;25(15):2042–8.

92. Alexander J, Watanabe T, Wu TT, et al. Histopathological identification of colon cancer with microsatellite instability. Am J Pathol 2001;158(2): 527–35.

93. Honore LH, Hanson J, Andrew SE. Microsatellite instability in endometrioid endometrial carcinoma: correlation with clinically relevant pathologic variables. Int J Gynecol Cancer 2006; 16(3):1386–92.

94. Shia J, Black D, Hummer AJ, et al. Routinely assessed morphological features correlate with microsatellite instability status in endometrial cancer. Hum Pathol 2008;39(1):116–25.

95. Westin SN, Lacour RA, Urbauer DL, et al. Carcinoma of the lower uterine segment: a newly described association with Lynch syndrome. J Clin Oncol 2008;26(36):5965–71.

96. Seiden MV, Patel D, O'Neill MJ, et al. Case records of the Massachusetts general hospital. Case 13-2007. A 46-year-old woman with gynecologic and intestinal cancers. N Engl J Med 2007;356(17): 1760–9.

97. Ollikainen M, Abdel-Rahman WM, Moisio AL, et al. Molecular analysis of familial endometrial carcinoma: a manifestation of hereditary nonpolyposis colorectal cancer or a separate syndrome? J Clin Oncol 2005;23(21):4609–16.

98. van Oijen MG, Slootweg PJ. Gain-of-function mutations in the tumor suppressor gene p53. Clin Cancer Res 2000;6(6):2138–45.

99. Roemer K. Mutant p53: gain-of-function oncoproteins and wild-type p53 inactivators. Biol Chem 1999;380(7–8):879–87.

100. Sherman ME, Bur ME, Kurman RJ. p53 in endometrial cancer and its putative precursors: evidence for diverse pathways of tumorigenesis. Hum Pathol 1995;26(11):1268–74.

101. Tashiro H, Isacson C, Levine R, et al. p53 gene mutations are common in uterine serous carcinoma and occur early in their pathogenesis. Am J Pathol 1997;150(1):177–85.

102. Trahan S, Tetu B, Raymond PE. Serous papillary carcinoma of the endometrium arising from endometrial polyps: a clinical, histological, and immunohistochemical study of 13 cases. Hum Pathol 2005; 36(12):1316–21.

103. Lax SF, Kendall B, Tashiro H, et al. The frequency of p53, K-ras mutations, and microsatellite instability differs in uterine endometrioid and serous carcinoma: evidence of distinct molecular genetic pathways. Cancer 2000;88(4):814–24.

104. Sakuragi N, Salah-eldin AE, Watari H, et al. Bax, Bcl-2, and p53 expression in endometrial cancer. Gynecol Oncol 2002;86(3):288–96.

105. Bancher-Todesca D, Gitsch G, Williams KE, et al. p53 protein overexpression: a strong prognostic factor in uterine papillary serous carcinoma. Gynecol Oncol 1998;71(1):59–63.

106. Salvesen HB, Iversen OE, Akslen LA. Prognostic significance of angiogenesis and Ki-67, p53, and p21 expression: a population-based endometrial carcinoma study. J Clin Oncol 1999; 17(5):1382–90.

107. Moll UM, Chalas E, Auguste M, et al. Uterine papillary serous carcinoma evolves via a p53-driven pathway. Hum Pathol 1996;27(12):1295–300.

108. Maxwell GL, Chandramouli GV, Dainty L, et al. Microarray analysis of endometrial carcinomas and mixed mullerian tumors reveals distinct gene expression profiles associated with different histologic types of uterine cancer. Clin Cancer Res 2005;11(11):4056–66.

109. Risinger JI, Maxwell GL, Chandramouli GV, et al. Microarray analysis reveals distinct gene expression profiles among different histologic types of endometrial cancer. Cancer Res 2003;63(1):6–11.

110. Zeisberg M, Neilson EG. Biomarkers for epithelial-mesenchymal transitions. J Clin Invest 2009; 119(6):1429–37.

111. Peinado H, Del Carmen Iglesias-de la Cruz M, Olmeda D, et al. A molecular role for lysyl oxidase-like 2 enzyme in snail regulation and tumor progression. EMBO J 2005;24(19):3446–58.

112. Yang AD, Fan F, Camp ER, et al. Chronic oxaliplatin resistance induces epithelial-to-mesenchymal transition in colorectal cancer cell lines. Clin Cancer Res 2006;12(14 Pt 1):4147–53.

113. Buck E, Eyzaguirre A, Barr S, et al. Loss of homotypic cell adhesion by epithelial-mesenchymal transition or mutation limits sensitivity to epidermal growth factor receptor inhibition. Mol Cancer Ther 2007;6(2):532–41.

114. Witta SE, Gemmill RM, Hirsch FR, et al. Restoring E-cadherin expression increases sensitivity to epidermal growth factor receptor inhibitors in lung cancer cell lines. Cancer Res 2006;66(2): 944–50.

115. Spoelstra NS, Manning NG, Higashi Y, et al. The transcription factor ZEB1 is aberrantly expressed in aggressive uterine cancers. Cancer Res 2006; 66(7):3893–902.

116. Singh M, Spoelstra NS, Jean A, et al. ZEB1 expression in type I vs type II endometrial cancers: a marker of aggressive disease. Mod Pathol 2008;21(7):912–23.

117. Blechschmidt K, Kremmer E, Hollweck R, et al. The E-cadherin repressor snail plays a role in tumor progression of endometrioid adenocarcinomas. Diagn Mol Pathol 2007;16(4):222–8.

118. Hipp S, Walch A, Schuster T, et al. Precise measurement of the E-cadherin repressor Snail in formalin-fixed endometrial carcinoma using protein lysate microarrays. Clin Exp Metastasis 2008;25(6): 679–83.

119. Kyo S, Sakaguchi J, Ohno S, et al. High Twist expression is involved in infiltrative endometrial cancer and affects patient survival. Hum Pathol 2006;37(4):431–8.

120. Yoshida H, Broaddus R, Cheng W, et al. Deregulation of the HOXA10 homeobox gene in endometrial carcinoma: role in epithelial-mesenchymal transition. Cancer Res 2006;66(2):889–97.

121. Xie R, Loose DS, Shipley GL, et al. Hypomethylation-induced expression of S100A4 in endometrial carcinoma. Mod Pathol 2007;20(10): 1045–54.

122. Xie R, Schlumbrecht MP, Shipley GL, et al. S100A4 mediates endometrial cancer invasion and is a target of TGF-beta1 signaling. Lab Invest 2009; 89(8):937–47.

ATYPICAL ENDOMETRIAL HYPERPLASIA AND WELL DIFFERENTIATED ENDOMETRIOID ADENOCARCINOMA OF THE UTERINE CORPUS

Anne M. Mills, MD, Teri A. Longacre, MD*

KEYWORDS

- Endometrial hyperplasia • Atypical endometrial hyperplasia
- Well differentiated endometrial adenocarcinoma • Endometrioid adenocarcinoma

ABSTRACT

The distinction between atypical endometrial hyperplasia and well differentiated adenocarcinoma of the endometrium is one of the more difficult differential diagnoses in gynecologic pathology. Different pathologists apply different histologic criteria, often with different individual thresholds for atypical endometrial hyperplasia and grade 1 adenocarcinoma. While some classifications are based on a series of molecular genetic alterations (which may or may not translate into biologically or clinically relevant risk lesions), almost all current diagnostic criteria use a series of histologic features – usually a combination of architecture and cytology - for diagnosing atypical hyperplasia and adenocarcinoma. This article presents evidence-based histologic criteria for atypical endometrial hyperplasia and low grade endometrial carcinoma (both FIGO grade 1 and 2) with emphasis on common and not so common histologic mimics. Grade 3 endometrioid carcinoma is discussed in the Oliva and Soslow article in this publication.

OVERVIEW

Endometrial carcinoma is the most common malignancy of the female genital tract.[1] The vast

Key Features
COMPLEX ATYPICAL HYPERPLASIA/ LOW-GRADE ENDOMETRIAL CARCINOMA

Uterine enlargement due to thickened endometrium often present, but not required

Voluminous endometrial tissue on curettage often present, but not required

Complex glandular architecture[a]: the degree of complexity distinguishes atypical hyperplasia from low grade endometrial carcinoma (see **Fig. 4**)

Cytologic atypia[b]: nuclear enlargement, nuclear hyperchromasia or clearing (vesicular appearance), nucleoli, loss of polarity, nuclear rounding, mitotic figures (can also be seen in non-atypical hyperplasia)

[a] Note: Rare low-grade endometrial carcinomas may have gland complexity in the range of hyperplasia, but harbor cells with marked cytologic atypia (prominent nucleoli and pleomorphism). This is typically a focal finding consisting of only scattered cells. If prominent and diffuse, a high grade serous or clear cell carcinoma should be considered.

[b] Note: The degree of cytologic atypia is often similar for both atypical hyperplasia and carcinoma, but rare low grade endometrial carcinomas may have deceptively bland nuclei – this is particularly true for mucinous carcinomas.

Department of Pathology, Stanford University, 300 Pasteur Drive, Stanford, CA 94305, USA
* Corresponding author. Stanford University School of Medicine, Room L235, 300 Pasteur Drive, Stanford, CA 94305.
E-mail address: longacre@stanford.edu

Surgical Pathology 4 (2011) 149–198
doi:10.1016/j.path.2010.12.007

majority (80%) of newly diagnosed endometrial carcinomas in the Western world exhibit endometrioid histology. Most endometrioid carcinomas of the uterus occur in perimenopausal and post-menopausal women under unopposed estrogen stimulation (Type I carcinoma). The unopposed estrogen may arise as a result of anovulatory cycles, estrogen administration, estrogen secreting-tumors, or conversion of androgens to estrone in adipose tissue in obese women. The average age of women with endometrioid carcinoma is approximately 63 years; most are low grade and confined to the uterine corpus at the time of diagnosis. Younger women with polycystic ovarian syndrome are also predisposed to endometrial carcinoma due to insulin resistance in peripheral tissues. These endometrioid tumors are frequently preceded by or coexist with atypical endometrial hyperplasia; most are low grade without deep myometrial invasion.

Women with an inherited predisposition to endometrial carcinoma tend to develop it ten years earlier than the general population. Most of these patients have Lynch syndrome/HNPCC (hereditary nonpolyposis colorectal carcinoma), an autosomal dominant disorder due to germline mutations in DNA mismatch repair genes. Although colorectal carcinoma is the dominant finding in this syndrome, approximately 30 to 60% of affected women also develop endometrial carcinoma and up to 50% of these women have endometrial or ovarian cancer diagnosed first as the sentinel cancer. In addition to microsatellite instability, characteristic molecular genetic abnormalities in low grade endometrioid adenocarcinoma of the uterus include alterations in *PTEN*, *KRAS*, *PIK3CA*, and *β-catenin*.[2]

ATYPICAL ENDOMETRIAL HYPERPLASIA: THE PRECURSOR LESION

Overview

The diagnosis of endometrial hyperplasia with atypia is one of the more problematic and arbitrary distinctions in gynecologic pathology. The most widely used criteria, adopted by the World Health Organization (WHO) in 1994, are derived from the outcome-based study by Kurman and colleagues[3] in 1985. However, these criteria are imperfect at predicting pre-cancer in the uterine corpus,[4] prompting the development of alternative systems, chief of which is the endometrial intraepithelial neoplasia system. The concept of endometrial intraepithelial neoplasia is derived from a number of carefully designed studies that have characterized expression of phosphatase and tensin homolog (*PTEN*) in the endometrium.[5-9] Like the p53

signature identified in the fallopian tube, the endometrium appears to exhibit a *PTEN* signature that may represent an early necessary, but insufficient step in endometrioid carcinogenesis.[10,11] However, as with the p53 signature in the fallopian tube, expression of *PTEN* in the endometrium is not a surrogate marker for precancer, as it can also be observed in a variety of non-precancer endometrial proliferations, including histologically normal secretory and proliferative phase endometrium.[12] Criteria used to make a diagnosis of endometrial intraepithelial neoplasia, like those used to make a diagnosis of atypical endometrial hyperplasia, are based on standard histologic features, but primarily reside in gland architecture and only secondarily in cytologic atypia. Since both systems appear to identify endometrioid lesions with a similar risk of progression to carcinoma, the diagnostic criteria for each are presented.[13] However, most treating physicians are unfamiliar with the endometrial intraepithelial neoplasia system and the utility (ie, value added) of this classification has not been fully established.

Gross Features

Hyperplastic endometrial tissue is generally more voluminous than normal cycling endometrium (with the exception of florid secretory phase or gestational endometrium). The endometrial tissue is pale tan and diffusely thickened throughout the uterus, although it may have a polypoid or diffuse and polypoid appearance. Foci of hemorrhage and/or necrosis may be present, especially if there is involvement of a polyp which has undergone secondary infarction. Since most women present with abnormal vaginal bleeding, the diagnosis is typically made on an endometrial biopsy or curettage specimen. The distinction between hyperplasia with atypia and hyperplasia without atypia can only be made on microscopic examination.

Microscopic Features

The WHO criteria for atypical endometrial hyperplasia are based on the presence of nuclear atypia in hyperplasic endometrial glands. Atypical hyperplasia is subdivided into simple hyperplasia with atypia and complex hyperplasia with atypia on the basis of the degree of architectural complexity, but most examples of atypical endometrial hyperplasia have complex architecture and it is the presence of atypia that denotes risk, not the degree of gland branching. Complex hyperplastic endometria typically exhibit a marked increase in glands (gland-to-stroma ratio is >3:1) with basic gland branching and budding and/or small villous or papillary infoldings and outpouchings (**Figs. 1–3**).

Fig. 1. Complex endometrial hyperplasia with atypia. (*A*) Budding and branching pattern is typical of complex hyperplasia, but this degree of glandular complexity is insufficient for a diagnosis of adenocarcinoma (see **Figs. 15**, and **17** for comparison). (*B*) The nuclei exhibit mild loss of polarity and enlarged nucleoli.

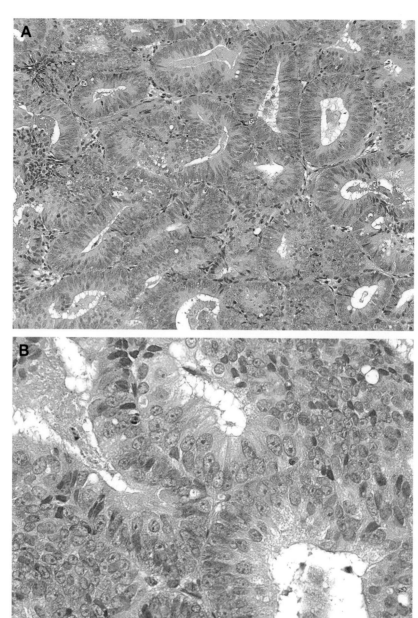

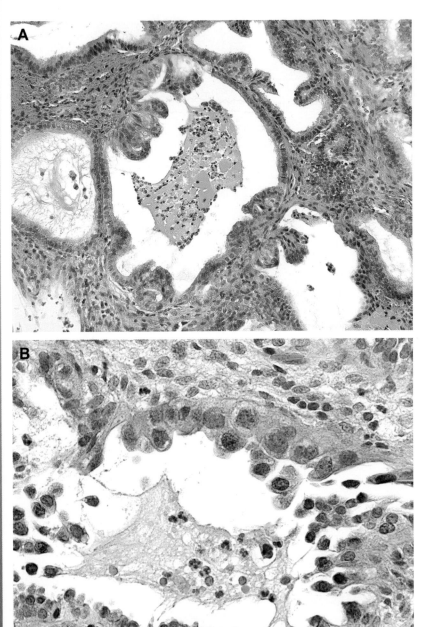

Fig. 2. Complex endometrial hyperplasia with atypia. (*A*) Macrogland pattern with small, non-branching intraglandular papillations (see **Figs. 16–18** for comparison). (*B*) Nuclei at top have distinct nucleoli and loss of polarity (compare with nuclei at bottom).

Fig. 3. Complex endometrial hyperplasia with atypia. (*A*) Macrogland pattern with simple villi/papillae. (*B*) The nuclei show mild loss of polarity; the nucleoli are minimally enlarged.

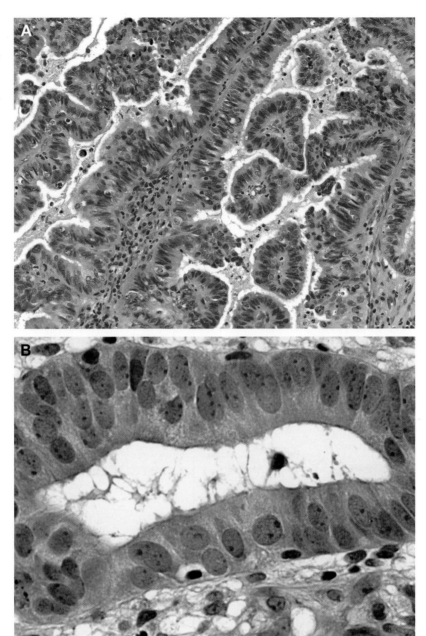

Features of nuclear atypia include: endometrioid proliferations, but does not sufficiently address the low level of atypia that can be seen in endometrial metaplasias, loss of polarity, enlarged nucleoli, nuclear rounding, and vesicular chromatin (see **Figs. 1–3**).[3] These cytologic changes should be present in the majority of the cells in any given gland. Mitotic figures and apoptotic figures are often present, but both may also be seen in hyperplasia without atypia.

Endometrial intraepithelial neoplasia is diagnosed on the basis of volume percentage stroma less than 55%, abnormal gland architecture greater than 1mm in linear extent, and cytologic features that differ from background endometrial glands.[14] The volume percentage stroma criterion is similar to the gland-to-stroma ratio criterion in the WHO system. The cytology criterion, while underspecified in comparison to the WHO criteria, emphasizes the importance of comparison to background endometrial tissue when making an assessment of nuclear atypia in these low grade endometrioid proliferations.

While it appears that both systems perform equally well at predicting increased risk for developing low grade endometrial adenocarcinoma, the WHO criteria are the most widely accepted and best understood amongst pathologists and gynecologists.

Diagnosis and Differential Diagnosis

The criteria for atypical endometrial hyperplasia include: loss of nuclear polarity, nuclear rounding, vesicular chromatin, and prominence of nucleoli. Mitotic figures are almost always present, but they are not a useful distinguishing criterion. The involved glands must be increased relative to surrounding stroma (gland-to-stroma ratio $\geq$3:1) and exhibit a complex architecture (= complex hyperplasia with atypia) or rarely, a simple architecture (= simple hyperplasia with atypia).

Atypical endometrial hyperplasia is distinguished from *well differentiated endometrial carcinoma* on the basis of architecture and cytology.[15] The architectural features of the glands usually inform the diagnosis. The degree of glandular complexity is higher in carcinoma than in hyperplasia (**Fig. 4**). Most low grade endometrial carcinomas exhibit cytologic atypia that is still in the range of that seen in atypical hyperplasia and so cytology is often not very useful in making this distinction; occasionally, well differentiated

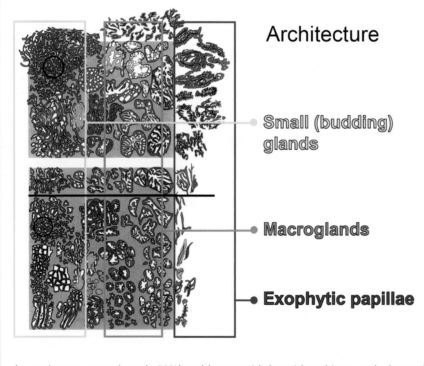

Architecture

Small (budding) glands

Macroglands

Exophytic papillae

Fig. 4. Architecture diagram for classification of low grade endometrial glandular proliferations. Gland patterns that map below the solid black line in the lower one-half of the diagram are classified as hyperplasia, while those that map to the upper one-half of the diagram are classified as carcinoma. A subset of gland patterns exhibit architecture that is intermediate between hyperplasia and carcinoma; this subset is represented by the zone immediately above the solid black line in the lower one-half of the diagram and is classified as borderline. Risk of myometrial invasion in the hysterectomy specimen is highest with high-risk architecture (= carcinoma, approximately 20%) and lowest with low-risk architecture (= hyperplasia, <0.05%). (*Data from* Longacre TA, Chung MH, Jensen DN, et al. Proposed criteria for the diagnosis of well-differentiated endometrial carcinoma. A diagnostic test for myoinvasion. Am J Surg Pathol 1995;19:371–406.)

endometrial carcinomas exhibit lesser degrees of atypia. However, there are occasional low-grade endometrial carcinomas that exhibit significant cytologic atypia beyond that which is accepted for atypical hyperplasia; this is most reproducibly recognized by the presence of prominent nucleoli and nuclear pleomorphism.[15] It is important to bear in mind that hyperplasia, particularly the atypical variant, is often coexistent with low grade endometrial cancer and samplings should be carefully examined in their entirety, often with level sections to exclude the presence of a higher risk lesion.

A variety of alternative epithelial types (metaplasias) may be present in the full spectrum of endometrial hyperplasia, including: ciliary (tubal) (**Fig. 5**), squamous (**Fig. 6**), eosinophilic (**Fig. 7**), mucinous (**Fig. 8**), papillary syncytial metaplasia

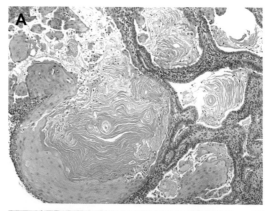

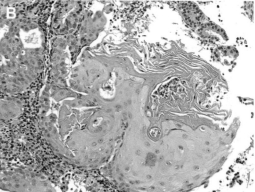

Fig. 6. Squamous metaplasia. (*A*) Continuity with the endometrial glands localizes this squamous proliferation to the endometrium. (*B*) Metaplastic squamous epithelium is cytologically banal. When extensive squamous epithelium is present in an endometrial sampling, the underlying glandular architecture cannot be assessed. In these instances, further evaluation is warranted to exclude an underlying carcinoma despite the apparent benignancy of the squamous elements.

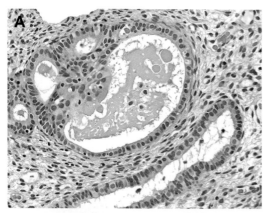

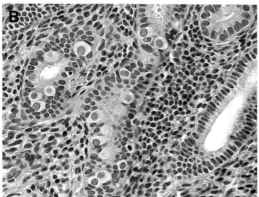

Fig. 5. Ciliated cell change/metaplasia. (*A*) Cilated cells are rounded, with fine chromatin. Eosinophilic cell change is also present. Most metaplasias are mixed. (*B*) Ciliated cell nuclei are rounded and often contain small nucleoli; these cytologic features do not warrant classification as "atypical" in this setting. Ciliated cell prominence is common in estrogenic states.

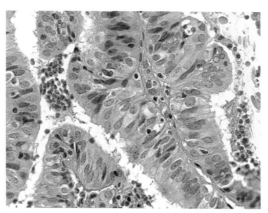

Fig. 7. Eosinophilic cell change is more prominent than the ciliated cell element in this example.

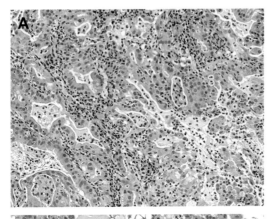

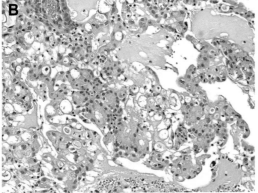

Fig. 8. Complex mucinous metaplasia with microglandular features (A) Low power appearance is similar to microglandular hyperplasia of the cervix (compare with Fig. 13). (B) A mixed microcystic and distended macrocystic appearance is common. Note copious mucin. Squamous component is absent.

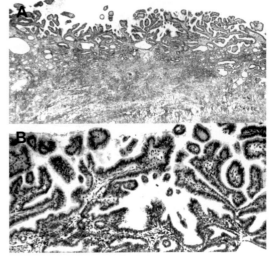

Fig. 9. Benign papillary change. (A) The papillae are short, non-branching or minimally branching. This pattern maps to the lower right quadrant of the architecture diagram in Fig. 4. (B) There is no cytologic atypia in benign papillary change/metaplasia.

(Fig. 9), and benign papillary change (Fig. 10).[16,17] Clear cell change may also be seen, typically in association with mucinous or squamous differentiation or in the context of hormonal influences. The chief reason to recognize these various metaplastic epithelia is to avoid misdiagnosis of atypical hyperplasia or carcinoma (eg, misdiagnosis of clear cell carcinoma in the presence of benign hobnail or clear cell change, misdiagnosis of serous carcinoma in the presence of benign papillary change or papillary syncytial metaplasia, etc). Once metaplastic epithelium is identified, it is important to remember to assess the background endometrial glandular proliferation independently of the superimposed metaplastic alteration(s) to determine whether there is atypia and if present, the degree of atypia (eg, atypical hyperplasia vs carcinoma).

Squamous metaplasia may be keratinizing or nonkeratinizing (forming morules). Squamous morules frequently show central necrosis (Fig. 11) and solid growth (Fig. 12); these features

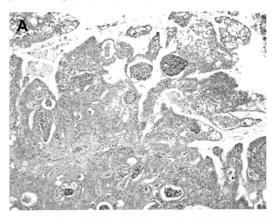

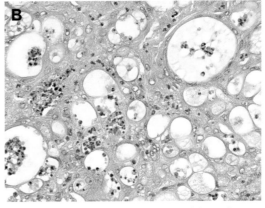

Fig. 10. Papillary syncytial metaplasia. (A) Papillae are formed by a syncytium of eosinophilic and mucinous epithelium. Neutrophils are prominent. This pattern is often encountered in endometria exhibiting glandular and stromal breakdown. (B) Microvacuoles are surrounded by pale-staining cells with indistinct cell membranes.

Fig. 11. Morular metaplasia. (*A*) Morular metaplasia with central luminal necrosis. (*B*) Necrosis is composed of necrotic epithelial cells, but the surrounding epithelium is benign.

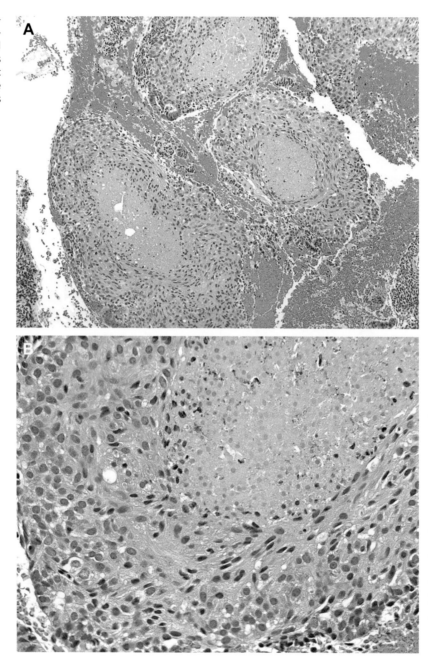

should not alter the interpretation of the background endometrial glandular pattern – in other words, a hyperplastic endometria composed of simple, tubular glands with morular metaplasia is classified or diagnosed as "simple endometrial hyperplasia with morular metaplasia." If the glands are complex, but not otherwise atypical, the appropriate diagnosis is "complex endometrial hyperplasia with morular metaplasia."

Often focal and mixed with other types of metaplastic epithelia, *mucinous metaplasia* may at times be quite prominent and pose significant differential diagnostic problems. The chief differential diagnosis is complex mucinous hyperplasia versus well differentiated mucinous carcinoma, but determining whether the lesion is arising in the endometrium or the cervix is also problematic. Since well differentiated mucinous carcinomas of

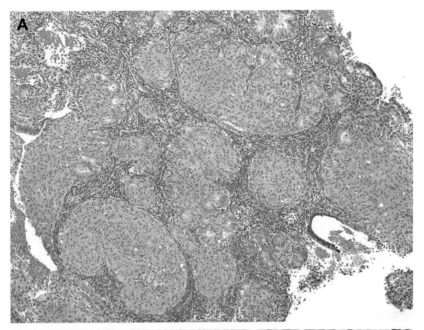

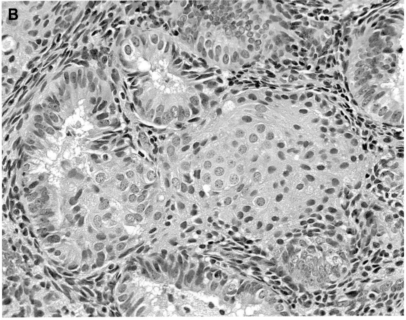

Fig. 12. Morular metaplasia, solid pattern.* (*A*) Morular metaplasia may extensively replace endometrial glands, forming coalescent sheets. (*B*) The morular nuclei may be rounder in configuration with small nucleoli when compared with the adjacent glandular epithelium. Solid areas of benign squamous or morular epithelium are not considered in endometrial cancer grading.

the endometrium may not always exhibit significant nuclear atypia, the decision between atypical mucinous hyperplasia and mucinous carcinoma rests on the assessment of the glandular architecture. However, a significant proportion of mucinous proliferations in the endometrium exhibit a glandular configuration that is borderline or intermediate to that of hyperplasia and carcinoma. In these cases, rather than err on one side or the other, a diagnosis of "complex mucinous proliferation, cannot exclude carcinoma" with a comment in the body of the report explaining the difficulty and raising the possibility that the lesion may also be arising in the cervix is prudent.

When the mucinous metaplastic epithelium is microglandular (see **Fig. 8**), the differential diagnostic possibilities include cervical microglandular hyperplasia and endometrial carcinoma with microglandular pattern.[18–20] *Cervical microglandular hyperplasia* is comprised of closely packed glands of variable size, shape, and internal cribriform complexity. The characteristic features include intraluminal mucin frequently admixed with neutrophils and variably shaped columnar, cuboidal, or flattened cells with prominent subnuclear vacuoles (**Fig. 13**). The nuclei are typically small, regular and often contain small nucleoli. Squamous metaplasia is frequently admixed, but mitotic figures are rare. In contrast, endometrial microglandular mucinous hyperplasia (with or without atypia) is architecturally similar, but generally features more attenuated epithelium imparting a mixed microcystic and

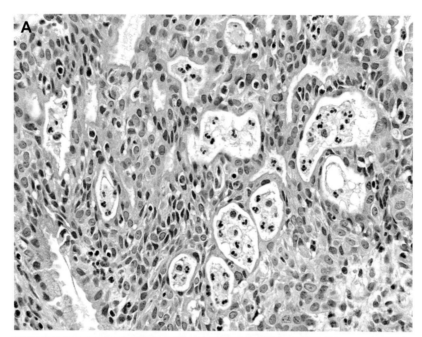
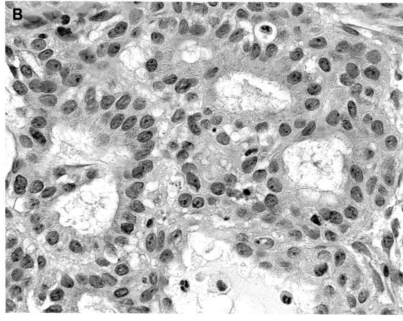

Fig. 13. Cervical microglandular hyperplasia. (*A*) Note closely packed glands of variable size, shape, and internal cribriform complexity. The characteristic features include intraluminal mucin with variably shaped columnar, cuboidal, or flattened cells with subnuclear vacuoles. A residual endocervical gland is present at bottom left. (*B*) The nuclei typically contain small nucleoli. Squamous metaplasia may be present, but mitotic figures are rare.

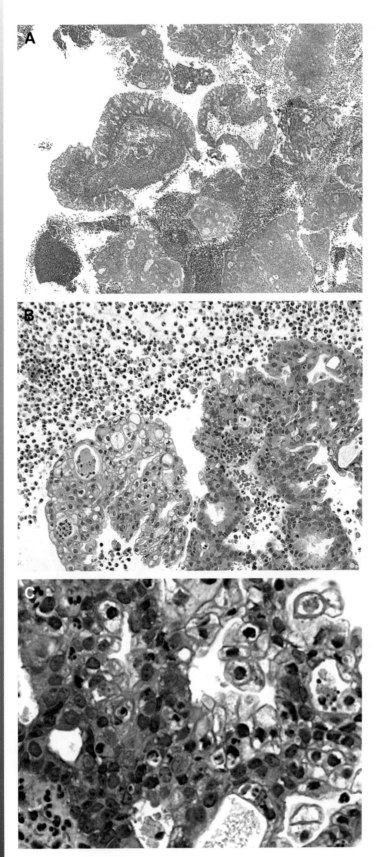

Fig. 14. Endometrial carcinoma with microglandular pattern (so-called microglandular hyperplasia-like carcinoma). (*A*) Diagnosis can be difficult and often requires identification of typical endometrial adenocarcinoma merging with the microglandular pattern or (*B, C*) the presence of significant nuclear atypia (nuclear pleomorphism and/or prominent nucleoli).

distended macrocystic appearance, more copious mucin and less pronounced squamous metaplasia (see **Fig. 8**). The diagnosis of endometrial carcinoma with microglandular pattern is based on identification of typical endometrial adenocarcinoma merging with the microglandular pattern or the presence of significant nuclear atypia (nuclear pleomorphism and/or prominent nucleoli) (**Fig. 14**). Identification of specific locational attributes (eg, stromal foam cells for endometrium) is an additional useful diagnostic maneuver; these are discussed more fully below.

Prognosis

In the 1985 study by Kurman and colleagues,[3] the risk of progression to adenocarcinoma among premenopausal women was 23% for atypical endometrial hyperplasia, whereas it was less than 2% for non-atypical hyperplasia. Subsequent studies have reported similar progression rates.[21] In addition, a recent study evaluating the WHO criteria for atypical hyperplasia and endometrial intraepithelial neoplasia found both to have similarly increased risks of progression to carcinoma.[13] However, a recent GOG study reported on the poor reproducibility amongst contributing institutions and a panel of experts in the diagnosis of atypical endometrial hyperplasia, with both underestimations and overestimations leading to misclassification of hyperplasia and carcinoma.[22] In a concurrent study, the prevalence of endometrial cancer in patients with diagnoses of atypical hyperplasia made by this same panel of experts was as high as 42.6%.[23] The importance of instituting a set of uniform, evidence-based criteria to be used by pathologists for the diagnosis of atypical endometrial hyperplasia and well differentiated endometrial adenocarcinoma cannot be overemphasized.[24]

Endometrial hyperplasia with atypia can be treated with progestins, but the response rate is poor compared with that of endometrial hyperplasia without atypia.[25] Nevertheless, a trial of progestin therapy is often recommended for premenopausal women who wish to preserve their uterus and for those postmenopausal women who are poor surgical candidates.[26] For all other patients, hysterectomy is indicated. Due to the poor reproducibility of the diagnosis of atypical hyperplasia amongst pathologists, the diagnosis should be confirmed by independent review before definitive therapy.

LOW GRADE ENDOMETRIAL ADENOCARCINOMA

Overview

Low grade endometrial carcinoma most commonly affects postmenopausal women (median age, 60 years) and is typically associated with pre-existing or concomitant endometrial hyperplasia. Premenopausal women may also develop endometrial carcinoma; almost all such

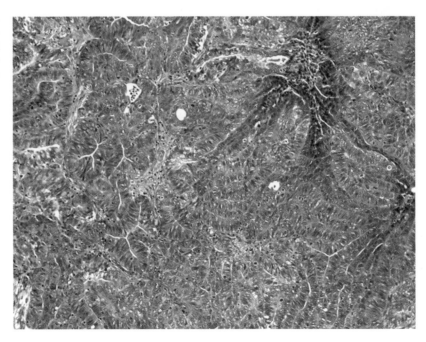

Fig. 15. Well differentiated endometrial adenocarcinoma. (*A*) Complex branching pattern (compare with **Figs. 1** and **4**).

patients have low grade tumors and evidence of excess estrogenic stimulation (obesity, diabetes, polycystic ovarian syndrome, etc).[1] Most patients present with abnormal vaginal bleeding. Indeed, any postmenopausal woman who presents with vaginal bleeding should undergo full evaluation, including an endometrial biopsy or curettage to exclude the presence of carcinoma. A small percentage of women do not present with vaginal bleeding; in some instances the diagnosis is raised due to uterine enlargement on clinical examination or abnormal endometrial thickening identified by radiologic imaging studies.

Gross Features

The uterus is typically enlarged and the uterine cavity is distended by low grade endometrial adenocarcinoma. The endometrial lining is thickened and polypoid projections into the cavity are often present. Rarely, low grade endometrial adenocarcinomas may directly invade the myometrium with minimal or no apparent exophytic

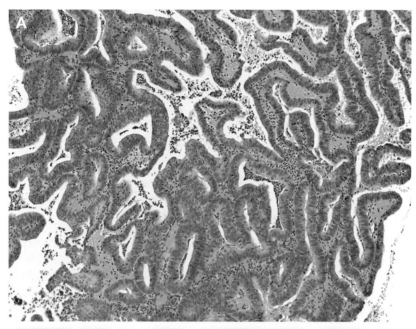

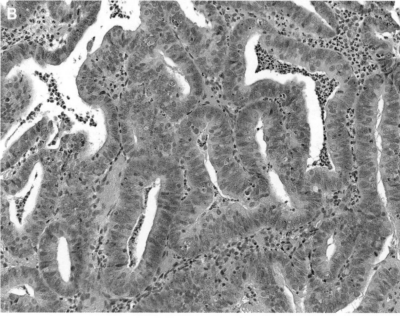

Fig. 16. Borderline endometrial glandular lesion. (*A*) Branching pattern is more prominent than in hyperplasia (see **Figs. 1** and **4**), but (*B*) not as well developed as in adenocarcinoma (see **Figs. 4** and **15**).

growth and are therefore not diagnosable on an endometrial sampling. These cases account for a very small proportion of endometrial adenocarcinoma in postmenopausal women and are often discovered at the time of hysterectomy for a diagnosis of hyperplasia on endometrial sampling.

Microscopic Features

The most clinically relevant approach to the diagnosis of low grade endometrial adenocarcinoma focuses on histologic features that predict myoinvasion in the paired hysterectomy specimen.[15,27] Only two diagnostic criteria with significant power aid in this distinction: complex glandular architectural patterns (glandular confluence, intraglandular complexity, and hierarchical papillary architecture) and marked cytologic atypia beyond that typically defined as atypical hyperplasia (= prominent nucleoli visible at low power and marked nuclear pleomorphism). Various lines of epithelial metaplasia (squamous, mucinous, ciliated, secretory/

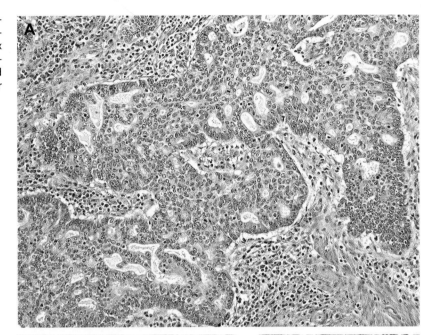

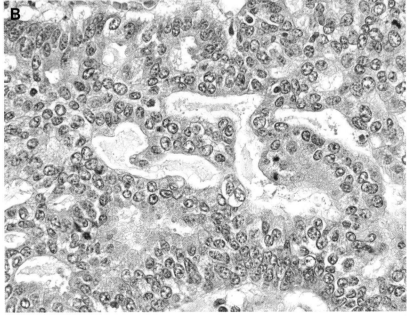

Fig. 17. Well differentiated endometrial adenocarcinoma. (*A*) Complex macrogland pattern (compare with **Figs. 2, 4,** and **18**). (*B*) Note nuclear rounding with nucleoli.

clear cell change) may on occasion pose specific problems in interpretation of these criteria, but this approach to diagnosis is not otherwise dependent on epithelial cell type.

The spectrum of architectural complexity that can be seen in low grade endometrioid proliferations (the hyperplasia-carcinoma spectrum) can be divided into three groups based on their associated risk of myoinvasion: Endometrial tissue specimens can be sorted into these 3 risk groups on the basis of three basic architectural patterns: small crowded glands, macroglands, and exophytic papillae, each of which may be admixed in a single biopsy specimen (see **Fig. 4**).[15,27]

Basic architectural pattern 1: small crowded (budding) glands

The proliferation of irregularly-shaped, small crowded glands with little intervening stroma is a common pattern seen in endometrial biopsies/

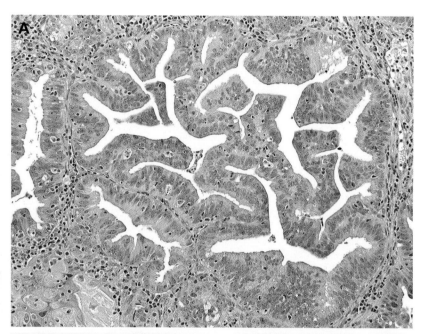

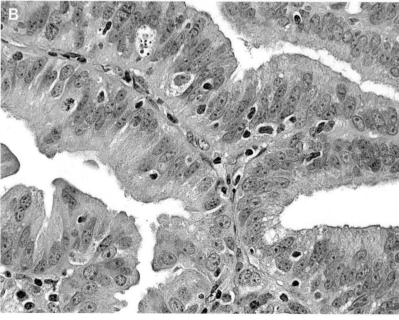

Fig. 18. Borderline endometrial glandular lesion. (*A*) Internal gland complexity is more prominent than in hyperplasia (see **Figs. 3** and **4**), but not as well developed as in adenocarcinoma (see **Figs. 1** and **17**). (*B*) Degree of cytologic atypia is similar to that seen in atypical hyperplasia as well as in well differentiated carcinoma.

curettings, and is generally the image pathologists associate with complex hyperplasia. The degree of glandular budding or confluence within this basic group can be stratified into three subgroups based on their associated risk of myoinvasion. The recognition of high-risk patterns involves glandular confluence <u>without intervening stroma</u> (**Fig. 15**). If a ×150 microscopic field (×10 objective and ×15 ocular) featuring this architectural pattern can be traversed in more than one direction without encountering stroma, then that focus represents a high-risk pattern (= adenocarcinoma). Cases showing an extreme, meandering or labyrinth pattern in any amount are also classified as adeno-carcinoma (see **Fig. 15**). Simple budding is equiv-alent to complex hyperplasia and is regarded as low risk when associated with cytologic atypia (see **Fig. 1**), whereas those proliferations that exhibit intermediate degrees of branching or only small foci of more complex branching are

Fig. 19. Well differentiated endometrial adenocarci-noma. (*A*) Villoglandular pattern. Note rigid, elon-gated, and branching villi. (*B*) The tips of the villi are typically pointed or angulated in villoglan-dular carcinoma; shorter, non-villous papillae are typically rounder.

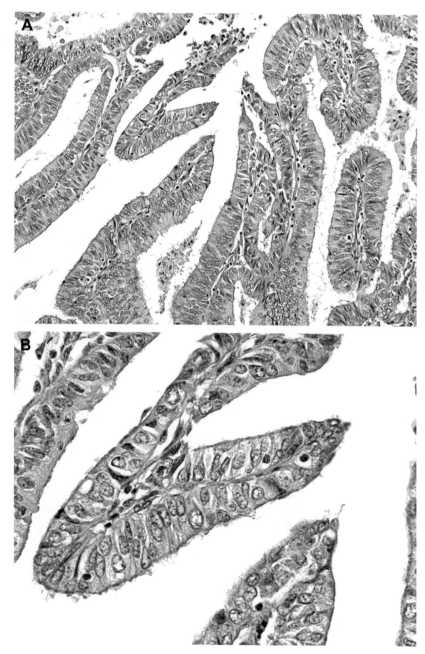

classified as borderline, cannot exclude adenocarcinoma (**Fig. 16**) and considered to be of intermediate risk for myoinvasion (approximately 5%).[15,27]

Basic architectural pattern 2: macroglands

Macroglands, defined as large caliber glands (often fivefold or more larger than normal glands) that may fill an entire low power field with varying amounts of intervening stroma, are another common pattern in biopsy specimens. They differ in their degree of intraglandular proliferation and are stratified into 3 risk groups depending on this internal structure. Low risk macroglandular proliferations may contain simple, non-branching non-villous papillae or minimal bridging arising from the lining epithelium (= complex atypical hyperplasia when associated with cytologic atypia) (see **Fig. 2**). The presence of well-developed secondary branching or multiple generations of bridging forming a cribriform pattern is associated

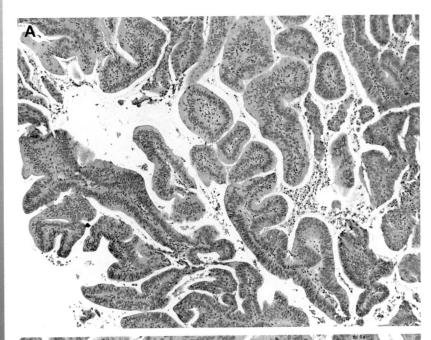

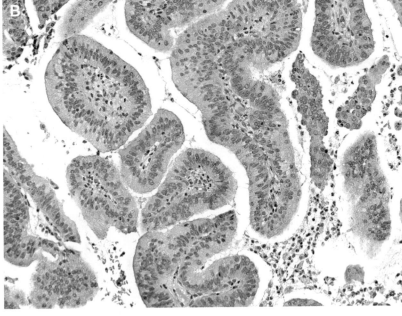

Fig. 20. Borderline endometrial glandular lesion. (*A*) The villi are more complex than in benign papillary change (see **Figs. 4** and **10**), but shorter and less angulated than in villoglandular carcinoma (see **Figs. 4** and **19**). (*B*) Some pathologists may interpret this degree of architectural complexity as representing carcinoma, but it falls short using the criteria discussed in this article.

with a significant risk of myometrial invasion (= adenocarcinoma) **(Fig. 17)**. Intermediate patterns containing focal secondary branching or focally mild increased complexity in a bridging architecture are classified as borderline (ie, complex atypical hyperplasia, cannot exclude well differentiated adenocarcinoma) and carry a low, but measurable and therefore intermediate risk for myometrial invasion (5%) **(Fig. 18)**.[15,27]

Basic architectural pattern 3: exophytic papillae

Exophytic papillary growth patterns fall into two broad groups: villous (or villoglandular) and short, nonvillous papillary patterns. As with the macro-glandular pattern, the degree of hierarchical complexity predicts the risk for myoinvasion. Simple non-branching villous and nonvillous papillae are in the low risk group (complex atypical hyperplasia, when associated with cytologic aty-pia) (see **Fig. 9**), while villous and nonvillous papillae containing second and third degree branching and/or cribriform budding are in the high risk group (ie, associated with myoinvasion) and classified as adenocarcinoma **(Fig. 19)**. As in the other patterns, intermediate forms may be encountered; these proliferations generally exhibit poorly developed or minimal second degree branching and are best classified as borderline lesions (ie, complex atypical hyperplasia, cannot exclude well differentiated adenocarcinoma) **(Fig. 20)**.[15,27] As noted in the atypical hyperplasia discussion above, it is important to exclude benign papillary change and papillary syncytial metaplasia when considering an exophytic papillary pattern.

Cytologic criteria

In some cases, the overall architecture of a clinically malignant endometrial glandular proliferation is not sufficiently complex to establish a diagnosis of well differentiated adenocarcinoma on architectural criteria alone. In most of these cases, the presence of marked nuclear pleomorphism and/or prominent nucleoli, identifiable at low power objective ($\times$150: $\times$10 objective with $\times$15 oculars) are sufficient to establish the diagnosis **(Fig. 21)**.[15,27] These nuclear changes may be present only focally within a given proliferation and are more pronounced than those typically designated as "atypical hyperplasia" (ie, approaching the degree of atypia seen in grade 2-3 adenocarcinoma). These criteria apply only to proliferations with non-serous and non-clear cell differentiation, almost all of which are endometrioid. Cases with simple gland architecture and serous or clear cell differentiation are designated as serous adenocarcinoma or clear cell adenocarcinoma, respectively, and are by definition high-grade (see Oliva and Soslow article in this publication).

Combining architectural and cytologic criteria

With the exception of the labyrinthine and complex nonvillous papillary patterns, a high risk pattern

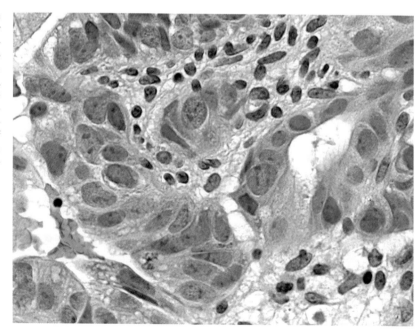

Fig. 21. Cytologic atypia in this architecturally simple endometrioid pro-liferation exceeds the degree of atypia seen in atypical hyperplasia. A small subset of FIGO grade 1 endometrioid ade-nocarcinomas are diag-nosed on the basis of marked cytologic atypia in the absence of archi-tectural complexity.

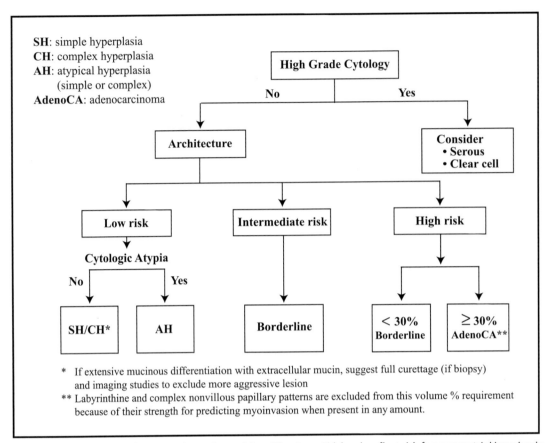

SH: simple hyperplasia
CH: complex hyperplasia
AH: atypical hyperplasia
  (simple or complex)
AdenoCA: adenocarcinoma

* If extensive mucinous differentiation with extracellular mucin, suggest full curettage (if biopsy) and imaging studies to exclude more aggressive lesion
** Labyrinthine and complex nonvillous papillary patterns are excluded from this volume % requirement because of their strength for predicting myoinvasion when present in any amount.

Fig. 22. Algorithm for classifying complex endometrial proliferations. Risk levels reflect risk for myometrial invasion in the hysterectomy specimen. Since the endometrial sampling is essentially a screening procedure, occasional false negative results will occur, particularly if the sampling is limited (ie, small volume and therefore non-representative, excessive fragmentation, extensive squamous differentiation, prominent surface mucinous micro-glandular hyperplasia). Since false positives may also occur, particularly when a complex lesion is present only focally, the presence of less than 30% of a high risk architecture pattern is usually insufficient to warrant a diagnosis of well differentiated adenocarcinoma, unless the lesion exhibits a papillary or labyrinthine growth pattern. (*Data from* Longacre TA, Chung MH, Jensen DN, et al. Proposed criteria for the diagnosis of well-differentiated endometrial carcinoma. A diagnostic test for myoinvasion. Am J Surg Pathol 1995;19:371–406.)

Table 1
Low grade endometrioid carcinoma variants

Variant	Description	Differential Diagnosis
Squamous	Rounded intraluminal morules or sheets of cells with sharp cell margins, intracellular or extracellular keratin; necrosis may be present	Primary cervical carcinoma Atypical polypoid adenomyoma
Villoglandular	Long, slender papillae with thin fibrovascular tissue cores	Serous carcinoma Primary cervical villoglandular carcinoma
Secretory	Subnuclear or supranuclear vacuoles due to glycogen accumulation, resembling secretory phase endometrium	Clear cell carcinoma
Ciliated	Extensive ciliated cell change (intracellular or membranous)	Endometrial hyperplasia, with or without atypia
Microglandular	Microglandular architecture with luminal secretions and neutrophils	Cervical microglandular hyperplasia Endometrial microglandular hyperplasia
Sertoliform	Hollow or solid tubules and/or cords of cells	Cervical adenocarcinoma
Spindled and corded	Spindled, corded or hyalinized stroma with or without osteoid-like or chondroid-like elements	Carcinosarcoma Adenosarcoma

should constitute 30% or greater of the abnormal glandular proliferation in an endometrial sampling to be classified as adenocarcinoma (**Fig. 22**).[15,27] If a high or intermediate risk pattern is present, but comprises 30% or less of the proliferation in the sampling, the lesion is designated as a borderline lesion. The 30% rule is not arbitrary, but optimizes the sensitivity and specificity (and hence, the reproducibility) of the biopsy as a screening test for the presence of underlying myoinvasion.[27]

Only tissue involved by the proliferation should be counted in the percentage estimate to prevent innocuous components of the sampling (eg, endocervix, disordered proliferative endometrium) from influencing the overall percentage.

Most low-grade carcinomas of endometrioid histology show a varied or polymorphous histologic appearance due to presence of metaplastic epithelium. Although the underlying glandular lesion is composed of columnar endometrioid

Fig. 23. Well differentiated mucinous endometrial adenocarcinoma. (*A*) The deceptively bland cytology in this subtype of endometrial carcinoma resembles its cervical adenoma malignum counterpart. (*B*) The epithelium resembles endocervical mucinous epithelium with basal nuclei. Extracellular mucin production is often abundant.

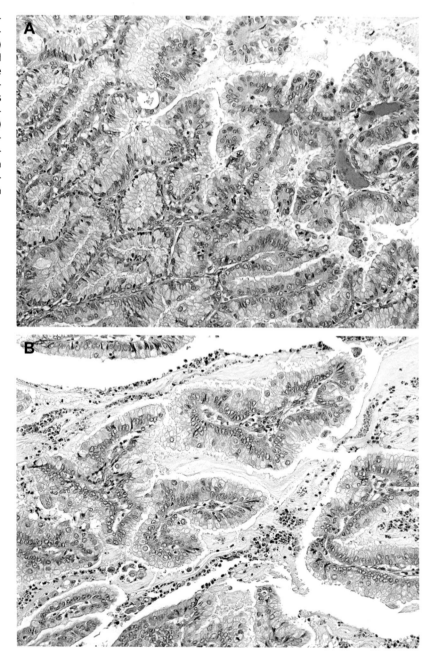

cells, squamous, mucinous, papillary syncytial, and eosinophilic epithelia are also common. When extensive, these metaplastic epithelia can mask the architecture of the underlying glands, making it difficult to determine whether a proliferation is endometrial or endocervical in origin and if endometrial, whether it is hyperplasia (simple or complex) or carcinoma; in these instances, resampling and/or differential curettage should be considered, especially if the specimen is a biopsy and not a complete curettage.

Low-grade endometrioid adenocarcinoma may exhibit several other variant histologic features which can also pose specific differential diagnostic problems (**Table 1**). However, low grade endometrial carcinomas with extensive mucinous differentiation (defined as the presence of intracellular mucin in 50% or more of the tumor cells) prove to be the most problematic. Mucinous carcinoma of the endometrium is uncommon, accounting for less than 10% of all low grade endometrial carcinomas. Most are low grade, but deep myoinvasion and even lymph node metastasis can be seen in these (often deceptively bland) tumors. Several authors have defined subtypes of mucinous endometrial carcinoma, based on variations in architecture and cytologic atypia, but these have not been tested in a large series.[28,29] Given the reported difficulty in diagnosing these low grade mucinous carcinomas, all cytologically bland mucinous epithelial proliferations should be diagnosed with caution in endometrial samplings. In particular, the presence of an endocervical-like mucinous epithelial process in association with voluminous extracellular mucin should prompt consideration for a minimal deviation (adenoma malignum-type) mucinous adenocarcinoma arising in the cervix or uterine corpus (**Fig. 23**).[30]

Diagnosis and Differential Diagnosis

The diagnosis of low grade (FIGO grade 1 or 2) endometrial carcinoma is based on architectural complexity (see **Fig. 4**) and/or cytologic atypia beyond that accepted for atypical endometrial hyperplasia.

Endometrial adenocarcinomas can exhibit a variety of unusual alterations that may pose considerable problems in differential diagnosis.

Table 2
Classification of complex endometrial proliferations based on risk of myometrial invasion

Diagnosis	Histology	Risk of Myometrial Invasion
Atypical Hyperplasia	Low Risk Cytology and Low Risk Architecture	<0.05%
Borderline Endometrial Proliferation[a]	Low Risk Cytology and Intermediate Risk Architecture	5.5%
Well-differentiated Endometrial Adenocarcinoma	High Risk Architecture (≥30%)[b] or Any Labyrinthine or Complex Non-Villus Papillary Architecture[b] or High Risk Cytology	20.4%

[a] Borderline is generally not sufficiently informative to the treating physician without further specification. Whenever possible, it is best to provide a diagnosis that identifies the reasons for the borderline diagnosis, ie, "[Complex] Atypical Hyperplasia, Cannot Exclude Well Differentiated Adenocarcinoma" for proliferations that feature diffuse, complex architecture bordering on, but not diagnostic of adenocarcinoma or "[Complex] Atypical Hyperplasia with Foci Bordering On (or Suspicious for) Well Differentiated Adenocarcinoma" for proliferations containing small (≤30% total volume of the problematic proliferation) foci that meet criteria for a high risk lesion but are too small to be diagnostically reproducible and so on.

[b] For this risk stratification, a high risk architectural pattern must comprise ≥30% of the glandular proliferation for a diagnosis of carcinoma (optimal sensitivity and specificity); labyrinthine and complex nonvillus papillary patterns are excluded from this requirement because of their strength for predicting myoinvasion.

Modified from McKenney JK, Longacre TA. Low-grade endometrial adenocarcinoma: a diagnostic algorithm for distinguishing atypical endometrial hyperplasia and other benign (and malignant) mimics. Adv Anat Pathol 2009;16:1–22.

Fig. 24. Atypical polypoid adenomyoma. (*A*) Irregular glands are embedded in a hybrid smooth muscle and fibrous stroma. (*B*) Morular metaplasia is present in most cases.

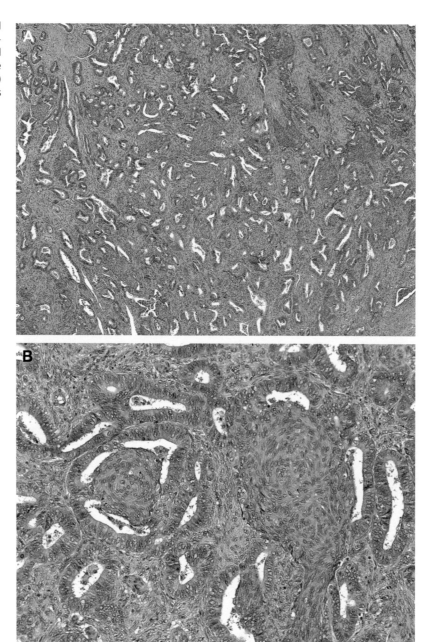

The chief alterations are that of hyperplasia and metaplasia. In addition, there are a variety of other proliferations that, because of their partial histologic overlap with endometrial carcinoma, may prove quite challenging when encountered in biopsy or curettage specimens. It is important to bear in mind that since many of these lesions are classified as "endometrioid" in differentiation, it should come as no surprise that tumors with overlapping features may be encountered.

Atypical hyperplasia exhibits lesser degrees of architectural complexity than low grade carcinoma (see **Figs. 1–3**). In most cases the degree of cytologic atypia is similar in atypical hyperplasia and low grade carcinoma; mitotic figures are present in both and are not useful in this distinction. In some endometrial sampling specimens, the architectural complexity appears to be too extreme for atypical hyperplasia, but does not clearly map into one of the high architectural patterns of carcinoma (see **Figs. 15, 17** and **19**); in these instances the distinction between atypical hyperplasia and carcinoma is not possible and the diagnosis of "atypical hyperplasia, cannot exclude carcinoma" is appropriate. This diagnosis serves to call attention to the estimated risk of invasive carcinoma in the uterus (more than atypical hyperplasia, but less than carcinoma, **Table 2**), and allows the treating physician the opportunity to tailor therapy accordingly.

Atypical polypoid adenomyoma is a localized, polypoid and complex endometrial proliferation set in a stroma composed of smooth muscle or more commonly, smooth muscle and fibrous tissue (**Fig. 24**).[31–33] The presence of complex and irregular glands within muscle can be mistaken for myoinvasive endometrial adenocarcinoma. The distinction between APA and well differentiated myoinvasive adenocarcinoma in an endometrial sampling is based on age (often <40

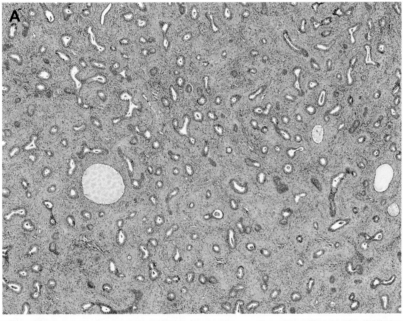

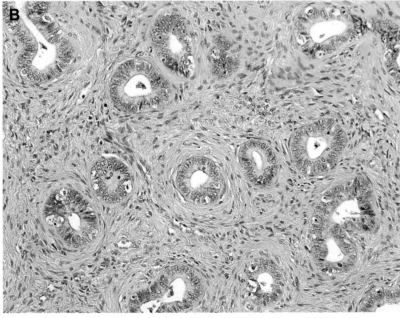

Fig. 25. Polypoid adenomyoma. (*A*) Glands are small or cystically dilated and regular in contour. (*B*) Morular metaplasia is typically absent.

Fig. 26. Clear cell change in endometrial adeno-carcinoma.

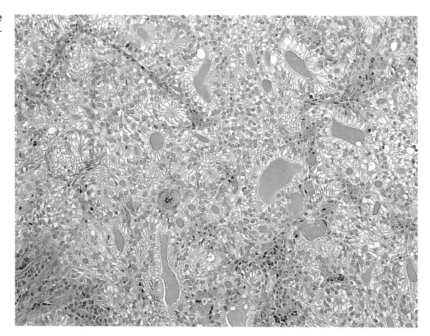

years for APA), hysteroscopic or microscopic evidence of a focal process, the presence of a biphasic glandular and fibromuscular stromal proliferation, absence of severe cytologic atypia and low architectural complexity.[31–33] Whereas most APA contain separate fragments of benign proliferative or secretory endometrium elsewhere in the endometrial sampling, most myoinvasive adenocarcinomas contain separate fragments of adenocarcinoma that are unassociated with the myoinvasive fragments elsewhere in the endometrial sampling.[34] Morular/squamous metaplasia is present in most APA and is often florid. Keratinization and necrosis within the areas of squamous

Fig. 27. Endometrial stromal tumor with glandular differentiation.

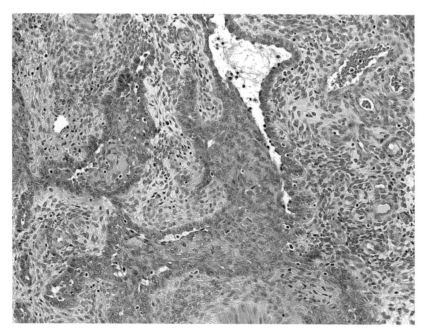

metaplasia are common. Many of the patients are nulliparous and a clinical history of infertility is not uncommon.

Polypoid adenomyomas or adenomyo*fibro*mas (PA) are circumscribed aggregates of fibromuscular tissue containing small, architecturally simple glands without branching or budding (**Fig. 25**).[35] The constituent cells are cytologically bland. Morules may be present but they are usually not prominent and endometrial stroma may be present. Polypoid adenomyomas are benign. They usually do not pose a significant diagnostic problem unless they are confused with atypical polypoid adenomyoma.

Clear cell carcinoma (see Oliva and Soslow article) is distinguished from endometrioid carcinoma with clear cell change by the presence of characteristic tubulocystic, solid, and papillary architecture in conjunction with high grade cytology.[16] Hobnail cells are often present. So-called secretory (endometrioid) carcinoma exhibits tubular architecture with prominent subnuclear or supranuclear vacuoles and low grade cytology. On occasion, higher grade cytology may be present, leading some pathologists to consider classifying these tumors as clear cell carcinoma (**Fig. 26**). However, this is usually an overdiagnosis as there are a variety of other processes that can

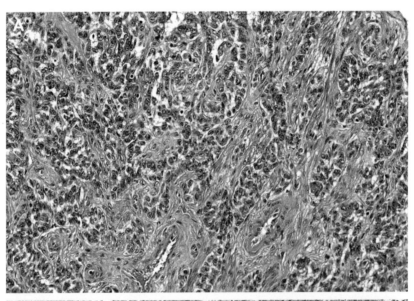

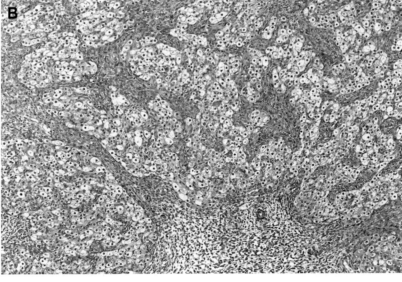

Fig. 28. Uterine tumor resembling ovarian sex cord stromal tumor (UTROSCT). (*A*) Glandular elements may be prominent and simulate an endometrial glandular process. (*B*) Luteinized cells and foam cells, if present, provide a histologic clue that the tumor is mesenchymal.

Fig. 29. Endometrioid adenocarcinoma with anastomosing cords and prominent trabecular pattern.

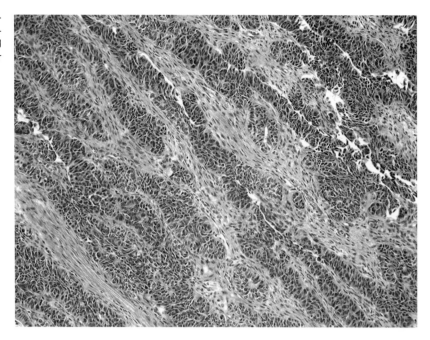

cause endometrioid proliferations to exhibit optically clear cytoplasm (eg, squamous glycogenization, lipid, artifact, etc).[36] Distinction from clear cell carcinoma is based on focality or mergence with other recognizable metaplastic epithelia, presence of columnar cells as opposed to cuboidal cells, and absence of marked nuclear atypia. The presence of squamous elements or areas elsewhere that are more diagnostic of endometrioid differentiation may help resolve this problem in endometrial samplings. If there is any uncertainty, it is better to diagnose the lower grade process, but mention the possibility of a clear cell component in the body of the report should this distinction translate into a different staging procedure. A definitive diagnosis of clear cell carcinoma in the uterus should be reserved for only those tumors that exhibit high grade cytology.

Serous carcinoma (see Oliva and Soslow article) is distinguished from villoglandular endometrioid

Fig. 30. Endometrioid adenocarcinoma with sertoliform pattern.

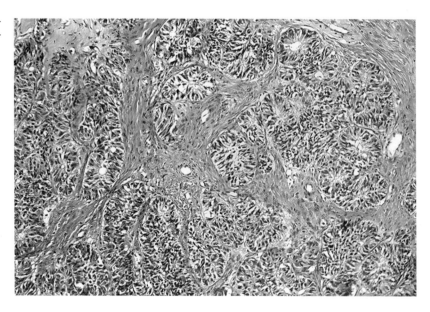

carcinoma on the basis of variable, complex papillae composed of broad connective tissue cores (or no cores at all), detached small aggregates or buds of cells with high grade nuclei and polyhedral (non-columnar) cells. Gland formation may be present, but the overall architecture is simple. Villoglandular endometrioid proliferations feature longer, more delicate, branching villi lined by columnar cells and low grade (nuclear grade 1 or 2) nuclei (see **Fig. 19**). Endometrioid carcinomas may feature smaller nonvillous papillae; these tumors typically feature grade 1 (or at most, grade 2) nuclei and can be recognized in larger samplings by their presence within typical endometrioid glands.[37] Rarely, endometrial carcinomas exhibit papillary or villoglandular architecture with only grade 2 nuclei. Whether these tumors represent endometrioid or serous histology has not been determined, but since they appear to exhibit clinical behavior intermediate to serous carcinoma

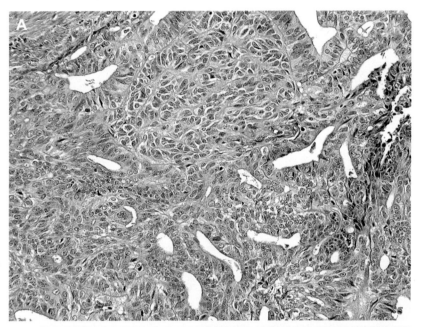

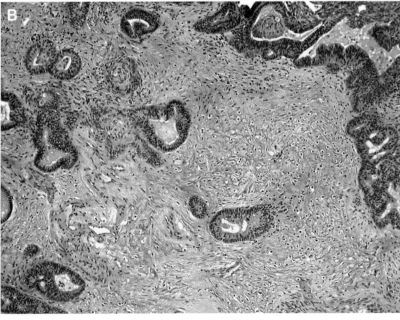

Fig. 31. (*A*) Endometrioid adenocarcinoma with corded pattern. (*B*) Endometrioid carcinoma with chondroid matrix. Both patterns may simulate a malignant mixed mullerian tumor. The presence of low grade endometrioid glands, abortive morular/squamous elements, and absence of significant atypia within the cords and matrix material are distinguishing features.

and villoglandular endometrioid carcinoma, they should be classified as FIGO grade 2 carcinomas.

Endometrial stromal tumors can show gland-like or sex cord-like elements that may be mistaken for an endometrial glandular proliferation (**Fig. 27**).[38] Recognition of the background endometrial stromal proliferation associated with a rich arteriolar network usually leads to the appropriate classification, but occasional cases may consist of predominantly sex cord-like elements and in these

instances, a trabecular and nested architecture often predominates, suggesting the diagnosis. The distinction may be especially difficult on small biopsies, where the border of the lesion cannot be appreciated. In hysterectomy specimens, the diagnosis of stromal neoplasms can usually be made on the basis of the pattern of myometrial infiltration (permeative with vascular intrusion in stromal sarcoma and circumscribed with no vascular invasion in stromal nodule), whereas

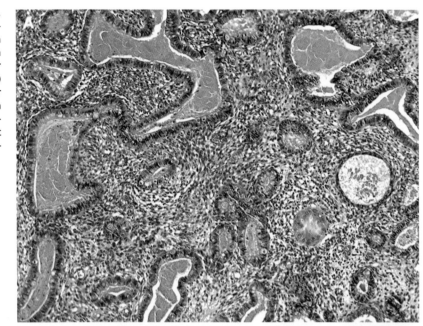
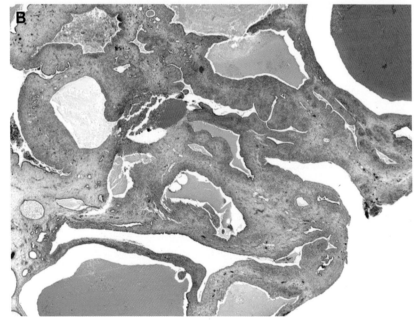

Fig. 32. Adenosarcoma. (*A*) Glandular component in adenosarcoma may exhibit metaplasia and architectural or cytologic atypia. (*B*) Attention to low power polyploid configuration and periglandular stromal condensation permit the appropriate classification.

Table 3
Features distinguishing endocervical and endometrial glandular lesions

Feature	Cervix	Endometrium
Clinical/Radiologic	Clinical examination Imaging studies Differential curettage/hysteroscopy with biopsy (to prove or exclude cervical involvement)	
Stromal	Eosinophilic, fibrotic	Endometrial stromal cells, foam cells
Epithelial	Adenocarcinoma in situ, especially with partial gland involvement; cervical intraepithelial neoplasia (CIN); carcinoma may merge with typical endocervical epithelium	Complex endometrial hyperplasia; carcinoma may merge with typical endometrial epithelium
Immunohistochemistry	ER-negative, vimentin-negative	ER-positive, vimentin-positive
HPV/p16^{INK4A}/ProEx C	HPV ISH-positive; p16^{INK4A} diffuse strong; ProEx C diffuse strong	HPV ISH-negative; p16^{INK4A} negative, weak or focal strong; ProEx C negative or focal strong

carcinoma is either confined to the endometrium or infiltrates myometrium in an irregular fashion, typically eliciting a host response. Immunohistochemistry is not useful in distinguishing stromal lesions with gland formation from endometrioid glandular processes, since both may express CD10 and keratin. However, desmin and/or inhibin or calretinin expression in glandular or sex cord-like areas, if present, favors a stromal process.[39]

Uterine tumor resembling ovarian sex cord tumor (UTROSCT) exhibits a variety of epithelial and stromal patterns that may mimic endometrial carcinoma (**Fig. 28**). Anastomosing cords (**Fig. 29**) and solid or hollow sertoliform tubules (**Fig. 30**) may be seen in low grade endometrial carcinoma, but the presence of prominent luteinized cells with foamy or eosinophilic cytoplasm (which must be distinguished from stromal foam

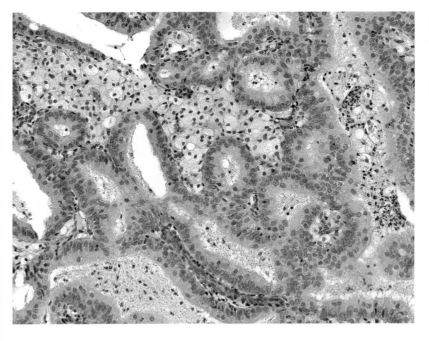

Fig. 33. Stromal foam cells are present in endometrial glandular proliferations, but are rarely, if ever, encountered in cervical glandular proliferations.

cells) in conjunction with desmin and inhibin expression on immunohistologic evaluation distinguish UTROSCT from adenocarcinoma.[39–41] Also, squamous differentiation is not present in UTROSCT.

Low grade endometrial carcinomas may contain a prominent spindled epithelial cell component, hyalinized osteoid-like stroma, or a cellular corded and hyalinized stromal pattern simulating a low grade *carcinosarcoma* (**Fig. 31**).[42] These tumors are distinguished from carcinosarcoma on the basis of low grade cytologic atypia and a lower degree of mitotic activity than that which is typically encountered in carcinosarcoma.[43] Additionally, they tend to occur at a comparatively younger age (mean, 52 years) than carcinosarcoma. A high frequency of associated squamous differentiation (70%) in these tumors has also been reported.

Rarely, *adenosarcoma* contains sex cord-like elements that mimic an endometrial glandular lesion. Adenosarcomas (and adenofibromas) can present with an exophytic papillary architecture simulating a carcinoma, but they typically have broader, more fibrotic to cellular stromal cores with intervening cleft-like epithelial-lined surfaces morphologically similar to phyllodes tumor of the breast.[44] The stromal predominance distinguishes these neoplasms from papillary endometrial epithelial proliferations. Like endometrial adenocarcinoma, the glandular cells in adenosarcoma may undergo complex squamous, eosinophilic or mucinous differentiation, but adenosarcoma also contains cystically enlarged glands and cleft-like spaces with intraglandular stromal projections (**Fig. 32**). Additionally, adenosarcomas contain a characteristic periglandular zone of stromal condensation. On occasion, adenosarcomas may contain foci of glandular atypia that meet criteria for carcinoma in situ or even focal adenocarcinoma. If the remaining glandular pattern is consistent with an adenosarcoma, the lesion should be diagnosed as such with a comment in the report that there are areas featuring carcinomatous epithelium. Such tumors are uncommon and so there is no outcome data (other than

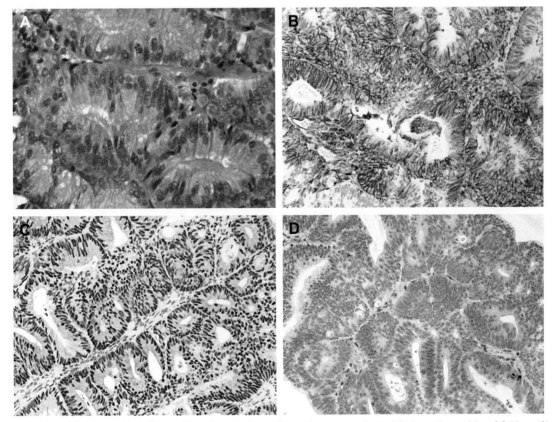

Fig. 34. (*A*) Mucinous glandular proliferations in the endometrium are typically (*B*) vimentin-positive, (*C*) ER- and/ or PR-positive, and (*D*) negative for p16 (or ProEx C, HPV in situ).

anecdotal) that supports this classification, but one would expect that such tumors would behave more like typical adenosarcoma unless there is associated high grade carcinoma, high grade sarcoma, or stromal overgrowth.

Distinction between primary endometrial and primary *endocervical adenocarcinoma* may be difficult, particularly in biopsy and curettage specimens. The distinction is important because the approach to therapy is different for carcinomas arising from each of these two sites. In many cases, a carefully performed physical examination with imaging studies and a differential curettage turn out to be the most useful diagnostic procedures. However, when the clinical, radiologic, and differential curettage data are indeterminate (**Table 3**), several histologic and immunohistologic strategies may be useful in determining the site of origin. The presence of stromal foam cells (**Fig. 33**) and background endometrial hyperplasia, in conjunction with a heterogeneous appearance of the neoplastic cells favor endometrial origin, while

partial gland involvement, adenocarcinoma in situ, and a more uniformly homogenous appearance with pronounced nuclear hyperchromasia and apoptotic nuclear debris, favor endocervical origin.[16] A panel of estrogen receptor, vimentin, and p16 (or ProExC or HPV ISH) is most useful for distinguishing low grade endometrioid adenocarcinoma from endocervical adenocarcinoma (**Figs. 34** and **35**).[45] Additional antibodies (eg, carcinoembryonic antigen or progesterone receptor) may also be used, but larger panels do not appear to add significant information beyond that of the three-marker panel.[45–50]

The most common sites of origin for *metastatic carcinoma* presenting in the uterus are breast, colon, stomach, and ovary.[51] Metastatic colon cancer (**Fig. 36**) may closely simulate endometrioid adenocarcinoma, while breast and gastric cancer are typically recognized by their lobular and/or signet ring histology (**Fig. 37**). Most patients have a prior history of carcinoma and the metastasis is not the first presentation of disease;

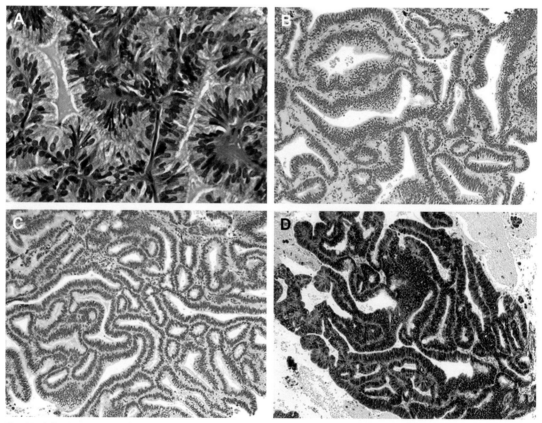

Fig. 35. (*A*) HPV-associated mucinous glandular neoplasms in the endocervix are typically (*B*) vimentin-negative, (*C*) ER- and/or PR-negative, and (*D*) positive for p16 (or ProEx C, HPV in situ).

Fig. 36. (*A*) Metastatic colorectal carcinoma. Note scattered goblet cells. (*B*) Distinction from endometrioid carcinoma is based on a (*B*) CK7-negative/CK20-positive phenotype.

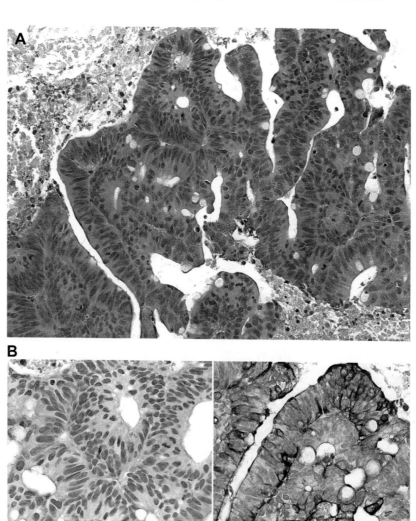

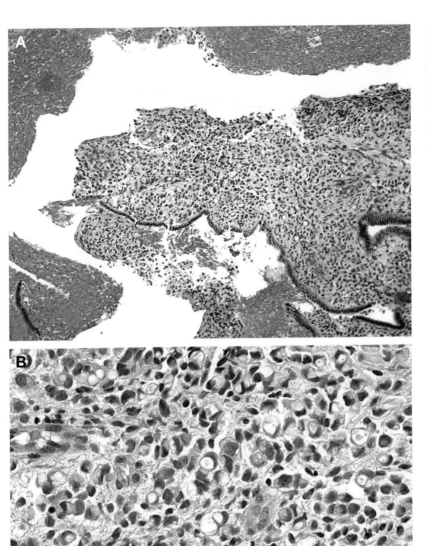

Fig. 37. Metastatic breast carcinoma. (*A*) Low power appearance may simulate a mesenchymal process. (*B*) Signet ring cells are typical of lobular carcinoma, gastric carcinoma, and rarely, metastasis from the appendix or colorectum.

however, not all treating clinicians and therefore, not all pathologists may be aware of this history at the time of evaluation. Use of a basic immuno-histochemical panel for undifferentiated tumors and a CK7/CK20 panel for gland-forming tumors in conjunction with a low threshold for suspecting metastasis will prevent most misclassifications.

Prognosis

Stage is the strongest prognostic feature for low grade endometrial adenocarcinoma (**Table 4**).[1] The FIGO staging system is a surgical-pathologic scheme that requires total hysterectomy, bilateral salpingo-oophorectomy, and assessment of any suspicious extrauterine lesions, as well as pelvic and para-aortic lymph nodes. Most low grade endo-metrial carcinomas are low stage and the overall prognosis is quite good. The 5-year survival rate for FIGO stage I grade 1 and grade 2 carcinoma is greater than 90% (92.9% and 89.9% for grade 1 and grade 2, respectively vs 79% for grade 3) and more than 80% for FIGO stage II (vs 66% for grade 3).[52] Recurrent disease, when it does occur, most commonly presents in the vaginal cuff, typically within 3 years following initial diagnosis and surgery. However, approximately 10% of patients develop recurrences beyond five years of initial treatment.[1]

Because of the overall favorable prognosis, patients with well differentiated endometrioid carcinoma are candidates for progestin treatment in lieu of hysterectomy. Although this therapy is typically reserved for younger women for whom reproductive conservation is an issue, older patients who wish to avoid surgery or who are poor candidates for surgery may also be treated with progestins. In younger women, successful pregnancy rates of 20 to 40% have been reported in patients so treated.[1] Success with this therapy is predicated on:

(1) Accurate diagnosis of the endometrial lesion to be treated
(2) Sufficiently high dose progestin delivered for a sufficiently prolonged period before re-evaluation
(3) Eradication of the lesion on follow up endome-trial biopsy and/or curettage.

Failures occur most often due to inadequate dosage, insufficient duration of treatment, and early or premature follow up evaluation of the treated endometrium. An additional source of failure is misdiagnosis of the initial lesion; for example, atypical polypoid adenomyoma may persist following adequate progestin treatment,

---

Table 4
International federation of gynecology and obstetrics (FIGO) surgical staging system for uterine corpus carcinoma

Stage	Definition
I	Tumor confined to uterine corpus
IA	Tumor limited to the endometrium or invades less than one-half of the myometrium
IB	Tumor invades one-half or more of the myometrium
II	Tumor invades stromal connective tissue of the cervix but does not extend beyond uterus (endocervical glandular involvement only should be considered as Stage I and not as Stage II)
III	
IIIA	Tumor involves serosa and/or adnexa (direct extension or metastasis)
IIIB	Vaginal involvement (direct extension or metastasis) or parametrial involvement
IIIC1	Regional lymph node metastasis to pelvic lymph nodes
IIIC2	Regional lymph node metastasis to para-aortic lymph nodes, with or without positive pelvic lymph nodes
IV	
IVA	Tumor invades bladder mucosa and/or bowel mucosa (bullous edema is not sufficient to classify a tumor as T4)
IVB	Distant metastasis (includes metastasis to inguinal lymph nodes, intra-peritoneal disease, or lung, liver, or bone. It excludes metastasis to para-aortic lymph nodes, vagina, pelvic serosa, or adnexa)

Data from Revised FIGO staging for carcinoma of the vulva, cervix, and endometrium. FIGO Committee on Gynecologic Oncology. Int J Gynecol Obstet 2009;105:103–4.

but this is not necessarily a warrant for hysterectomy since it is a focal lesion, poses minimal risk if carefully followed and is not incompatible with successful pregnancy.

When the pathologist receives a follow up uterine sampling in a patient who has undergone progestin therapy for hyperplasia or carcinoma, the prior lesion(s) should be compared to determine degree of response. The glandular complexity, gland-to-stroma ratio, and degree of atypia present, if any should be commented on. Complete response is manifested by diffuse stromal decidual-like reaction with inactive or weakly proliferative appearing glands. Often, there may be a more pronounced mucinous, squamous or eosinophilic metaplastic change than was evident in the initial biopsy (**Fig. 38**), since many of these metaplasias appear to be hormonally

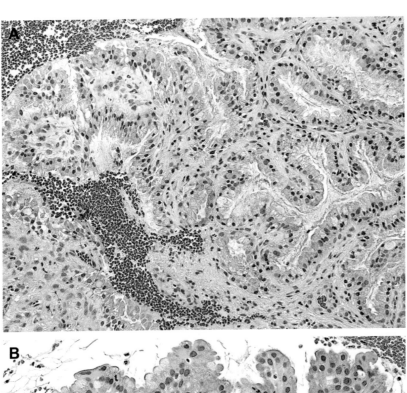

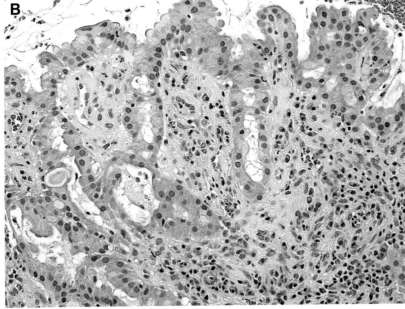

Fig. 38. Progestin treated adenocarcinoma. (*A*) There is more pronounced mucinous and eosinophilic metaplastic change than was evident in the initial biopsy (not shown here). (*B*) Note bland cytology and absence of mitotic figures.

Fig. 39. Endometrioid adenocarcinoma, FIGO grade 2. Solid component is greater than 5%, but significantly less than 50% of the tumor.

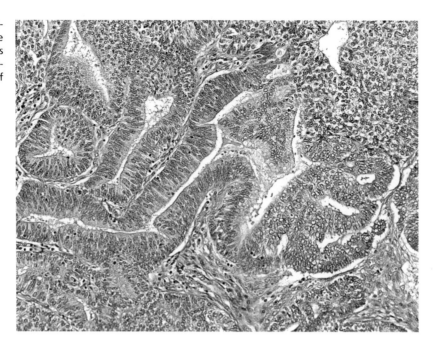

driven.[53] In some instances, partial response, followed by progression occurs and so all biopsies should ideally be reviewed.

ENDOMETRIAL CARCINOMA GRADING

The 1988 revised FIGO/ISGP (GOG) three-tiered scheme for endometrioid carcinoma relies primarily on architecture (**Fig. 39**) and secondarily on cytologic atypia (**Table 5**).[54] By definition, squamous or morular elements are not considered in the assessment of the solid component; however malignant spindled cell elements may occur in low grade endometrioid carcinoma and these latter elements do contribute to the overall FIGO grade (**Fig. 40**). Cytologic atypia can be subjective, but generally requires the presence of marked nuclear atypia (manifested by nuclear pleomorphism and large, prominent nucleoli) in a substantial proportion of the cells to warrant an upgrade (either from grade 1 to grade 2 or from grade 2 to grade 3) (**Fig. 41**). The degree of atypia required to upgrade is that which is seen in grade 3 carcinomas (= grade 3 nuclear atypia). Serous and clear cell variants of endometrial carcinoma are not assigned a FIGO grade, and are considered high grade, by definition.

There have been several proposals to move to a two-tiered grading scheme for endometrial carcinoma in recent years.[55–57] The desire to simplify grading is driven in part by the desire to improve the reproducibility of diagnosis. To date, these alternative schemes have not proven to be advantageous in terms of reproducibility or prognostic significance over simple dichotomization of the FIGO grading scheme (grade 1 and 2 vs grade 3) and have not been widely adopted.[55–59]

Table 5
International federation of gynecology and obstetrics (FIGO) grading system for uterine corpus carcinoma

Grade[a]	Criteria[b]
Grade 1	<5% solid component[c]
Grade 2	5%–50% solid component[c]
Grade 3	>50% solid component[c]

[a] Serous and clear cell carcinomas are high grade, by definition.
[b] High grade nuclear atypia in architecturally grade 1 or grade 2 carcinomas increases the overall FIGO grade by one.
[c] Squamous (including morular) elements are not included in the assessment of the solid component.

Data from Announcements: FIGO stages - 1988 revisions. Gynecol Oncol 1989;35:125–7.

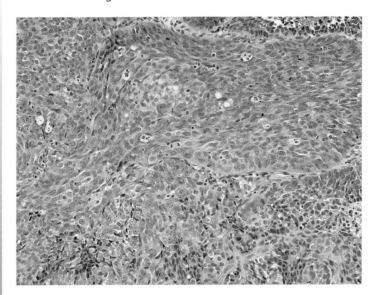

Fig. 40. Endometrioid adenocarcinoma, FIGO Grade 3. Solid component is spindled, but is distinguished from morular metaplasia by the presence of cytologic atypia and increased mitotic figures (compare with **Fig. 12**).

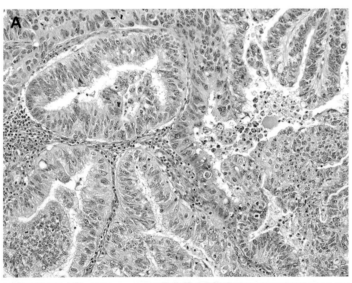

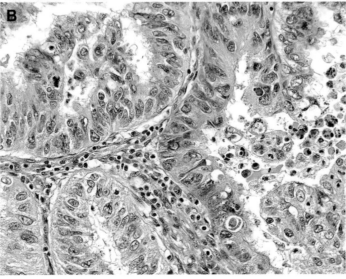

Fig. 41. Endometrioid adenocarcinoma, FIGO grade 2. (*A*) There is no solid architectural component, but (*B*) the degree and extent of cytologic atypia exceeds that which is typically seen in low grade endometrioid adenocarcinoma.

ENDOMETRIAL CARCINOMA STAGING

Overview

Endometrial carcinoma is staged and treated on the basis of the pathologic evaluation of the uterus and adnexa, and for more advanced or high grade tumors, peritoneal biopsies and lymph nodes. In many institutions, the pathologist assists in the determination of the extent of the surgical staging procedure, based on findings in the endometrial sampling and/or the uterus at the time of hysterectomy. Most of the diagnostic difficulties posed by these evaluations are centered on assessment for the presence and depth of myometrial invasion, the presence of cervical stromal involvement and the presence and type of ovarian involvement (metastases vs simultaneous primary ovarian tumors).[16]

Fig. 42. (*A*) Myoinvasive endometrial adenocarcinoma. (*B*) Typical granulation tissue-like pattern.

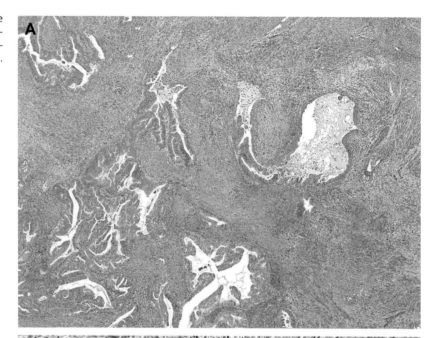

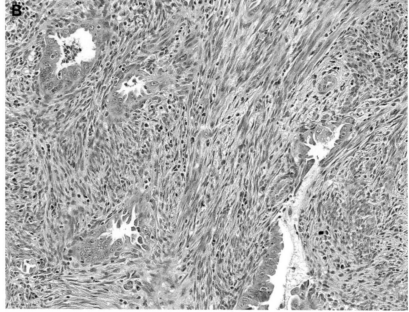

PATTERNS OF MYOMETRIAL INVASION

The most common pattern of myoinvasion by endometrial carcinoma is characterized by irregularly shaped, jagged glands dispersed in the underlying myometrium in an infiltrative pattern and separated from the myometrial tissue by a zone of edematous and inflamed fibroblastic or fibromyxoid tissue (so-called granulation tissue-type host response) (**Fig. 42**). In some instances, the glands at the leading front of invasion may be attenuated, forming microcystic, elongated or fragmented structures (so-called MELF pattern); these foci may be subtle and escape notice on a cursory, low power evaluation (**Fig. 43**).[60] The inflammatory cells consist of a mix of lymphocytes, neutrophils and macrophages.

A more diagnostically challenging pattern of myometrial invasion is the adenoma malignum pattern (so-called diffusely infiltrating or "melter" pattern).[61,62] The adenoma malignum pattern features widely dispersed single glands, often with minimal branching, throughout the myometrium with little or no host response (**Fig. 44**). The individual glands may show only minimal cytologic atypia in areas, although a scrupulous search often discloses cytologic features of carcinoma and at least some glands with a more characteristic, but blunted fibromyxoid host response. This condition almost always manifests as massive myometrial infiltration in the involved areas. Although

an early report suggested that this pattern may represent a more clinically aggressive form of endometrial carcinoma, this was not substantiated in the larger Stanford series when controlled for grade and stage of disease.[61,63]

Cancerous involvement of foci of adenomyosis does not qualify as myometrial invasion (**Fig. 45**) However, cases that demonstrate extensive involvement of adenomyosis with focal unequivocal invasion from one or more of these foci are diagnosed as "focal (or multifocal) invasion from adenomyosis" and the depth of the invasive focus (ie, whether it is arising in superficial or deep adenomyosis) is specified. Whether invasion from deep adenomyosis (outer one-half of myometrium) confers the same risk as deep myometrial invasion from the surface endometrium is unknown.

PATTERNS OF CERVICAL STROMAL INVASION

To qualify as cervical involvement by endometrial carcinoma, the 2009 FIGO (FIGO stage II) and the 7th edition of the AJCC staging manual require the presence of cervical stromal invasion.[64,65] The most important strategy in making this determination is adequate sectioning of the hysterectomy specimen. Sections of the corpus should be obtained in a cross-sectional manner to obtain the most complete view of the myometrium, but commencing in the lower uterine segment, sections should be taken longitudinally to visualize

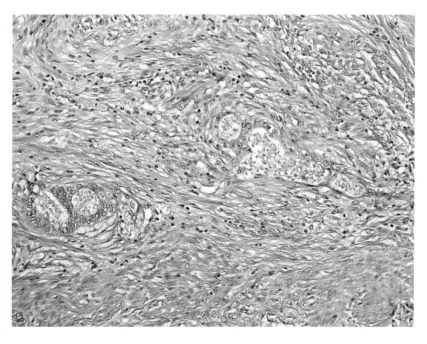

Fig. 43. Microcystic elongated and fragmented glands at the leading front of invasion (so-called MELF pattern) may be subtle and escape notice on a cursory, low power evaluation.

Fig. 44. "Melting" pattern (or so-called adenoma malignum pattern) of myometrial invasion simulates invasive pattern seen in adenoma malignum of the uterine cervix. (*A*) The uterus is diffusely permeated by small glands with minimal or no stromal response. (*B*) Despite the architectural simplicity, the cytology is atypical in this deeply myoinvasive well differentiated adenocarcinoma.

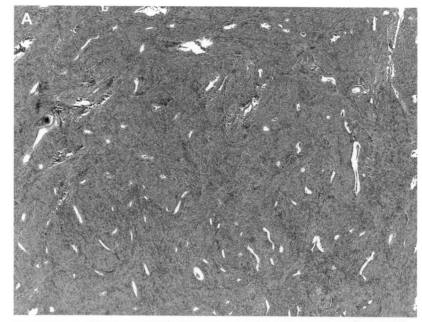

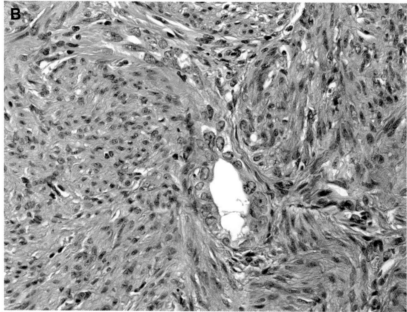

the transition from lower uterine segment to endocervix. Clear involvement of stromal tissue bearing endocervical glands is definitive evidence of cervical stromal involvement. Care must be taken to ensure the glandular process is histologically malignant. Foci of atypical endometriosis

(**Fig. 46**), tubo-endometrial metaplasia (**Fig. 47**), florid endosalpingiosis, and superficial cervical extension of hyperplastic endometrium should be excluded. As some metastases of low grade endometrioid carcinoma may appear more mature (ie, are better differentiated than the primary tumor),

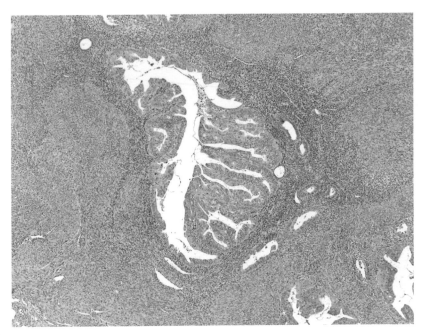

Fig. 45. Adenocarcinoma involving adenomyosis is not considered to be a pattern of myometrial invasion. It is recognized by its smooth contour, residual benign endometrial glands or stroma (often compressed along one edge), and presence of concentric smooth muscle hypertrophy typical of adenomyosis.

this distinction can be quite difficult on frozen section.

Occasionally, endometrial carcinoma may infiltrate the endocervical stroma in a pattern that is reminiscent of a primary endocervical process – either endocervical carcinoma, when the glands are histologically malignant or endocervical hyperplasia (particularly mesonephric hyperplasia), when the glands exhibit deceptively bland architectural and cytologic features (**Fig. 48**).[66] In these cases, the invasive front tends to exhibit a burrowing pattern, sparing the superficial glandular portion of the cervix, and often extending deeper into the cervix than in the myometrium (in some cases, little or no myometrial invasion is present, despite deep cervical stromal involvement). The constituent glands are smaller or more cystic, exhibit lesser degrees of atypia than the uterine component, often exhibit little or no stromal response and probably represent a variant of the diffusely infiltrating "melter" pattern of invasion seen in the myometrium. Mergence of the endometrial and endocervical components is almost always present, but may require additional sectioning.

Rarely, low grade endometrioid carcinoma exhibits cervical stromal involvement with no apparent myometrial invasion. This is an uncommon finding, for which there is little clinical outcome information.

LYMPHATIC VESSEL INVASION

Most, but not all studies suggest the presence of lymphatic vessel invasion (LVI) in the myometrium is a poor prognostic indicator. Since LVI may increase the probability of lymph node metastasis, the presence or absence of LVI should be reported for all patients undergoing a staging procedure for endometrial carcinoma. LVI can be subtle, consisting of pale staining "histiocytoid" tumor cells that in some cases are masked by admixed intravascular inflammatory cells (**Fig. 49**).[67] A perivascular lymphoid infiltrate may also "flag" areas of possible intravascular invasion. LVI often occurs along the base of the advancing tumor front, but may be scattered widely throughout the uterus. When encountered near the invasive tumor, it may be very difficult to distinguish LVI from stromal retraction. Use of D2-40 to highlight lymphatic endothelium and cytokeratin to highlight intralymphatic tumor cells can be helpful in problematic cases (see **Fig. 49**).

There are a variety of mimics of LVI. Just as menstrual endometrium may occasionally become displaced into myometrial blood vessels, so too can

Fig. 46. (*A*) Endometriosis may mimic metastatic endometrioid adenocarcinoma in biopsies obtained for staging or possible recurrence. (*B*) The presence of endometrial stroma, and hemosiderin, as well as a history of endometriosis help differentiate the two processes.

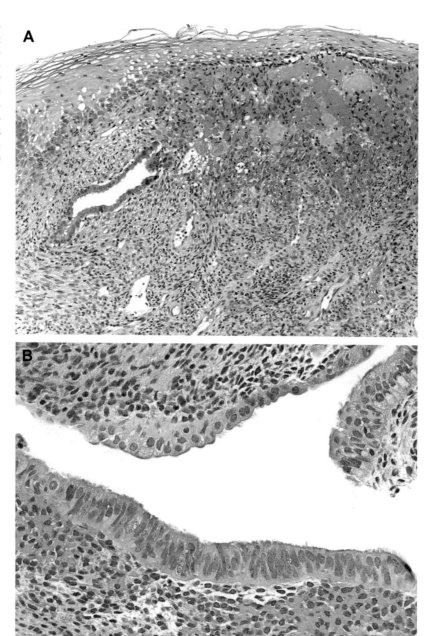

tumor plugs. This pseudoinvasion of vascular spaces is encountered most commonly in laparoscopic and robotic-assisted hysterectomy specimens and has been variously attributed to an artifact of the procedure itself as well as to manipulation by the pathologist.[68,69] Key distinguishing features are the presence of widespread pseudovascular involvement in a well differentiated carcinoma with minimal or no myometrial invasion, preferential involvement of thick-walled vessels in the outer myometrium or ectatic vessels anywhere in the myometrium, tumor fragments in artifactual tissue clefts elsewhere in the myometrium, absence of attachment to the vessel wall, and absence of an inflammatory cell infiltrate in the myometrium surrounding the involved vessel walls (**Fig. 50**).

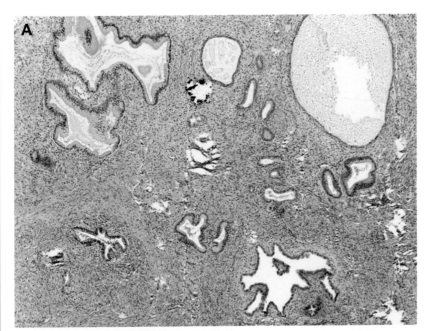

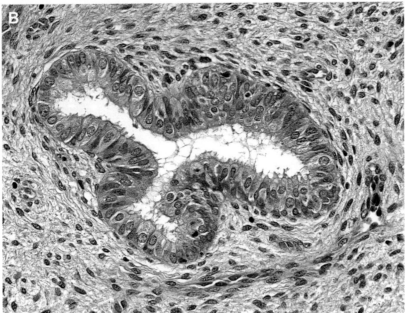

Fig. 47. (*A*) Tuboendo-metrioid metaplasia of the uterine cervix is distin-guished from endome-trioid carcinoma by (*B*) bland cytology, simple architecture, and absence of stromal response.

SIMULTANEOUS OVARIAN (OR TUBAL) PRIMARY

Low grade endometrioid carcinomas are associated with synchronous endometrioid borderline tumors and low-grade endometrioid carcinomas of the ovary (and occasionally, of the fallopian tube) in 15 to 20% of cases.[70] In some cases,

the tumors exhibit mucinous histology. A variety of molecular approaches have been used to determine whether these concurrent tumors are independent primary tumors or metastases from one organ to the other, with variable results.[71–77] However, provided these low-grade tumors are (1) confined to the uterus and are minimally invasive (inner one-half of the myometrium, with no

Fig. 48. (*A*) Rarely, endo-metrioid adenocarcinoma may invade the cervix with a deceptively bland appearance, often simu-lating endocervical meso-nephric hyperplasia. (*B*) The constituent glands are smaller, exhibit lesser degrees of atypia than the uterine component, often exhibit little or no stromal response and pro-bably represent a variant of the diffusely infil-trating "melter" pattern of invasion seen in the myometrium.

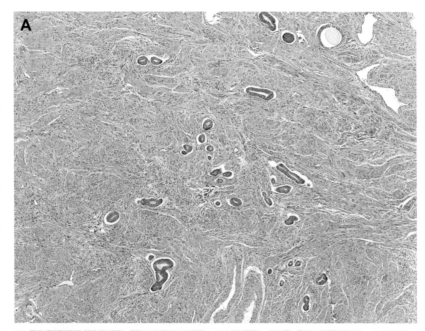

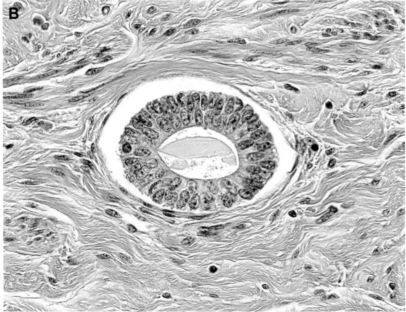

LVI and no cervical stromal involvement) and (2) confined to the ovary (with no hilar LVI, and no predominant surface or parenchymal nodular distribution), the prognosis is highly favorable and similar to that of low grade carcinoma restricted to one or the other organ.[78] In the pres-ence of deep myoinvasion (outer one-half of myometrium with or without prominent LVI) and nodular surface involvement of one or both ovaries (with or without hilar LVI), ovarian metastasis(es) from a uterine primary should be considered. Synchronous primary carcinomas of the ovary and endometrium are unlikely to be part of the Lynch syndrome in absence of a family history.[79]

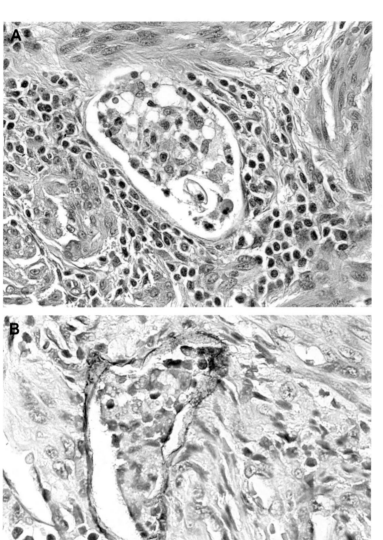

Fig. 49. (*A*) Lymph-vascular space involvement (LVI) in low grade adenocarcinoma is often associated with an inflammatory response in the adjacent myometrium. (*B*) Lymphatic endothelium can be confirmed in problematic cases by positive reaction with D2-40.

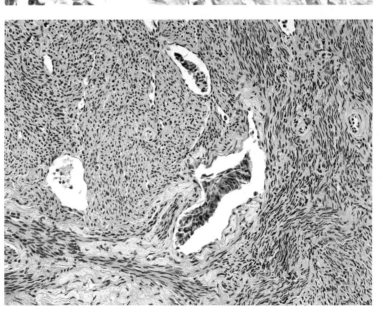

Fig. 50. Pseudovascular invasion is due to artifactual displacement, either at the time of the procedure or during sectioning of the hysterectomy specimen. Note the vessels are ectatic, there is no attachment to the vascular endothelium and there is no inflammatory response.

⚠ Pitfalls
COMPLEX ATYPICAL HYPERPLASIA/
LOW-GRADE ENDOMETRIAL CARCINOMA

! Fragments of atypical polypoid adenomyoma can be misinterpreted as atypical hyperplasia and carcinoma, but are recognized on the basis of focality, morular/squamous metaplasia, and normal cycling endometrium elsewhere in the specimen

! Prominent squamous metaplasia can mask glandular tissue, preventing assessment for overall complexity. Rebiopsy or curettage should be performed to exclude an underlying endometrial lesion. If there is doubt about the source of the squamous epithelium (cervix vs endometrium), differential curettage should resolve this problem

! Mucinous hyperplasia and carcinomas can be deceptively bland and should be viewed with caution, particularly if associated with voluminous extracellular mucin. Consider diagnosis of "complex mucinous proliferation, cannot exclude mucinous carcinoma" for borderline cases

! Scant specimens with fragmented or disrupted glandular tissue may not be representative. Suggest rebiopsy or curettage, especially when there is strong clinical suspicion for an underlying endometrial process

! Extensive necrosis in a uterine sampling should prompt consideration for further study – either rebiopsy and/or curettage or hysterectomy if there is strong clinical suspicion for malignancy

! Papillary architecture can be seen in a variety of benign metaplastic and hyperplastic processes, but cytologic atypia is minimal or absent in most cases

! Ciliated cells may contain small nucleoli but are recognized on the basis of ovoid or polyhedral configuration and presence of apical cilia on adjacent cells

! Endocervical carcinoma can mimic atypical endometrial hyperplasia or carcinoma, but can be identified using immunohistochemical panel consisting of ER, vimentin, and p16/HPV in situ/ProEx C

! Metastasis, particularly colorectal, can mimic endometrial carcinoma, but can be recognized by presence of goblet cells, excess necrosis, and garland pattern. Clinical history, if available, is most useful.

PERITONEAL WASHINGS

The newly adopted FIGO staging system no longer includes positive cytology to determine stage, but cytology results of peritoneal washings should be reported, when available.[64]

REFERENCES

1. Hacker N. Uterine cancer. In: Berek JS, Hacker NF, editors. Gynecologic oncology. Philadelphia: Lippincott Williams and Wilkins; 2009. p. 36.
2. Prat J, Gallardo A, Cuatrecasas M, et al. Endometrial carcinoma: pathology and genetics. Pathology 2007;39:72–87.
3. Kurman RJ, Kaminski PF, Norris HJ. The behavior of endometrial hyperplasia. A long-term study of "untreated" hyperplasia in 170 patients. Cancer 1985;56:403–12.
4. Kendall BS, Ronnett BM, Isacson C, et al. Reproducibility of the diagnosis of endometrial hyperplasia, atypical hyperplasia, and well-differentiated carcinoma. Am J Surg Pathol 1998;22:1012–9.
5. Mutter GL. Endometrial intraepithelial neoplasia (EIN): will it bring order to chaos? The Endometrial Collaborative Group. Gynecol Oncol 2000;76: 287–90.
6. Mutter GL, Baak JP, Crum CP, et al. Endometrial precancer diagnosis by histopathology, clonal analysis, and computerized morphometry. J Pathol 2000;190: 462–9.
7. Mutter GL, Ince TA, Baak JP, et al. Molecular identification of latent precancers in histologically normal endometrium. Cancer Res 2001;61:4311–4.
8. Mutter GL, Lin MC, Fitzgerald JT, et al. Altered PTEN expression as a diagnostic marker for the earliest endometrial precancers. J Natl Cancer Inst 2000; 92:924–30.
9. Mutter GL, Lin MC, Fitzgerald JT, et al. Changes in endometrial PTEN expression throughout the human menstrual cycle. J Clin Endocrinol Metab 2000;85: 2334–8.
10. Folkins AK, Jarboe EA, Saleemuddin A, et al. A candidate precursor to pelvic serous cancer (p53 signature) and its prevalence in ovaries and fallopian tubes from women with BRCA mutations. Gynecol Oncol 2008;109:168–73.
11. Jarboe EA, Pizer ES, Miron A, et al. Evidence for a latent precursor (p53 signature) that may precede serous endometrial intraepithelial carcinoma. Mod Pathol 2009;22:345–50.
12. Lacey JV Jr, Mutter GL, Ronnett BM, et al. PTEN expression in endometrial biopsies as a marker of progression to endometrial carcinoma. Cancer Res 2008;68:6014–20.
13. Lacey JV Jr, Mutter GL, Nucci MR, et al. Risk of subsequent endometrial carcinoma associated with

endometrial intraepithelial neoplasia classification of endometrial biopsies. Cancer 2008;113:2073–81.

14. Mutter GL. Histopathology of genetically defined endometrial precancers. Int J Gynecol Pathol 2000;19:301–9.

15. Longacre TA, Chung MH, Jensen DN, et al. Proposed criteria for the diagnosis of well-differentiated endometrial carcinoma. A diagnostic test for myoinvasion. Am J Surg Pathol 1995;19:371–406.

16. Longacre TA, Atkins KA, Kempson RL, et al. The uterine corpus. In: Sternberg S, Mills S, editors. Diagnostic surgical pathololgy. New York: Raven Press; 2009. p. 2184–277.

17. Hendrickson M, Kempson R. Endometrial epithelial metaplasias: proliferations frequently misdiagnosed as adenocarcinoma. Report of 89 cases and proposed classification. Am J Surg Pathol 1980;4:525–42.

18. Young RH, Clement PB. Pseudoneoplastic glandular lesions of the uterine cervix. Semin Diagn Pathol 1991;8:234–49.

19. Young RH, Scully RE. Atypical forms of microglandular hyperplasia of the cervix simulating carcinoma. A report of five cases and review of the literature. Am J Surg Pathol 1989;13:50–6.

20. Young R, Scully R. Uterine carcinomas simulating microglandular hyperplasia. A report of six cases. Am J Surg Pathol 1992;16:1092–7.

21. Huang S, Amparo E, Fu Y. Endometrial hyperplasia: histologic classification and behavior. Surg Pathol 1988;1:215–29.

22. Zaino RJ, Kauderer J, Trimble CL, et al. Reproducibility of the diagnosis of atypical endometrial hyperplasia: a Gynecologic Oncology Group study. Cancer 2006;106:804–11.

23. Trimble CL, Kauderer J, Zaino R, et al. Concurrent endometrial carcinoma in women with a biopsy diagnosis of atypical endometrial hyperplasia: a Gynecologic Oncology Group study. Cancer 2006;106:812–9.

24. Soslow RA. Problems with the current diagnostic approach to complex atypical endometrial hyperplasia. Cancer 2006;106:729–31.

25. Ferenczy A, Gelfand M. The biologic significance of cytologic atypia in progestogen-treated endometrial hyperplasia. Am J Obstet Gynecol 1989;160:126–31.

26. Ushijima K, Yahata H, Yoshikawa H, et al. Multicenter phase II study of fertility-sparing treatment with medroxyprogesterone acetate for endometrial carcinoma and atypical hyperplasia in young women. J Clin Oncol 2007;25:2798–803.

27. McKenney JK, Longacre TA. Low-grade endometrial adenocarcinoma: a diagnostic algorithm for distinguishing atypical endometrial hyperplasia and other benign (and malignant) mimics. Adv Anat Pathol 2009;16:1–22.

28. Nucci MR, Prasad CJ, Crum CP, et al. Mucinous endometrial epithelial proliferations: a morphologic spectrum of changes with diverse clinical significance. Mod Pathol 1999;12:1137–42.

29. Vang R, Tavassoli FA. Proliferative mucinous lesions of the endometrium: analysis of existing criteria for diagnosing carcinoma in biopsies and curettings. Int J Surg Pathol 2003;11:261–70.

30. Fujiwara M, Longacre TA. Low-grade mucinous adenocarcinoma of the uterine corpus: a rare and deceptively bland form of endometrial carcinoma. Am J Surg Pathol 2011, in press.

31. Longacre TA, Chung MH, Rouse RV, et al. Atypical polypoid adenomyofibromas (atypical polypoid adenomyomas) of the uterus. A clinicopathologic study of 55 cases. Am J Surg Pathol 1996;20: 1–20.

32. Mazur M. Atypical polypoid adenomyomas of the endometrium. Am J Surg Pathol 1981;5:473–82.

33. Young R, Treger T, Scully R. Atypical polypoid adenomyoma of the uterus. A report of 27 cases. Am J Clin Pathol 1986;86:139–45.

34. Soslow RA, Chung MH, Rouse RV, et al. Atypical polypoid adenomyofibroma (APA) versus well-differentiated endometrial carcinoma with prominent stromal matrix: an immunohistochemical study. Int J Gynecol Pathol 1996;15:209–16.

35. Gilks CB, Young RH, Clement PB, et al. Adenomyomas of the uterine cervix of of endocervical type: a report of ten cases of a benign cervical tumor that may be confused with adenoma malignum [corrected]. Mod Pathol 1996;9:220–4.

36. Silva EG, Young RH. Endometrioid neoplasms with clear cells: a report of 21 cases in which the alteration is not of typical secretory type. Am J Surg Pathol 2007;31:1203–8.

37. Murray SK, Young RH, Scully RE. Uterine Endometrioid Carcinoma with Small Nonvillous Papillae: An Analysis of 26 Cases of a Favorable-Prognosis Tumor To Be Distinguished from Serous Carcinoma. Int J Surg Pathol 2000;8:279–89.

38. Clement P, Scully R. Mullerian adenosarcomas of the uterus with sex cord-like elements. A clinicopathologic analysis of eight cases. Am J Clin Pathol 1989;91:664–72.

39. Baker RJ, Hildebrandt RH, Rouse RV, et al. Inhibin and CD99 (MIC2) expression in uterine stromal neoplasms with sex-cord-like elements. Hum Pathol 1999;30:671–9.

40. Clement P, Scully R. Uterine tumors resembling ovarian sex-cord tumors. A clinicopathologic analysis of fourteen cases. Am J Clin Pathol 1976;66:512–25.

41. Irving JA, Carinelli S, Prat J. Uterine tumors resembling ovarian sex cord tumors are polyphenotypic neoplasms with true sex cord differentiation. Mod Pathol 2006;19:17–24.

42. Murray SK, Clement PB, Young RH. Endometrioid carcinomas of the uterine corpus with sex cord-like formations, hyalinization, and other unusual

morphologic features: a report of 31 cases of a neoplasm that may be confused with carcinosarcoma and other uterine neoplasms. Am J Surg Pathol 2005;29:157–66.

43. Soslow RA. Mixed müllerian tumors of the female genital tract. Surgical Pathology Clinics 2009;2: 707–30.

44. Clement P, Scully R. Mullerian adenosarcoma of the uterus: a clinicopathologic analysis of 100 cases with a review of the literature. Hum Pathol 1990;21: 363–81.

45. Kong C, Beck A, Longacre T. A panel of three markers including p16, ProEx C, or HPV ISH is optimal for distinguishing between primary endometrial and endocervical adenocarcinomas. Am J Surg Pathol 2010;34(7):915–26.

46. Alkushi A, Irving J, Hsu F, et al. Immunoprofile of cervical and endometrial adenocarcinomas using a tissue microarray. Virchows Arch 2003;442: 271–7.

47. Kamoi S, AlJuboury MI, Akin MR, et al. Immunohistochemical staining in the distinction between primary endometrial and endocervical adenocarcinomas: another viewpoint. Int J Gynecol Pathol 2002;21: 217–23.

48. Staebler A, Sherman ME, Zaino RJ, et al. Hormone receptor immunohistochemistry and human papillomavirus in situ hybridization are useful for distinguishing endocervical and endometrial adenocarcinomas. Am J Surg Pathol 2002;26:998–1006.

49. McCluggage WG, Sumathi VP, McBride HA, et al. A panel of immunohistochemical stains, including carcinoembryonic antigen, vimentin, and estrogen receptor, aids the distinction between primary endometrial and endocervical adenocarcinomas. Int J Gynecol Pathol 2002;21:11–5.

50. Castrillon DH, Lee KR, Nucci MR. Distinction between endometrial and endocervical adenocarcinoma: an immunohistochemical study. Int J Gynecol Pathol 2002;21:4–10.

51. Kumar A, Schneider V. Metastases to the uterus from extrapelvic primary tumors. Int J Gynecol Pathol 1983;2:134–40.

52. Creasman WT, Odicino F, Maisonneuve P, et al. Carcinoma of the corpus uteri. FIGO 6th Annual Report on the Results of Treatment in Gynecological Cancer. Int J Gynaecol Obstet 2006;95(Suppl 1): S105–43.

53. Wheeler DT, Bristow RE, Kurman RJ. Histologic alterations in endometrial hyperplasia and well-differentiated carcinoma treated with progestins. Am J Surg Pathol 2007;31:988–98.

54. Announcements: FIGO stages - 1988 revisions. Gynecol Oncol 1989;35:125–7.

55. Lax SF, Kurman RJ, Pizer ES, et al. A binary architectural grading system for uterine endometrial endometrioid carcinoma has superior reproducibility compared with FIGO grading and identifies subsets of advance-stage tumors with favorable and unfavorable prognosis. Am J Surg Pathol 2000;24: 1201–8.

56. Alkushi A, Abdul-Rahman ZH, Lim P, et al. Description of a novel system for grading of endometrial carcinoma and comparison with existing grading systems. Am J Surg Pathol 2005;29:295–304.

57. Taylor RR, Zeller J, Lieberman RW, et al. An analysis of two versus three grades for endometrial carcinoma. Gynecol Oncol 1999;74:3–6.

58. Scholten AN, Smit VT, Beerman H, et al. Prognostic significance and interobserver variability of histologic grading systems for endometrial carcinoma. Cancer 2004;100:764–72.

59. Gemer O, Uriev L, Voldarsky M, et al. The reproducibility of histological parameters employed in the novel binary grading systems of endometrial cancer. Eur J Surg Oncol 2009;35:247–51.

60. Murray SK, Young RH, Scully RE. Unusual epithelial and stromal changes in myoinvasive endometrioid adenocarcinoma: a study of their frequency, associated diagnostic problems, and prognostic significance. Int J Gynecol Pathol 2003;22:324–33.

61. Longacre TA, Hendrickson MR. Diffusely infiltrative endometrial adenocarcinoma: an adenoma malignum pattern of myoinvasion. Am J Surg Pathol 1999;23:69–78.

62. Kalyanasundaram K, Ganesan R, Perunovic B, et al. Diffusely infiltrating endometrial carcinomas with no stromal response: report of a series, including cases with cervical and ovarian involvement and emphasis on the potential for misdiagnosis. Int J Surg Pathol 2010;18(2):138–43.

63. Mittal K, Barwick K. Diffusely infiltrating adenocarcinoma of the endometrium. A subtype with poor prognosis. Am J Surg Pathol 1988;12:754–8.

64. Revised FIGO staging for carcinoma of the vulva, cervix, and endometrium. FIGO Committee on Gynecologic Oncology. Int J Gynecol Obstet 2009; 105:103–4.

65. Edge SB, Byrd DR, Compton CC, et al, editors. AJCC cancer staging manual. New York: Springer; 2010. p. 404.

66. Tambouret R, Clement PB, Young RH. Endometrial endometrioid adenocarcinoma with a deceptive pattern of spread to the uterine cervix: a manifestation of stage IIb endometrial carcinoma liable to be misinterpreted as an independent carcinoma or a benign lesion. Am J Surg Pathol 2003;27: 1080–8.

67. McKenney JK, Kong CS, Longacre TA. Endometrial adenocarcinoma associated with subtle lymphvascular space invasion and lymph node metastasis: a histologic pattern mimicking intravascular and sinusoidal histiocytes. Int J Gynecol Pathol 2005;24:73–8.

68. Logani S, Herdman AV, Little JV, et al. Vascular "pseudo invasion" in laparoscopic hysterectomy specimens: a diagnostic pitfall. Am J Surg Pathol 2008;32:560–5.

69. Kitahara S, Walsh C, Frumovitz M, et al. Vascular pseudoinvasion in laparoscopic hysterectomy specimens for endometrial carcinoma: a grossing artifact? Am J Surg Pathol 2009;33:298–303.

70. Culton LK, Deavers MT, Silva EG, et al. Endometrioid carcinoma simultaneously involving the uterus and the fallopian tube: a clinicopathologic study of 13 cases. Am J Surg Pathol 2006;30: 844–9.

71. Brinkmann D, Ryan A, Ayhan A, et al. A molecular genetic and statistical approach for the diagnosis of dual-site cancers. J Natl Cancer Inst 2004;96: 1441–6.

72. Emmert-Buck MR, Chuaqui R, Zhuang Z, et al. Molecular analysis of synchronous uterine and ovarian endometrioid tumors. Int J Gynecol Pathol 1997;16:143–8.

73. Fujita M, Enomoto T, Wada H, et al. Application of clonal analysis. Differential diagnosis for synchronous primary ovarian and endometrial cancers and metastatic cancer. Am J Clin Pathol 1996;105: 350–9.

74. Lin WM, Forgacs E, Warshal DP, et al. Loss of heterozygosity and mutational analysis of the PTEN/MMAC1 gene in synchronous endometrial and ovarian carcinomas. Clin Cancer Res 1998;4: 2577–83.

75. Matias-Guiu X, Lagarda H, Catasus L, et al. Clonality analysis in synchronous or metachronous tumors of the female genital tract. Int J Gynecol Pathol 2002; 21:205–11.

76. Moreno-Bueno G, Gamallo C, Perez-Gallego L, et al. beta-Catenin expression pattern, beta-catenin gene mutations, and microsatellite instability in endometrioid ovarian carcinomas and synchronous endometrial carcinomas. Diagn Mol Pathol 2001;10:116–22.

77. Shenson DL, Gallion HH, Powell DE, et al. Loss of heterozygosity and genomic instability in synchronous endometrioid tumors of the ovary and endometrium. Cancer 1995;76:650–7.

78. Ramus SJ, Elmasry K, Luo Z, et al. Predicting clinical outcome in patients diagnosed with synchronous ovarian and endometrial cancer. Clin Cancer Res 2008;14:5840–8.

79. Shannon C, Kirk J, Barnetson R, et al. Incidence of microsatellite instability in synchronous tumors of the ovary and endometrium. Clin Cancer Res 2003; 9:1387–92.

HIGH-GRADE ENDOMETRIAL CARCINOMAS

Esther Oliva, MD[a], Robert A. Soslow, MD[b],*

KEYWORDS

- FIGO grade 3 endometrioid carcinoma • High-grade endometrioid carcinoma • Serous carcinoma
- Clear cell carcinoma • Undifferentiated carcinoma • Malignant mixed müllerian tumor
- High grade endometrial carcinoma

ABSTRACT

High-grade endometrial carcinomas are a heterogeneous group of clinically aggressive tumors. They include FIGO grade 3 endometrioid carcinoma, serous carcinoma, clear cell carcinoma, undifferentiated carcinoma, and malignant mixed Müllerian tumor (MMMT). Epidemiologic, genetic, biologic prognostic and morphologic differences between these entities are striking in prototypic cases, yet substantial overlap exists and diagnostic criteria and therapeutic approaches that account for the group's diversity are currently insufficient. FIGO grade 3 endometrioid carcinoma demonstrates solid, trabecular or nested growth and may resemble poorly differentiated squamous cell carcinoma. Endometrioid glandular differentiation is usually focally present. Serous carcinoma usually displays papillary architecture but glandular and solid patterns may predominate. Tumor cells typically display diffuse and severe atypia. Clear cell carcinoma should be diagnosed by recognizing characteristic papillary or tubulocystic architecture with cuboidal tumor cells showing atypical but uniform nuclei. Cells with clear cytoplasm are frequently but not always present. On the other hand, clear cells may be encountered in endometrioid and serous carcinomas. Immunohistochemical stains for p53, p16, ER, PR, mib-1, hepatocyte nuclear factor 1β and pan-cytokeratin can be helpful in classifying these high-grade carcinomas. They should be used in concert with thorough morphologic examination, as part of rational panel of markers and only in specific circumstances. Although these tumors may appear clinically and even morphologically similar, demographic and epidemiologic features as well as patterns of spread and treatment modalities differ.

OVERVIEW

High-grade endometrial carcinomas are a heterogeneous group of tumors that are clinically aggressive. The following tumor types are currently recognized as part of this group of neoplasms: FIGO grade 3 endometrioid carcinoma; serous carcinoma; clear cell carcinoma; undifferentiated carcinoma; and MMMT (malignant mixed Müllerian tumor or carcinosarcoma), details about which can be found in "Mixed Mullerian Tumors of the Female Genital Tract" in *Mesenchymal tumors of the gynecologic tract* in this series.

Epidemiologic, genetic, prognostic and morphologic differences between these entities are striking in prototypic cases (**Table 1; Fig. 1**), yet substantial overlap exists and diagnostic criteria and a therapeutic approaches that account for the group's diversity are currently insufficient. A recent unpublished study by experienced gynecologic pathologists on diagnostic reproducibility of consecutive cases coded as "high-grade endometrial carcinoma" found diagnostic agreement in only 31 of 59 of them. The discrepancies included 5 cases that were not uniformly interpreted as

[a] Pathology Department, Massachusetts General Hospital, 55 Fruit Street WRN 2, Boston, MA 02114-2696, USA
[b] Department of Pathology, Memorial Sloan-Kettering Cancer Center, 1275 York Avenue, New York, NY 10065, USA
* Corresponding author.
E-mail address: soslowr@MSKCC.ORG

Surgical Pathology 4 (2011) 199–241
doi:10.1016/j.path.2010.12.008

surgpath.theclinics.com

Table 1
High-grade endometrial carcinomas[a]

	Age (% Older than 65 yrs)	Stage (% FIGO Stage III/IV)	Metastatic Site (% Peritoneal)	Median Survival	Pathogenetic Pathway
FIGO 3 endometrioid	50%	40%	10%	50 months	PIK3CA/PTEN; MSI; p53
Serous and MMMT	70%	70%	40%	40 months	P53; PIK3CA; EMT
Clear cell	60%	60%	10%	30 months	PIK3CA; MSI
Undifferentiated	60%	60%	10%[b]	<30 months	EMT; MSI

Abbreviations: EMT, epithelial-mesenchymal transitions; MSI, microsatellite instability.
[a] Values estimated from review of several references[1,68,164]; survival data are for treated patients.
[b] Present only with nodal, pelvic soft tissue or parenchymal disease.

"high grade" and 31 where there was disagreement about tumor type.

GROSS PATHOLOGY

Gross differences between these tumors tend to be minor, with only a few exceptions. FIGO grade 3 endometrioid and undifferentiated carcinomas that arise in the setting of a differentiated endometrioid neoplasm (complex atypical hyperplasia or FIGO grade I endometrioid carcinoma) may be found in large uteri containing obvious tumor (**Fig. 2**), but uteri harboring serous carcinomas tend to be small, may contain atrophic endometrial polyps and lack the hyperplastic thickened endometrium that is more characteristic of endometrioid adenocarcinomas (**Fig. 3**). MMMTs are

frequently polypoid tumors with extensive areas of necrosis and/or hemorrhage. Uterine serous carcinomas and MMMTs have a predilection for peritoneal dissemination.

HISTOPATHOLOGIC FEATURES

FIGO Grade 3 Endometrioid Carcinoma

FIGO grade 3 endometrioid carcinomas are typified by solid growth that usually manifests as sheets or large nests of cohesive cells that may resemble a poorly differentiated non-keratinizing squamous cell carcinoma (**Fig. 4**). Only approximately 20% of FIGO grade 3 endometrioid carcinomas are accompanied by complex atypical hyperplasia.[1] Many of these tumors overgrow this precursor lesion and/or arise from other

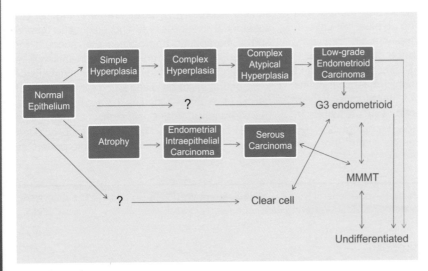

Fig. 1. Endometrial tumorigenesis. This diagram is meant to illustrate that apart from serous carcinoma, high grade endometrial carcinomas are not easily accommodated by models of endometrial tumorigenesis that recognize only two types of carcinomas. Type 1 carcinomas, displayed along the top, may progress to high grade endometrial carcinomas of several types and mechanisms that account for the development of clear cell carcinoma, for example, are not well understood.

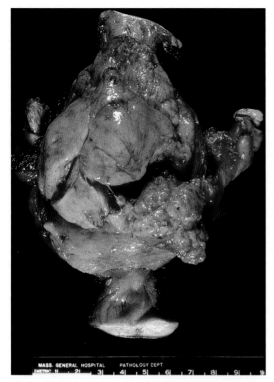

Fig. 2. FIGO grade 3 endometrioid carcinoma. A large polypoid mass fills and distends the endometrial cavity. It has a yellow appearance with small areas of hemorrhage.

Key Features
FIGO GRADE 3 ENDOMETRIOID CARCINOMA

Solid, nested or trabecular architecture

Cohesive cells that may resemble poorly differentiated squamous carcinoma

Moderately or severely atypical nuclei

Usually present in a background of a gland-forming endometrioid carcinoma

Serous, clear cell and undifferentiated carcinomas should be excluded first

precursors (**Fig. 5**), including low-grade endometrioid carcinoma. Most tumors contain a small number of glands (**Fig. 6**), which aids in recognizing such a tumor as endometrioid. Tumors that are predominantly solid may show either

moderately or severely atypical nuclear features (**Fig. 7**). Severe, diffuse nuclear atypia should be present when glandular architecture predominates although this pattern should suggest an alternative diagnosis, either serous or clear cell carcinoma.

Immunohistochemistry can be used to confirm a diagnosis of FIGO grade 3 endometrioid carcinoma, especially when serous carcinoma with a solid growth pattern and undifferentiated carcinoma are under consideration. All high-grade endometrial carcinomas except undifferentiated carcinoma typically express pan-cytokeratins, EMA, CA125, Ber EP4, B72.3, CK7, and vimentin. They do not show diffuse CK20 labeling and lack diffuse, strong CEA cytoplasmic expression. ER and PR are detected in about 50% of cases. Approximately 20% of these tumors overexpress p53[2–5] although higher rates have been reported,[6,7] and many display p16 positivity (**Fig. 8**), although typically not to the degree seen in serous carcinoma.[5,8] When admixed with a serous

Fig. 3. Serous carcinoma. Uteri containing serous carcinoma are frequently atrophic. In this example, the tumor presents as a diffuse irregularity of the endometrial lining without an obvious mass.

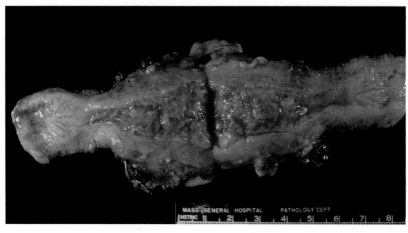

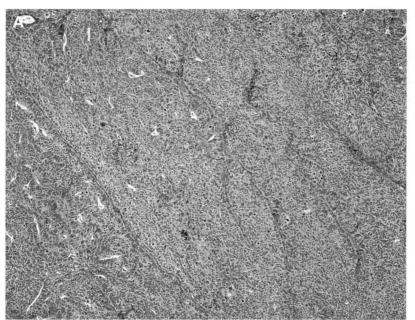

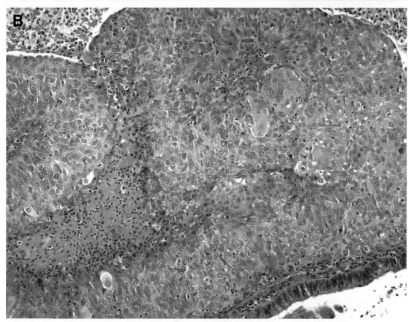

Fig. 4. (*A*) FIGO grade 3 endometrioid carcinoma. The tumor cells grow in sheets and large solid nests with minimal gland formation. (*B*) FIGO grade 3 endometrioid carcinoma. The tumor exhibits solid architecture. Geographic necrosis in this setting imparts the appearance of broad papillae, features that are shared with transitional cell carcinoma (see **Fig. 47**). Gland formation, found elsewhere, supports classification as endometrioid carcinoma (see **Fig. 46**).

Fig. 5. FIGO grade 3 endometrioid carcinoma. This high-grade endometrioid carcinoma (*right*) is associated with a FIGO grade 1 endometrioid carcinoma component (*left*), which suggests evolution to high-grade carcinoma from a low-grade substrate. Classification as FIGO grade 3 endometrioid carcinoma is justified when the solid component predominates (>50%).

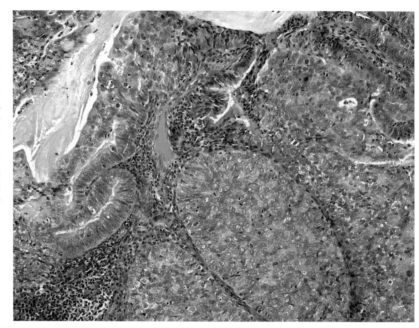

Fig. 6. FIGO grade 3 endometrioid carcinoma. This mostly solid tumor can be recognized as endometrioid by the focal presence of endometrioid-type glandular differentiation.

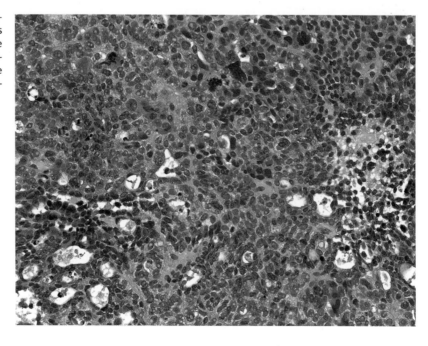

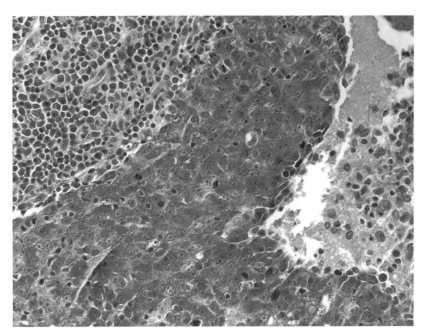

Fig. 7. FIGO grade 3 endometrioid carcinoma. This tumor displays moderately atypical nuclear features.

component the most common alterations include p53 overexpression and activating *PIK3CA* mutations, followed by *PTEN* mutations,[2] which result in loss of PTEN expression. Her-2/neu and

occasional WT1 expression have been reported.[7,9] They may also show evidence of DNA mismatch repair abnormalities[5] and can occur in the setting of Lynch syndrome/Hereditary nonpolyposis colorectal carcinoma syndrome.[10–12]

Serous Carcinoma

These tumors are almost always present in a background of atrophic endometrium and atrophic endometrial polyps (**Fig. 9**).[13–17] A diagnosis of

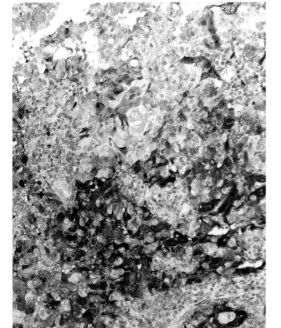

Fig. 8. Grade 3 endometrioid carcinoma. The neoplastic cells show multifocal and strong p16 expression.

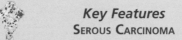

Key Features
SEROUS CARCINOMA

Irregular papillae with micropapillae (but glandular and solid architecture can predominate)

Large, tufted and non-cohesive cells with irregular luminal contours

Large nuclei with bizarre forms, dark, smudged chromatin or macronucleoli

Mitotic rate >10/10 high power fields

Gaping gland myometrial invasion

Lymphovascular invasion common

Intraepithelial carcinoma

P53 and p16 overexpression with high Ki-67 labeling

Low or undetectable ER and PR

Fig. 9. Endometrial polyp involved by serous carcinoma. The complex and papillary architecture of the tumor contrasts with the uninvolved atrophic appearing endometrial glands.

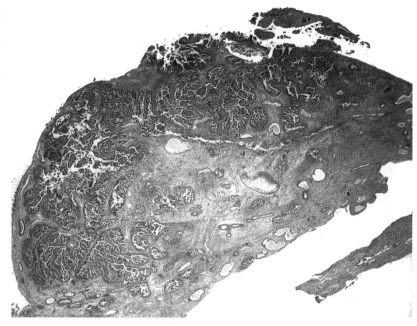

serous carcinoma should be questioned if the non-neoplastic endometrium is secretory, proliferative or hyperplastic.

Serous carcinomas typically have papillae and micropapillae (**Figs. 10** and **11**) lined by large, tufted and non-cohesive cells (**Figs. 12** and **13**) with large nuclei containing macronucleoli (**Fig. 14**). Bizarre nuclear forms, multinucleated cells and nuclei with dark, smudged chromatin are also typical (**Fig. 15**). Architecturally, serous carcinomas feature slit-like spaces that result from compact micropapillae (see **Fig. 11**), but some serous carcinomas demonstrate glandular architecture (**Figs. 16** and **17**) and some are solid. This, unfortunately, leads to diagnostic problems that involve endometrioid carcinoma in particular.

Fig. 10. Serous carcinoma. The tumor shows striking papillary architecture.

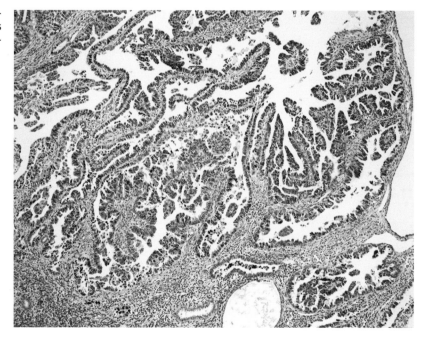

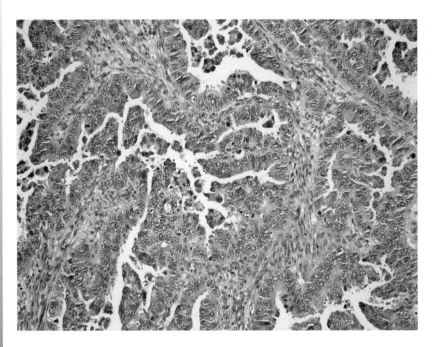

Fig. 11. Serous carcinoma. The neoplastic glands show irregular and complex outlines with prominent branching and micropapillae.

Occasional tumors mimic clear cell carcinoma because of cytoplasmic clearing[18] and hobnail cells. Psammoma bodies are seen in approximately one third of the neoplasms and in general are less common than in their ovarian counterpart. The mitotic rate almost always exceeds 10 per 10 high power fields. A gaping gland appearance when serous carcinomas invade myometrium (Figs. 18 and 19) is typical, but not invariable. Extensive lymphovascular invasion and extrauterine extension are common even when there is limited or absent myometrial invasion.[13,19–22] Serous carcinomas may occasionally coexist with an endometrioid, clear cell or even neuroendocrine carcinoma, with endometrioid carcinoma being perhaps the most

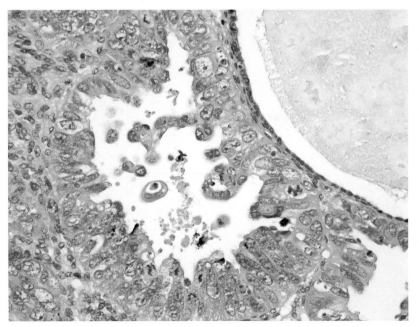

Fig. 12. Intraepithelial serous carcinoma. The tumor cells show nuclear pseudostratification, loss of nuclear polarity and budding, high nuclear to cytoplasmic ratios, and prominent nuclear pleomorphism.

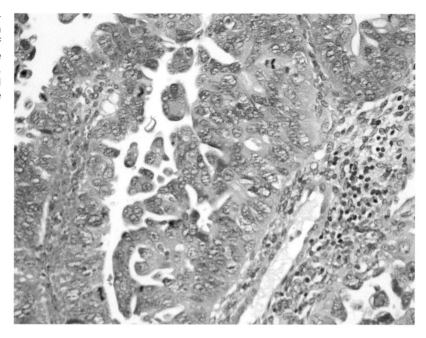

Fig. 13. Serous carcinoma. Micropapillae with apparent detachment of tumor cell clusters are typical of this tumor type. Note the highly atypical nuclear features and the evident mitotic activity.

common.[23–26] Trophoblastic differentiation has also been reported.[27]

Many serous carcinomas include a non-invasive component that replaces non-neoplastic atrophic endometrium.[16,19,28–30] This lesion, endometrial intraepithelial carcinoma or, preferably, intraepithelial serous carcinoma, is fully malignant as it has the ability to metastasize even when endometrial stromal or myometrial invasion is lacking.[30] Intraepithelial serous carcinoma is occasionally present without an adjacent invasive component. Because it replaces non-neoplastic endometrial epithelium and fails to form a mass, intraepithelial serous carcinoma usually shows architectural

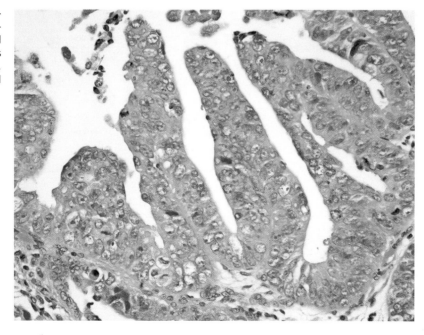

Fig. 14. Serous carcinoma. Thin and elongated papillae are lined by highly atypical cells showing large nuclei, prominent nucleoli, and brisk mitotic rate.

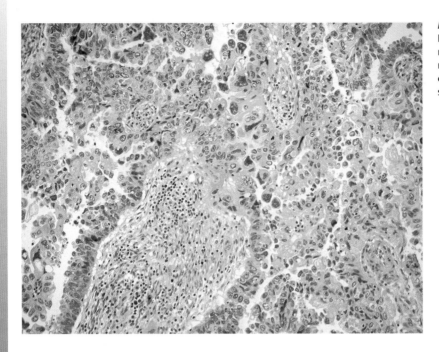

Fig. 15. Serous carcinoma. Bizarre nuclear forms, multinucleated cells and nuclei with dark, smudged chromatin are commonly seen.

preservation of the preexisting endometrial glands (see **Figs. 12, 16** and **17**). As such, it may be mistaken for complex atypical hyperplasia or well-differentiated adenocarcinoma at low-power magnification, but these latter neoplasms generally display architectural complexity, with cribriformed and fused glands. The presence of intraepithelial serous carcinoma at low-power magnification may be suggested by the presence of a dark-staining, sharply defined proliferation of tall columnar cells that colonizes the luminal surface of flat or polypoid endometrium. The

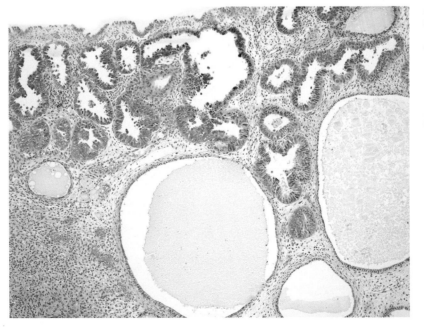

Fig. 16. Intraepithelial serous carcinoma. The preexisting glandular architecture is preserved but most of the endometrial glands appear thickened and "dark blue" as they have been replaced by serous carcinoma cells. Tumor cell budding is appreciable at this low-power magnification. No stromal invasion is appreciated.

Fig. 17. Intraepithelial serous carcinoma. The cytologic features of serous carcinoma are present, but stromal invasion is lacking. This leads to the impression of a gland-forming tumor.

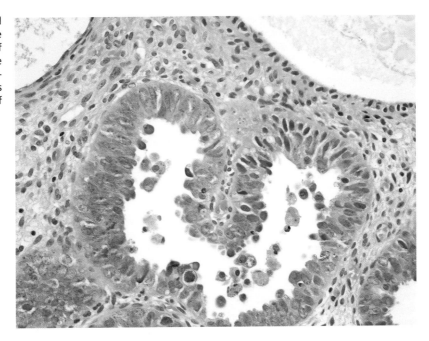

cytologic features are identical to those of invasive serous carcinoma.

Immunohistochemistry can be used to assist in the diagnosis of serous carcinoma, especially when another type of endometrial carcinoma is under consideration (**Table 2**). The vast majority of serous carcinomas (up to 90%), show *p53* over-expression (intense expression in greater than 50 to 75% of tumor cell nuclei),[31–35] which results from *p53* mutation and the accumulation of mutant protein (**Figs. 20** and **21**). Many of the remaining tumors, some of which lack p53 expression,

Fig. 18. Serous carcinoma. The tumor shows diffuse permeation of the myometrium by irregularly oriented gaping glands showing focal branching and slit-like spaces.

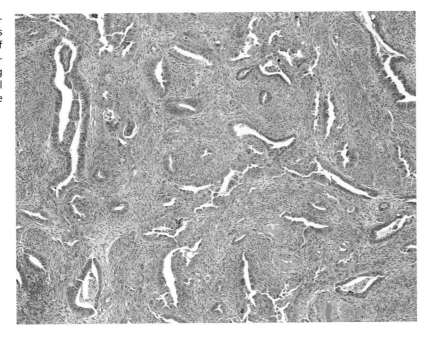

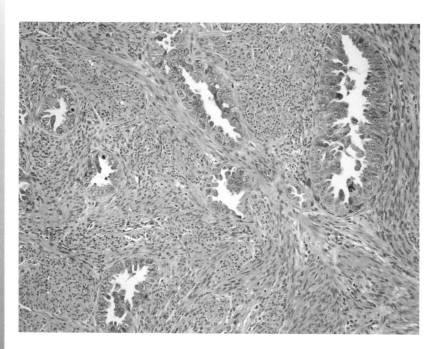

Fig. 19. Serous carcinoma. Gaping glands are unassociated with a desmoplastic reaction; they vary in size and shape, and lack nuclear polarization and smooth luminal outlines.

harbor *p53* mutations that produce a protein that cannot be detected using commercially available antibodies.[31,36] Proliferative activity, estimated with the Ki-67 antibody, is extremely high (ie, >75% of tumor cell nuclei) regardless of p53 overexpression. Diffuse p16 overexpression is also typical of serous carcinoma[8,36] (**Fig. 22**) and may be a more sensitive marker of serous differentiation as compared with p53.[36] This finding is not related to HPV infection, but it may be secondary to disturbances in the cell cycle that promote high levels of proliferative activity. ER may be only weakly and focally positive, in contrast to ovarian serous carcinoma, and PR is even less frequently expressed than ER (**Fig. 23**).[8,37,38] Unlike tubal, ovarian and peritoneal serous carcinomas, WT1 expression in endometrial serous carcinomas is seen in at most 20 to 30% of

Table 2
Immunohistochemical summary

	P53 or p16 (Overexpression)	ER/PR	HNF 1β	Pankeratin
FIGO 3 endometrioid	<30%	<50%	rare	>90%
Serous and MMMT	>90%	<20%	rare	>90%
Clear cell	<30%	<10%	>80%	>90%
Undifferentiated	NK	0	NK	<10%

Abbreviation: NK, not known.
Table lists approximate percentages of tumors expressing each marker in each category.

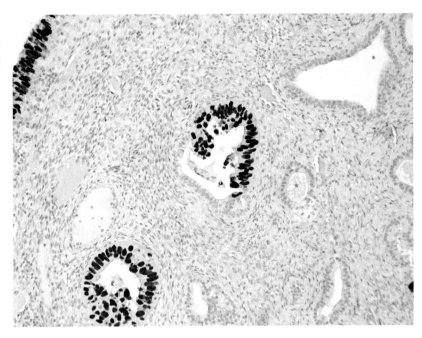

Fig.   20. Intraepithelial serous carcinoma. Preexisting atrophic endometrial glands (p53 negative) are partially replaced by neoplastic cells showing strong p53 positivity.

tumors.[9,35,39] They also may express HER2/neu (related to resistance to chemotherapy and poor prognosis when overexpressed)[37] and rarely D2-40.[38] Uterine serous carcinomas also frequently show loss of p27, bcl-2, and E-cadherin expression[37,40,41] while they are positive for Cyclin E and retain PTEN expression in all but exceptional cases.[37,42]

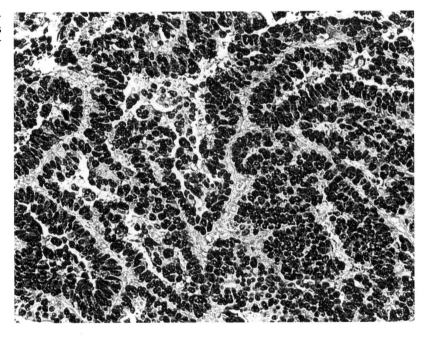

Fig.   21. Serous carcinoma. The tumor cells display strong p53 nuclear staining.

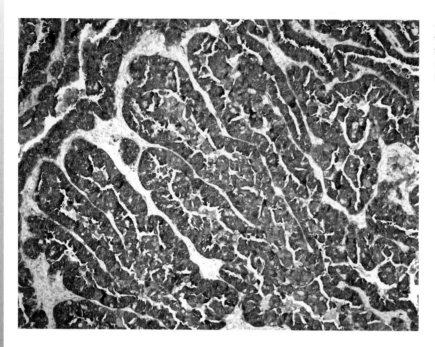

Fig. 22. Papillary serous carcinoma. The tumor cells show strong and diffuse nuclear and cytoplasmic p16 immunoreactivity.

Clear Cell Carcinoma

Clear cell carcinoma of the endometrium is an enigmatic entity. Due to the presence of clear cytoplasm, this tumor was classified in the past within the group of secretory endometrial carcinomas.[43] The morphologic features overlap significantly with serous carcinoma and FIGO grade 3 endometrioid carcinoma.[44–46] Many high-grade endometrial carcinomas contain clear cells and papillary architecture, but only rare

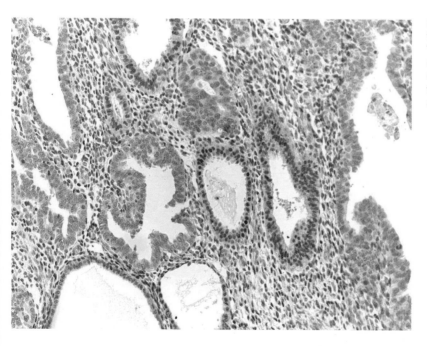

Fig. 23. Endometrial intraepithelial carcinoma. The background atrophic endometrial glands show diffuse ER positivity while the serous carcinoma cells are ER negative.

examples resemble the prototypic ovarian clear cell carcinoma. When clear cell carcinoma mimics and mixed epithelial carcinomas are excluded, pure clear cell carcinoma remains a very infrequent tumor type.[47]

Clear cell carcinoma should be diagnosed based on the architectural appearance of the tumor, rather than by focusing on the presence of tumor cells with clear cytoplasm. Clear cell carcinoma of the endometrium often shows a papillary (**Fig. 24**), glandular (**Figs. 25 and 26**) and/or solid growth patterns (**Fig. 27**). Tubulocystic architecture is less commonly seen than in ovarian clear cell carcinoma (**Fig. 28**). The papillae tend to be small and round with only one or two layers of cuboidal cells lining the fibrovascular cores (**Fig. 29**; see **Fig. 24**). Some cores display hyaline material, which is typical of this tumor (see **Figs. 24 and 29**). Solid clear cell carcinomas are composed of sheets of cuboidal cells with a cobblestone appearance (see **Fig. 27**). The typical neoplastic cell contains clear cytoplasm with a round nucleus that frequently features a large nucleolus (see **Fig. 26**). Hobnail cells may be present (**Fig. 30**). Some clear cell carcinomas, however, have eosinophilic cytoplasm (ie, oxyphilic variant) (Soslow and Han review Fig. 44) or scant, nondescript cytoplasm (see **Fig. 28**), Most clear cell carcinomas contain large nuclei of uniform size (see **Fig. 26**), although some cells have wrinkled and hyperchromatic

nuclei, and scattered bizarre and enlarged nuclei may be apparent (**Fig. 31**). Mitotic figures are typically sparse, with rates less than 10 per 10 high power fields. Necrosis is common and can be extensive (see **Fig. 30**). Intra- and extracellular hyaline bodies may be seen (targetoid bodies)[48,49] as can psammoma bodies, particularly in papillary neoplasms. Some tumors may have a prominent lymphoplasmacytic infiltrate.[48] Myometrial and lymphovascular invasion occur in approximately 80% and 25% of clear cell carcinomas respectively.[47,50]

> ### *Key Features*
> #### CLEAR CELL CARCINOMA
>
> Papillary, tubulocystic, or solid architecture
>
> Round papillae, sometimes with hyaline cores, lined by one or two layers of tumor cells
>
> Uniform, but highly atypical nuclei, sometimes with prominent nucleoli
>
> Mitotic rate <10/10 high power fields
>
> Hepatocyte nuclear factor 1β positive
>
> No p53 or p16 overexpression
>
> ER/PR negative

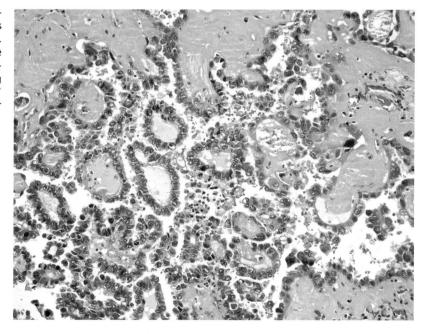

Fig. 24. Clear cell carcinoma. The tumor shows a papillary architecture. Most of the papillae are relatively small and rounded, some of them showing edematous "open rings" or hyalinized fibrovascular cores.

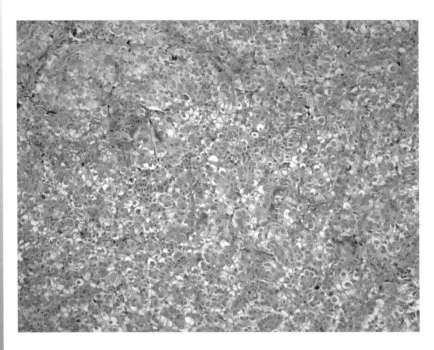

Fig. 25. Clear cell carcinoma. The tumor shows closely packed papillae and tubules separated by scant hyalinized stroma.

Like serous carcinoma, clear cell carcinoma usually arises in the setting of atrophic endometrium and may be associated with endometrial polyps.[48,49,51] Clear cell carcinoma may also be associated with a component of serous or endometrioid carcinoma[48,51–53] but the true incidence of this second component must be lower than that previously reported. Recently, a precursor to

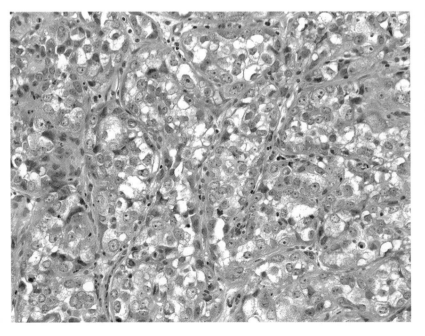

Fig. 26. Clear cell carcinoma. The compressed tubules are lined by tumor cells with relatively abundant clear cytoplasm and uniformly enlarged and atypical nuclei with visible nucleoli.

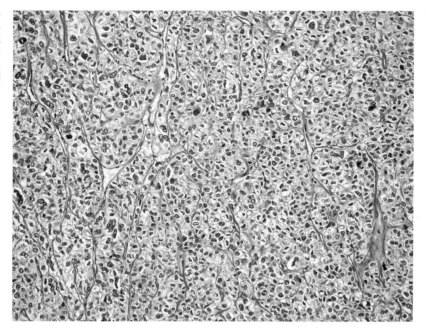

Fig. 27. Clear cell carcinoma. Tumor cells are arranged in large nests separated by scant, compressed stroma, leading to the appearance of a solid neoplasm.

clear cell carcinoma of the endometrium has been reported in which isolated glands or surface epithelium within an otherwise normal endometrial region display cytoplasmic clarity and/or eosinophilia with varying degrees of cytologic atypia.[54]

Some of these lesions may show focally hobnail nuclei with mitotic figures and apoptotic bodies.

Using immunohistochemistry, most clear cell carcinomas (see **Table 2**) express CK7, CAM5.2, 34βE12, CEA, Leu-M1, vimentin and CA-125,

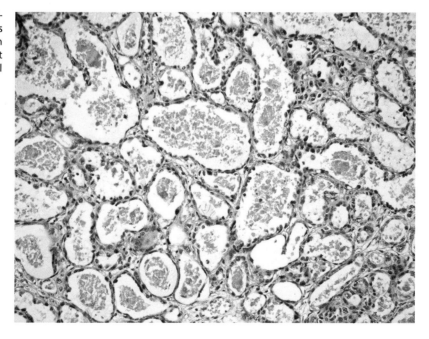

Fig. 28. Clear cell carcinoma. The tumor shows striking tubulocystic growth associated with abundant eosinophilic intraluminal secretions.

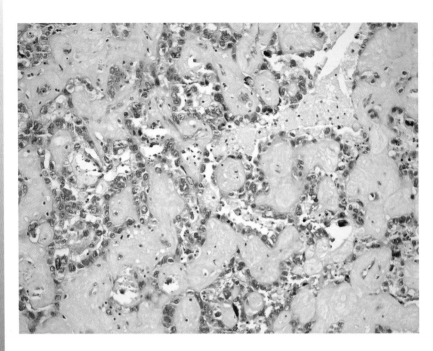

Fig. 29. Clear cell carcinoma. The papillae show striking hyalinization of the fibrovascular cores and are lined by a single layer of neoplastic cells.

and a small percentage may be CEA positive but they are CK20 negative.[8,55] ER and PR expression is uncommon (**Figs. 32** and **33**) and, when present, is weak and focal.[8,46,56] p53 overexpression can be seen, but in general there is no diffuse and strong expression as seen in serous carcinoma.[46,56,57] Only few studies have looked at WT1 expression in clear cell carcinoma with variable results. Among all tested tumors, 12/43 clear cell carcinomas were positive for this marker.[9,39,58] p16 expression is more common than in endometrioid carcinomas but less frequent

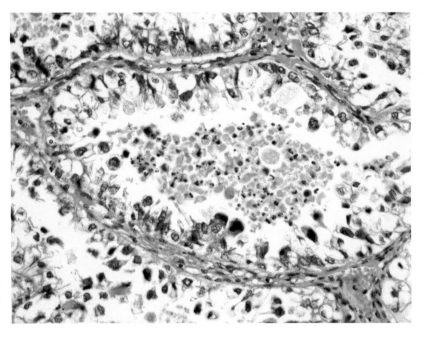

Fig. 30. Clear cell carcinoma. Hobnail cells with hyperchromatic nuclei located toward the lumen are prominent.

Fig. 31. Clear cell carcinoma. Scattered, bizarre and enlarged nuclei may be apparent.

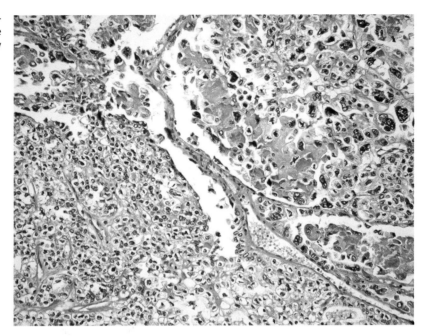

than in serous carcinomas.[8] HER-2/neu seems to be more frequently observed in clear cell carcinoma than in the other endometrial carcinoma subtypes, but when correlated with clinical features it is not associated with stage or outcome.[59,60] HNF-1β is frequently positive in clear cell carcinoma and may help to distinguish it from other endometrial tumors,[61,62] as has been reported in the ovary.[63] Low-level or no expression of cyclin E and loss of e-cadherin expression is common in contrast to endometrioid carcinoma.[41,56] Finally, recent studies have shown

Fig. 32. Clear cell carcinoma. This solid tumor is uniformly ER negative.

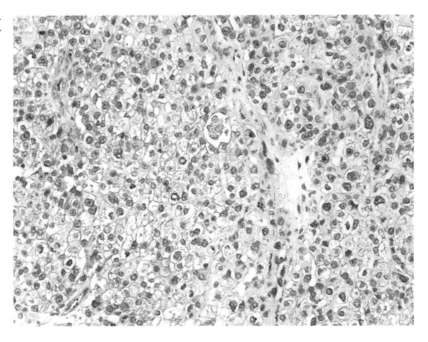

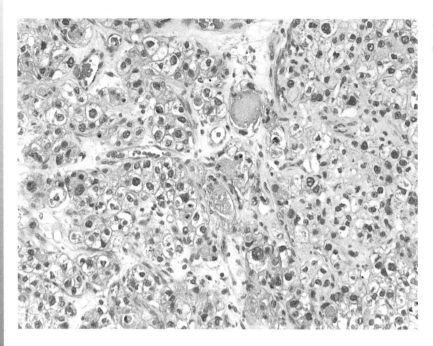

Fig. 33. Clear cell carcinoma. The neoplastic cells showing solid growth lack PR expression.

that the gene expression profile for clear cell carcinoma is quite distinct from uterine serous carcinoma.[64–66] Loss of expression of one or more DNA mismatch repair proteins (ie, MLH1, MSH2, MSH6) can be encountered, particularly in the setting of Lynch Syndrome.[56,67]

Undifferentiated Carcinoma

Undifferentiated carcinoma is diagnosed in the setting of a tumor with solid architecture and cytologic features that lack distinguishing characteristics. When the tumor exhibits a combination of

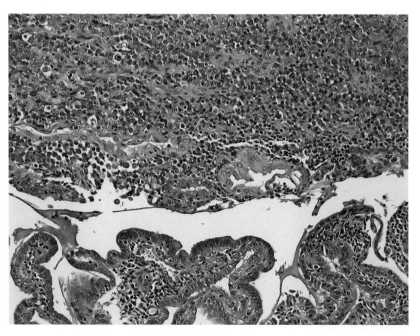

Fig. 34. Dedifferentiated carcinoma. Undifferentiated cells with a rhabdoid appearance are seen juxtaposed to a well-differentiated endometrioid carcinoma.

Fig. 35. Undifferentiated carcinoma. The loosely cohesive tumor cells have a diffuse growth pattern without gland formation.

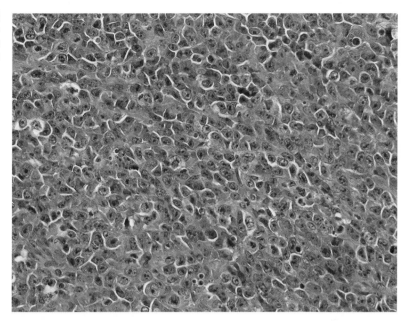

Key Features
UNDIFFERENTIATED CARCINOMA

Solid, non-nested, non-trabecular architecture

Non-cohesive tumor cells of uniform appearance

Myxoid stroma and rhabdoid appearance may be present

EMA and CK18 expression only focally present

ER, PR, e-cadherin negative

Synaptophysin and chromogranin either focally positive or negative

undifferentiated component and well-differentiated endometrioid carcinoma it can be diagnosed as dedifferentiated endometrial carcinoma (**Fig. 34**), provided that the undifferentiated component does not resemble FIGO grade 3 endometrioid carcinoma. Areas that appear undifferentiated may be found in the setting of other carcinomas, particularly serous carcinoma, but many pathologists currently classify these latter tumors as serous carcinomas with focally solid architecture.

A specific type of undifferentiated carcinoma has been described recently.[68,69] This tumor is

Fig. 36. Undifferentiated carcinoma. The tumor cells have high nuclear to cytoplasmic ratios, eosinophilic cytoplasm (some with a plasmacytoid appearance), and large nuclei with irregular outlines containing one or more nucleoli. The tumor cells are seen in an extensive background of single cell apoptosis.

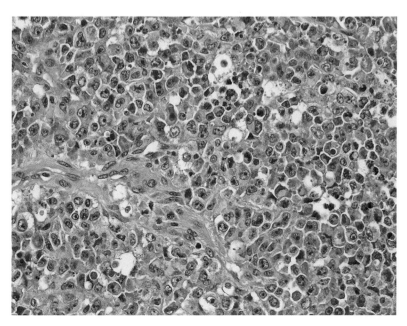

composed of diffuse sheets of loosely cohesive tumor cells (**Fig. 35**) that usually resemble lymphoma or plasmacytoma (**Fig. 36**). Many of these tumors have also been misdiagnosed as "high-grade endometrial stromal sarcoma" or the mesenchymal component of a MMMT. Glandular, nested or trabecular architecture excludes the diagnosis of undifferentiated carcinoma. Myxoid stroma with rhabdoid tumor cells may be apparent focally (**Fig. 37**) and tumor infiltrating lymphocytes may be prominent.

Given the solid architecture seen in this tumor and its resemblance to lymphoma or sarcoma, it is important to verify epithelial differentiation. However, most undifferentiated carcinomas display only focal, limited expression of epithelial-associated proteins (see **Table 2**). Evidence of AE1/3 expression is usually minimal at most, with

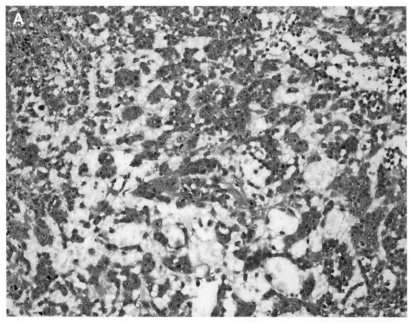

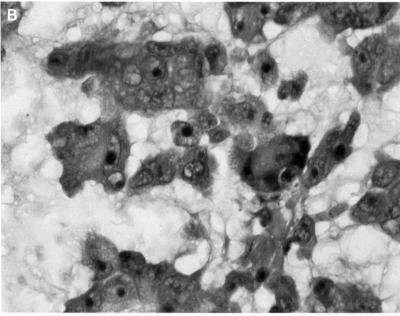

Fig. 37. Undifferentiated carcinoma. The tumor cells are arranged in small nests associated with a prominent myxoid background (*A*) and show a high degree of pleomorphism (*B*).

Fig. 38. Dedifferentiated carcinoma. Only scattered tumor cells are positive for CK18.

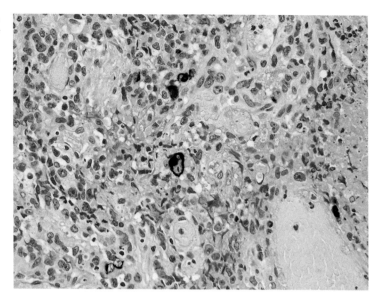

Fig. 39. Dedifferentiated carcinoma. Areas of well-differentiated carcinoma show strong E-cadherin membranous staining (*A*) in contrast to lack of staining in the dedifferentiated component (*B*).

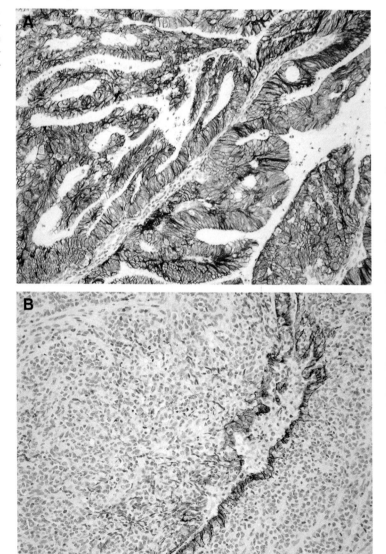

most neoplasms being negative. EMA and CK18 are characteristically expressed in only rare, scattered tumor cells, although the expression tends to be of strong intensity (**Fig. 38**).[68,69] They lack ER and PR as well as e-cadherin expression (**Fig. 39**). Neuroendocrine markers such as synaptophysin and chromogranin may be expressed in rare cells[68]; thus diffuse expression should prompt consideration for a neuroendocrine carcinoma. CD138 can be expressed weakly,[69] but not other hematolymphoid-associated markers. Desmin is negative despite the rhabdoid appearance of the tumor cells. p16 and p53 staining patterns are currently unknown. Some neoplasms demonstrate DNA mismatch repair abnormalities (see "Familial Tumors of the Corpus" article).[12,69]

Mixed Epithelial Carcinomas

Mixed epithelial carcinoma (ie, mixed endometrioid and serous carcinoma) should only be diagnosed when 2 or more types of carcinoma are present and the minor component(s) constitute at least 10% of the overall tumor. Only components with absolutely distinctive features should be recognized as parts of a mixed epithelial tumor (ie, a tumor with easily separable endometrioid and serous components). Tumors with overlapping features (ie, tumors with glandular features and high-nuclear grade) should not be considered mixed epithelial carcinomas (see below). Mixed epithelial carcinomas are, in fact, likely to be unusual when rigorous criteria are applied. Mixed epithelial tumors should be graded based on the highest grade component, but it is acknowledged that this approach has not been formally codified. Applying FIGO grading resulting in an "average" grade of the two components is likely to underestimate a tumor's potential for metastasis and recurrence.

High-Grade Endometrial Carcinoma, not Otherwise Specified

It can sometimes be impossible to subcategorize an endometrial carcinoma with an aggressive appearance (see Fig. 9A in Garg and Soslow article in this publication). This is particularly true for neoplasms that display some features of one tumor type with overlapping features of another tumor type. If clinical, morphologic and immunohistochemical correlation fails to solve the diagnostic problem, it will remain important to establish a tumor grade. The Gilks' grading system is a prognostically informative and reproducible scheme that can be applied to endometrial cancer regardless of histologic subtype.[70] "High-grade" tumors show 2 of the 3 following characteristics: severe

nuclear atypia; solid or papillary architecture; more than 6 mitotic figures per 10 high power fields. It is reasonable to report these tumors as high-grade endometrial carcinomas as it has been shown that even different histologic subtypes treated in an individualized manner are associated with similar clinical outcomes.[1] In a small curettage or biopsy specimen, it is probably sufficient to indicate that a serous component cannot be excluded, which will encourage the gynecologist to perform a comprehensive staging surgery.

DIFFERENTIAL DIAGNOSIS

Non-Neoplastic Lesions

Severe cytologic atypia due to reparative changes or secondary to radiation therapy may cause concern for serous carcinoma (**Figs. 40** and **41**). In most cases, however, cells with reactive changes alternate with more normal appearing endometrial cells. In changes associated with radiation, cells maintain their nuclear to cytoplasmic ratio and the nuclei have a smudged appearance.[71,72] Similarly, papillary eosinophilic metaplasia[73,74] and atypical tubal metaplasia may enter in the differential diagnosis with uterine serous carcinoma (**Fig. 42**). Eosinophilic metaplasia is typically associated with stromal breakdown. The metaplastic cells form a syncytium without discernible cell membranes and show overlapping nuclei. Ki-67 and PHH3 may be helpful in distinguishing this reactive process from serous carcinoma.[74] Tubal metaplasia is one of the most common metaplasias of the endometrium, with cells displaying abundant eosinophilic cytoplasm, enlarged nuclei and relatively prominent nucleoli. A clue to the diagnosis is the presence of cilia.[73] Tubal metaplasia may be prominent in curettage or biopsy specimens from postmenopausal women, causing concern for serous carcinoma. p16 is not helpful in this differential diagnosis as tubal metaplasia is typically

Differential Diagnosis
NON NEOPLASTIC LESIONS

Reparative changes

Radiation therapy induced atypia

Atypical tubal metaplasia

Papillary eosinophilic metaplasia (especially with stromal breakdown)

Arias-Stella reaction

Infarcted endometrial polyps

Fig. 40. Radiation atypia involving endometrial glands. The lining cells show high nuclear to cytoplasmic ratios, prominent nucleoli, and some nuclei with degenerative-type atypia (*upper right*).

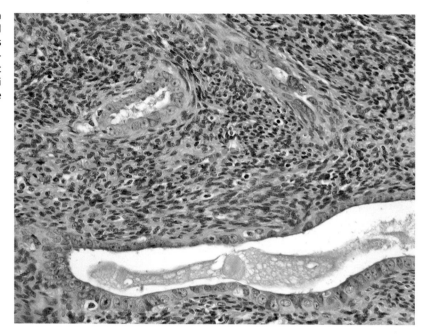

positive for this marker.[75] Features in favor of serous carcinoma include a mitotically active, cytologically atypical proliferation with high nucleus-to-cytoplasmic ratio, lacking cilia and stromal breakdown. p53 and Ki-67 can also be helpful. It is important to be aware that some atypical metaplastic and reactive epithelium can display a large percentage of p53 positive cells (see **Fig. 41**); the proliferative rate in these conditions, however, typically remains below 50% in contrast to serous carcinoma.[76,77]

The Arias-Stella reaction (**Fig. 43**) can be confused with clear cell carcinoma. Its main characteristic is nucleomegaly with cellular enlargement to double or many times the normal nuclear size.[78] There is a form of Arias-Stella characterized by the presence of giant and bizarre nuclei, which when involving all the cells in the glands, may

Fig. 41. Radiation atypia involving endometrial glands. The cells show weak to moderate and multifocal p53 positivity.

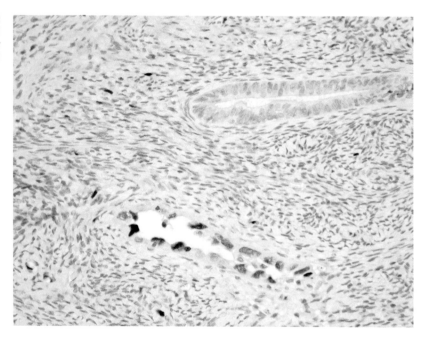

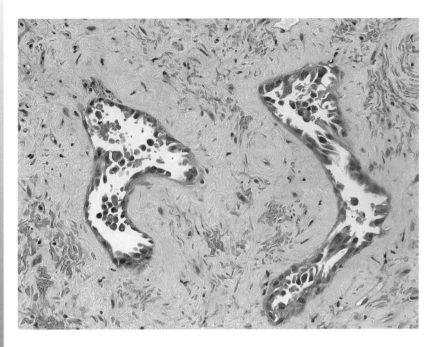

Fig. 42. Hobnail change involving an infarcted endometrial polyp. This finding may resemble serous or clear cell carcinoma at first glance.

cause even more concern for malignancy. However, in general, Arias Stella reaction typically preserves the normal architecture of secretory-phase glands with retention of endometrial stroma. Additional features in favor of Arias Stella reaction include partial gland involvement, a degenerative appearance featuring round nuclei with smudged chromatin, and the absence of mitotic activity[34] (although occasional cases may contain rare mitoses). Infarcted endometrial polyps or stromal breakdown may be associated with clear or hobnail cells as well. However, this change is usually focal and may be associated with syncytial metaplasia.[45] When present in this context, avoiding a malignant diagnosis should be straightforward (see **Fig. 42**).

Tumors with Solid Architecture

The prototypic high-grade endometrial carcinoma with solid architecture is FIGO grade 3

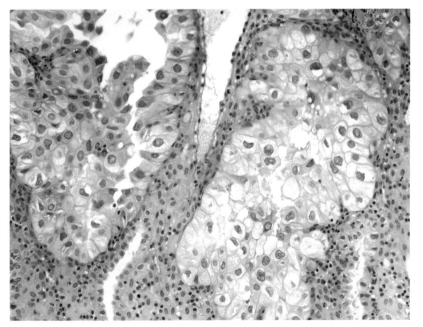

Fig. 43. Arias-Stella reaction. The endometrial glands are lined by cells with abundant clear cytoplasm. The nuclei have pale chromatin and small nucleoli. Scattered nuclei with a smudgy, degenerated appearance are present.

△△ **Differential Diagnosis**
SOLID ARCHITECTURE

FIGO grade 3 endometrioid carcinoma

FIGO grades 1 and 2 carcinoma with squamous differentiation and/or spindle cell features

Serous carcinoma

Clear cell carcinoma

Undifferentiated carcinoma

Squamous cell carcinoma

Transitional cell carcinoma

Neuroendocrine carcinoma

Malignant mixed müllerian tumor

Sarcomas and PEComa

Placental site and epithelioid trophoblastic tumors

Primitive neuroectodermal tumor

Metastatic lobular carcinoma

---

endometrioid carcinoma. FIGO grade 1 or 2 carcinoma with squamous differentiation should display no more than moderate nuclear atypia and lack a predominant pattern of solid, nonsquamous growth. Most examples of squamous differentiation that accompany these tumors are cytologically low grade and, frequently, keratinizing (see Fig. 6B and Fig. 12B in Mills and Longacre review on Atypical Endometrial Hyperplasia and Well Differentiated Endometrioid Adenocarcinoma of the Uterine Corpus). Low-grade endometrioid

adenocarcinoma with spindle cell elements (See Fig. 31A in Mills and Longacre article in this publication) may be confused at low power with a FIGO grade 3 endometrioid carcinoma as these may show extensive solid areas. However, the spindle cell component does not show high-grade cytologic features and it merges with both conventional areas of squamous metaplasia and endometrioid glands.[79,80]

Distinguishing solid clear cell carcinoma and endometrioid carcinoma can be challenging, especially in a tumor that gives the impression of having a predominance of immature squamous metaplasia with cytoplasmic glycogenation. If such a tumor also had papillary or tubulocystic components lacking columnar cells and were ER and PR negative, the diagnosis of clear cell carcinoma would be favored.

Pure squamous carcinomas of the endometrium (**Fig. 44**) are extremely rare[81–87] Endometrial squamous carcinoma can only be diagnosed when a clinical history of cervical squamous carcinoma *and* concurrent histologic evidence of cervical high-grade squamous dysplasia and squamous cell carcinoma (**Fig. 45**) are absent. Any endometrioid differentiation in the form of glands must also be lacking. The potential association between HPV and squamous cell carcinoma of the endometrium is contradictory. Some investigators have reported these tumors to be HPV positive[85] but most lack HPV expression.[82,86,88,89] Some studies have looked at p16 expression and its relation to HPV status in these tumors with inconclusive results.[87–89] Thus, p16 cannot be used to separate squamous cell carcinoma of the endometrium from other high-grade endometrial carcinomas.

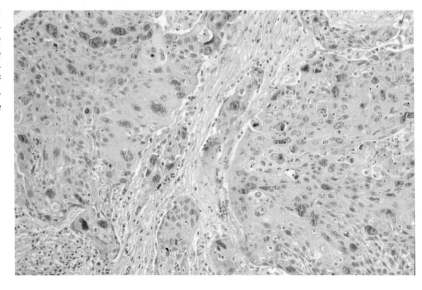

Fig. 44. Squamous cell carcinoma of endometrium. This exceedingly rare tumor can only be diagnosed when endometrioid carcinoma of endometrium and squamous neoplasms of the cervix are excluded.

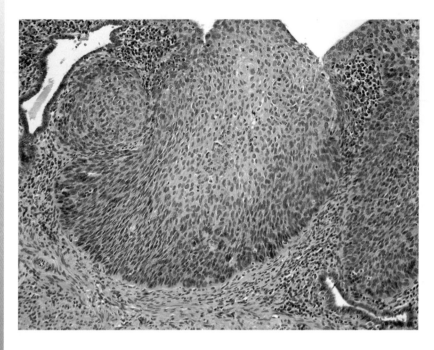

Fig. 45. Cervical squamous carcinoma in situ (high-grade squamous intraepithelial lesion/CIN 3) is colonizing the surface and glands of the lower uterine segment.

Occasional endometrioid adenocarcinomas demonstrate exophytic, broad papillae lined by multiple layers of stratified cells with squamo-transitional features. These tumors should be classified as endometrioid if they retain some evidence of glandular differentiation (**Fig. 46**), but they can also be classified as transitional cell carcinoma (**Fig. 47**)[90–92] if those features are absent. Rare transitional cell carcinomas of the urinary tract secondarily involve the uterine corpus, but most of these show vaginal and cervical involvement

as well[93] (see **Fig. 11** in Park, Neoplastic Lesions of the Cervix).

Pure neuroendocrine carcinomas of the endometrium[94] are extraordinary rare, but there are also occasional reports of combined neuroendocrine carcinoma and adenocarcinoma.[25,95] A solid architecture in these tumors inevitably leads to consideration of a FIGO grade 3 endometrioid carcinoma (**Fig. 48**). Tumors with a large cell neuroendocrine component are probably more commonly encountered and more prone to

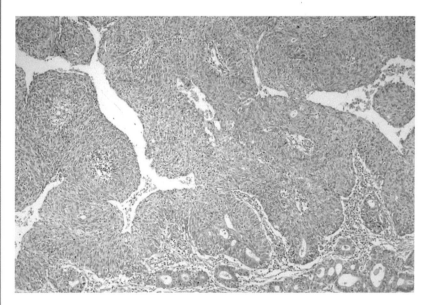

Fig. 46. FIGO grade 3 endometrioid carcinoma resembling transitional cell carcinoma. Glandular architecture suggests endometrioid differentiation.

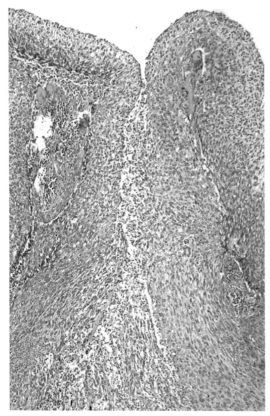

Fig. 47. Transitional cell carcinoma. The tumor shows a papillary architecture with multiple layers of neoplastic cells.

confusion than those with a small cell component. Diagnostic criteria for these tumors are the same as those used in other organs. Small cell neuroendocrine carcinomas should be composed of small cells, with a high nucleus-to-cytoplasm ratio, nuclear molding, but no nucleoli, with an extremely high proliferative rate and numerous apoptotic bodies. Large cell neuroendocrine carcinomas show a nested or trabecular growth with large cells containing nuclei with nucleoli and high proliferative indices. Although many pathologists do not require immunohistochemical stains to establish a diagnosis of small cell neuroendocrine carcinoma, many rely on immunohistochemistry to diagnose the large cell variant. The latter should show convincing expression of a neuroendocrine marker such as chromogranin in at least 20% of tumor cells. Of note, many endometrioid carcinomas contain a significant percentage of neoplastic cells that stain positively for neuroendocrine markers, but in general, these tumors neither resemble neuroendocrine carcinomas nor exhibit widespread immunohistochemical evidence of neuroendocrine differentiation.

Primitive neuroectodermal tumors (PNETs) also occasionally arise in the uterus.[96,97] The presence of scattered rosettes may mimic endometrioid glands and the solid growth can suggest a FIGO grade 3 endometrioid carcinoma. The correct diagnosis can be suggested by the presence of true rosettes and confirmed with immunohistochemical stains and molecular testing. PNETs, particularly

Fig. 48. Undifferentiated neuroendocrine carcinoma. The tumor cells grow in cords and nests and have a monotonous appearance.

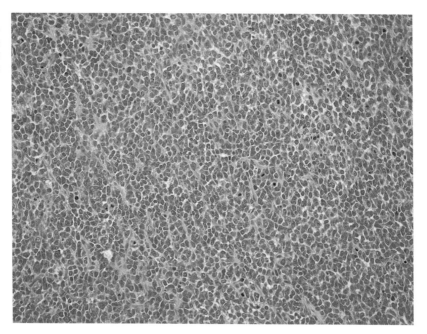

those of the peripheral variety (ie, part of the spectrum of Ewing Sarcoma), express CD99 (membranous pattern) and Fli-1 diffusely and are usually, but not always, cytokeratin negative. The vast majority of peripheral PNETs harbor t(11;22)(q24;q12), involving the *EWS* and *FLI1* genes.

Serous carcinomas may display a solid architecture, but this is almost always only one component of a tumor that elsewhere exhibits papillary and/or glandular features. Solid areas of serous carcinoma tend to be cytologically similar to papillary areas. Although both FIGO grade 3 endometrioid and serous carcinomas may overexpress p53, some investigators have proposed that p53 and p16 overexpression along with loss of PR and retention of PTEN immunohistochemical stains favor serous over endometrioid differentiation in a solid tumor.[98]

Undifferentiated carcinoma fails to show nested and trabecular architecture and, unlike FIGO grade 3 endometrioid carcinoma, is composed of non-cohesive cells (see **Figs. 35** and **36**). Undifferentiated carcinoma shows only minimal to no evidence of epithelial differentiation with focal EMA and/or CK18 staining and lacks expression of e-cadherin.[69] The epithelial immunophenotype, while limited in most cases, along with absent expression of muscle markers, are sufficient to exclude undifferentiated sarcoma or epithelioid leiomyosarcoma given a high-grade tumor composed of uniform epithelioid cells. Undifferentiated carcinoma should not be confused with MMMT as pleomorphic spindle cells, typical of MMMT, are lacking. Lymphoma and plasmacytoma are also in the differential diagnosis of undifferentiated carcinoma, but immunohistochemistry usually solves this problem. Metastatic lobular carcinoma from the breast typically replaces the endometrial stroma with sheets and infiltrative cords of uniform, small neoplastic cells. The distribution of tumor and its cytologic features are distinctive (**Fig. 49**).

Epithelioid smooth muscle tumors, either benign or malignant, PEComa, and rarely other tumors including endometrial stromal tumors, placental site trophoblastic tumor, and alveolar soft part sarcoma may enter the differential diagnosis with solid carcinomas, particularly clear cell carcinoma. Epithelioid smooth muscle tumors can cause even more confusion as they are frequently positive for keratins, EMA[99] and p16. However, most of these tumors show focal spindle areas, lack the typical architectural patterns of clear cell and endometrioid carcinomas, and frequently display some degree of positivity for smooth muscle markers.[100–104] Although PEComas may have clear cells with an epithelioid appearance, they not infrequently also have a spindle cell component. These tumors react with HMB-45 and Melan-A, and are often also positive for smooth muscle markers, but not for keratins.[105,106] Endometrial stromal tumors may have clear cells but the tumor shows the typical appearance reminiscent of the proliferative-phase of endometrium.[107] Placental site trophoblastic tumor may have a striking component of clear cells and it is

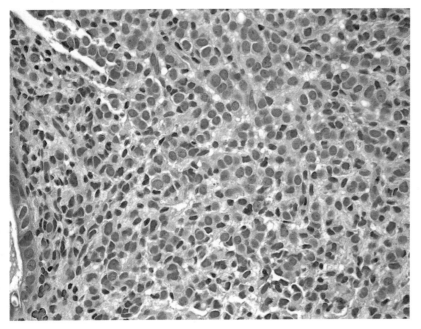

Fig. 49. Metastatic lobular carcinoma to the endometrium. The tumor is composed of uniform cells with scant cytoplasm and round nuclei arranged in cords and trabeculae mimicking an undifferentiated carcinoma.

frequently keratin positive, but it also stains for inhibin and HPL.[108–111] Finally, alveolar soft part sarcoma contains clear cells, forms solid or open tubules, and the cells may have a hobnail appearance. However, the cytoplasm of these tumors contain PAS-positive, diastase-resistant granules and they are positive for TFE-3.[112,113]

Tumors with Papillary Architecture

The prototypic high-grade endometrial carcinoma with papillary architecture is serous carcinoma. Distinction from almost all of the entities in the differential diagnosis of papillary tumor centers on the presence of cellular tufting, multilayering and detachment of tumor cells in the presence of diffuse and marked nuclear pleomorphism and a high-mitotic rate in serous carcinoma.

Extrauterine serous carcinoma (ie, tubal, ovarian and/or peritoneal primary tumors) may secondarily involve the endometrium, leading to difficulty in distinguishing them from primary endometrial serous carcinoma. The latter may display overlapping clinical features with extrauterine serous carcinoma because of its tendency to metastasize to ovaries and peritoneum without forming a mass in the uterus. In premenopausal patients, extrauterine serous carcinomas may be present in a background of cycling endometrium, unlike that seen in the typical postmenopausal patient with endometrial serous carcinoma. In curettage specimens, there may be only scanty evidence of tumor and it may be distributed in minute clusters and single, detached cells, admixed with non-neoplastic native endometrium. The presence of low-grade serous carcinoma in a curettage should be regarded as metastasis because this tumor exclusively arises in extrauterine sites. In hysterectomy specimens, drop metastases from high-grade extrauterine serous carcinoma frequently involve the endometrium only superficially, may be multifocal, and fail to demonstrate the almost invariable relationship with endometrial polyps as seen in primary endometrial serous carcinoma. Many of such neoplasms also show intraepithelial serous carcinoma of the fallopian tube fimbriae.[114] In general, extrauterine serous carcinoma tends to be more frequently positive for ER, PR and WT1, less frequently positive for vimentin and slightly less frequently overexpress p53.[38,39,115,116] It is not currently considered standard practice to use this immunophenotype to separate uterine and extrauterine serous carcinomas partly because as many as 30% of uterine serous carcinomas have been reported to be WT1 positive[9,35,39,117] and 20%–30% of ovarian, tubal and peritoneal carcinomas are WT1 negative.[35,39,117]

Endometrioid carcinomas with papillae (ie, villoglandular carcinoma and carcinomas with non-villous papillae (**Figs. 50 and 51**) or surface pseudopapillae have smooth luminal contours without prominent micropapillae or tufting.[45] They show marked nuclear atypia only exceptionally. In general, features that favor a diagnosis of endometrioid carcinoma (including papillary variants) over serous carcinoma include:

1. Gland formation with smooth luminal borders, rounded contours lacking cellular dyshesion or extensive budding
2. Retained nuclear polarity
3. Homogeneous nuclear features
4. Unequivocal squamous metaplasia (including morules)
5. Intracytoplasmic mucin
6. Cilia.

In contrast, the papillae in serous carcinoma are often irregular and short and lined by markedly atypical, pseudostratified cells with single cell budding (**Fig. 52**).[45,118,119] As such, these two tumors can be distinguished in most cases without the use of immunohistochemistry. When immunohistochemistry is employed, p53 and p16 overexpression are lacking or minimally expressed in papillary variants of FIGO grades 1 and 2 endometrioid carcinoma with retention of ER and PR expression in contrast to serous carcinoma.

As discussed earlier, clear cell carcinoma (see **Fig. 24**) can be separated from serous carcinoma (see **Fig. 52**) by finding short, round papillae lined by only one or two layers of cuboidal to flat cells with a low mitotic rate; tufting, budding and obvious dyshesion of cells are unusual findings. Although the nuclear features are highly atypical, the nuclear appearance tends to be substantially more uniform in clear cell than in serous carcinoma.[45] In contrast to serous carcinoma,

Differential Diagnosis
PAPILLARY ARCHITECTURE

Serous carcinoma

Endometrioid carcinoma (NOS, villoglandular and non-villous papillary variants)

Clear cell carcinoma

Malignant mixed müllerian tumor

Endocervical adenocarcinoma

Metastatic serous carcinoma

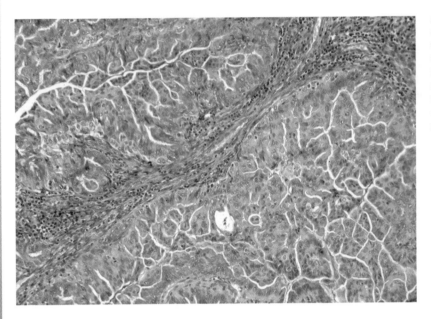

Fig. 50. Endometrioid carcinoma with small non-villous papillae. Tumors with small, back-to-back intraglandular papillae superficially resemble serous carcinoma. Luminal contours, however, are smooth.

clear cell carcinoma expresses HNF-1β[61] and fails to overexpress p53[46,56,57] and p16.[8] ER and PR are negative[8,46,56] in most tumors.

HPV-associated endocervical adenocarcinoma may show notable nuclear atypia in the context of a papillary neoplasm. Affected patients are substantially younger and both cytologic features and immunophenotype differ from that of serous carcinoma. In endocervical adenocarcinoma, the nuclei tend to be long, thin, darkly stained and pseudostratified. Mucinous differentiation is usually, but not always, apparent. Extensive tufting and dyshesion are not typical findings. While both serous and HPV-associated endocervical adenocarcinoma show overexpression of p16, only serous carcinoma shows p53 overexpression[36,104,120–124] Most pathologists tend to agree that serous carcinomas of the endocervix represent either misclassified HPV-associated papillary endocervical carcinomas or serous

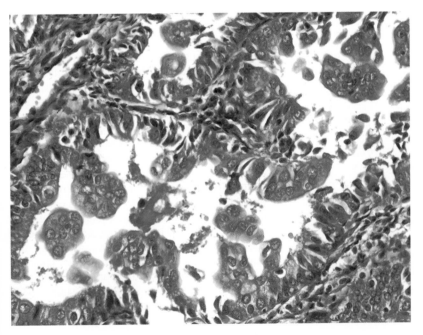

Fig. 51. Endometrioid carcinoma with small non-villous papillae. Small pseudopapillae lacking central fibrovascular cores have cells with eosinophilic cytoplasm and small round nuclei with tiny nucleoli. This is in contrast to the high-grade nuclear features seen in serous carcinoma.

Fig. 52. Papillary serous carcinoma. The tumor is composed of irregularly shaped and sized papillae associated with prominent budding of pleomorphic cells.

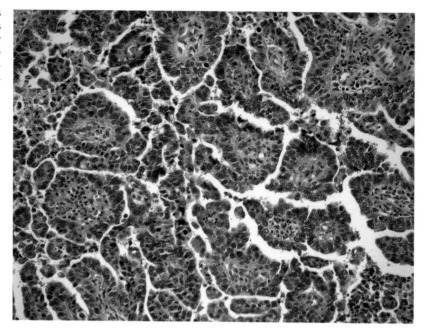

carcinomas that have secondarily extended to the cervix or metastasized from another site.

Tumors with Glandular Architecture

The usual default diagnosis for a gland-forming neoplasm in the endometrium is either hyperplasia or differentiated endometrioid adenocarcinoma. It cannot be emphasized strongly enough that, with only one exception, the presence of diffuse severe nuclear atypia is sufficient to invalidate these diagnoses. It is still permissible, in theory, to "upgrade" an architecturally well-differentiated tumor with severe nuclear atypia from FIGO grade 1 to FIGO grade 2 (See Fig. 41B in Mills and Longacre review on Atypical Endometrial Hyperplasia and Well Differentiated Endometrioid Adenocarcinoma of the Uterine Corpus); however, it should be noted that many of these neoplasms are significantly more clinically aggressive than other FIGO grade

▲▲ **Differential Diagnosis**
    Glandular Architecture

Complex and simple atypical hyperplasia

Endometrioid carcinoma

Serous carcinoma

Clear cell carcinoma

Endocervical adenocarcinoma

Metastatic colorectal adenocarcinoma

2 tumors and at least some of them may represent in fact the glandular variant of serous carcinoma. This suggests that a diagnosis of serous, clear cell or HPV-associated endocervical adenocarcinoma should be seriously considered before making an erroneous diagnosis of a differentiated endometrioid neoplasm.

Gland forming endometrial tumors with severe nuclear atypia that show very high mitotic rates, serrated luminal contours, micropapillae, tufting and dyshesion of the tumor cells, with or without intraepithelial carcinoma, should be considered serous carcinomas until proven otherwise, especially when the proliferation appears centered in an endometrial polyp (see **Fig. 9**). Unlike differentiated endometrioid neoplasms, these tumors diffusely overexpress p53[31,125] and p16[8,36] and tend to lack diffuse ER and PR expression. Gland forming tumors with cuboidal to flat cells showing severe nuclear atypia and without high mitotic rate, budding and dyshesion, are likely to be clear cell carcinomas (see **Fig. 26**) whereas tumors composed of columnar cells with oval or elongate nuclei lacking nucleoli are likely endometrioid (**Figs. 53** and **54**). These tumors lack ER and PR expression. Metastatic colorectal carcinoma may occasionally present as a primary endometrial carcinoma. Many of these tumors are relatively mucin-depleted, leading to a superficial resemblance to endometrioid carcinoma. However, the nuclear features are usually severely atypical, mitotic rate is very high, and necrosis is common. These features, in addition

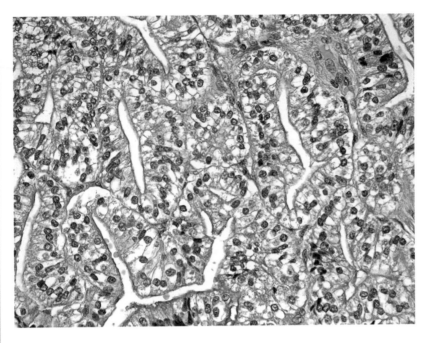

Fig. 53. Endometrioid carcinoma, secretory variant. The neoplastic glands show prominent subnuclear vacuoles. Note the low-grade nuclear features and columnar cell shape, which contrast with the high-grade features of clear cell carcinoma.

to the presence of elongate, darkly stained nuclei and goblet cells, should be clues that the tumor is not endometrioid. Metastatic colorectal carcinomas (See Fig. 36A in Mills and Longacre review on Atypical Endometrial Hyperplasia and Well Differentiated Endometrioid Adenocarcinoma of the Uterine Corpus) are CK20 positive and CK7, ER and PR negative. As both endometrioid and colorectal carcinomas can express CDX2, the use of this marker should be avoided when

metastatic colorectal carcinoma is in the differential diagnosis.[126–130]

CLINICAL FEATURES AND PROGNOSIS

FIGO Grade 3 Endometrioid Carcinoma

This tumor is a distinct, biologically aggressive endometrioid carcinoma subtype that has a higher risk of both locoregional and distant relapse and overall poor survival when compared

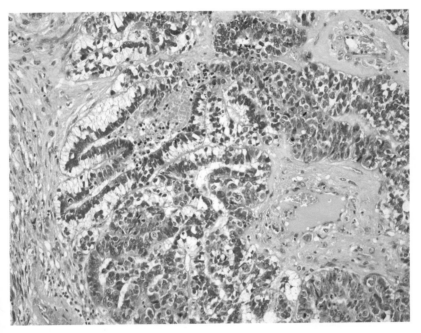

Fig. 54. Endometrioid carcinoma with focal secretory changes. Large subnuclear vacuoles, as seen in secretory endometrium day 17, are present in a component of the tumor showing pseudopapillary architecture (*left*), mimicking mixed endometrioid and clear cell carcinoma.

with differentiated endometrioid carcinoma. It is associated with deep myometrial invasion, cervical involvement and lymphovascular invasion.[131] Thus, patients with FIGO grade 3 endometrioid carcinoma should be offered comprehensive surgical staging similar to serous carcinoma and clear cell carcinoma. Overall survival for patients with FIGO grade 3 endometrioid carcinoma can be estimated to be approximately 40%–60%,[1] but valid figures cannot be ascertained at present because of different approaches to therapy and difficulties in distinguishing FIGO grade 3 carcinoma from other high-grade endometrial carcinomas. In populations that are suboptimally staged and where chemotherapy is used infrequently, FIGO grade 3 endometrioid carcinoma appears clinically more favorable when compared with serous carcinoma.[132] However, when staging is comprehensive and chemotherapy is used, most of these apparent differences in survival become muted.[1] Like differentiated endometrioid carcinoma, they typically demonstrate pelvic recurrence, but in contrast to low-grade endometrioid carcinomas, they also can spread to para-aortic lymph nodes and lungs. In one study, the overall recurrence rate for patients with surgical stage IA-IC FIGO grade 3 endometrioid carcinoma was 8 to 13% but when patients with stage IB/IC were separated from stage IA, the patients had a significant risk for extra-pelvic recurrence independent of the treatment modality used with most patients dying secondary to their disease,[133] usually within 2 years of diagnosis.[134] In contrast to serous carcinoma, patients who appear to have tumor confined to the uterus much less frequently have occult peritoneal metastases.[1] Therefore, patients with stage I disease, particularly when it is non-invasive, have an excellent outcome. Currently, chemotherapy is reserved for patients with extrauterine disease. However, some evolving treatment protocols mandate chemotherapy for patients with risk factors that include advanced age, lymphovascular invasion or deep myometrial invasion (see article by Leitao and Barakat in this publication). Patients are generally offered vaginal brachytherapy to decrease the risk of vaginal apex recurrence and may be offered pelvic external beam radiation if they have not been comprehensively staged.

Serous Carcinoma

Despite the fact that there are some morphologic similarities between endometrial and extrauterine serous carcinoma, their epidemiologic features are distinct.[135] Uterine serous carcinomas lack associations with nulliparity and oral contraceptives that are typical of ovarian serous carcinoma patients, and in North America, patients with endometrial serous carcinoma are more frequently African American and are significantly older than the typical patient with extrauterine serous carcinoma. Uterine serous carcinomas are associated with endometrial atrophy and endometrial polyps.[13,14,33,52,136,137] Many of these tumors occur in breast cancer patients, including those treated with tamoxifen,[138] and in rectal or cervical carcinoma patients treated with pelvic radiation therapy.[139,140] Rare serous carcinomas occur in a background of well- or moderately differentiated endometrioid carcinoma and only occasional examples have been reported in the setting of BRCA1 or 2 mutations[141,142] or in association with hereditary non-polyposis colorectal carcinoma (Lynch syndrome).[10]

Uterine serous carcinoma patients may present with uterine bleeding and frequently have an abnormal cervicovaginal pap test.[143,144] Serum CA-125 levels are often elevated[145] and rare patients may present with paraneoplastic hypercalcemia.[146] Serous carcinoma is a highly aggressive tumor that disseminates widely, early in its evolution,[147] sometimes without obvious clinical evidence of metastasis. It frequently exhibits peritoneal spread and lymphovascular invasion in the absence of demonstrable myometrial invasion. This can be explained by the observation that serous carcinomas are composed of non-cohesive cells which are prone to retrograde displacement through the fallopian tubes or shedding into the cervix.

Overall survival estimates for serous carcinoma are approximately 30 to 40%. FIGO stage I carcinoma patients have the best survival, in the range of 70 to 80%, but qualifying for favorable prognosis stage I serous carcinoma involves surgical staging with formal lymph node dissection, omentectomy and peritoneal biopsies. This meticulous staging is important because as many as one-half of patients without obvious extrauterine tumor have metastasis demonstrable only after comprehensive staging.[148–151] Bona fide stage I serous carcinoma patients with tumor confined to the endometrium have survivals estimated at 90%.[13,15,152–156] "Minimal uterine serous carcinoma" (<1 cm of carcinoma in the endometrium)[2] and patients without residual tumor on hysterectomy and staging, after curettage,[3] have superior prognoses. Chemotherapy and radiotherapy are usually offered to all patients with serous carcinoma except those with FIGO stage I carcinoma limited to the endometrium.

Clear Cell Carcinoma

Little is known about the epidemiologic risk factors for developing clear cell carcinoma. Patient age at presentation is intermediate between FIGO grade 3 carcinoma and serous carcinoma, approximately 65 years, although rare tumors may be seen in young patients with Lynch syndrome (see Garg and Soslow review on Familial Tumors of the Uterine Corpus). They tend to present with non-specific signs, with postmenopausal or dysfunctional uterine bleeding being most common.[49,51] No association with diethylstilbestrol has been reported in contrast to clear cell carcinoma arising in the uterine cervix or vagina.[157] These tumors may be clinically associated with paraneoplastic hypercalcemia, which in some cases has been related to PTH-rP expression.[158,159] This tumor also displays a high rate of venous thromboembolism.[160]

As with FIGO grade 3 endometrioid carcinoma, valid survival figures are impossible to quote because of difficulties in distinguishing clear cell carcinoma from other high-grade endometrial carcinomas. Pure clear cell carcinoma of the endometrium is also an exceedingly uncommon tumor. Assumptions about similarities between clear cell and serous carcinoma are largely inaccurate. In contrast to the peritoneal spread seen in ovarian and uterine serous carcinoma, the distribution of recurrent disease in uterine clear cell carcinoma includes intra-abdominal and retroperitoneal structures as well as distant sites, but not peritoneal metastases (similar to FIGO grade 3 endometrioid carcinoma).[1,161] Patients with stage I tumors have a significantly better prognosis than that reported for stage I uterine serous carcinoma[48,161] even more if tumors lack myometrial invasion.[47] Some studies have shown that patients with uterine serous and clear cell carcinoma have a significantly poorer prognosis compared with those with FIGO grade 3 endometrioid carcinoma[132]; however, other studies have shown that high-grade endometrial cancers of different histologic subtypes treated in an individualized manner are associated with similar clinical outcomes.[1] Some oncologists advocate treating almost all clear cell carcinoma patients with chemotherapy (like serous carcinoma), whereas others treat only in the presence of other risk factors (advanced age, lymphovascular invasion or deep myometrial invasion) or high stage disease.

Undifferentiated Carcinoma

Undifferentiated carcinoma is a very aggressive tumor with almost all patients experiencing recurrence or tumor-related death[68] with metastases to pelvic structures, lymph nodes and parenchymal organs.[69] The degree of lymphadenopathy and elevated serum LDH levels sometime raise clinical suspicion of lymphoma or a germ cell tumor when the patient is young.[69] Some tumors arise in patients with Lynch syndrome (see Garg and Soslow article on Hereditary Endometrial Cancer in this publication).

Mixed Epithelial Carcinomas

There are only limited data regarding the prognosis and treatment of patients with mixed epithelial carcinomas. It has been suggested that the presence of a serous or undifferentiated component likely drives prognosis. It is important to emphasize that any component of serous carcinoma should be noted in the pathology report as the presence of even a 10% serous component has significant therapeutic and prognostic implications.[162] One study in abstract form reports that mixed epithelial carcinomas with a clear cell component (many of which were mixed serous and clear cell carcinomas) are significantly more aggressive than pure clear cell carcinomas.[53] So-called de-differentiated endometrial carcinomas (combined differentiated and undifferentiated carcinomas) disseminate widely and aggressively despite the presence of a low grade component.[163]

Pitfalls
HIGH-GRADE ENDOMETRIAL CARCINOMA

! Many solid endometrial tumors are NOT endometrioid carcinomas

! Not every papillary endometrial carcinoma is of serous subtype

! Not every glandular endometrial carcinoma is of endometrioid subtype

! Failing to use immunohistochemical panels that are precisely tailored for specific differential diagnoses may lead to misdiagnosis

! p53 immunoexpression in isolation from other clinical, pathologic and immunohistochemical features is not diagnostic of serous carcinoma. p53 and p16 *overexpression* refers, specifically, to expression in more than 75% of tumor cells, which is typically seen in serous carcinoma

! Do not assume that all high-grade endometrial carcinomas are clinically similar; overall survivals are similar in some studies, but demographic and epidemiologic features as well as patterns of spread and treatment modalities differ

REFERENCES

1. Soslow RA, Bissonnette JP, Wilton A, et al. Clinicopathologic analysis of 187 high-grade endometrial carcinomas of different histologic subtypes: similar outcomes belie distinctive biologic differences. Am J Surg Pathol 2007;31(7):979–87.

2. Catasus L, Gallardo A, Cuatrecasas M, et al. Concomitant PI3K-AKT and p53 alterations in endometrial carcinomas are associated with poor prognosis. Mod Pathol 2009;22(4):522–9.

3. Soslow RA, Shen PU, Chung MH, et al. Distinctive p53 and mdm2 immunohistochemical expression profiles suggest different pathogenetic pathways in poorly differentiated endometrial carcinoma. Int J Gynecol Pathol 1998;17:129–34.

4. Lax SF, Kendall B, Tashiro H, et al. The frequency of p53, K-ras mutations, and microsatellite instability differs in uterine endometrioid and serous carcinoma - evidence of distinct molecular genetic pathways. Cancer 2000;88(4):814–24.

5. Alvarez T, Bhan AK, Miller E, et al. Molecular profile of grade 3 endometrial endometrioid carcinoma: is it a type I or type II endometrial carcinoma? [abstract 820]. Mod Pathol 2005;18(Suppl 1):177A.

6. Feng YZ, Shiozawa T, Horiuchi A, et al. Intratumoral heterogeneous expression of p53 correlates with p53 mutation, Ki-67, and cyclin A expression in endometrioid-type endometrial adenocarcinomas. Virchows Arch 2005;447(5):816–22.

7. Halperin R, Zehavi S, Habler L, et al. Comparative immunohistochemical study of endometrioid and serous papillary carcinoma of endometrium. Eur J Gynaecol Oncol 2001;22(2):122–6.

8. Reid-Nicholson M, Iyengar P, Hummer AJ, et al. Immunophenotypic diversity of endometrial adenocarcinomas: implications for differential diagnosis. Mod Pathol 2006;19(8):1091–100.

9. Dupont J, Wang X, Marshall DS, et al. Wilms Tumor Gene (WT1) and p53 expression in endometrial carcinomas: a study of 130 cases using a tissue microarray. Gynecol Oncol 2004;94(2):449–55.

10. Carcangiu ML, Radice P, Casalini P, et al. Lynch syndrome–related endometrial carcinomas show a high frequency of nonendometrioid types and of high FIGO grade endometrioid types. Int J Surg Pathol 2010;18(1):21–6.

11. Garg K, Leitao MM Jr, Kauff ND, et al. Selection of endometrial carcinomas for DNA mismatch repair protein immunohistochemistry using patient age and tumor morphology enhances detection of mismatch repair abnormalities. Am J Surg Pathol 2009;33(6):925–33.

12. Broaddus RR, Lynch HT, Chen LM, et al. Pathologic features of endometrial carcinoma associated with HNPCC: a comparison with sporadic endometrial carcinoma. Cancer 2006;106(1):87–94.

13. Carcangiu ML, Tan LK, Chambers JT. Stage IA uterine serous carcinoma. A study of 13 cases. Am J Surg Pathol 1997;21(12):1507–14.

14. McCluggage WG, Sumathi VP, McManus DT. Uterine serous carcinoma and endometrial intraepithelial carcinoma arising in endometrial polyps: report of 5 cases, including 2 associated with tamoxifen therapy. Hum Pathol 2003;34(9):939–43.

15. Hui P, Kelly M, O'Malley DM, et al. Minimal uterine serous carcinoma: a clinicopathological study of 40 cases. Mod Pathol 2005;18(1):75–82.

16. Wheeler DT, Bell KA, Kurman RJ, et al. Minimal uterine serous carcinoma: diagnosis and clinicopathologic correlation. Am J Surg Pathol 2000;24(6):797–806.

17. Silva EG, Jenkins R. Serous carcinoma in endometrial polyps. Mod Pathol 1990;3(2):120–8.

18. Sherman ME, Bitterman P, Rosenshein NB, et al. Uterine serous carcinoma: a morphologically diverse neoplasm with unifying clinicopathologic features. Am J Surg Pathol 1992;16:600–10.

19. Ambros RA, Sherman ME, Zahn CM, et al. Endometrial intraepithelial carcinoma: a distinctive lesion specifically associated with tumors displaying serous differentiation. Hum Pathol 1995;26:1260–7.

20. Goff BA, Kato D, Schmidt RA, et al. Uterine papillary serous carcinoma: patterns of metastatic spread [see comments]. Gynecol Oncol 1994;54:264–8.

21. Hendrickson M, Martinez A, Ross J, et al. Uterine papillary serous carcinoma: a highly malignant form of endometrial adenocarcinoma. Am J Surg Pathol 1982;6:93–108.

22. Lee KR, Belinson JL. Recurrence in noninvasive endometrial carcinoma: relationship to uterine papillary serous carcinoma. Am J Surg Pathol 1991;15:965–73.

23. Williams KE, Waters ED, Woolas RP, et al. Mixed serous-endometrioid carcinoma of the uterus: pathologic and cytopathologic analysis of a high-risk endometrial carcinoma. Int J Gynecol Cancer 1994;4:7–18.

24. Carcangiu ML, Chambers JT. Uterine papillary serous carcinoma: a study on 108 cases with emphasis on the prognostic significance of associated endometrioid carcinoma, absence of invasion, and concomitant ovarian carcinoma. Gynecol Oncol 1992;47:298–305.

25. Posligua L, Malpica A, Liu J, et al. Combined large cell neuroendocrine carcinoma and papillary serous carcinoma of the endometrium with pagetoid spread. Arch Pathol Lab Med 2008;132(11):1821–4.

26. Jordan LB, Abdul-Kader M, Al-Nafussi A. Uterine serous papillary carcinoma: histopathologic

changes within the female genital tract. Int J Gynecol Cancer 2001;11(4):283–9.

27. Horn LC, Hanel C, Bartholdt E, et al. Mixed serous carcinoma of the endometrium with trophoblastic differentiation: analysis of the p53 tumor suppressor gene suggests stem cell origin. Ann Diagn Pathol 2008;12(1):1–3.

28. Sherman ME, Bur ME, Kurman RJ. p53 in endometrial cancer and its putative precursors: evidence for diverse pathways of tumorigenesis. Hum Pathol 1995;26:1268–74.

29. Spiegel GW. Endometrial carcinoma in situ in postmenopausal women. Am J Surg Pathol 1995;19:417–32.

30. Soslow RA, Pirog E, Isacson C. Endometrial intraepithelial carcinoma with associated peritoneal carcinomatosis. Am J Surg Pathol 2000;24(5):726–32.

31. Tashiro H, Isacson C, Levine R, et al. p53 gene mutations are common in uterine serous carcinoma and occur early in their pathogenesis. Am J Pathol 1997;150(1):177–85.

32. Chiesa-Vottero AG, Malpica A, Deavers MT, et al. Immunohistochemical overexpression of p16 and p53 in uterine serous carcinoma and ovarian high-grade serous carcinoma. Int J Gynecol Pathol 2007;26(3):328–33.

33. Trahan S, Tetu B, Raymond PE. Serous papillary carcinoma of the endometrium arising from endometrial polyps: a clinical, histological, and immunohistochemical study of 13 cases. Hum Pathol 2005; 36(12):1316–21.

34. Vang R, Barner R, Wheeler DT, et al. Immunohistochemical staining for Ki-67 and p53 helps distinguish endometrial Arias-Stella reaction from high-grade carcinoma, including clear cell carcinoma. Int J Gynecol Pathol 2004;23(3):223–33.

35. Egan JA, Ionescu MC, Eapen E, et al. Differential expression of WT1 and p53 in serous and endometrioid carcinomas of the endometrium. Int J Gynecol Pathol 2004;23(2):119–22.

36. Yemelyanova A, Ji H, Shih IeM, et al. Utility of p16 expression for distinction of uterine serous carcinomas from endometrial endometrioid and endocervical adenocarcinomas: immunohistochemical analysis of 201 cases. Am J Surg Pathol 2009; 33(10):1504–14.

37. Alkushi A, Clarke BA, Akbari M, et al. Identification of prognostically relevant and reproducible subsets of endometrial adenocarcinoma based on clustering analysis of immunostaining data. Mod Pathol 2007;20(11):1156–65.

38. Nofech-Mozes S, Khalifa MA, Ismiil N, et al. Immunophenotyping of serous carcinoma of the female genital tract. Mod Pathol 2008;21(9):1147–55.

39. Acs G, Pasha T, Zhang PJ. WT1 is differentially expressed in serous, endometrioid, clear cell, and

40. Schmitz MJ, Hendricks DT, Farley J, et al. p27 and cyclin D1 abnormalities in uterine papillary serous carcinoma. Gynecol Oncol 2000;77(3):439–45.

41. Holcomb K, Delatorre R, Pedemonte B, et al. E-cadherin expression in endometrioid, papillary serous, and clear cell carcinoma of the endometrium. Obstet Gynecol 2002;100(6):1290–5.

42. Cassia R, Moreno-Bueno G, Rodriguez-Perales S, et al. Cyclin E gene (CCNE) amplification and hCDC4 mutations in endometrial carcinoma. J Pathol 2003;201(4):589–95.

43. Silverberg SG, De Giorgi LS. Clear cell carcinoma of the endometrium. Clinical, pathologic, and ultrastructural findings. Cancer 1973;31:1127–40.

44. Silva EG, Young RH. Endometrioid neoplasms with clear cells: a report of 21 cases in which the alteration is not of typical secretory type. Am J Surg Pathol 2007;31(8):1203–8.

45. Clement PB, Young RH. Non-endometrioid carcinomas of the uterine corpus: a review of their pathology with emphasis on recent advances and problematic aspects. Adv Anat Pathol 2004;11(3):117–42.

46. Lax SF, Pizer ES, Ronnett BM, et al. Clear cell carcinoma of the endometrium is characterized by a distinctive profile of p53, Ki-67, estrogen, and progesterone receptor expression. Hum Pathol 1998;29(6):551–8.

47. Abeler VM, Kjorstad KE. Clear cell carcinoma of the endometrium: a histopathological and clinical study of 97 cases. Gynecol Oncol 1991;40:207–17.

48. Malpica A, Tornos C, Burke TW, et al. Low-stage clear-cell carcinoma of the endometrium. Am J Surg Pathol 1995;19:769–74.

49. Kanbour-Shakir A, Tobon H. Primary clear cell carcinoma of the endometrium: a clinicopathologic study of 20 cases. Int J Gynecol Pathol 1991;10:67–78.

50. Abeler VM, Vergote IB, Kjorstad KE, et al. Clear cell carcinoma of the endometrium. Prognosis and metastatic pattern. Cancer 1996;78(8):1740–7.

51. Kurman RJ, Scully RE. Clear cell carcinoma of the endometrium: an analysis of 21 cases. Cancer 1976;37:872–82.

52. Prat J, Oliva E, Lerma E, et al. Uterine papillary serous adenocarcinoma: a 10-case study of p53 and c-erbB-2 expression and DNA content. Cancer 1994;74:1778–83.

53. Logani S, Soslow RA, Oliva E, et al. Is pure uterine clear cell carcinoma clinically distinct from endometrioid/serous carcinoma with a clear cell component? [abstract 896]. Mod Pathol 2005;18(Suppl 1):193A.

mucinous carcinomas of the peritoneum, fallopian tube, ovary, and endometrium. Int J Gynecol Pathol 2004;23(2):110–8.

54. Fadare O, Liang SX, Cagnur UE, et al. Precursors of endometrial clear cell carcinoma. Am J Surg Pathol 2006;30(12):1519–30.

55. Vang R, Whitaker BP, Farhood AI, et al. Immunohistochemical analysis of clear cell carcinoma of the gynecologic tract. Int J Gynecol Pathol 2001; 20(3):252–9.

56. Arai T, Watanabe J, Kawaguchi M, et al. Clear cell adenocarcinoma of the endometrium is a biologically distinct entity from endometrioid adenocarcinoma. Int J Gynecol Cancer 2006;16(1):391–5.

57. An HJ, Logani S, Isacson C, et al. Molecular characterization of uterine clear cell carcinoma. Mod Pathol 2004;17(5):530–7.

58. Coosemans A, Moerman P, Verbist G, et al. Wilms' tumor gene 1 (WT1) in endometrial carcinoma. Gynecol Oncol 2008;111(3):502–8.

59. Rolitsky CD, Theil KS, McGaughy VR, et al. HER-2/neu amplification and overexpression in endometrial carcinoma. Int J Gynecol Pathol 1999;18(2): 138–43.

60. Khalifa MA, Mannel RS, Haraway SD, et al. Expression of EGFR, HER-2/neu, P53, and PCNA in endometrioid, serous papillary, and clear cell endometrial adenocarcinomas. Gynecol Oncol 1994;53:84–92.

61. Yamamoto S, Tsuda H, Aida S, et al. Immunohistochemical detection of hepatocyte nuclear factor 1beta in ovarian and endometrial clear-cell adenocarcinomas and nonneoplastic endometrium. Hum Pathol 2007;38(7):1074–80.

62. Han G, DeLair D, Gilks CB, et al. Endometrial adenocarcinoma with clear cell morphology: interovserver variability and immunohistochemical analysis using hepatocyte nuclear factor-1 β [abstract 1097]. Mod Pathol 2010;23(Suppl 1):245A.

63. Kobel M, Kalloger SE, Carrick J, et al. A limited panel of immunomarkers can reliably distinguish between clear cell and high-grade serous carcinoma of the ovary. Am J Surg Pathol 2009;33(1): 14–21.

64. Risinger JI, Maxwell GL, Chandramouli GV, et al. Microarray analysis reveals distinct gene expression profiles among different histologic types of endometrial cancer. Cancer Res 2003;63(1):6–11.

65. Maxwell GL, Chandramouli GV, Dainty L, et al. Microarray analysis of endometrial carcinomas and mixed mullerian tumors reveals distinct gene expression profiles associated with different histologic types of uterine cancer. Clin Cancer Res 2005;11(11):4056–66.

66. Zorn KK, Bonome T, Gangi L, et al. Gene expression profiles of serous, endometrioid, and clear cell subtypes of ovarian and endometrial cancer. Clin Cancer Res 2005;11(18):6422–30.

67. Garg K, Shih K, Barakat R, et al. Endometrial carcinomas in women aged 40 years and younger: tumors associated with loss of DNA mismatch repair proteins comprise a distinct clinicopathologic subset. Am J Surg Pathol 2009;33(12): 1869–77.

68. Altrabulsi B, Malpica A, Deavers MT, et al. Undifferentiated carcinoma of the endometrium. Am J Surg Pathol 2005;29(10):1316–21.

69. Tafe LJ, Garg K, Chew I, et al. Endometrial and ovarian carcinomas with undifferentiated components: clinically aggressive and frequently underrecognized neoplasms. Mod Pathol 2010;23(6): 781–9.

70. Alkushi A, bdul-Rahman ZH, Lim P, et al. Description of a novel system for grading of endometrial carcinoma and comparison with existing grading systems. Am J Surg Pathol 2005;29(3):295–304.

71. Silverberg SG, DeGiorgi LS. Histopathologic analysis of preoperative radiation therapy in endometrial carcinoma. Am J Obstet Gynecol 1974; 119(5):698–704.

72. Kraus FT. Irradiation changes in the uterus. Baltimore (MD): Williams & Wilkins; 1973.

73. Hendrickson MR, Kempson RL. Endometrial epithelial metaplasias: proliferations frequently misdiagnosed as adenocarcinoma. Report of 89 cases and proposed classification. Am J Surg Pathol 1980;4:525–42.

74. Shah SS, Mazur MT. Endometrial eosinophilic syncytial change related to breakdown: immunohistochemical evidence suggests a regressive process. Int J Gynecol Pathol 2008;27(4):534–8.

75. Horree N, Heintz AP, Sie-Go DM, et al. p16 is consistently expressed in endometrial tubal metaplasia. Cell Oncol 2007;29(1):37–45.

76. Shimizu K, Norimatsu Y, Kobayashi TK, et al. Expression of immunoreactivity and genetic mutation in eosinophilic and ciliated metaplastic changes of endometrial glandular and stromal breakdown: cytodiagnostic implications. Ann Diagn Pathol 2009;13(2):89–95.

77. Quddus MR, Sung CJ, Zheng W, et al. p53 immunoreactivity in endometrial metaplasia with dysfunctional uterine bleeding. Histopathology 1999;35(1):44–9.

78. Arias-Stella J. The Arias-Stella reaction: facts and fancies four decades after. Adv Anat Pathol 2002; 9(1):12–23.

79. Tornos C, Silva EG, Ordonez NG, et al. Endometrioid carcinoma of the ovary with a prominent spindle-cell component, a source of diagnostic confusion. A report of 14 cases. Am J Surg Pathol 1995;19:1343–53.

80. Murray SK, Clement PB, Young RH. Endometrioid carcinomas of the uterine corpus with sex cord-like formations, hyalinization, and other unusual morphologic features: a report of 31 cases of a neoplasm that may be confused with

carcinosarcoma and other uterine neoplasms. Am J Surg Pathol 2005;29(2):157–66.

81. Goodman A, Zukerberg LR, Rice LW, et al. Squamous cell carcinoma of the endometrium: a report of eight cases and a review of the literature. Gynecol Oncol 1996;61:54–60.

82. Zidi YS, Bouraoui S, Atallah K, et al. Primary in situ squamous cell carcinoma of the endometrium, with extensive squamous metaplasia and dysplasia. Gynecol Oncol 2003;88(3):444–6.

83. Rodolakis A, Papaspyrou I, Sotiropoulou M, et al. Primary squamous cell carcinoma of the endometrium. A report of 3 cases. Eur J Gynaecol Oncol 2001;22(2):143–6.

84. Kondis A, Liapis A, Kairi E, et al. Primary squamous cell carcinoma of the endometrium. Immunopathological study of a case. Eur J Gynaecol Oncol 1999;20(3):235–6.

85. Kataoka A, Nishida T, Sugiyama T, et al. Squamous cell carcinoma of the endometrium with human papillomavirus type 31 and without tumor suppressor gene p53 mutation. Gynecol Oncol 1997;65:180–4.

86. Im DD, Shah KV, Rosenshein NB. Report of three new cases of squamous carcinoma of the endometrium with emphasis in the HPV status. Gynecol Oncol 1995;56:464–9.

87. Chew I, Post MD, Carinelli SG, et al. p16 expression in squamous and trophoblastic lesions of the upper female genital tract. Int J Gynecol Pathol 2010;29(6):513–22.

88. Horn LC, Richter CE, Einenkel J, et al. p16, p14, p53, cyclin D1, and steroid hormone receptor expression and human papillomaviruses analysis in primary squamous cell carcinoma of the endometrium. Ann Diagn Pathol 2006;10(4):193–6.

89. Giordano G, Azzoni C, D'Adda T, et al. P16(INK4a) overexpression independent of Human Papilloma Virus (HPV) infection in rare subtypes of endometrial carcinomas. Pathol Res Pract 2007;203(7):533–8.

90. Spiegel GW, Austin RM, Gelven PL. Transitional cell carcinoma of the endometrium. Gynecol Oncol 1996;60:325–30.

91. Lininger RA, Ashfaq R, Albores-Saavedra J, et al. Transitional cell carcinoma of the endometrium and endometrial carcinoma with transitional cell differentiation. Cancer 1997;79(10):1933–43.

92. Marino-Enriquez A, Gonzalez-Rocha T, Burgos E, et al. Transitional cell carcinoma of the endometrium and endometrial carcinoma with transitional cell differentiation: a clinicopathologic study of 5 cases and review of the literature. Hum Pathol 2008;39(11):1606–13.

93. Park KJ, Lamb C, Oliva E, et al. Unusual endocervical adenocarcinomas: an immunohistochemical analysis with molecular detection of human papillomavirus [abstract 993]. Mod Pathol 2008;21(Suppl 1):217A.

94. Albores-Saavedra J, Martinez-Benitez B, Luevano E. Small cell carcinomas and large cell neuroendocrine carcinomas of the endometrium and cervix: polypoid tumors and those arising in polyps may have a favorable prognosis. Int J Gynecol Pathol 2008;27(3):333–9.

95. Mulvany NJ, Allen DG. Combined large cell neuroendocrine and endometrioid carcinoma of the endometrium. Int J Gynecol Pathol 2008;27(1):49–57.

96. Odunsi K, Olatinwo M, Collins Y, et al. Primary primitive neuroectodermal tumor of the uterus: a report of two cases and review of the literature. Gynecol Oncol 2004;92(2):689–96.

97. Daya D, Lukka H, Clement PB. Primitive neuroectodermal tumors of the uterus: a report of four cases. Hum Pathol 1992;23:1120–9.

98. Alkushi A, Kobel M, Kalloger SE, et al. High grade endometrial carcinoma: Serous and grade 3 endometrioid carcinoma have different immunophenotypes and outcomes [abstract 934]. Mod Pathol 2009;22(Suppl 1):206A.

99. Oliva E, Young RH, Amin MB, et al. An immunohistochemical analysis of endometrial stromal and smooth muscle tumors of the uterus. A study of 54 cases emphasizing the importance of using a panel because of overlap in immunoreactivity for individual antibodies. Am J Surg Pathol 2002;26(4):403–12.

100. Kurman RJ, Norris HJ. Mesenchymal tumors of the uterus. VI. Epithelioid smooth muscle tumors including leiomyoblastoma and clear cell leiomyoma: a clinical and pathological analysis of 26 cases. Cancer 1976;37:1853–65.

101. Prayson RA, Goldblum JR, Hart WR. Epithelioid smooth-muscle tumors of the uterus. A clinicopathologic study of 18 patients. Am J Surg Pathol 1997;21(4):383–91.

102. Silva EG, Tornos C, Ordóñez NG, et al. Uterine leiomyosarcoma with clear cell areas. Int J Gynecol Pathol 1995;14:174–8.

103. Iwata J, Fletcher CD. Immunohistochemical detection of cytokeratin and epithelial membrane antigen in leiomyosarcoma: a systematic study of 100 cases. Pathol Int 2000;50(1):7–14.

104. O'Neill CJ, McCluggage WG. p16 expression in the female genital tract and its value in diagnosis. Adv Anat Pathol 2006;13(1):8–15.

105. Vang R, Kempson RL. Perivascular epithelioid cell tumor ('PEComa') of the uterus: a subset of HMB-45-positive epithelioid mesenchymal neoplasms with an uncertain relationship to pure smooth muscle tumors. Am J Surg Pathol 2002;26(1):1–13.

106. Folpe AL, Mentzel T, Lehr HA, et al. Perivascular epithelioid cell neoplasms of soft tissue and

gynecologic origin: a clinicopathologic study of 26 cases and review of the literature. Am J Surg Pathol 2005;29(12):1558–75.

107. Lifschitz-Mercer B, Czernobilsky B, Dgani R, et al. Immunocytochemical study of an endometrial diffuse clear cell stromal sarcoma and other endometrial stromal sarcomas. Cancer 1987;59:1494–9.

108. Baergen RN, Rutgers JL, Young RH, et al. Placental site trophoblastic tumor: a study of 55 cases and review of the literature emphasizing factors of prognostic significance. Gynecol Oncol 2006;100(3):511–20.

109. Shih IM, Kurman RJ. Immunohistochemical localization of inhibin-alpha in the placenta and gestational trophoblastic lesions. Int J Gynecol Pathol 1999;18(2):144–50.

110. Pelkey TJ, Frierson HF Jr, Mills SE, et al. Detection of the alpha-subunit of inhibin in trophoblastic neoplasia. Hum Pathol 1999;30(1):26–31.

111. Shih IM, Seidman JD, Kurman RJ. Placental site nodule and characterization of distinctive types of intermediate trophoblast. Hum Pathol 1999;30(6):687–94.

112. Nielsen GP, Oliva E, Young RH, et al. Alveolar soft-part sarcoma of the female genital tract: a report of nine cases and review of the literature. Int J Gynecol Pathol 1995;14:283–92.

113. Roma AA, Yang B, Senior ME, et al. TFE3 immunoreactivity in alveolar soft part sarcoma of the uterine cervix: case report. Int J Gynecol Pathol 2005;24(2):131–5.

114. Jarboe EA, Miron A, Carlson JW, et al. Coexisting intraepithelial serous carcinomas of the endometrium and fallopian tube: frequency and potential significance. Int J Gynecol Pathol 2009;28(4):308–15.

115. Wong KK, Lu KH, Malpica A, et al. Significantly greater expression of ER, PR, and ECAD in advanced-stage low-grade ovarian serous carcinoma as revealed by immunohistochemical analysis. Int J Gynecol Pathol 2007;26(4):404–9.

116. Halperin R, Zehavi S, Hadas E, et al. Immunohistochemical comparison of primary peritoneal and primary ovarian serous papillary carcinoma. Int J Gynecol Pathol 2001;20(4):341–5.

117. Euscher ED, Malpica A, Deavers MT, et al. Differential expression of WT-1 in serous carcinomas in the peritoneum with or without associated serous carcinoma in endometrial polyps. Am J Surg Pathol 2005;29(8):1074–8.

118. Ambros RA, Ballouk F, Malfetano JH, et al. Significance of papillary (villoglandular) differentiation in endometrioid carcinoma of the uterus. Am J Surg Pathol 1994;18:569–75.

119. Ambros RA, Malfetano JH. Villoglandular adenocarcinoma of the endometrium. Am J Surg Pathol 2000;24(1):155–6.

120. Alkushi A, Irving J, Hsu F, et al. Immunoprofile of cervical and endometrial adenocarcinomas using a tissue microarray. Virchows Arch 2003;442(3):271–7.

121. Kamoi S, AlJuboury MI, Akin MR, et al. Immunohistochemical staining in the distinction between primary endometrial and endocervical adenocarcinomas: another viewpoint. Int J Gynecol Pathol 2002;21(3):217–23.

122. McCluggage WG, Sumathi VP, McBride HA, et al. A panel of immunohistochemical stains, including carcinoembryonic antigen, vimentin, and estrogen receptor, aids the distinction between primary endometrial and endocervical adenocarcinomas. Int J Gynecol Pathol 2002;21(1):11–5.

123. McCluggage WG. Immunohistochemistry as a diagnostic aid in cervical pathology. Pathology 2007;39(1):97–111.

124. McCluggage WG, Jenkins D. p16 immunoreactivity may assist in the distinction between endometrial and endocervical adenocarcinoma. Int J Gynecol Pathol 2003;22(3):231–5.

125. Garg K, Leitao MM Jr, Wynveen CA, et al. p53 overexpression in morphologically ambiguous endometrial carcinomas correlates with adverse clinical outcomes. Mod Pathol 2010;23(1):80–92.

126. Kumar A, Schneider V. Metastases to the uterus from extrapelvic primary tumors. Int J Gynecol Pathol 1983;2(2):134–40.

127. Zannoni GF, Vellone VG, Fadda G, et al. Colonic carcinoma metastatic to the endometrium: the importance of clinical history in averting misdiagnosis as a primary endometrial carcinoma. Int J Surg Pathol 2009. [Epub ahead of print].

128. Park KJ, Bramlage MP, Ellenson LH, et al. Immunoprofile of adenocarcinomas of the endometrium, endocervix, and ovary with mucinous differentiation. Appl Immunohistochem Mol Morphol 2009;17(1):8–11.

129. Wani Y, Notohara K, Saegusa M, et al. Aberrant Cdx2 expression in endometrial lesions with squamous differentiation: important role of Cdx2 in squamous morula formation. Hum Pathol 2008;39(7):1072–9.

130. Houghton O, Connolly LE, McCluggage WG. Morules in endometrioid proliferations of the uterus and ovary consistently express the intestinal transcription factor CDX2. Histopathology 2008;53(2):156–65.

131. Nofech-Mozes S, Ghorab Z, Ismiil N, et al. Endometrial endometrioid adenocarcinoma: a pathologic analysis of 827 consecutive cases. Am J Clin Pathol 2008;129(1):110–4.

132. Hamilton CA, Cheung MK, Osann K, et al. Uterine papillary serous and clear cell carcinomas predict for poorer survival compared to grade 3 endometrioid corpus cancers. Br J Cancer 2006;94(5):642–6.

133. Rasool N, Fader AN, Seamon L, et al. Stage I, grade 3 endometrioid adenocarcinoma of the endometrium: an analysis of clinical outcomes and patterns of recurrence. Gynecol Oncol 2010; 116(1):10–4.

134. van Wijk FH, van der Burg ME, Burger CW, et al. Management of recurrent endometrioid endometrial carcinoma: an overview. Int J Gynecol Cancer 2009;19(3):314–20.

135. Soslow RA, Slomovitz BM, Saqi A, et al. Tumor suppressor gene, cell surface adhesion molecule, and multidrug resistance in Mullerian serous carcinomas: clinical divergence without immunophenotypic differences. Gynecol Oncol 2000; 79(3):430–7.

136. Sherman ME, Sturgeon S, Brinton LA, et al. Risk factors and hormone levels in patients with serous and endometrioid uterine carcinomas. Mod Pathol 1997;10:963–8.

137. Dotto J, Tavassoli FA. Serous intraepithelial carcinoma arising in an endometrial polyp: a proposal for modification of terminology. Int J Surg Pathol 2008;16(1):8–10.

138. Carcangiu ML. Uterine pathology in tamoxifen-treated patients with breast cancer. Anat Pathol 1997;2:53–70.

139. Pothuri B, Ramondetta L, Eifel P, et al. Radiation-associated endometrial cancers are prognostically unfavorable tumors: a clinicopathologic comparison with 527 sporadic endometrial cancers. Gynecol Oncol 2006;103(3):948–51.

140. Pothuri B, Ramondetta L, Martino M, et al. Development of endometrial cancer after radiation treatment for cervical carcinoma. Obstet Gynecol 2003;101(5 PT 1):941–5.

141. Lavie O, Barnett-Griness O, Narod SA, et al. The risk of developing uterine sarcoma after tamoxifen use. Int J Gynecol Cancer 2008;18(2):352–6.

142. Lavie O, Ben-Arie A, Pilip A, et al. BRCA2 germline mutation in a woman with uterine serous papillary carcinoma–case report. Gynecol Oncol 2005; 99(2):486–8.

143. Gu M, Shi WJ, Barakat RR, et al. Pap smears in women with endometrial carcinoma. Acta Cytol 2001;45(4):555–60.

144. Park JY, Kim HS, Hong SR, et al. Cytologic findings of cervicovaginal smears in women with uterine papillary serous carcinoma. J Korean Med Sci 2005;20(1):93–7.

145. Tseng PC, Sprance HE, Carcangiu ML, et al. CA 125, NB/70K, and lipid-associated sialic acid in monitoring uterine papillary serous carcinoma. Obstet Gynecol 1989;74(3 Pt 1):384–7.

146. Sachmechi I, Kalra J, Molho L, et al. Paraneoplastic hypercalcemia associated with uterine papillary serous carcinoma. Gynecol Oncol 1995;58: 378–82.

147. Ng JS, Han AC, Edelson MI, et al. Uterine papillary serous carcinoma presenting as distant lymph node metastasis. Gynecol Oncol 2001;80(3):417–20.

148. Cirisano FD Jr, Robboy SJ, Dodge RK, et al. Epidemiologic and surgicopathologic findings of papillary serous and clear cell endometrial cancers when compared to endometrioid carcinoma. Gynecol Oncol 1999;74(3):385–94.

149. Chambers JT, Merino M, Kohorn EI, et al. Uterine papillary serous carcinoma. Obstet Gynecol 1987;69:109–13.

150. Gitsch G, Friedlander ML, Wain GV, et al. Uterine papillary serous carcinoma: a clinical study. Cancer 1995;75:2239–43.

151. Rosenberg P, Boeryd B, Simonsen E. A new aggressive treatment approach to high-grade endometrial cancer of possible benefit to patients with stage I uterine papillary cancer. Gynecol Oncol 1993;48:32–7.

152. Lim P, Al Kushi A, Gilks B, et al. Early stage uterine papillary serous carcinoma of the endometrium. Effect of adjuvant whole abdominal radiotherapy and pathologic parameters on outcome. Cancer 2001;91(4):752–7.

153. Abeler VM, Kjorstad KE. Serous papillary carcinoma of the endometrium: a histopathological study of 22 cases. Gynecol Oncol 1990;39: 266–71.

154. Aquino-Parsons C, Lim P, Wong F, et al. Papillary serous and clear cell carcinoma limited to endometrial curettings in FIGO stage 1a and 1b endometrial adenocarcinoma: treatment implications. Gynecol Oncol 1998;71:83–6.

155. Bancher-Todesca D, Neunteufel W, Williams KE, et al. Influence of postoperative treatment on survival in patients with uterine papillary serous carcinoma. Gynecol Oncol 1998;71:344–7.

156. Gallion HH, von Nagel JR, Powell D, et al. Stage I serous papillary carcinoma of the endometrium. Cancer 1989;63:2224–8.

157. Verloop J, van Leeuwen FE, Helmerhorst TJ, et al. Cancer risk in DES daughters. Cancer Causes Control 2010;21(7):999–1007.

158. Hiller N, Sonnenblick M, Hershko C. Paraneoplastic hypercalcemia in endometrial carcinoma. Oncology 1989;46(1):45–8.

159. Savvari P, Peitsidis P, Alevizaki M, et al. Paraneoplastic humorally mediated hypercalcemia induced by parathyroid hormone-related protein in gynecologic malignancies: a systematic review. Onkologie 2009;32(8–9):517–23.

160. Lee L, Garrett L, Lee H, et al. Association of clear cell carcinoma of the endometrium with a high

rate of venous thromboembolism. J Reprod Med 2009;54(3):133–8.

161. Carcangiu ML, Chambers JT. Early pathologic stage clear cell carcinoma and uterine papillary serous carcinoma of the endometrium: comparison of clinicopathologic features and survival. Int J Gynecol Pathol 1995;14:30–8.

162. Tavassoli FA, Devilee P, International Agency for Research on C, World Health O. Pathology and genetics of tumours of the breast and female genital organs. Lyon (France): International Agency for Research on Cancer; 2003.

163. Silva EG, Deavers MT, Bodurka DC, et al. Association of low-grade endometrioid carcinoma of the uterus and ovary with undifferentiated carcinoma: a new type of dedifferentiated carcinoma? Int J Gynecol Pathol 2006;25(1):52–8.

164. Tafe L, Garg K, Tornos C, et al. Undifferentiated carcinoma of the endometrium and ovary: a clinicopathologic correlation. Mod Pathol 2009;22(1):238A.

FAMILIAL TUMORS OF THE UTERINE CORPUS

Karuna Garg, MD*, Robert A. Soslow, MD

KEYWORDS

- Familial endometrial carcinoma • Lynch syndrome • HNPCC

ABSTRACT

Women with Lynch syndrome are at considerable risk for developing endometrial carcinoma, but current screening guidelines for detection of Lynch syndrome focus almost exclusively on colorectal carcinoma. Lynch syndrome associated colorectal and endometrial carcinomas have some important differences with implications for screening strategies. These differences are discussed in this review, along with the most effective screening criteria and testing methods for detection of Lynch syndrome in endometrial carcinoma patients.

OVERVIEW

The vast majority of endometrial carcinomas are sporadic, with familial conditions accounting for only a minority (approximately 5%) of these tumors. Most hereditary endometrial carcinomas are associated with Lynch syndrome (LS).[1,2] The term "hereditary non polyposis colorectal cancer" (HNPCC) is used synonymously. Muir Torre syndrome is a subtype of Lynch syndrome and represents the association of sebaceous tumors or keratoacanthomas with a visceral malignancy, frequently in the setting of *hMSH2* mutation.[3] Other syndromes that predispose to endometrial carcinomas include Cowden syndrome, which is an autosomal dominant disorder caused by germline *PTEN* mutations.[4,5] Although some authors

Key Features
PATHOLOGIC FEATURES OF ENDOMETRIAL CARCINOMAS ASSOCIATED WITH MISMATCH REPAIR DEFECTS

Gross features:

1. Lower uterine segment localization.

2. Multicentricity (more than 1 tumor).

Microscopic features:

1. Peritumoral lymphocytes and tumor infiltrating lymphocytes.

2. Tumor heterogeneity.

3. Dedifferentiated/undifferentiated endometrial carcinomas

4. Morphologically ambiguous ("hard to classify") endometrial carcinomas.

5. Non endometrioid carcinomas (serous, clear cell, carcinosarcoma) in young patients (younger than age 60 years).

have raised the possibility of a relationship between uterine papillary serous carcinomas and *BRCA1* mutations,[6] most studies have found no such association[7,8] and it is likely that the increased incidence of endometrial carcinoma in this setting is related to tamoxifen therapy or drop metastasis from occult fallopian tube carcinomas.[7]

Editor's Comment: Portions of content in Familial Tumors of the Uterine Corpus are addressed by Bojana Djordjevic and Russell Broaddus in Selected Topics in the Molecular Pathology of Endometrial Carcinoma in the discussions of microsatellite instability. Factual information discussed there complements parts of this article, but differs in point of view and presentation.

Department of Pathology, Memorial Sloan-Kettering Cancer Center, 1275 York Avenue, New York, NY 10065, USA
* Corresponding author.
E-mail address: gargk@mskcc.org

Surgical Pathology 4 (2011) 243–259
doi:10.1016/j.path.2010.12.002

LYNCH SYNDROME AND ENDOMETRIAL CARCINOMA

Lynch syndrome, an autosomal dominant syndrome, results from germline mutations in the DNA mismatch repair genes, which frequently but not always lead to microsatellite instability.[9,10] Poorly understood mechanisms involve constitutive epimutation, which may be inherited, or overexpression of certain miRNAs. The most frequently affected genes are *hMLH1*, *hMSH2*, *hMSH6* and rarely *hPMS2*. Microsatellites are DNA sequences that are widely dispersed throughout the genome. They are prone to replication errors due to their repetitive nature. Normally, these replication errors are corrected by the DNA mismatch repair system. Microsatellite instability (MSI) results from defects in the DNA mismatch repair system.[9,10] Defects in mismatch repair system can be epigenetic (sporadic), resulting from *hMLH1* promoter methylation, or hereditary due to germline mutations in the DNA mismatch repair genes. The overall prevalence of microsatellite instability in endometrial carcinomas is 20 to 25%. In most cases (75%), this is sporadic and results from epigenetic *hMLH1* promoter methylation.[11,12] Lynch syndrome, an autosomal dominant syndrome, accounts for most of the remaining cases. The mechanism of tumorigenesis in the setting of MSI appears to involve frameshift mutations of microsatellite repeats within coding regions of genes including tumor suppressor genes. Affected genes such as these are well characterized in MSI-associated colorectal carcinomas, but not in endometrial carcinomas.

Patients with Lynch syndrome are at increased risk for multiple malignancies, including colon and endometrial carcinomas.[1,2] Other, less frequent cancers include those of the ovary, stomach, urinary tract, hepatobiliary tract, small intestine and brain. The frequency of LS associated germline mutations in endometrial carcinomas is 1.8 to 2.1%, similar to that in colon cancer.[13–15] In younger patients with endometrial carcinoma, the prevalence increases to approximately 9%.[16,17]

Lynch syndrome has traditionally been perceived as a colorectal carcinoma dominated syndrome, and the focus on screening strategies have focused almost exclusively on colon cancer (**Box 1**).[18] The lifetime risk for development of endometrial carcinoma in these patients is 20 to 60%, and the risk is particularly high for patients with *hMSH6* mutations.[1,2,19–23] Moreover, more than half of these patients present with a gynecologic malignancy as their sentinel cancer.[24] Recognition of these patients at presentation is important since they and their family members

---

Box 1

Revised Bethesda Guidelines for testing colorectal tumors for microsatellite instability (MSI)

Tumors from individuals should be tested for MSI in the following situations:

1. Colorectal cancer diagnosed in a patient who is less than age 50 years.

2. Presence of synchronous, metachronous colorectal, or other HNPCC-associated tumors, regardless of age.

3. Colorectal cancer with the MSI-H histology diagnosed in a patient who is less than age 60 years.

4. Colorectal cancer diagnosed in one or more first-degree relatives with an HNPCC-related tumor, with one of the cancers being diagnosed under age 50 years.

5. Colorectal cancer diagnosed in two or more first- or second-degree relatives with HNPCC-related tumors, regardless of age.

---

are at increased risk for multiple cancers, especially colon cancer. These patients and their family members could benefit from genetic counseling and testing. Implementation of appropriate screening and prevention guidelines can substantially decrease the risk of other LS-associated tumors.

The association between Lynch syndrome and endometrial carcinoma is important but under recognized. Women with Lynch syndrome are at equal, if not higher, risk for development of gynecologic malignancies compared with their risk for colon cancer.[2]

Since testing for mismatch repair abnormalities cannot be performed on every endometrial carcinoma, effective screening guidelines are required to maximize detection of EC patients at risk for LS. Implementation of the revised Bethesda guidelines has substantially decreased the morbidity and mortality from LS associated colorectal carcinoma,[25] but similar guidelines are lacking for endometrial carcinoma.

Specific screening guidelines directed toward EC patients are important since there are significant differences between LS associated colorectal and endometrial carcinomas that may have impact on screening criteria and methodology.[19–23] LS associated colorectal carcinomas frequently harbor *hMLH1* and *hMSH2* mutations, while *hMSH6* mutations are rare. LS associated endometrial carcinomas on the other hand, frequently

Table 1
Lynch syndrome characteristics

	Typical Lynch Syndrome (*hMLH1/hMSH2* Mutations)	Atypical Lynch Syndrome (*hMSH6* Mutations)
Risk for LS-associated tumors	Colon greater risk than Endometrium	Endometrium greater risk than Colon
Median age of onset of LS associated tumors	43 years	51 years
Family history of LS associated tumors	Frequently present	Frequently absent
MSI analysis results	MSI-high	MSI-low or MS-stable moreso than MSI-high

demonstrate mutations in *hMSH6* and women with *hMSH6* mutations appear to have a particular risk for endometrial carcinoma that is significantly higher than their risk for colon cancer. LS due to mutations in *hMSH6* is associated with unique characteristics, which are in general referred to as "atypical Lynch syndrome" (**Table 1**). The median age of presentation for these patients, both with colorectal cancer and endometrial cancer, is significantly higher compared with those who have mutations in *hMLH1* or *hMSH2*. Patients with *hMSH6* mutations also fail to have significant family history suggestive of LS and usually do not meet revised Amsterdam criteria. It has also been observed that endometrial carcinomas with *hMSH6* mutations can often be MSI-low or microsatellite stable (MSS), and could therefore remain undetected by MSI analysis alone. All of these factors have an impact on screening criteria for LS associated ECs and must be considered while establishing screening guidelines.

SCREENING ENDOMETRIAL CARCINOMA PATIENTS FOR LYNCH SYNDROME

Various screening criteria have been proposed to enhance detection of LS in EC patients. These include patient age, personal and family history and body mass index (BMI). While helpful, none of these criteria is sufficiently sensitive. While presentation with endometrial carcinoma at a young age may be indicative of LS, many EC patients with LS, particularly those with *hMSH6* mutations, present at older ages.[19–23] A significant proportion of LS patients with EC do not meet the Amsterdam criteria and do not have personal or family history suggestive of LS.[13] In the study by Hampel and colleagues,[13] six of ten EC patients with LS would have remained undetected using the age criteria and seven of ten did not meet the Amsterdam criteria or Bethesda guidelines. It has

been observed that young EC patients with LS are often thin with low BMI, in contrast with sporadic ECs in this age group.[17,26–28] However, occasional overweight or obese young EC patients with LS have been reported.[17,28]

Therefore, more sensitive screening criteria are required for detection of LS in EC patients. In the revised Bethesda guidelines, morphologic features in colorectal carcinoma have been integrated as one of the criteria to initiate testing for mismatch repair defects. Accumulating data suggests that similarly, endometrial carcinomas associated with mismatch repair defects may show certain gross and histologic characteristics that may enhance their detection (see Key Features Box).[29–34]

GROSS FEATURES

Endometrial carcinomas associated with mismatch repair deficiency appear to have a predilection for the lower uterine segment (LUS). In the study by Westin and Broaddus,[29] 29% of LUS tumors were associated with LS. Our group has also made similar observations.[28,30]

MICROSCOPIC FEATURES

Lynch syndrome associated endometrial carcinomas can show a wide spectrum of histologic subtypes. While endometrioid carcinomas predominate,[32] it appears that young LS patients may be at increased risk for developing non-endometrioid endometrial carcinomas.[34,35]

The presence of certain histologic features in endometrioid carcinomas has been shown to be suggestive of mismatch repair abnormalities,[30,31] although this remains controversial.[36,37] These include the presence of prominent peritumoral lymphocytes (apparent at scanning magnification), increased tumor infiltrating lymphocytes (TILs

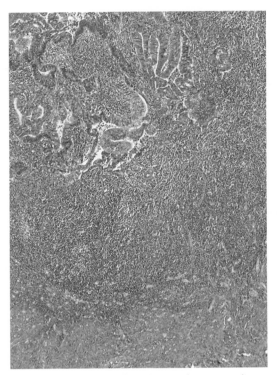

Fig. 1. This endometrial carcinoma shows prominent peritumoral lymphocytes that are visible at scanning magnification.

greater than 42 per 10 high power fields), tumor heterogeneity and dedifferentiated/undifferentiated histology. When these tumor characteristics were incorporated in a screening algorithm along with age and personal/family history, application of this algorithm enhanced detection of mismatch repair abnormalities in endometrial carcinoma patients by approximately 3-fold.[30]

Dense lymphocytic infiltrates surrounding the tumor cells, visible at low magnification, are considered evidence of peritumoral lymphocytes (**Fig. 1**). TILs are lymphocytes located within the boundary of tumor cell nests or glands, and the score is expressed as the number of lymphocytes per ten high power fields (**Fig. 2**). TILs should be counted in lymphocyte dense areas. Tumor heterogeneity is defined as two juxtaposed, morphologically distinct tumor populations, each constituting at least 10% of the tumor volume. Most tumors showing these features are dedifferentiated endometrial carcinomas, as described by Silva and colleagues.[38] These tumors are composed of FIGO grade 1 or grade 2 endometrioid carcinoma associated with undifferentiated carcinoma (**Fig. 3**).

Undifferentiated carcinoma exhibits solid, dyshesive sheets of round or polygonal cells with vesicular nuclei and prominent nucleoli, without any evidence of gland formation (**Fig. 4**).[39] Foci within some of these tumors may display myxoid matrix and cells with eosinophilic cytoplasm and

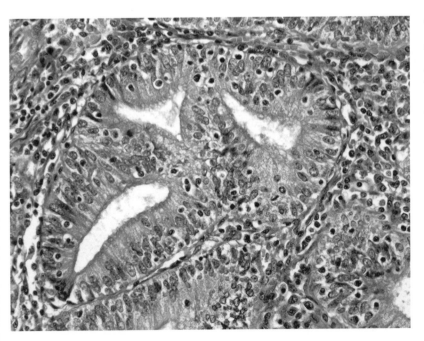

Fig. 2. Tumor infiltrating lymphocytes (TILs) are defined specifically as lymphocytes located within cell boundaries. TILs should be counted in the most lymphocyte dense areas of the tumor.

Fig. 3. Dedifferentiated endometrial carcinomas are composed of well differentiated endometrioid carcinoma with abrupt transition into undifferentiated carcinoma.

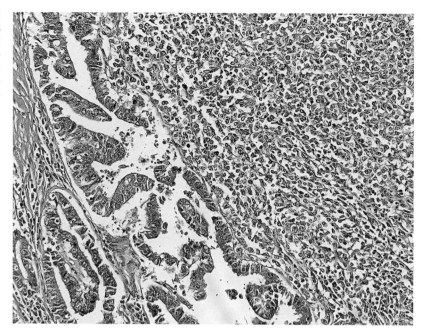

eccentrically located nuclei with prominent central nucleoli (rhabdoid cells) (**Fig. 5**). Some of these tumors can show lymphoepithelioma-like areas, defined as sheets of undifferentiated cells with a prominent lymphocytic infiltrate (**Fig. 6**).

Undifferentiated/dedifferentiated endometrial carcinomas have been shown to have mismatch repair abnormalities. Some are sporadic and associated with *MLH1* promoter methylation,[35] while others are LS associated.[30] Patients with undifferentiated endometrial carcinoma that display IHC loss of MLH1/PMS2 must be investigated for the possibility of Lynch syndrome. For example, our group recently diagnosed a 52-year old woman with dedifferentiated endometrial carcinoma that showed IHC loss of MLH1/PMS2. The patient underwent genetic counseling and was noted to have a significant family history of LS associated tumors. A deleterious *hMLH1* mutation was detected, and subsequent colonoscopy showed tubular and tubulovillous adenomas.

The presence of nonendometrioid endometrial carcinomas in young women, including clear cell carcinoma (**Fig. 7**), serous carcinoma and carcinosarcoma (malignant mixed Mullerian tumor) have been reported in LS.[34,35] We have noted that carcinosarcomas in young patients in this setting may have an unusual morphologic appearance. Unlike typical MMMTs that are

composed of serous carcinomas with a high grade sarcoma component, these carcinosarcomas show low grade endometrioid carcinoma and undifferentiated carcinoma, with focal transition to a high grade spindle cell component (**Fig. 8**). Endometrial carcinomas with mismatch repair abnormalities can also be difficult to sub-classify, as they can show overlapping morphologic features of serous, clear cell or endometrioid carcinomas (**Fig. 9**). Further studies are needed to determine whether particular tumor types or histologic features are associated with mutations in different genes, but it has been observed that *MSH2* mutations may be associated with nonendometrioid endometrial carcinomas.[34,35] Our group has noted more carcinomas with endometrioid and undifferentiated histology in patients with *hMLH1* mutations, while endometrial clear cell carcinomas are more often associated with abnormalities in *hMSH2* or *hMSH6*. The presence of synchronous endometrial endometrioid carcinoma with ovarian clear cell carcinoma may also be indicative of LS[28,30]; ovarian clear cell carcinomas, particularly in young women, have been shown to be LS associated.[40–43] Synchronous endometrioid carcinomas of the endometrium and ovary on the other hand, appear unrelated to mismatch repair abnormalities.[28,44,45]

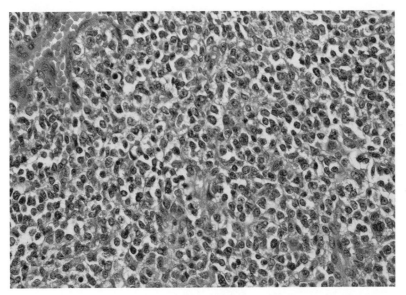

Fig. 4. Undifferentiated endometrial carcinomas are composed of sheets of dyshesive, round to ovoid cells, and often do not display overt nuclear pleomorphism.

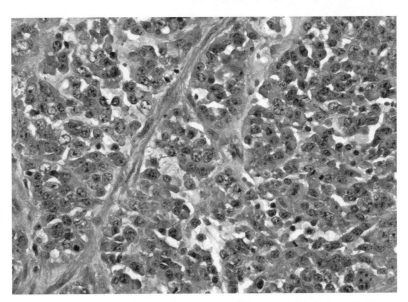

Fig. 5. Undifferentiated carcinomas can show foci with myxoid matrix and rhabdoid cells.

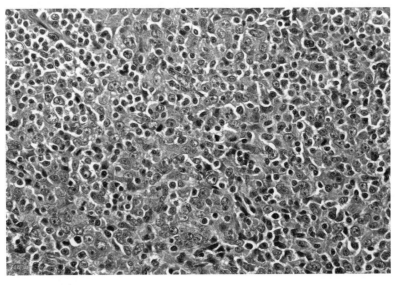

Fig. 6. When undifferentiated carcinomas are associated with a prominent lymphocytic infiltrate, they evoke a lymphoepithelioma like appearance.

Fig. 7. (*A*) This endometrial clear cell carcinoma with oxyphilic features, presented in a 55-year old woman. (*B*) The tumor showed loss of MSH6 staining by IHC.

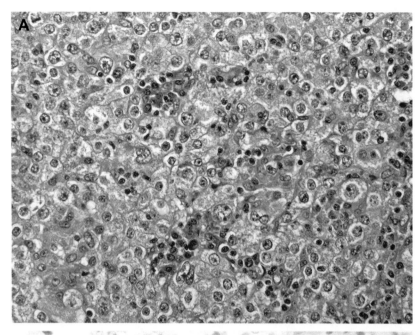

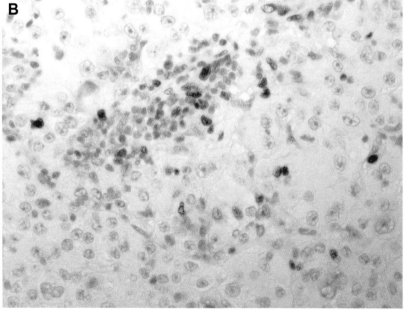

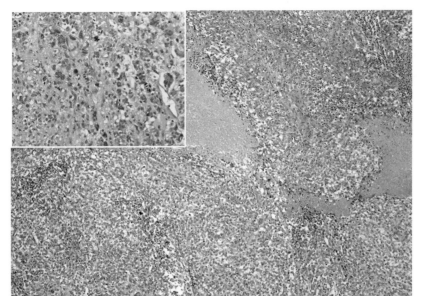

Fig. 8. This endometrial tumor was composed predominantly of dedifferentiated endometrioid carcinoma (undifferentiated carcinoma component present at bottom right of image) with focal evolution into high grade sarcoma (inset). This 52 year old woman was found to have a deleterious *MLH1* mutation.

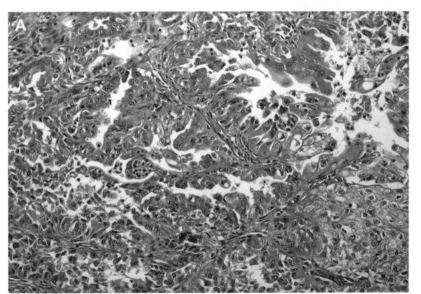

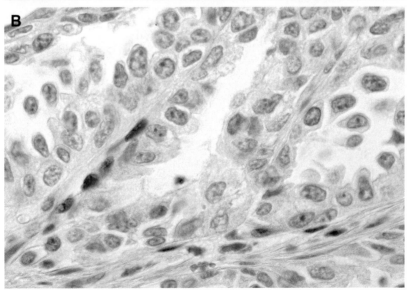

Fig. 9. This endometrial carcinoma in a 50 year old woman showed histologic features of endometrioid, clear cell and serous carcinoma (*A*). Many such tumors can be difficult to subclassify. The tumor showed loss of MSH2 and MSH6 by IHC (*B*).

METHODS FOR DETECTION OF LYNCH SYNDROME IN ENDOMETRIAL CARCINOMA

Since Lynch syndrome is defined by the presence of germline mutations in DNA mismatch repair genes, mutation analysis is the definitive test to establish the diagnosis. However, this is an expensive and time consuming test due to the heterogeneity of mutation spectrum in Lynch syndrome, and cannot be performed on every endometrial carcinoma patient. Moreover, germline testing is complicated by ethical and regulatory issues related to patient consent. Germline testing is therefore best used as a confirmatory test. Other simpler and less expensive tests should be performed first for screening. These include immunohistochemistry (IHC) for DNA mismatch repair proteins, microsatellite instability analysis by PCR and *MLH1* promoter methylation analysis.

IMMUNOHISTOCHEMISTRY (IHC) FOR DNA MISMATCH REPAIR PROTEINS

IHC for DNA mismatch repair proteins has been shown to be a sensitive and specific test for detection of mismatch repair abnormalities in endometrial carcinoma.[46] When all 4 antibodies (MLH1, PMS2, MSH2 and MSH6) are used, IHC has a sensitivity of 91% and specificity of 83% for detecting MSI-H.[46] The lower specificity is likely due to mutations in *hMSH6* (indirectly detectable with IHC), that can result in MSI-low or MS-stable tumors. The mismatch repair proteins can be lost in isolation or in pairs. In their functional state, the mismatch repair proteins form dimers; MLH1 dimerizes with PMS2 while MSH2 dimerizes with MSH6. Since MLH1 and MSH2 are the obligatory partners in these dimers, mutations in *hMLH1* lead to concurrent loss of PMS2, while mutations in *hMSH2* lead to concurrent loss of MSH6. Some *hMLH1* mutations result in isolated loss of PMS2, without abnormal MLH1 expression patterns. *hPMS2* and *hMSH6* mutations can lead to isolated IHC loss of PMS2 and MSH6 respectively. Loss of more than 2 proteins or loss of mismatch repair proteins in other combinations is extremely rare and should be interpreted with caution (**Box 2**).

hMLH1 promoter methylation or mutation will both result in IHC loss of MLH1 and PMS2. Since IHC loss of MLH1 and PMS2 may be due to *hMLH1* promoter methylation or germline mutations in MLH1 or PMS2, further testing is required to differentiate between the two mechanisms of loss. Loss of MSH2 and/or MSH6 on the other hand, is virtually diagnostic of Lynch syndrome.

> **Box 2**
>
> **Immunohistochemistry for mismatch repair proteins**
>
> *Expected patterns of IHC loss*
>
> Loss of MLH1 and PMS2
>
>   Sporadic as a result of MLH1 promoter methylation
>
>   or
>
>   LS-associated
>
> Loss of MSH2 and MSH6
>
>   LS-associated
>
> Loss of MSH6 alone
>
>   LS-associated
>
> Loss of PMS2 alone
>
>   Likely LS-associated

Advantages of IHC as a screening test include its availability and simplicity. It is also relatively inexpensive. A recent paper suggests that IHC with only two proteins (PMS2 and MSH6) may be as effective in detecting MMR deficient colorectal carcinomas when compared with the 4 marker panel.[47] Such studies on endometrial carcinomas are currently lacking. IHC can also direct gene sequencing efforts, which can be focused on only one or two genes based on the pattern of IHC loss. It has been shown that IHC followed by directed gene sequencing is the most cost effective strategy for detection of LS in EC patients.[48] IHC for MMR proteins may be particularly advantageous in endometrial carcinomas. LS associated ECs not infrequently harbor *hMSH6* mutations, and since these tumors may be MSI-low or MS-stable on MSI analysis by PCR, they would remain undetected using this technique alone.[19–23]

Although IHC has many advantages, its interpretation can sometimes be problematic.[49] To establish IHC loss of an MMR protein, one should see complete loss of staining in all tumor cells in the presence of internal positive control (stromal cells, lymphocytes, normal endometrium) (**Fig. 10**). Nuclear staining of tumor cells, even when focal and weak, is evidence of retained staining (**Fig. 11**). Interpretation of the MLH1 stain can be particularly challenging. This can occur when the tumor cells are negative but the surrounding stromal cells and lymphocytes are also negative (**Fig. 12**). Another problem that can be encountered with the MLH1 stain is the presence of extremely weak and equivocal staining (**Fig. 13**). In these situations, evaluation of the PMS2 stain can be helpful. If there is unequivocal

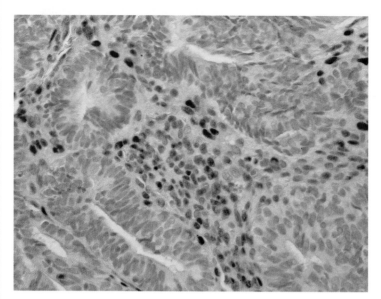

Fig. 10. To interpret IHC for DNA mismatch repair proteins as abnormal, one should see complete loss of staining in all tumor cells in the presence of internal positive controls such as stromal cells and lymphocytes.

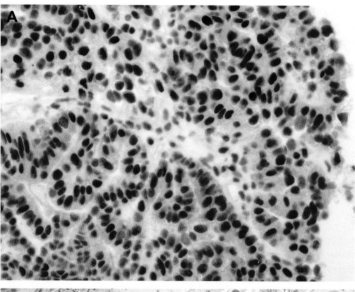

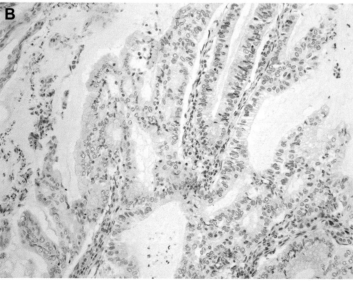

Fig. 11. (*A*) Cases that display strong diffuse staining for mismatch repair proteins are easy to interpret. (*B*) Sometimes, staining for mismatch repair proteins, particularly MLH1, can be focal and weak, as in this case.

Fig. 12. The tumor shows only rare, nonspecific staining for mismatch repair proteins in the tumor cells. However, notice the complete absence of an internal positive control. This result is inconclusive.

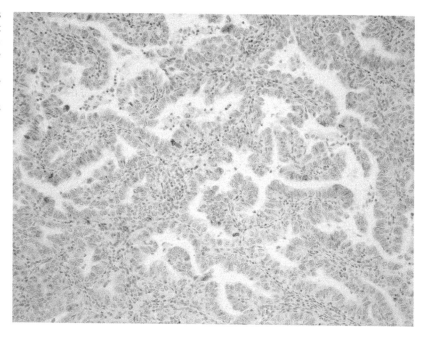

loss of PMS2, equivocal MLH1 staining probably indicates staining loss. In difficult situations, the slide should be reviewed with another pathologist with experience in interpretation of MMR stains or the stain may be repeated. If it continues to be problematic, the stain should be interpreted as inconclusive. If there is clinical suspicion for LS, an alternative testing method can be pursued. IHC fails to detect germline mutations in approximately 10% of cases, mainly missense mutations.[13]

Since IHC loss can be epigenetic, it is not considered a germline test; however, since it can indicate the presence of LS, the issue of patient

Fig. 13. The MLH1 stain can sometimes show granular, equivocal nuclear staining. Repeating the stain and assessment of the PMS2 stain may be helpful.

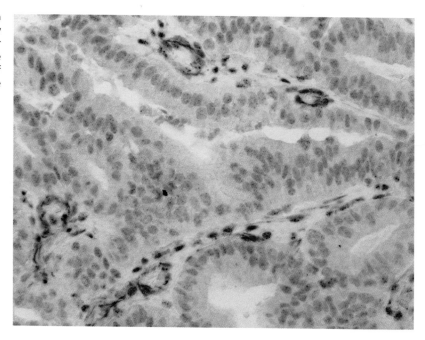

consent should be addressed. In some hospitals, specific consent is required while in others, this is part of the general consent signed by the patient at time of surgery and no separate consent is needed. If no consent is required, it is important that the pathologists, surgeons and oncologists communicate with each other and reach consensus about the medical necessity of performing such tests. It should be ensured that all patients with an abnormal result receive appropriate counseling and further testing as required.

MICROSATELLITE INSTABILITY (MSI) ANALYSIS

MSI analysis by PCR uses dinucleotide and mononucleotide markers.[50,51] DNA from tumor and normal tissue is isolated and tested, most commonly with 5 microsatellite markers as recommended by NCI (BAT25, BAT26, D2S123, D5S346 and D17S250),[50] although it has since been noted that a panel composed of mononucleotide markers is more sensitive and specific (BAT-25, BAT-26, NR-21, NR-24 and MONO-27).[18,51] When a tumor shows MSI at 2 or more loci, it is considered MSI-high; MSI at one locus is interpreted as MSI-low and if no instability is detected, it is considered MS-stable (**Fig. 14**). This test has some disadvantages when compared with IHC:

- It requires a molecular laboratory set up and staff and is relatively more expensive.
- Endometrial carcinomas with *hMSH6* mutations may be MSI-low or MS-stable, and could potentially remain undetected using this test.
- This test also does not distinguish between epigenetic and genetic causes for MSI.

Some authors still advocate a combination of both IHC and MSI analysis to maximize detection of mismatch repair abnormalities.

hMLH1 PROMOTER METHYLATION ASSAY

This test detects the presence of *hMLH1* promoter methylation, which is usually an acquired phenomenon that results in inactivation of *hMLH1* and an inability to detect the protein by IHC. The presence of *hMLH1* promoter methylation indicates that the tumor is likely unrelated to LS.[52,53] On the other hand, the absence of *hMLH1* promoter methylation in a tumor that is MSI-high or shows IHC loss of MLH1/PMS2 is likely to be Lynch syndrome related.

All the aforementioned tests have their advantages and disadvantages and are best used in combination. We generally prefer IHC as a screening test in the presence of suggestive clinical history or tumor morphology (see following). If the IHC is abnormal, further testing depends on the pattern of IHC loss (**Fig. 15**). In the event of MLH1/PMS2 loss, *hMLH1* promoter methylation analysis can be the next step, particularly in patients under 60 years of age. If methylation is present, the tumor is likely sporadic. In the absence of methylation, *hMLH1* mutation analysis should be pursued. *hPMS2* mutations are rare, therefore *hPMS2* mutation analysis should be reserved for patients with no detectable *hMLH1* mutation. If there is IHC loss of MSH2 and MSH6, mutation analysis for *hMSH2* and *hMSH6* should follow. With isolated MSH6 loss, *hMSH6* gene mutation analysis should be pursued.

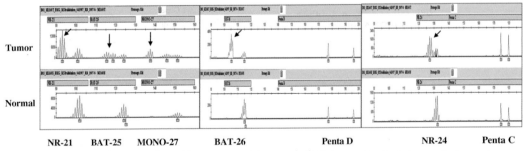

Fig. 14. The shifted alleles are indicated by an arrow. The tumor DNA (upper tracing) demonstrates an increased number of peaks compared with normal DNA from the same patient (lower tracing). Therefore, the tumor is MSI-high with allelic shift in 5 of 5 microsatellites. (*Courtesy of* Liying Zhang, MD, Memorial Sloan Kettering Cancer Center.)

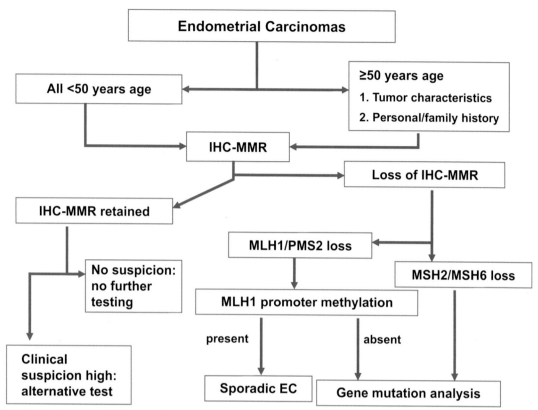

Fig. 15. In the event of abnormal IHC results for DNA mismatch repair proteins, this testing algorithm may be most efficient and cost-effective.

SCREENING ALGORITHM FOR DETECTION OF LS IN ENDOMETRIAL CARCINOMA PATIENTS

A combination of patient factors (age, personal and family history and body mass index), tumor characteristics (gross and microscopic) and IHC for DNA mismatch repair proteins may be the most effective strategy for detection of LS in endometrial carcinoma patients.

We would consider performing immunohistochemical stains for the four DNA mismatch repair proteins in the following patients with endometrial cancer:

1. All patients younger than age 50 years
2. Patients of any age whose tumors show the following characteristics:
   Lower uterine segment origin
   Multicentric uterine tumors
   Peritumoral lymphocytes and tumor infiltrating lymphocytes (TILs greater than 42 per 10 high power fields)
   Tumor heterogeneity

   De-differentiated or undifferentiated endometrial carcinomas
   Non-endometrioid carcinomas (clear cell, serous and carcinosarcomas) in patients younger than age 60 years
   High grade endometrial carcinoma with overlapping features of different histologic subtypes
   Synchronous endometrial endometrioid and ovarian clear cell carcinomas
3. Patients of any age with suggestive personal or family history of LS associated tumors.

PROGNOSTIC AND THERAPEUTIC IMPLICATIONS

MICROSATELLITE INSTABILITY IN ENDOMETRIAL CARCINOMA

The prognostic and therapeutic impact of mismatch repair status on endometrial carcinoma is not clear. Some studies, mostly using MSI as an endpoint instead of LS, have found no association with prognosis while others have showed improved or worse clinical outcomes.[54–57] Many studies, including some from our group, have noted that LS associated ECs are often associated with adverse prognostic indicators, including higher FIGO grade and stage and more frequent lymphovascular invasion.[28,30,34,57,58] This suggests that sporadic MSI-H EC might be prognostically favorable, in contrast to LS associated EC.

Whether defects in the mismatch repair system should have an impact on therapeutic decision making in endometrial carcinoma patients is currently not known. Type I or differentiated endometrioid carcinomas of the uterus are related to estrogen excess and selected young EC patients may be treated conservatively with progesterones. The relationship between estrogens and mismatch repair abnormalities is interesting and deserves further exploration. It has been suggested that one or more MMR genes may be estrogen responsive, with loss of estrogens resulting in loss of MMR function.[59–61] Endometrial carcinomas with mismatch repair abnormalities often occur in young patients with low body mass index, in contrast with sporadic ECs in this age group. ECs associated with MMR defects in these patients also show lower levels of ER/PR expression, particularly PR.[28] PR status has been shown to correlate with prognosis and therapeutic response to progesterone therapy.[62–66] This raises the possibility that relationships between hormonal milieu and development of EC may differ in sporadic and LS-associated ECs, and may suggest that young EC patients with MMR defects may not be appropriate candidates for conservative management. Further studies are required to elucidate the relationship between hormones and mismatch repair defects and the impact on treatment strategies. Larger studies with long term clinical follow up are required to definitively assess the impact of mismatch repair status on therapy and outcome in endometrial carcinoma patients.

RISK REDUCING STRATEGIES FOR ENDOMETRIAL CARCINOMA IN LYNCH SYNDROME

Colonoscopy has been shown to decrease mortality from colorectal carcinomas in Lynch syndrome. The efficacy of surveillance methods for endometrial carcinoma, including annual pelvic examination, transvaginal and pelvic ultrasound and endometrial biopsy, is not well established.[67] The effect of chemoprevention such as with oral contraceptives is currently not known. Small studies have shown that prophylactic hysterectomy and bilateral salpingo-oophorectomy can prevent development of endometrial and ovarian cancer in women with LS.[68,69]

SUMMARY

The association between endometrial carcinoma and Lynch syndrome is important and should be recognized. Women with Lynch syndrome can present with a gynecologic malignancy as their sentinel cancer. These patients and their family members are at risk for multiple malignancies and would benefit from screening and surveillance measures. Along with patient age and family history, gross and microscopic tumor characteristics of endometrial carcinomas may be suggestive of mismatch repair defects. Immunohistochemistry for DNA mismatch repair proteins is an effective tool for detection of Lynch Syndrome in endometrial carcinomas. Large long term studies are required to assess the prognostic and therapeutic impact of this association.

REFERENCES

1. Vasen HF, Offerhaus GJ, den Hartog Jager FC, et al. The tumor spectrum in hereditary nonpolyposis colorectal cancer: a study of 24 kindreds in the Netherlands. Int J Cancer 1990;46(1):31–4.

2. Aarnio M, Sankila R, Pukkala E, et al. Cancer risk in mutation carriers of DNA-mismatch repair genes. Int J Cancer 1999;81:214–8.

3. Graham R, McKee P, McGibbon D, et al. Torre-Muir syndrome: an association with isolated sebaceous carcinoma. Cancer 1985;55(12):2868–73.

4. Eng C. Will the real Cowden syndrome please stand up: revised diagnostic criteria. J Med Genet 2000; 37:828–30.

5. Blumenthal GM, Dennis PA. Germline PTEN mutations as a cause of early-onset endometrial cancer. J Clin Oncol 2007;25(33):2234.

6. Hornreich G, Beller U, Lavie O, et al. Is uterine papillary serous carcinoma a BRCA1-related disease? Case report and review of literature. Gynecol Oncol 1999;75(2):300–4.

7. Benier ME, Finch A, Rosen B, et al. The risk of endometrial cancer in women with BRCA1 and BRCA2 mutations. A prospective study. Gynecol Oncol 2007;104:7–10.

8. Levine DA, Barakat RR, Robson ME, et al. Risk of endometrial carcinoma associated with BRCA mutation. Gynecol Oncol 2001;80(3):445.

9. Loeb LA. Microsatellite instability: marker of a mutator phenotype in cancer. Cancer Res 1994;54: 5059–63.

10. Peltomaki P, Lothe RA, Aaltonen L, et al. Microsatellite instability is associated with tumors that

characterize the hereditary non polyposis colorectal carcinoma syndrome. Cancer Res 1993;53(24): 5853–5.

11. Esteller M, Levine R, Baylin SB, et al. MLH1 promoter hypermethylation is associated with the microsatellite instability phenotype in sporadic endometrial carcinomas. Oncogene 1998;17(18): 2413–7.

12. Gurin CC, Federici MG, Kang L, et al. Causes and consequences of microsatellite instability in endometrial carcinoma. Cancer Res 1999;59:462–6.

13. Hampel H, Frankel W, Panescu J, et al. Screening for Lynch syndrome (Hereditary Nonpolyposis Colorectal Cancer) among endometrial carcinoma patients. Cancer Res 2006;66(15):7810–7.

14. Ollikainen M, Abdel-Rahman WM, Moisio AL, et al. Molecular analysis of familial endometrial carcinoma: a manifestation of hereditary nonpolyposis colorectal cancer or separate syndrome? J Clin Oncol 2005;23:4609–16.

15. Hampel H, Frankel WL, Martin E, et al. Screening for the Lynch syndrome (Herediatry Nonpolyposis Colorectal Cancer). N Engl J Med 2005;352:1851–60.

16. Berends MJ, Wu Y, Sijmons RH, et al. Toward new strategies to select young endometrial cancer patients for mismatch repair gene mutation analysis. J Clin Oncol 2003;21:4364–70.

17. Lu KH, Schorge JO, Rodabaugh KJ, et al. Prospective determination of prevalence of Lynch syndrome in young women with endometrial cancer. J Clin Oncol 2007;25(33):5158–64.

18. Umar A, Boland CR, Terdiman JP, et al. Revised bethesda guidelines for hereditary nonpolyposis colorectal cancer (Lynch syndrome) and microsatellite instability. J Natl Cancer Inst 2004;96(4): 961–8.

19. Plaschke J, Engel C, Kruger S, et al. Lower incidence of colorectal cancer and later age of disease onset in 27 families with pathogenic MSH6 germline mutations compared with families with MLH1 or MSH2 mutations: the German Hereditary Nonpolyposis colorectal cancer consortium. J Clin Oncol 2004;22:4486–94.

20. Goodfellow PJ, Buttin BM, Herzog TJ, et al. Prevalence of defective DNA mismatch repair and MSH6 mutation in an unselected series of endometrial cancers. Proc Natl Acad Sci U S A 2003;100(10): 5908–13.

21. Baglietto L, Lindor NM, Dowty JG, et al. Risks of Lynch syndrome cancers for MSH6 mutation carriers. J Natl Cancer Inst 2009;102:1–9.

22. Berends MJW, Wu Y, Sijmons RH, et al. Molecular and clinical characteristics of MSH6 variants: an analysis of 25 index carriers of a germline variant. Am J Hum Genet 2002;70:26–37.

23. Ramsoekh D, Wagner A, van Leerdam ME. Cancer risk in MLH1, MSH2 and MSH6 mutation carriers: different risk profiles may influence clinical management. Hered Cancer Clin Pract 2009;7:17.

24. Lu KH, Dinh M, Kohlmann W, et al. Gynecologic cancer as a "sentinel cancer" for women with Hereditary Nonpolyposis Colorectal cancer syndrome. Obstet Gynecol 2005;105:569–74.

25. Jarvinen HJ, Aarnio M, Mustonen H, et al. Controlled 15-year trial on screening for colorectal cancer in families with Hereditary Non Polyposis Colorectal Cancer. Gastroenterology 2000;118:829–34.

26. McCourt CK, Mutch DG, Gibb RK, et al. Body mass index: relationship to clinical, pathologic and features of microsatellite instability in endometrial cancer. Gynecol Oncol 2007;104:535–9.

27. Schmeler KM, Soliman PT, Sun CC, et al. Endometrial cancer in young, normal-weight women. Gynecol Oncol 2005;99:388–92.

28. Garg K, Shih K, Barakat R. Endometrial carcinomas in women age 40 years and younger: tumors associated with loss of DNA mismatch repair proteins comprise a distinct clinicopathologic subset. Am J Surg Pathol 2009;33(12):1869–77.

29. Westin S, Broaddus R. Adenocarcinoma of the lower uterine segment: a unique subset of endometrial carcinoma. J Clin Oncol 2008;26(36): 5965–71.

30. Garg K, Leitao M, Kauff N, et al. Selection of endometrial carcinomas for DNA mismatch repair protein immunohistochemistry using patient age and tumor morphology enhances detection of mismatch repair abnormalities. Am J Surg Pathol 2009;33(6):925–33.

31. Shia JS, Black DB, Hummer AJ, et al. Routinely assessed morphologic features correlate with microsatellite instability status in endometrial cancer. Hum Pathol 2008;39:116–25.

32. van den Bos M, van den Hoven M, Jongejan E, et al. More differences between HNPCC-related and sporadic carcinomas from the endometrium as compared to the colon. Am J Surg Pathol 2004; 28(6):706–11.

33. Walsh MD, Cummings MC, Buchanan DD, et al. Molecular, pathologic and clinical features of early onset endometrial cancer: Identifying presumptive Lynch syndrome patients. Clin Cancer Res 2008; 14(6):1692–700.

34. Carcangiu ML, Radice P, Casalini P, et al. Lynch syndrome related endometrial carcinomas show a high frequency of non-endometrioid types and of high FIGO grade endometrioid types. Int J Surg Pathol 2010;18(1):21–6.

35. Broaddus RR, Lynch HT, Chen LM, et al. Pathologic features of endometrial carcinoma associated with HNPCC. Cancer 2006;106:87–94.

36. Honore LH, Hanson J, Andrew SE. Microsatellite instability in endometrioid endometrial carcinoma: correlation with clinically relevant pathologic variables. Int J Gynecol Cancer 2006;16:1386–92.

37. Toledo G, Growdon WB, Dias-Santagata D, et al. Microsatellite instability status and clinicopathologic profile of endometrial cancer in young women [abstract number 1036]. Mod Pathol 2008;21(Suppl 1).

38. Silva EG, Deavers MT, Bodurka DC, et al. Association of low-grade endometrioid carcinoma of the uterus and ovary with undifferentiated carcinoma: a new type of dedifferentiated carcinoma? Int J Gynecol Pathol 2006;25(1):52–8.

39. Altrabulsi B, Malpica A, Deavers MT, et al. Undifferentiated carcinoma of the endometrium. Am J Surg Pathol 2005;29(10):1316–21.

40. Jensen KC, Mariappan MR, Putcha GV, et al. Microsatellite instability and mismatch repair protein defects in ovarian epithelial neoplasms in patients 50 years of age or younger. Am J Surg Pathol 2008;32(7):1029–37.

41. Cai KQ, Albarracin C, Rosen D, et al. Microsatellite instability and alteration of the expression of MLH1 and MSH2 in ovarian clear cell carcinoma. Hum Pathol 2004;35(5):552–9.

42. Bewtra C, Watson P, Conway T, et al. Hereditary ovarian cancer: a clinicopathologic study. Int J Gynecol Pathol 1992;11(3):180–8.

43. Watson P, Butzow R, Lynch HT, et al. The clinical features of ovarian cancer in hereditary nonpolyposis colorectal cancer. Gynecol Oncol 2001;82(2):223–8.

44. Shannon C, Kirk J, Barnetson R, et al. Incidence of microsatellite instability in synchronous tumors of the ovary and endometrium. Clin Cancer Res 2003;9:1387–92.

45. Soliman PT, Broaddus RR, Schmeler KM, et al. Women with synchronous primary cancers of the endometrium and ovary: do they have lynch syndrome? J Clin Oncol 2005;23:9344–50.

46. Modica I, Soslow RA, Black D, et al. Utility of immunohistochemistry in predicting microsatellite instability in endometrial carcinoma. Am J Surg Pathol 2007;31:744–51.

47. Shia J, Tang LH, Vakiani E, et al. Immunohistochemistry as first line screening for detection of colorectal carcinoma patients at risk for hereditary non polyposis colorectal cancer: A 2 antibody panel may be as predictive as a 4 antibody panel. Am J Surg Pathol 2009;33(11):1639–45.

48. Kwon JS, Sun CC, Peterson SK. Cost-effectiveness analysis of prevention strategies for gynecologic cancers in Lynch syndrome. Cancer 2008;113:326–35.

49. Shia J. Immunohistochemistry versus microsatellite instability testing for screening colorectal cancer patients at risk for HNPCC. J Mol Diagn 2008;10:293–300.

50. Boland CR, Thibodeau SN, Hamilton SR, et al. A National Cancer Institute workshop on microsatellite instability for cancer detection and familial predisposition: development of international criteria for the determination of microsatellite instability in colorectal cancer. Cancer Res 1998;58(22):5248–57.

51. Laghi L, Bianchi P, Malesci A. Differences and evolution of the methods for the assessment of microsatellite instability. Oncogene 2008;27:6313–21.

52. Whelan AJ, Babb S, Mutch DG, et al. MSI in endometrial carcinoma: absence of MLH1 promoter methylation is associated with increased familial risk for cancers. Int J Cancer 2002;99(5):697–704.

53. Buttin BM, Powell MA, Mutch DG, et al. Increased risk for hereditary non polyposis colorectal cancer-associated synchronous and metachronous malignancies in patients with microsatellite instability positive endometrial carcinoma lacking MLH1 promoter methylation. Clin Cancer Res 2004;10(2):481–90.

54. Black D, Soslow RA, Levine DA, et al. Clinicopathologic significance of defective DNA mismatch repair in endometrial carcinoma. J Clin Oncol 2006;24:1745–53.

55. Basil JB, Goodfellow PJ, Rader JS, et al. Clinical significance of microsatellite instability in endometrial carcinoma. Cancer 2000;89:1758–64.

56. Zighelboim I, Goodfellow PJ, Gao F, et al. Microsatellite instability and epigenetic inactivation of MLH1 and outcome of patients with endometrial carcinomas of the endometrioid type. J Clin Oncol 2007;25:2042–8.

57. Fiumicino S, Ercoli A, Ferrandina G, et al. Microsatellite instability is an independent indicator of recurrence in sporadic stage I-II endometrial adenocarcinoma. J Clin Oncol 2001;19(4):1008–14.

58. Jung An H, Kim KI, Kim JY, et al. Microsatellite instability in endometrioid type endometrial adenocarcinoma is associated with poor prognostic indicators. Am J Surg Pathol 2007;31:846–53.

59. Natarnicola M, Gristina R, Messa C, et al. Estrogen receptors and microsatellite instability in colorectal carcinoma patients. Cancer Lett 2001;168:65–70.

60. Slattery ML, Potter JD, Curtin K, et al. Estrogens reduce and withdrawal of estrogens increase risk of microsatellite instability positive colon cancer. Cancer Res 2001;61:126–30.

61. Ferreira AM, Westers H, Albergaria A, et al. Estrogens, MSI and Lynch syndrome associated tumors. Biochim Biophys Acta 2009;1796(2):194–200.

62. Gehrig PA, Van Le L, Olatidoye B, et al. Estrogen receptor status, determined by immunohistochemistry, as a predictor of the recurrence of stage I endometrial carcinoma. Cancer 1999;86:2083–9.

63. Ingram SS, Rosenman J, Heath R, et al. The predictive value of progesterone receptor levels in endometrial cancer. Int J Radiat Oncol Biol Phys 1989;17(1):21–7.

64. Jeon YT, Park IA, Kim YB, et al. Steroid receptor expressions in endometrial cancer: clinical significance and epidemiologic implication. Cancer Lett 2006;239:198–204.

65. Jongen V, Briet J, de Jong R, et al. Expression of estrogen receptor alpha and beta and progesterone receptor A and B in a large cohort of patients with endometrioid endometrial cancer. Gynecol Oncol 2009;112:537–42.

66. Thigpen JT, Brady MF, Alvarez RD, et al. Oral medroxyprogesterone acetate in the treatment of advanced or recurrent endometrial carcinoma: a dose-response study by the Gynecology Oncology group. J Clin Oncol 1999;17(6): 1736–44.

67. Renkonen-Sinisalo L, Butzow R, Lehtovirta P, et al. Surveillance for endometrial cancer in hereditary nonpolyposis colorectal cancer syndrome. Int J Cancer 2006;120:821–4.

68. Schmeler KM, Lynch HT, Chen LM, et al. Prophylatic surgery to reduce the risk of gynecologic cancers in the Lynch syndrome. N Engl J Med 2006;354:261–9.

69. Pistorius S, Kruger S, Hohl R, et al. Occult endometrial cancer and decision making for prophylactic hysterectomy in hereditary nonpolyposis colorectal cancer patients. Gynecol Oncol 2006;102(2):189–94.

CLINICAL APPROACH TO DIAGNOSIS AND MANAGEMENT OF OVARIAN, FALLOPIAN TUBE, AND PERITONEAL CARCINOMA

David F. Silver, MD[a],*, Dennis S. Chi, MD[b], Nadim Bou-Zgheib, MD[a]

KEYWORDS

- Ovarian cancer • Fallopian tube cancer • Primary peritoneal cancer • Genetic screening
- Epidemiology • Staging procedures • Cytoreductive surgery • Chemotherapy

ABSTRACT

Ovarian, fallopian tube and peritoneal carcinomas make up the deadliest group of malignancies of the female genital tract. Ovarian carcinoma is the second most common malignancy of the female reproductive tract in developed countries and the sixth most common cancer diagnosed in women in the United States. While signs and symptoms of ovarian carcinoma related to the mass-effect of advanced disease are used for diagnosis, no reliable signs or symptoms are seen in patients with early ovarian carcinoma. The diagnosis can only be made by surgical removal and pathologic evaluation of a suspicious mass. This review details staging procedures and surgical and chemotherapeutic techniques for management of various stages of ovarian cancer. The authors present an overview of the disease, discussion of genetic predisposition, screening and prevention and diagnosis of ovarian cancer, cancer of fallopian tube, and peritoneal carcinoma.

OVERVIEW

Ovarian, fallopian tube and peritoneal carcinomas make up the deadliest group of malignancies of the female genital tract. While peritoneal and fallopian tube cancers are rare, ovarian carcinoma, as currently defined, is the second most common malignancy of the female reproductive tract in developed countries and the sixth most common cancer diagnosed in women in the United States affecting 1 in 70 women in their lifetime.[1] The highest incidence is found in Northern European countries, the United Kingdom, and the United States. Native Japanese have the lowest incidence.[2] Although the primary anatomic sites of fallopian tube and peritoneal carcinomas appear to differ, their histologic characteristics resemble those of ovarian carcinoma. Similarly, issues surrounding detection, treatment and outcomes reflect a commonality within this group of diseases. Therefore, ovarian carcinoma is used as the model for the following discussion on their detection and treatment.

[a] The Women's Institute for Gynecologic Cancer & Special Pelvic Surgery, 755 Memorial Parkway, Phillipsburg, NJ 08865, USA
[b] Gynecologic Service, Department of Surgery, Memorial Sloan-Kettering Cancer Center, 1275 York Avenue, New York, NY 10065, USA
* Corresponding author.
E-mail address: dsilver@upthevolume.org

Surgical Pathology 4 (2011) 261–274
doi:10.1016/j.path.2010.12.003
1875-9181/11/$ – see front matter © 2011 Published by Elsevier Inc.

It is increasingly recognized that ovarian carcinoma is heterogenous, not only from a clinical standpoint, but also morphologically, biologically and genetically. An appreciation of these specific features has led to the recognition that each type is distinctive and constitutes a unique disease entity. These include: low grade serous carcinoma, high grade serous carcinoma, low grade endometrioid carcinoma, high grade endometrioid carcinoma, clear cell carcinoma and mucinous carcinoma.

High-grade (grades 2 and 3) serous carcinoma, the prototypic "ovarian cancer," represents between 80 and 85% of ovarian carcinomas in North America. Almost all diagnostic and therapeutic efforts in the clinical realm have been developed with the mistaken assumption that lessons learned from studying this prototype can be generalized to less common ovarian cancer types. This will undoubtedly change in the coming years. All of the details concerning diagnosis and treatment in this review address high-grade serous carcinomas specifically, unless otherwise noted. One should remain hesitant to assume that these generalities are applicable across the ovarian carcinoma spectrum. Details regarding diagnosis and treatment of the less common entities will be covered in the relevant articles.

EPIDEMIOLOGY

Ovarian carcinoma is typically a postmenopausal disease identified in women with a median age of 63. Although the etiology of ovarian carcinoma is still unclear, several theories have been hypothesized. The previously, the most popular causation theory was associated with ovulation. It was postulated that ovulation resulted in epithelial damage and subsequent repair. With repeated cyclical injuries to the ovarian epithelium there may be an increased rate of chromosomal aberration leading to an increased likelihood of oncogenic mutation and carcinogenesis. This theory was supported by the known protective effects of multiple pregnancies, oral contraceptives, and lactation. Conversely, early menarche, late menopause and nulliparity are risk factors and the use of ovulation induction agents has been associated with an increased incidence of ovarian cancer.[3–5]

There are accumulating data that suggest that some, if not most, high grade ovarian serous carcinomas derive from intraepithelial neoplasms of the fimbriated end of the fallopian tube. If these neoplastic cells become incorporated into the ovarian cortex through disruptions in the ovarian surface that occur during ovulation, this hypothesis would account for both the protective effects of multiple pregnancies, oral contraceptives, lactation, tubal ligation, and also the presence of fimbrial intraepithelial serous carcinoma in an appreciable number of risk-reducing salpingectomy specimens and in the fimbria of patients with established ovarian cancer. This is discussed in detail in this publication by Shaw, in Hereditary Carcinomas of the Ovary, Fallopian Tube, and Peritoneum.

There are conflicting reports that implicate dietary, environmental and carcinogen exposures (such as talc, asbestos, and radiation) as risk factors of ovarian cancer. It is theorized that their direct exposure to the peritoneal cavity through the endometrial canal and fallopian tubes may result in a carcinogenic effect to the surface of the ovary. The theory that ovarian carcinogenesis is a result of exogenous toxins is supported by studies that have demonstrated a decreased incidence of ovarian cancer in women who have undergone prior tubal ligation.[6]

A known genetic predisposition is associated with 8 to 13% of ovarian carcinomas, specifically high-grade serous carcinoma.[7–9] BRCA1 and BRCA2 (chromosomes 17q and 13q) genes code for DNA repair proteins. While BRCA mutations are strongly associated with breast cancer, BRCA1 gene mutations also result in a 35% to 60% lifetime risk of ovarian cancer. Mutations in BRCA2 result in a lifetime risk of 10% to 20%.[10–13] Hereditary Nonpolyposis Colon Cancer (HNPCC) or Lynch Syndrome is a result of inherited defects in the mismatch repair genes MLH1, MLH2, and MSH6. Women with Lynch syndrome have a 12% lifetime risk of developing ovarian cancer in addition to being at increased lifetime risk for colon, endometrial, and gastric cancers among others.[14] Even without genetic information available, a family history of early onset breast or ovarian cancers increases the relative risk of developing ovarian cancer by 3- to 5-fold.[15]

SCREENING AND PREVENTION

The single most important change that must occur in the discipline of curing ovarian carcinoma is the development of an accurate and reproducible method to screen or detect the disease at its earliest stages. Difficulties in identifying a reliable screening tool are multifactorial. The adnexa and peritoneal surfaces are internal structures, not easily accessible to an examining physician; and the heterogeneity of the disease makes it difficult to pinpoint a single marker. High-grade serous carcinoma, the most common and most lethal type of ovarian carcinoma does not likely evolve from a clinically detectable precursor lesion. In contrast, some of the less common and less aggressive ovarian carcinomas arise from longstanding precursors that form clinically detectable masses. A recently proposed model of ovarian carcinogenesis posits that low-grade ovarian carcinomas (low-grade serous, low-grade endometrioid, mucinous and some clear cell carcinomas) arise from mass-forming precursor lesions such as endometriosis or borderline tumor, unlike high-grade serous carcinoma, which might arise from microscopic precursors in an anatomically normal fallopian tube.[16]

A large investment in effort and funds has been directed to the discovery of an effective screening modality.[17] Serum CA-125 levels and transvaginal ultrasounds have been the most evaluated methods in screening for adnexal cancers. However, these methods are not of sufficient accuracy for the screening of asymptomatic women and are only of modest benefit in high risk populations known to have a genetic predisposition.[18] The United Kingdom Collaborative Trial of Ovarian Cancer Screening (UKCTOCS) is an ongoing randomized trial evaluating the use of transvaginal ultrasound and CA-125 as screening tools in women with average risk of ovarian cancer. Final results are anticipated in 2012.[19] The American Cancer Society (ACS), American College of Obstetricians and Gynecologists (ACOG), Society of Gynecologic Oncologists (SGO) and the National Comprehensive Cancer Network (NCCN) all endorse ultrasounds and CA-125 screening of women at high risk of ovarian cancer who have not undergone risk-reducing (or prophylactic) salpingo-oophorectomy.[20–23] It is hopeful that a panel of tests will demonstrate the accuracy and reliability needed to successfully screen for ovarian cancer in the future. If further discovery results in reliable screening tests for the general public, the treatment and outcomes for ovarian cancer would be revolutionized, changing it from a late staged disease with little chance for long-term survival, to an early staged disease with expected high rates of cure.

Until then, high risk patients are encouraged to consider risk-reducing surgery. Risk-reducing salpingo-oophorectomy has demonstrated a high rate of protection against the development of ovarian, tubal and even breast cancers.[24,25] Risk-reducing surgery offers a greater than 90% reduction in the risk of developing ovarian cancer in high-risk patients with BRCA mutations. It should be recognized that despite the use of risk-reducing surgery, 4% may develop primary

---

Box 1
Epidemiology and screening for ovarian cancer

- Genetic predisposition is responsible for 8 to 13% of ovarian cancer cases.

- *BRCA1, BRCA2, MLH1, MLH2,* and *MSH6* are the most common mutations.

- A universal screening method is not available for ovarian cancer.

- CA 125 and transvaginal ultrasounds are recommended for high risk patients that have not undergone a risk reducing salpingoophorectomy,[20–23] although this may not be effective.

- Risk reducing salpingoophorectomy offers greater than 90% reduction in the incidence of "ovarian" cancer in high risk patients.[26]

- Prophylactic salpingo-oophorectomy is recommended at age 35 to 40 or after childbearing for patients with *BRCA1* mutation, and around perimenopause for *BRCA2* patients.[27,28]

---

peritoneal cancer.[26] While the preventative effect has been demonstrated in numerous studies, the age at which prophylactic surgery should be performed and the balance between early menopause and cancer prevention are questions that have not been entirely answered. The NCCN recommends prophylactic salpingo-oophorectomy for women with *BRCA1* mutations at age 35 through 40 or after childbearing.[27] Since *BRCA2* related ovarian carcinoma occurs at the expected age of sporadic cancers, it may be reasonable to delay risk-reducing surgery until the perimenopausal period (**Box 1**).

DIAGNOSIS

Signs and symptoms of ovarian carcinoma are related to the mass-effect of advanced disease. These include: palpable mass, ascites, abdominal distention, bloating, changes in bowel and bladder function, early satiety, dyspepsia, and shortness of breath. No reliable signs or symptoms are seen in patients with early ovarian carcinoma. The diagnosis can only be made by surgical removal and pathologic evaluation of a suspicious mass. The surgical management of ovarian carcinoma is maximized by appropriate referral to a gynecologic oncologist.[28–30] ACOG and SGO issued a Joint Committee Opinion in 2002 regarding the role of referral of suspicious ovarian masses to gynecologic oncologists.[31] These recommendations are listed in **Box 2**.

> **Box 2**
> **ACOG diagnostic criteria for referral to a gynecologic oncologist**
>
> Pelvic mass in postmenopausal woman that is suspicious for an ovarian malignancy, as suggested by at least one of the following:
>
> - Elevated CA 125 concentration
> - Ascites
> - Nodular or fixed pelvic mass
> - Evidence of abdominal or distant metastasis
> - Family history of one or more first-degree relatives with ovarian or breast cancer
>
> Premenopausal women who have a pelvic mass that is suspicious for a malignant ovarian neoplasm, as suggested by at least one of the following indicators:
>
> - Very elevated CA 125 concentration (eg, exceeding 200 U/mL)
> - Ascites
> - Evidence of abdominal or distant metastasis
> - Family history of one or more first-degree relatives with ovarian or breast cancer

TREATMENT

LOW-STAGE (FIGO STAGES I AND II) OVARIAN AND FALLOPIAN TUBE CARCINOMA

Early epithelial malignancies of the ovary and fallopian tube are confined to the pelvis without spread to the retroperitoneum, abdomen or distant sites. By convention, primary peritoneal cancers are staged based on ovarian carcinoma criteria and are therefore, by definition, almost always stage III or IV at the time of diagnosis. Therefore, our discussion of treatment for early cancers will be limited to ovarian and fallopian tube carcinomas.

STAGING PROCEDURES

Surgical staging for ovarian carcinoma established in the 1970s and revised by FIGO in 1985 remains the mainstay of identifying the extent of disease spread in epithelial ovarian malignancies.[32] **Box 3** outlines the FIGO surgical staging system. The procedures required for complete surgical staging include:

1. Exploration of all peritoneal surfaces
2. Aspiration of peritoneal ascites or washings for cytologic analysis
3. Bilateral salpingo-oophorectomy
4. Total hysterectomy
5. Subcolic omentectomy
6. Bilateral pelvic and periaortic lymph node dissection
7. Random biopsies of the peritoneal surfaces of the pelvis, paracolic gutters, diaphragms, and any bands of adhesion.

For those with radiologic evidence of pleural effusions, cytologic confirmation of metastatic cells is required. Nearly one-third of patients who are thought to have early ovarian cancer by clinical criteria are upstaged by surgical staging.[33,34] Those with metastatic disease are selected out as individuals who will truly benefit from the use of adjuvant chemotherapy.

Postoperative chemotherapy is the standard of care in the United States and most other countries for high-risk, low-stage ovarian carcinomas including: stage I grade 3, stage IC and stage II. The Gynecologic Oncology Group (GOG) compared three versus six cycles of postoperative paclitaxel/carboplatin for high-risk, low-stage ovarian carcinoma and found no survival advantage and higher toxicity with six cycles compared with three.[35] However, when Gynecologic Oncologists were subsequently surveyed about their practice patterns, the majority still give 6 cycles after surgical staging for high-risk, low-stage ovarian carcinomas.

Two large, randomized trials comparing observation versus chemotherapy for low-stage ovarian cancer were performed simultaneously in 2003 (EORTC-ACTION Trial, ICON 1 Trial). These studies and their long-term follow-up have provided a broad base of knowledge for the treatment of low-stage ovarian carcinoma.[36–38] Although ICON 1 demonstrated a survival advantage with the use of adjuvant chemotherapy (83% vs 74%, $P = .03$), the ACTION trial reveal that the benefit of adjuvant chemotherapy was limited to patients with inadequate surgical staging. Analysis of the combined populations from both the ACTION and ICON 1 trials confirmed the survival benefit offered by adjuvant chemotherapy; however, a subset analysis on the adequacy of staging versus survival was not done since ICON-1 did not collect data on surgical staging.[39] The information gleaned from these trials emphasizes the importance of complete surgical staging. While it is understood that surgically staged IC, IIA and grade 3 ovarian carcinoma patients have an increased risk for recurrence,

---

Box 3
International Federation of Gynecology and Obstetrics (FIGO) staging system for ovarian cancer stage characteristics

I. Growth limited to the ovaries

   IA Growth limited to one ovary; no ascites; no tumor on the external surface; capsule intact.

   IB Growth limited to both ovaries; no ascites; no tumor on the external surfaces; capsule intact.

   IC Tumor either Stage IA or IB, but with tumor on the surface of one or both ovaries; or with capsule ruptured; or with malignant cells in ascites or peritoneal washings.

II. Growth involving 1 or both ovaries with pelvic extension.

   IIA Extension and/or metastases to the uterus and/or tubes.

   IIB Extension to other pelvic tissues.

   IIC Tumor either Stage IIA or IIB, but with tumor on the surface of one or both ovaries; or capsule ruptured; or with malignant cells in ascites or peritoneal washings.

III. Tumor involving 1 or both ovaries with peritoneal implants outside the pelvis and/or positive retroperitoneal or inguinal lymph nodes.

   IIIA Tumor grossly limited to the true pelvis but with histologically confirmed microscopic involvement of abdominal peritoneal surfaces. Nodes are negative.

   IIIB Tumor involving one or both ovaries with histologically confirmed implants of abdominal peritoneal surfaces, none exceeding 2 cm in diameter. Nodes are negative.

   IIIC Abdominal implants greater than 2 cm in diameter and/or positive retroperitoneal or inguinal nodes.

IV. Growth involving one or both ovaries with distant metastases.

   Pleural effusion with positive cytology, parenchymal liver disease.

---

there is little definitive evidence to substantiate a survival benefit from postoperative chemotherapy. As we learn more about the clinical biology of ovarian carcinoma subtypes we might clarify a subset of low-stage ovarian carcinoma patients that would benefit from adjuvant chemotherapy and another in which avoiding adjuvant chemotherapy is optimal. A Cochrane meta-analysis[40] using randomized trials comparing adjuvant chemotherapy to no treatment in low-stage ovarian carcinoma demonstrated no significant survival or disease-specific survival advantage to chemotherapy for those women who underwent optimal staging surgery. A survival advantage for adjuvant chemotherapy was obtained for women who were suboptimally staged.[36,37,39,41,42]

HIGH STAGE (FIGO STAGES III AND IV) OVARIAN, FALLOPIAN TUBE, AND PERITONEAL CARCINOMAS

Due to the lack of reliable early signs, symptoms or screening tests, the majority of ovarian carcinomas are detected after metastatic extension to surfaces throughout the peritoneal cavity and, at times, to distant sites - most commonly the thorax. Treatment for advanced disease must include the combination of surgical resection and chemotherapy if a curative intent is the goal. Treatment with surgery or chemotherapy alone should only be used for palliation. Although there is universal agreement that both modalities are required for a therapeutic effect, the sequencing of surgery and chemotherapy as well as the route of chemotherapy administration are not firmly established or agreed upon around the world or within given regions.[43]

Controversial issues with respect to primary treatment of high-stage ovarian carcinoma include the following:

1. While the standard of care is primary cytoreductive surgery (PCS) followed by adjuvant chemotherapy, a recent randomized trial suggests that sequencing neoadjuvant chemotherapy (NCT) before cytoreductive surgery

decreases morbidity without decreasing survival.[44] Hence, many institutions are considering a paradigm shift to the use of NCT for primary treatment of high-stage disease.

2. While intraperitoneal (IP) chemotherapy has demonstrated survival superiority over intravenous (IV) chemotherapy in multiple large randomized trials,[45–47] the majority of patients with high-stage disease continue to receive chemotherapy via the intravenous route. Below we will define what is meant by cytoreductive surgery and delineate standard options for chemotherapy. A discussion about the various options for sequencing surgery and chemotherapy will follow.

CYTOREDUCTIVE SURGERY

Cytoreductive surgery was established in the 1970s after the Griffiths publication described improved survival in high-stage ovarian carcinoma patients after surgical resection of visible disease to residual nodules no larger than 1.5 cm in diameter.[48] The definition of cytoreductive surgery is simply, the resection of primary and metastatic disease. The degree of resection, by convention, is described as a measurement of the largest nodule of disease remaining upon completion of surgery. Unlike other solid tumors that require wide excision with free pathologic margins to impact survival, in ovarian carcinoma residual microscopic or small volume disease can be treated with relative effectiveness using postoperative chemotherapy. Hoskins and colleagues[49] reviewed randomized GOG chemotherapy trials on patients who had undergone primary surgery for high-stage ovarian carcinoma. Subgroup analysis based on measurements of residual disease clearly established an inverse relationship between the amount of residual disease and (1) response to chemotherapy, (2) progression-free survival, and (3) overall survival (**Fig. 1**). A multitude of nonrandomized studies have substantiated these results.[50–55]

Three descriptive terms have been linked to cytoreductive surgery: (1) complete, (2) optimal, and (3) suboptimal. Complete cytoreduction describes the result of a surgical procedure that leaves no visible residual tumor within the peritoneal cavity and leads to the highest rates of survival.[50,51] Optimal cytoreduction describes a surgical effort that results in low volume residual disease. The specific definition for "optimal" residual disease has evolved to include nodules no larger than 10 mm in largest dimension.[54] Suboptimal cytoreduction, therefore, is defined as surgery that results in bulky residual disease with nodules greater than 10 mm. Patients with suboptimal residual disease demonstrate the lowest rates of survival.[49,51]

Within the last decade, techniques required to accomplish maximal cytoreduction have been thoroughly described. While pelvic procedures such as modified posterior exenterations used to resect advanced regional disease are well established,[56] more recently, techniques to cytoreduce upper abdominal and thoracic disease have been described in the literature. These procedures are inclusive of but not limited to:

Colon resection[57,58]
Small bowel resection[59,60]
Bladder resection[61]

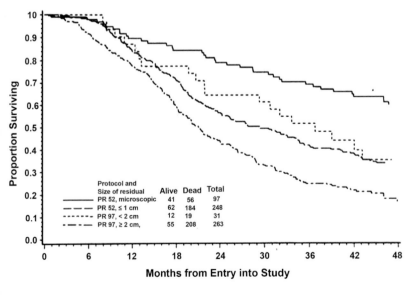

Fig. 1. The effect of diameter of largest residual disease on survival. (*From* Hoskins WJ, McGuire WJ, Brady MF, et al. The effect of diameter of largest residual disease on survival after primary cytoreductive surgery in patients with suboptimal residual epithelial ovarian carcinoma. Am J Obstet Gynecol 1994;170:974–80.)

Ureteric resection[62]
Nephrectomy[63]
Splenectomy[64,65]
Partial gastrectomy[66]
Distal pancreatectomy[65]
Liver resection[65,66]
Diaphragmatic stripping or resection[65,67]
Peritonectomy[68]
Extended lymphadenectomy[69]
Video-Assisted Thoracic Surgery (VATS) procedures to resect pleural and parenchymal thoracic metastases[70]

Spirtos and Eisenkop analyzed data on a large cohort of consecutive patients who underwent complete cytoreductive surgeries. Survival was stratified against each individual procedure required to attain complete cytoreduction. They found that the requirement for aggressive techniques to accomplish complete cytoreduction did not negatively impact the duration of survival in patients with high-stage disease[71] suggesting that the extent of metastatic disease can be overcome by the appropriate use of maximal cytoreductive surgery. Therefore, cytoreductive surgery should be planned with care to balance the completeness of tumor resection and surgical safety.

CHEMOTHERAPY FOR PRIMARY ADNEXAL OR PERITONEAL CARCINOMAS

Over the past 15 years several landmark trials have altered our view of the most appropriate use of platinum-based chemotherapy for primary stage III and IV disease. McGuire and colleagues[72] (GOG111) demonstrated a 14-month survival advantage (38 months vs 24 months) for 24-hour paclitaxel/cisplatin over cyclophosfamide/cisplatin in suboptimally cytoreduced patients in 1996. Ozols and colleagues[73] (GOG158) demonstrated the non-inferiority of 3-hour paclitaxel/carboplatin compared with 24-hour paclitaxel/cisplatin with less renal and neurotoxicity in optimally cytoreduced patients in 2003. In 2005 Armstrong and colleagues[45] reported the results of GOG172 demonstrating a 16 month survival advantage (66 months vs 50 months) for patients treated with a combination of IP/IV paclitaxel/cisplatin over those treated with standard IV paclitaxel/platinum. Two previously reported randomized trials also demonstrated the superiority of IP/IV chemotherapy.[46,47] Despite the survival advantage achieved with the use of IP/IV therapy, the oncology community-at-large has not widely accepted its use as standard of care for multiple reasons including concerns related to its toxicity. Therefore, though there is continued interest and investigation

in the use of IP/IV chemotherapy, most patients with high-stage disease are currently being treated with IV paclitaxel/carboplatin.

Several promising changes in recommendations for primary treatment of advanced ovarian cancer are anticipated to occur in the near future. In June of 2009 GOG218, a randomized trial comparing standard paclitaxel/carboplatin to paclitaxel/carboplatin/ bevacizumab closed to accrual. When outcomes from this trial mature it is anticipated that bevacizumab will be the first biologically targeted agent added to the standard primary treatment of high-stage ovarian carcinoma. Results of this trial will be compared with ICON 7, a similar trial with a slightly lower dose of bevacizumab which recently closed to accrual in Europe. The Japanese Gynecologic Oncology Group (JGOG) has demonstrated that the use of dose-dense IV paclitaxel combined with carboplatin resulted in a 13-month progression-free survival advantage over standard intravenous paclitaxel/carboplatin.[74] This has stimulated interest within the GOG for further clinical investigation to incorporate dose-dense chemotherapy into primary therapies. These potential additions to our upfront treatment of ovarian carcinoma promise to extend the duration of survival for this group of patients in the future.

PRIMARY CYTOREDUCTIVE SURGERY (PCS) FOLLOWED BY ADJUVANT CHEMOTHERAPY

A plethora of nonrandomized data has accumulated to substantiate the role of PCS followed by adjuvant chemotherapy.[50-55] Theories behind the benefit of performing PCS before chemotherapy suggest that the effects of surgical cytoreduction:

1. Removes chemo-resistant clones
2. Decreases the amount of hypoxic tumor mass
3. Results in smaller tumor masses with higher growth fractions expected to be more sensitive to chemotherapy
4. Reduces the immunosuppressive effect of large volume tumor burden.

Aletti and colleagues[75] at the Mayo Clinic compared surgeons who commonly used aggressive techniques to accomplish maximal cytoreduction versus surgeons who were less likely to use aggressive techniques within the same institution. They demonstrated higher rates of both optimal cytoreduction (87% vs 63%) and median survival (2 vs 3.5 years) among patients treated by the more aggressive surgeons. Bristow and colleagues[76] demonstrated that PCS survival benefit is not exclusive to patients who have advanced intraperitoneal spread of disease. Its benefit is also demonstrated in patients with stage IV disease.

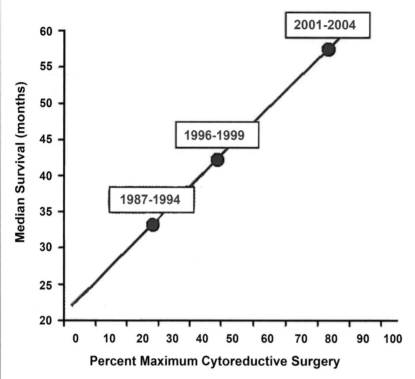

Fig. 2. Median overall survival as a function of percent maximum or optimal cytoreductive surgery. Memorial Sloan Kettering Cancer Center advanced ovarian cancer survival 1987–2004. (*Adapted from* Chi DS, Schwartz PE. Cytoreduction vs neoadjuvant chemotherapy for ovarian cancer. Gynecol Oncol 2008; 111:391–9; with permission.)

Chi[43] demonstrated that over a period of time in which the paradigm at Memorial Sloan Kettering Cancer Center shifted toward the use of more extensive cytoreductive techniques, the institution's rates of optimal cytoreduction, progression free, and overall survival all increased (**Fig. 2**).

If optimal cytoreduction is not achieved at the time of PCS, clinical investigators have evaluated the role of a subsequent interval cytoreductive surgery (ICS) following the demonstration of responsiveness to several cycles of adjuvant chemotherapy. Van der Burg and colleagues,[77] in a large European randomized trial, compared the use of ICS versus chemotherapy alone in patients who underwent suboptimal primary surgical procedures. They demonstrated a survival benefit (median survival = 26 months vs 20 months) with the use of ICS. In a subsequent trial designed to address the same question, GOG152 compared ICS to chemotherapy alone in suboptimal ovarian carcinoma.[78] In this trial all surgical procedures were performed by fellowship-trained gynecologic oncologists. No survival advantage was offered by the addition of ICS. The conclusion was that if the initial surgical cytoreduction is performed by a gynecologic oncologist and results in suboptimal residual disease, it is unlikely that chemotherapy would improve the likelihood of subsequent optimal resection or improve survival. Therefore, ICS is not recommended to patients who undergo a suboptimal PCS performed by a fellowship-trained gynecologic oncologist. On the other hand, if a patient demonstrates a response to chemotherapy after a suboptimal PCS performed by a non-gynecologic oncologist, consideration for ICS is reasonable.

NEOADJUVANT CHEMOTHERAPY (NCT) FOLLOWED BY CYTOREDUCTIVE SURGERY

In patients with poor performance status or significant comorbidities, NCT has been used in an effort to decrease tumor burden in the hope that a subsequent cytoreductive surgery could be made less morbid. Anecdotal findings of complete responses to NCT prompted the question of whether sequencing NCT before surgery could be a more appropriate treatment option for all patients with high-stage ovarian carcinoma. Findings from nonrandomized trials have demonstrated reduced surgical morbidity, higher optimal cytoreduction rates, less cost, and better chemotherapy tolerability with the use of NCT.[79–83] The survival rates in these studies are consistently no greater than those attained in patients who underwent suboptimal PCS followed by adjuvant chemotherapy. Bristow and Chi reported results from a meta-analysis on NCT. Their findings suggest that NCT is inferior to PCS. For every 10% increase in the rate of maximal cytoreduction in a given cohort, there was a 2 months increase in median survival; and for every incremental increase in the number of preoperative chemotherapy cycles, there was a 4 months decrease in median survival.[84]

The first large, international, randomized trial comparing NCT followed by ICS to PCS followed by adjuvant chemotherapy was reported in 2008 (EORTC-GCG/NCIC). The outcomes of this trial demonstrate the non-inferiority of the NCT strategy to PCS with a median progression-free survival of 12 months and an overall median survival of approximately 30 months (**Fig. 3**).[44] Interestingly, optimal cytoreduction remained the strongest independent prognostic factor for survival in multivariate analysis whether it was performed before chemotherapy as PCS or following chemotherapy as ICS. While some have changed their recommendations for upfront treatment of high-stage ovarian carcinoma based on this report, most await results from ongoing confirmatory trials.

RECURRENT OVARIAN CARCINOMA

Although advanced carcinomas of the ovary have a high rate of response to primary chemotherapy, over 80% will develop recurrence of disease. Recurrences can be divided into two broad categories based on the interval of time between completion of primary platinum-based chemotherapy and recurrence of disease. If the platinum-free interval is less than 6 months, patients are classified as "platinum-resistant." Conversely, if the platinum-free interval is longer than 6 months then they are "platinum-sensitive." The treatment-free intervals have been correlated with response to subsequent chemotherapy and overall survival.[85] It is unlikely that recurrent disease can be cured and it is expected that the platinum-free interval will decrease with each subsequent recurrence, ultimately resulting in resistant disease.

PLATINUM-RESISTANT RECURRENT DISEASE

Patients with platinum-resistant recurrent ovarian carcinoma have a 15 to 30% response rate to second-line chemotherapy and median survival of 10 to 15 months.[86] In choosing the most appropriate chemotherapy regimen, toxicities from prior chemotherapy and overall performance status must be considered. With short treatment-free intervals and potentially cumulative toxicities, single-agent therapy is often used in this group of patients (**Table 1**).

PLATINUM-SENSITIVE RECURRENT DISEASE

Patients with platinum-sensitive recurrence are expected to respond to chemotherapy 30 to 60% of the time and have a median survival of 18 to 29 months.[86] Since their treatment-free interval is longer it is expected that patients in this group will have a better performance status

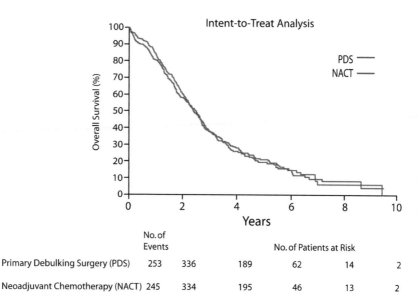

Fig. 3. Overall survival in patients treated with neoadjuvant chemotherapy vs primary cytoreductive (debulking) surgery. (*From* Vergote I, Tropé CG, Amant F, et al. Neoadjuvant chemotherapy or primary surgery in stage IIIC or IV ovarian cancer. N Engl J Med 2010;363: 943–53; with permission. Copyright © 2010, Massachusetts Medical Society.)

	No. of Events		No. of Patients at Risk			
Primary Debulking Surgery (PDS)	253	336	189	62	14	2
Neoadjuvant Chemotherapy (NACT)	245	334	195	46	13	2

Table 1
Common chemo regimens for platinum-resistant recurrent ovarian cancer

Regimens	Response	Median Overall Survival (mo)
Topotecan[87]	6.5%	10
Doxil[87]	12.3%	9
Gemcitabine[88]	16%	7
Docetaxel[89]	35%	8

and tolerate combination chemotherapy relatively well (**Table 2**).

Similar to discussions about the utility of PCS for primary ovarian carcinoma, there is a significant body of nonrandomized data in the gynecologic oncology literature that supports the use of secondary cytoreductive surgery (SCS) for a select group of patients with recurrent, platinum-sensitive disease.[93–95] Bristow and colleagues[96] performed a meta-analysis on SCS and found that for every 10% increase in the rate of complete cytoreduction, there was a 3 months increase in the median survival. The best candidates for SCS include patients who have good performance status, long platinum-free intervals, and who have recurrent tumors deemed to be amenable to complete resection. In the Memorial Sloan Kettering Cancer Center experience, Chi and colleagues[95] delineate a reasonable set of selection criteria for SCS that can be seen in **Table 3**. Those who question the value of SCS, argue that the reported benefits are solely a result of selection bias. An ongoing randomized GOG trial comparing chemotherapy alone versus SCS plus chemotherapy is currently accruing and is anticipated to shed light on this controversial topic.

Table 2
Common chemo regimens for platinum-sensitive recurrent ovarian cancer

Regimens	Response	Median Overall Survival (mo)
PLD[a]+ Carboplatinum[90]	63%	32
Carboplatinum[91]	54%	24
Paclitaxel+ Carboplatinum[91]	66%	29
Gemcitabine+ Carboplatinum[92]	47%	18

[a] Pegylated Liposomal Doxorubicin.

Table 3
Selection criteria for secondary cytoreductive surgery (SCS)

Disease-free Interval (DFI) (mo)	One Site	Multiple Sites, No Carcinomatosis	Carcinomatosis
6–12	Offer SC	Consider SC	No SC
12–30	Offer SC	Offer SC	Consider SC
Over 30	Offer SC	Offer SC	Offer SC

Data from Chi DS, McCaughty K, Diaz JP, et al. Guidelines and selection criteria for secondary cytoreductive surgery in patients with recurrent, platinum-sensitive epithelial ovarian carcinoma. Cancer 2006;106:1933–9.

SUMMARY

Carcinomas of the ovary, fallopian tube, and peritoneum make up a group of relatively rare cancers that account for an inordinately high rate of mortality that can be accounted for by the lack of reliable early signs, symptoms, or screening tests. In the 20% who are diagnosed with early staged disease, surgical staging is critically important as a prognostic and therapy-directing tool. For a select group of patients with early disease, chemotherapy options should be considered. Overall, survival rates greater than 80% are expected.

With advanced disease, the standard of care remains PCS followed by platinum-based chemotherapy. This standard is being challenged by recent randomized data that supports the use of NCT followed by ICS to reduce the morbidities related to primary surgery. Further confirmatory randomized data will be forthcoming in the near future. The expected 5-year survival for this group of patients is 20% to 50% and is most influenced by the degree of maximal cytoreductive surgery performed.

It is expected that the majority of patients with high-stage primary disease will undergo several courses of chemotherapy for recurrences that will ultimately become resistant to treatments. Platinum-free intervals, performance status, and quality of life play an important role in their prognoses and treatment options. The option of SCS for a select group of platinum-sensitive patients should be considered.

It is an exciting time with respect to the treatment of high-stage ovarian carcinoma. Many nuances of standard recommendations are changing and some of these are likely to become new dictums in the future. These changes may include the use of bevacizumab or other biologic agents, dose-dense chemotherapy, and new variations of IP/IV chemotherapy. With future advances it is anticipated that we will continue to improve upon the length and quality of the lives of our patients with ovarian, fallopian tube and peritoneal carcinomas.

REFERENCES

1. Jemal A, Siegel R, Ward E, et al. Cancer statistics, 2006. CA Cancer J Clin 2006;56:106–30.
2. Ferlay J, Bray F, Pisani P, et al. GLOBOCAN 2002: cancer incidence, mortality and prevalence worldwide. IARC CancerBase No. 5, version 2.0. Lyon (France): IARCPress; 2004.
3. Ozols RF, Bookman MA, Connolly DC, et al. Focus on epithelial ovarian cancer. Cancer Cell 2004;5: 19–24.
4. Rish HA. Hormonal etiology of epithelial ovarian cancer, with a hypothesis concerning the role of androgens and progesterone. J Natl Cancer Inst 1998;90:1774–86.
5. Rossing MA, Daling JR, Weiss NS, et al. Ovarian tumors in a cohort of infertile women. N Engl J Med 1994;331:771–6.
6. Hankinson SE, Hunter DJ, Colditz GA, et al. Tubal ligation, hysterectomy, and risk of ovarian cancer: a prospective study. JAMA 1993;270:2813–8.
7. Rish HA, Mclaughlin JR, Cole DE, et al. Prevalence and penetrance of germline BRCA1 and BRCA2 mutations in a population series of 649 women with ovarian cancer. Am J Hum Genet 2002;68:700–10.
8. Pal T, Remuth-Wey J, Betts JA, et al. BRCA1 and BRCA2 mutations account for a large proportion of ovarian carcinoma cases. Cancer 2005;104:2807–16.
9. Rubin SC, Blackwood MA, Bandera C, et al. BRCA1, BRCA2 and hereditary nonpoliposis colorectal cancer gene mutations in an unselected ovarian cancer population: relationship to family history and implications for genetic testing. Am J Obstet Gynecol 1998;178:670–7.
10. King MC, Marks JH, Mandell JB, New York Breast Cancer Study Group. Breast and ovarian cancer risks due to inherited mutations in BRCA1 and BRCA2. Science 2003;302:643–6.
11. Struewing JP, Hartge P, Wacholder S, et al. The risk of cancer associated with specific mutations of BRCA1 and BRCA2 among Ashkenasi Jews. N Engl J Med 1997;336:1401–8.
12. Ford D, Easton DF, Bishop DT, et al. Risks of cancer in BRCA1-mutation carriers. Breast Cancer Linkage Consortium. Lancet 1994;343:692–5.
13. Antoniou A, Pharoah PD, Narod S, et al. Average risks of breast and ovarian cancer associated with BRCA1 or BRCA2 mutations detected in case series unselected fro family history: a combined analysis of 22 studies. Am J Hum Genet 2003;72:1117–30.
14. Aarnio M, Sankila R, Pukkala E, et al. Cancer risk in mutation carriers of DNA-mismatch repair genes. Int J Cancer 1999;81:214–8.
15. Bergfeldt K, Rydh B, Granath F, et al. Risk of ovarian cancer in breast-cancer patients with a family history of breast or ovarian cancer: a population-based cohort study. Lancet 2002;360:891–4.
16. Singer G, Kurman RJ, Chang HW, et al. Diverse tumorigenic pathways in ovarian serous carcinoma. Am J Pathol 2002;160(4):1223–8.
17. Vang R, Shih IeM, Kurman RJ. Ovarian low-grade and high-grade serous carcinoma: pathogenesis, clinicopathologic and molecular biologic features, and diagnostic problems. Adv Anat Pathol 2009; 16(5):267–82.
18. Rosenthal AN, Menon U, Jacobs IJ. Screening for ovarian cancer. Clin Obstet Gynecol 2006;49:433–47.
19. Menon U, Gentry-Maharaj A, Hallett R, et al. Sensitivity and specificity of multimodal and ultrasound screening for ovarian cancer, and stage distribution of detected cancers: results of the prevalence screen of the UK Collaborative Trial of Ovarian Cancer Screening (UKCTOCS). Lancet Oncol 2009;10:327–40.
20. U.S. Preventive Services Task Force. Screening for ovarian cancer: recommendation statement. U.S. Preventive Services Task Force. Am Fam Physician 2005;71:759–62.
21. American Cancer Society. Detailed guide: ovarian cancer – can ovarian cancer be found early? Available at: http://www.cancer.org/docroot/CRI/content/CRI_2_4_3X_Can_ovarian_cancer_be_found_early_33.asp?rnav=cri. Accessed June 12, 2009.
22. ACOG Committee on Gynecologic Practice. The role of the generalist obstetrician-gynecolgist in the early detection of ovarian cancer. Gynecol Oncol 2002;87: 237–9.
23. National Comprehensive Cancer Network Practice Guidelines in oncology: ovarian cancer and genetic screening. Available at: http://www.nccn.org/professionals/physician_gls/PDF/genetics_screening.pdf. V. 1. 2010. Accessed December 13, 2010.
24. Rebbeck TR, Lynch HT, Neuhausen SL, et al, Prevention and Observation of Surgical End points Study Group. Prophylactic oophorectomy in carriers BRCA1 or BRCA2 mutations. N Engl J Med 2002; 346:1616–22.
25. Kauff ND, Satagopan JM, Robson ME, et al. Risk-reducing salpingo-oophorectomy in women with BRCA1 or BRCA2 mutation. N Engl J Med 2002; 346:1609–15.
26. Finch A, Beiner M, Lubinski J, et al, Hereditary Ovarian Cancer Clinical Study Group. Salpingo-oophorectomy and the risk of ovarian, fallopian

tube, and peritoneal cancers in women with BRCA 1 or BRCA2 mutation. JAMA 2006;296:185–92.

27. NCCN Clinical Practice Guidelines in Oncology. Hereditary breast and or ovarian cancer. Version 1.2006, December 14, 2005. Jenkintown (PA): National Comprehensive Cancer Network; 2005.

28. Dowdy SC, Stefanek M, Hartmann LC. Surgical risk reduction: prophylactic salpingo-oophorectomy and prophylactic mastectomy. Am J Obstet Gynecol 2004;191:1113–23.

29. Eisenkop SM, Spirtos NM, Montag TW, et al. The impact of the subspecialty training on the management of advanced ovarian cancer. Gynecol Oncol 1992;47:203–9.

30. Mayer AR, Chambers SK, Graves E, et al. Ovarian cancer staging: does it require a gynecologic oncologist? Gynecol Oncol 1992;47:223–7.

31. American College of Obstetricians and Gynecologists. ACOG Committee Opinion No. 280, December 2002. The role of the generalist obstetrician-gynecologist in the early detection of ovarian cancer. Obstet Gynecol 2002;100:1413–6.

32. Staging announcement: FIGO cancer committee. Gynecol Oncol 1986;25:383–5.

33. Young RC, Decker DG, Wharton JT, et al. Staging laparotomy in early ovarian cancer. JAMA 1983; 250:3072–6.

34. Bushsbaum HJ, Brady MF, Delgado G, et al. Surgical staging of carcinoma of the ovaries. Surg Gynecol Obstet 1989;169:226–32.

35. Bell F, Brady MF, Young RC, et al. Randomized phase III trial of three versus six cycles of adjuvant carboplatin and paclitaxel in early stage epithelial ovarian carcinoma: a Gynecologic Oncology Group study. Gynecol Oncol 2006;102:432–9.

36. Trimbos JB, Vergote I, Bolis G, et al, EORTC-ACTION collaborators, European Organisation for Research and Treatment of Cancer-Adjuvant Chemotherapy in Ovarian Neoplasm. Impact of adjuvant chemotherapy and surgical staging in early-stage ovarian carcinoma: European Organisation for Research and Treatment of Cancer-Adjuvant Chemotherapy in Ovarian Neoplasm trail. J Natl Cancer Inst 2003;95(2):113–25 4.

37. Colombo N, Guthrie D, Chiari S, et al. International Collaborative Ovarian Neoplasm trial 1: a randomized trial of adjuvant chemotherapy in women with early-stage ovarian cancer. J Natl Cancer Inst 2003;95(2):125–32.

38. Swart AC, on behalf of ICON collaborators. Long-term follow-up of women enrolled in a randomized trial of adjuvant chemotherpay for early stage ovarian cancer (ICON1). J Clin Oncol 2007; 25(18S):5509.

39. Trimbos JB, Parmar M, Vergote I, et al. International Collaborative Ovarian Neoplasm trial 1 and Adjuvant Chemotherapy in Ovarian Neoplasm trial: two parallel randomized phase III trials of adjuvant chemotherapy in patients with early-stage ovarian carcinoma. J Natl Cancer Inst 2003;95:105–12.

40. Winter-Roach BA, Kitchener HC, Dickinson HO. Adjuvant (post-surgery) chemotherapy for early stage epithelial ovarian cancer. Cochrane Database Syst Rev 2009;3:CD004706. DOI:10.1002/14651858. CD004706.pub3.

41. Bolis G, Colombo N, Pecorelli S, et al. Adjuvant treatment for early epithelial ovarian cancer: results of two randomised clinical trials comparing cisplatin to no further treatment or chromic phosphate (32P). G.I.C.O.G.: Gruppo Interregionale Collaborativo in Ginecologia Oncologica. Ann Oncol 1995;6(9): 887–93.

42. Trope C, Kaern J, Hogberg T, et al. Randomized study on adjuvant chemotherapy in stage I high risk ovarian cancer with evaluation of DNA-ploidy as prognostic instrument. Ann Oncol 2000;11(3): 281–8.

43. Chi DS, Schwartz PE. Cytoreduction vs neoadjuvant chemotherapy for ovarian cancer. Gynecol Oncol 2008;111:391–9.

44. Vergote I, Trope CG, Amant F, et al. EORTC-GCG/NCIC-CTG Randomised trial comparing primary debulking surgery with neoadjuvant chemotherapy in stage IIIC-IV ovarian, fallopian tube and peritoneal cancer (OVCA). Presented at the 12th Biennial meeting International Gynecologic Cancer Society-IGCS. Bangkok (Thailand), October 25–28, 2008.

45. Armstrong DK, Bundy B, Wenzel L, et al. Intraperitoneal cisplatin and paclitaxel in ovarian cancer. N Engl J Med 2006;354:34–43.

46. Alberts DS, Liu PY, Hannigan EV, et al. Intraperitoneal cisplatin plus intravenous cyclophosphamide versus intravenous cisplatin plus intravenous cyclophosphamide for stage III ovarian cancer. N Engl J Med 1996;335:1950–5.

47. Markman M, Bundy BN, Alberts DS, et al. Phase III trial of standard-dose intravenous cisplatin plus paclitaxel versus moderately high-dose carboplatin followed by intravenous paclitaxel and intraperitoneal cisplatin in small-volume stage III ovarian carcinoma: an intergroup study of the Gynecologic Oncology Group, South-western Oncology Group, and Eastern Cooperative Oncology Group. J Clin Oncol 2001;19:1001–7.

48. Griffiths CT. Surgical resection of tumor bulk in the primary treatment of ovarian carcinoma. Natl Cancer Inst Monogr 1975;42:101–4.

49. Hoskins WJ, McGuire WJ, Brady MF, et al. The effect of diameter of largest residual disease on survival after primary cytoreductive surgery in patients with suboptimal residual epithelial ovarian carcinoma. Am J Obstet Gynecol 1994;170:974–80.

50. Eisenkop SM, Friedman RL, Wang HJ. Complete cytoreductive surgery is feasible and maximizes

survival in patients with advanced epithelial ovarian cancer: a prospective study. Gynecol Oncol 1998; 69:103–8.

51. Bristow RE, Tamacruz RS, Armstrong DK, et al. Survival effect of maximal cytoreductive surgery for advanced ovarian carcinoma during the platinum era: a meta-analysis. J Clin Oncol 2002;20:1248–59.

52. Michel G, De Iaco P, Castaigne D, et al. Extensive cytoreductive surgery in advanced ovarian carcinoma. Eur J Gynaecol Oncol 1997;18:9–15.

53. Dauplat J, Le Bouedec G, Pomel C, et al. Cytoreductive surgery for advanced stages of ovarian cancer. Am J Obstet Gynecol 1992;166:843–6.

54. Chi DS, Eisenhauer EL, Lang J, et al. What is the optimal goal of primary cytoreductive surgery for bulky stage IIIC epithelial ovarian carcinoma? Gynecol Oncol 2006;103:559–64.

55. Aletti GD, Dowdy SC, Gostout BS, et al. Aggressive surgical effort and improved survival in advanced-stage ovarian cancer. Obstet Gynecol 2006;107: 77–85.

56. Eisenkop SM, Natlick RH, Teng NNH. Modified posterior exenteration for ovarian cancer. Obstet Gynecol 1991;78:879–85.

57. Hoffman MS, Zervose E. Colon resection for ovarian cancer: intraoperative decisions. Gynecol Oncol 2008;111:S56–65.

58. Silver DF, Bou Zgheib N. Extended left colon resections as part of complete cytoreduction for ovarian cancer: tips and considerations. Gynecol Oncol 2009;114:427–30.

59. Gillette-Cloven N, Burger RA, Monk BJ, et al. Bowel resection at the time of primary cytoreduction for epithelial ovarian cancer. J Am Coll Surg 2001;193: 626–32.

60. Cai HB, Zhou YF, Chen HZ, et al. The role of bowel surgery with cytoreduction for epithelial ovarian cancer. Clin Oncol 2007;19:757–62.

61. Berek JS, Hacker NF, Lagasse LD, et al. Lower urinary tract resection as part of cytoreductive surgery for ovarian cancer. Gynecol Oncol 1982; 13:87–92.

62. Hoffman MS, Tebes SJ. Ureteral surgery performed by a university gynecologic oncology service. Am J Obstet Gynecol 2006;195:562–6.

63. Guidozzi F, Ball JH. Extensive primary cytoreductive surgery for advanced epithelial ovarian cancer. Gynecol Oncol 1994;53:326–30.

64. Eisenkop SM, Spirtos NM, Lin WC. Splenectomy in the context of primary cytoreductive operations for advanced epithelial ovarian cancer. Gynecol Oncol 2006;100:344–8.

65. Kehoe SM, Eisenhauer EL, Chi DS. Upper abdominal surgical procedures: liver mobilization and diaphragm peritonectomy/resection, splenectomy, and distal pancreatectomy. Gynecol Oncol 2008;111: S51–5.

66. Hoffman MS, Tebes SJ, Sayer RA, et al. Extended cytoreduction of intraabdominal metastatic ovarian cancer in the left upper quadrant utilizing en bloc resection. Am J Obstet Gynecol 2007;197:209.e1–5.

67. Silver DF. Full-thickness diaphragmatic resection with simple and secure closure to accomplish complete cytoreductive surgery for patients with ovarian cancer. Gynecol Oncol 2004;95:384–7.

68. Aletti GD, Podratz KC, Jones MB, et al. Role of rectosigmoidectomy and stripping of pelvic peritoneum in outcomes of patients with advanced ovarian cancer. J Am Coll Surg 2006;203:521–6.

69. Aletti GD, Dowdy S, Podratz KC, et al. Role of lymphadenectomy in the management of grossly apparent advanced stage epithelial ovarian cancer. Am J Obstet Gynecol 2006;195:1862–8.

70. Juretzka MM, Abu-Rustum NR, Sonoda Y. The impact of video-assisted thoracic surgery (VATS) in patients with suspected advanced ovarian malignancies and pleural effusions. Gynecol Oncol 2007;104:670–4.

71. Eisenkop SM, Spirtos NM. Procedures required to accomplish complete cytoredution of ovarian cancer: is there a correlation with "Biological Aggressiveness" and survival? Gynecol Oncol 2001;82:435–41.

72. McGuire WP, Hoskins WJ, Brady MF, et al. Cyclophosphamide and cisplatin compared with paclitaxel and cisplatin in patients with stage III and stage IV ovarian cancer. N Engl J Med 1996;334:1–6.

73. Ozols RF, Bundy BN, Greer BE, et al. Phase III trial of carboplatin and paclitaxel compared with cisplatin and paclitaxel in patients with optimally resected stage III ovarian cancer: a Gynecologic Oncology Group study. J Clin Oncol 2003;21:3194–200.

74. Katsumata N, Yasuda M, Takahashi F. Dose-dense paclitaxel once a week in combination with carboplatin every 3 weeks for advanced ovarian cancer: a phase 3, open-label, randomised controlled trial. Lancet 2009;374:1331–8.

75. Aletti GD, Gostout BS, Podratz KC, et al. Ovarian cancer surgical resectability: relative impact of disease, patient status, and surgeon. Gynecol Oncol 2006;100:33–7.

76. Bristow RE, Montz FJ, Lagasse L, et al. Survival impact of surgical cytoreduction in stage IV epithelial ovarian cancer. Gynecol Oncol 1999;72:278–87.

77. Van Der Burg ME, van Lent M, Buyse M, et al. The effect of debulking surgery after chemotherapy on the prognosis in advanced epithelial ovarian cancer. N Engl J Med 1995;332:629–34.

78. Rose PG, Nerenstone S, Brady M, et al. A phase III randomised study of interval secondary surgery in patients with advanced stage ovarian carcinoma with suboptimal residual disease: a Gynecologic Oncology Group study. Proc Amer Soc Clin Oncol 2002;21(Pt 1):201a.

79. Kumar L, Janga D, Berge S, et al. Neoadjuvant chemotherapy in stage III & IV epithelial ovarian carcinoma (EOC). J Int Med Soc Acad 2003;16(2): 89–92.

80. Swartz PE, Rutherford TJ, Chambers JT, et al. Neoadjuvant chemotherapy for advanced ovarian cancer: long-term survival. Gynecol Oncol 1999;72:93–9.

81. Vergote I, De Wever I, Tjalma W, et al. Neoadjuvant chemotherapy or primary debulking surgery in advanced ovarian carcinoma: a retrospective analysis of 285 patients. Gynecol Oncol 1998;71:431–6.

82. Lim JT, Green JA. Neoadjuvant carboplatin and Ifosfamide chemotherapy for inoperable FIGO stage III and IV ovarian carcinoma. Clin Oncol 1993;5:198–202.

83. Jacob JH, Gershenson DM, Morris M, et al. Neoadjuvant chemotherapy and interval debulking for advanced epithelial ovarian cancer. Gynecol Oncol 1991;42:146–50.

84. Bristow RE, Chi DS. Platinum-based neoadjuvant chemotherapy and interval surgical cytoreduction for advanced ovarian cancer: a meta-analysis. Gynecol Oncol 2006;103:1070–6.

85. Markman M, Hoskins W. Responses to salvage chemotherapy in ovarian cancer: a critical need for precise definitions of the treated population. J Clin Oncol 1992;10:513–4.

86. Sonoda Y, Spriggs D. Ovarian cancer. Oncology 2007;52:903b–27b.

87. Gordon A, Fleagle J, Guthrie D, et al. Recurrent epithelial ovarian carcinoma: a randomized phase III study of pegylated liposomal doxorubicin versus topotecan. J Clin Oncol 2001;19:3312–22.

88. Markman M, Webster K, Zanotti K, et al. Phase II trial of single-agent gemcitabine in platinum-paclitaxel refractory ovarian cancer. Gynecol Oncol 2003;90: 593–6.

89. Francis P, Schneider J, Hann L, et al. Phase II trial of Docetaxel in patients with platinum-refractory advanced ovarian cancer. Clin Oncol 1994;12: 2301–8.

90. Ferrero JM, Weber B, Geay J-F, et al. Second-line chemotherapy with pegylated liposomal doxorubicin and carboplatinum is highly effective in patients with advanced ovarian cancer in late relapse: a GINECO phase II trial. Ann Oncol 2007;18:263–8.

91. The ICON and AGO Collaborators. Paclitaxel plus platinum-based chemotherapy versus conventional platinum-based chemotherapy in women with relapsed ovarian cancer; the ICON4/AGO-OVAR-2.2 trial. Lancet 2003;361:2099–106.

92. Ago-Ovar Ncic Ctg & EORTC GCG. Combination therapy with gemcitabine and carboplatinum in recurrent ovarian cancer. Int J Gynecol Cancer 2005;15(Suppl 1):36–41.

93. Bristow RE, Peiretti M, Gerardi M, et al. Secondary cytoreductive surgery including rectosigmoid colectomy for recurrent ovarian cancer: operative technique and clinical outcome. Gynecol Oncol 2009; 114:173–7.

94. Salani R, Santillan A, Zahurak M, et al. Secondary cytoreductive surgery for localized recurrent epithelial ovarian cancer. Analysis of prognostic factors and survival outcome. Cancer 2007;109: 685–91.

95. Chi DS, McCaughty K, Diaz J, et al. Guidelines and selection criteria for secondary cytoreductive surgery in patients with recurrent, platinum-sensitive epithelial ovarian carcinoma. Cancer 2006;106:1933–9.

96. Bristow RE, Puri I, Chi DS. Cytoreductive surgery for recurrent ovarian cancer: a meta-analysis. Gynecol Oncol 2009;112:265–74.

MOLECULAR PATHOLOGY OF OVARIAN CARCINOMAS

Martin Köbel, MD[a],*, David Huntsman, MD[b]

KEYWORDS
- Molecular pathology • Ovarian cancer • Prognostic markers • Molecular therapeutic targets
- Cell of origin

ABSTRACT

This is a review of the molecular pathology of ovarian carcinoma. Over the past ten years it has become evident that serous carcinomas represent two distinct diseases, high-grade and low-grade serous carcinomas.[3] TP53 mutations and chromosomal instability (CIN) are characteristic of high-grade but are rarely seen in low-grade serous carcinomas.[4] Defects in genes encoding proteins involved in double-stranded DNA repair causing CIN, are also seen in high-grade but not low-grade serous carcinomas.[5] After decades of research, credible precursor lesions for high-grade serous carcinomas have been identified within the distal fallopian tube; these are not associated with low-grade serous carcinomas.[6,7]

OVERVIEW

Gynecologic tumors are traditionally classified according to their putative site of origin, clinical stage, degree of differentiation and histologic type. It has now become clear that ovarian carcinoma histotypes are associated with distinct precursor lesions at their site of origin. Histologic type is also strongly associated with grade, stage at presentation and specific molecular alterations.[1] The classification system proposed by the Vancouver group can accurately assign greater than 98% of tumors to one of the five major types: high-grade serous (68%), clear cell (12%), endometrioid (11%), mucinous (3%) and low-grade serous (3%).[2]

Over the past ten years it has become evident that serous carcinomas represent two distinct diseases, high-grade and low-grade serous carcinomas.[3] TP53 mutations and chromosomal instability (CIN) are characteristic of high-grade but are rarely seen in low-grade serous carcinomas.[4] Defects in genes encoding proteins involved in double-stranded DNA repair causing CIN, are also seen in high-grade but not low-grade serous carcinomas.[5] After decades of research, credible precursor lesions for high-grade serous carcinomas have been identified within the distal fallopian tube; these are not associated with low-grade serous carcinomas.[6,7]

Mouse models for ovarian carcinomas are also subtype specific, re-enforcing the notion that these are distinct diseases. Carcinomas that recapitulate high grade serous morphology were induced in mice by mutational changes of genes controlling proliferation (RB1 or MYC) in a TP53−/− background.[8,9] In contrast, endometrioid and clear cell carcinomas have been shown to be associated with endometriosis as a putative precursor lesion.[10] A mouse model for

[a] Department of Pathology, University of Calgary and Calgary Laboratory Services, Foothills Medical Centre, 1403 29 ST NW, Calgary, Alberta, Canada T2N 2T9
[b] Faculty of Medicine, Department of Pathology and Laboratory Medicine, University of British Columbia, BC Cancer Agency, #3427-600 West 10th Avenue, Vancouver, British Columbia V5Z 4E6, Canada
* Corresponding author.
E-mail address: Martin.Kobel@cls.ab.ca

Surgical Pathology 4 (2011) 275–296
doi:10.1016/j.path.2010.12.009

surgpath.theclinics.com

Table 1
Mutational landscape of ovarian carcinomas

Gene	HGSC	LGSC	MC	EC G1/G2	CCC
TP53	119/123 (97%)[4]	1/13 (8%)[12]	5/19 (26%)[25]	15/42 (36%)[11]	4/38 (10%)[13]
BRCA1	37/341 (11%)[14]	0/2[15]		0/5[15]	0/4[15]
BRCA1 epi genetic	9/38 (24%)[15]	0/2		0/5	0/4
BRCA2	19/341 (6%)[14]				
PTEN	2/51 (4%)[16]			8/42 (19%)[11]	1/18[17]
PI3KCA	0/51 (0%)[16]			5/42 (12%)[11]	32/97 (33%)[18]
ARID1A				10/33 (30%)	55/119 (46%)[26]
CTNNB1	0/51 (0%)[16]			18/42 (43%)[11]	3/87 (3%)[18]
KRAS	0/72 (0%)[3]	12/22 (54%)[19]	11/22 (50%)[20]	5/42 (12%)[11]	4/97 (4%)[18]
BRAF	0/72 (0%)[3]	7/21 (33%)[3]	0/22[20]		0/87[18]
ERBB2 amplification	3/105 (3%)[21]		6/33 (18%)[22]		
MSI-H	1/38 (3%)[15]			15/74 (20%)[23]	6/42 (14%)[4]

Shading indicates aberrations that are characteristic of each entity.
Abbreviations: CCC, clear cell carcinoma; EC G1/G2, endometrioid carcinoma low grade (grade 1 and 2) where possible; HGSC, high-grade serous carcinoma; LGSC, low-grade serous carcinoma; MC, mucinous carcioma.

endometrioid carcinomas has been established by inducing alterations in the PI3K/PTEN and Wnt/CTNNB1 pathway.[11] An overview of the mutational landscape of ovarian carcinomas as known today is given in **Table 1**.

With the advent of high throughput techniques such as oligonucleotide microarrays to analyze mRNA profiles and tissue microarrays for immuno-histochemistry it has become clear that the mRNA and protein expression patterns are in keeping with morphologic classification.[27–29] Importantly, biomarker expression reflects histopathological type and not stage.[29] Expression profiles of the histologic types resemble normal tissue:

Table 2
Protein expression and selected differentially expressed markers assessed by immunohistochemistry

Marker	HGSC	LGSC	EC	CCC	MC
MUC16/CA125	88%	100%	81%	67%	7%
ESR/ER	76%	80%	77%	10%	3%
WT1	80%	70%	2%	4%	0
TP53/p53	88%		32%	24%	
CDKN2A/p16	60%		27%	0	0
PTEN	14%		33%		
CTNNB1/β-catenin	0		45%		
HNF1B/HNF1-β	5%			83%	
Ki67 median (95%CI)	22% (3%–70%)	2.5% (0.5%–20%)	8% (1%–49%)	8% (1%–45%)	13% (2%–71%)

Shading indicates characteristic of each entity expression. The definition of positive staining includes any staining for MUC16, ER, WT1, HNF1β, diffuse staining in more than 50% of tumor cell nuclei or complete absence of staining for p53, no staining for PTEN, and nuclear expression for β-catenin. Ki67 index was assessed by quantitative image analysis.
Abbreviations: CCC, clear cell carcinoma; EC, endometrioid carcinoma; HGSC, high-grade serous carcinoma; LGSC, low-grade serous carcinoma; MC, mucinous carcioma.
Data from Refs.[29,60,114,143,144]

serous/fallopian tube, endometroid and clear cell/endometrium and mucinous/colon but not ovarian surface epithelium.[30] For any given subtype of ovarian carcinoma the diagnostic expression patterns consist of a combination of distinct cell lineage markers (eg, WT1 as a marker for serous lineage) and markers specific for oncogenic pathways (eg, p53 for high-grade serous carcinoma) (**Tables 2** and **3**).

On the basis of shared clinical and molecular features, a binary classification system for all ovarian carcinomas has been proposed that splits these tumors into type I (low-grade serous, mucinous, endometrioid, clear cell) and type II (high-grade serous).[31] This model clearly delineates genomically unstable tumors from other types and provides a framework for the study of ovarian carcinogenesis, but does not replace standard histopathological typing. Notably, it obscures some of the significant differences and potential therapeutic opportunities of the different type I tumors. The histopathological types differ with respect to grade, precursor lesions, genetic risk factors, molecular alterations, pattern of spread, stage at presentation, response to chemotherapy and outcome (**Fig. 1**). Since the histologic subtypes have distinct molecular abnormalities, our evolving understanding of the mutational landscape of these cancers will likely add context and granularity rather than changing the framework. For instance, the upcoming publication of The

Cancer Genome Atlas Project (TCGA) comprehensive analysis of high-grade serous cancers could help fill in many of the gaps in our understanding of this disease. As our knowledge improves, there will be opportunities to incorporate novel biomarkers to assist in the diagnosis of problematic cases and predict response to therapy.

Table 3
Suggested immunohistochemical marker panel to support subtype diagnosis of ovarian carcinomas based on expression frequencies in Table 2

Ovarian Carcinomas	Marker Panel
HGSC versus LGSC	p53, p16
HGSC versus EC	WT1, p53, p16, VIM, PR
HGSC versus CCC	WT1, p53, p16, HNF-1β
HGSC versus MC	WT1, p53, p16
EC versus MC/CCC	PR, VIM
EC versus LGSC	WT1
LGSC versus MC/CCC	WT1, PR, VIM

Abbreviations: CCC, clear cell carcinoma; EC, endometrioid; HGSC, high-grade serous; LGSC, low-grade serous; MC, mucinous.

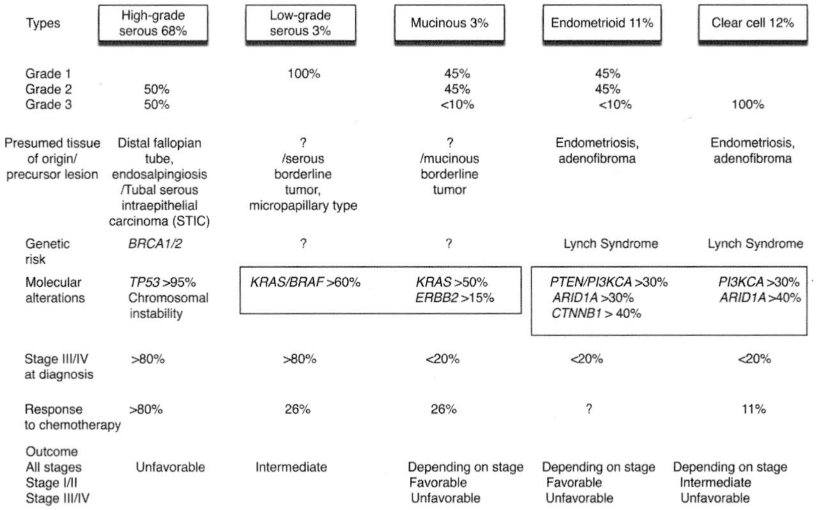

Fig. 1. Overview about the five major subtypes of ovarian carcinomas.

Types	High-grade serous 68%	Low-grade serous 3%	Mucinous 3%	Endometrioid 11%	Clear cell 12%
Grade 1		100%	45%	45%	
Grade 2	50%		45%	45%	
Grade 3	50%		<10%	<10%	100%
Presumed tissue of origin/ precursor lesion	Distal fallopian tube, endosalpingiosis /Tubal serous intraepithelial carcinoma (STIC)	? /serous borderline tumor, micropapillary type	? /mucinous borderline tumor	Endometriosis, adenofibroma	Endometriosis, adenofibroma
Genetic risk	BRCA1/2	?	?	Lynch Syndrome	Lynch Syndrome
Molecular alterations	TP53 >95% Chromosomal instability	KRAS/BRAF >60%	KRAS >50% ERBB2 >15%	PTEN/PI3KCA >30% ARID1A >30% CTNNB1 > 40%	PI3KCA >30% ARID1A >40%
Stage III/IV at diagnosis	>80%	>80%	<20%	<20%	<20%
Response to chemotherapy	>80%	26%	26%	?	11%
Outcome All stages Stage I/II Stage III/IV	Unfavorable	Intermediate	Depending on stage Favorable Unfavorable	Depending on stage Favorable Unfavorable	Depending on stage Intermediate Unfavorable

HIGH-GRADE SEROUS CARCINOMAS

High-grade Serous Carcinomas Key Molecular Features	
Molecular Pathology Features	1. *TP53* mutation (97% of cases) 2. Chromosomal instability due to *BRCA* loss of function (~50%), *BRCA1/2* germline mutation (16%), *BRCA1* promoter hypermethylation (25%) 3. High proliferation
Key Molecular Diagnostic Markers	1. WT1 expression >80% 2. Aberrant p53 expression 88% 3. P16 over-expression >50%
Key Molecular Prognostic Markers	1. Intraepithelial CD8-positive lymphocytes are associated with favorable prognosis 2. Loss of *BRCA* indicates favorable prognosis
Key Molecular Therapeutic Target	1. *TP53* mutation – platinum based chemotherapy 2. High proliferation – paclitaxel chemotherapy 3. BRCA deficiencies - PARP inhibitors, platinum based chemotherapy
Knowledge deficiencies	1. What is the natural history of the proposed fallopian tube precursor lesions? 2. Are these lesions distinct enough from normal fallopian tube epithelium to be detected by screening tests? 3. What is the basis of chromosomal instability in HGSCs without detectable *BRCA* abnormalities? 4. Will PARP inhibitors be effective in all HGSCs regardless of the presence of germline or somatic *BCRA* mutations? 5. Means to identify cancers with *BCRA* like defects in DNA repair as a predictive tool for PARP inhibitor based therapy

MOLECULAR PATHOLOGY FEATURES OF HIGH-GRADE SEROUS CARCINOMAS

High-grade serous carcinomas (HGSCs) are characterized by three features: *TP53* mutation, chromosomal instability, and high proliferation rate.[32,33] High-grade serous carcinomas account for 67% of all ovarian carcinomas and 88% of tumors diagnosed as stage III/IV.[2]

RISK FACTORS

Pregnancy and breastfeeding as well as the use of oral contraceptives, particularly those with high progestin content, reduce ovarian cancer risk by 50%,[34,35] possibly through reduced ovulation.[36]

Women who inherit a deleterious mutation in *BRCA1/BRCA2* have a very high risk of developing high-grade serous carcinoma. The lifetime risk is estimated to be up to 39%.[37] The frequency of *BRCA1/BRCA2* germline mutation of women diagnosed with high-grade serous carcinoma is 15–20%.[14] Testing for *BRCA1/BRCA2* germline mutations is widely available and prophylactic salpingo-oophorectomy can reduce the risk of high-grade serous carcinoma in mutation carriers by 80%.[38]

There have been recent efforts to identify more common, low penetrance genetic polymorphisms that affect ovarian carcinoma risk both by candidate gene approaches and genome wide association studies.[39] Candidate single nucleotide variants (SNPs) within *TP53* were investigated in 2829 serous carcinomas and 8790 controls. The SNP rs2287498 was associated with a slight increased risk of serous carcinomas.[40] A genome wide association study (GWAS) identified a tagged SNP at 9p22 that is associated with a 23% decreased risk of serous carcinoma.[41]

CELL LINEAGE

The 'cell of origin' of these tumors has been intensely disputed,[42] mainly because there was no recognizable precursor lesion. Proposed cells of origin include:

1. Mesothelium (the ovarian surface epithelium) or inclusion cysts, which undergo metaplasia to become Müllerian epithelium[43]
2. "Secondary Müllerian system," Müllerian epithelium in paraovarian or paratubar location[42]
3. Epithelium directly derived from the fallopian tube or endometrium.[44,45]

Diligent histologic examinations of salpingo-oophorectomy specimens from prophylactic surgeries have identified putative precursor lesions within the distal fallopian tube but not within the ovaries.[6,7,46] This precursor lesion is usually referred to as serous tubal intraepithelial carcinoma (STIC). This is not the only possible precursor lesion for this cancer as occult carcinoma within the ovaries has been reported in women undergoing risk reducing salpingo-oophorectomy.[47] Nevertheless, the distal fallopian tube is by far the most common site of STIC in BRCA mutation carriers. Further studies showing that STIC and HGSCs often co-exist[48] led to the conclusion that the majority of HGSCs may arise from the fallopian tube,[49,50] which is in sharp contrast to the traditional view that classified the vast majority of HGSCs as ovarian in origin.[32] STIC associated with a concomitant HGSC share not only morphologic features but also identical TP53 mutations indicating a clonal relationship.[51]

Some HGSCs cannot be linked to the fallopian tube.[48] Normal tubal cells from the fimbriated end may be dislodged and implanted within the ovary and on peritoneal surfaces giving rise to the development of endosalpingiosis. Thus, some HGSCs may develop from ectopic fallopian tube tissue rather than from metaplasia of ovarian surface epithelium.[44] Given the uncertainty about the primary site in routine practice in most cases, the term "pelvic HGSC" has been proposed to refer to HGSCs that arise from the fallopian tube, ovary or peritoneum, exclusive of those arising from within the uterus.[49]

A type specific classification irrespective of localization has started to fundamentally change our perspective, ie, HGSC presumed to arise in the fallopian tube, ovary or peritoneum share more in common than tumors that just happen to occur in the same location, eg, other types of ovarian carcinoma.[52] Even if the exact site of origin remains elusive, HGSCs share the cell lineage characteristics of fallopian tube, which should be considered in the choice of normal control tissue in molecular studies.

TP53 MUTATION

FUNCTION

The hallmark mutation of high-grade serous carcinomas is the somatic mutation of TP53 in 97% of cases (see **Table 1**). Genetically engineered mouse models developed serous carcinomas exclusively in TP53 mutated background, but TP53 mutation alone was not sufficient to generate serous carcinomas; a second oncogenic mutation in a proliferation pathway such as RB1 or MYC was required.[8,9]

p53 is a multitargeted transcription factor that is expressed in response to cellular stress such as DNA damage. Under normal conditions, DNA damage causes p53 to arrest the cell cycle at the G_1/S regulation point on recognition of DNA damage. p53 also activates DNA repair proteins to fix the damage. If this fails, p53 initiates apoptosis. Under conditions of mutated TP53, p53 deficiency compromises cell cycle control by impairing repair of DNA damage or induction of apoptosis thereby permitting cell survival even with chromosomal instability.

'P53 SIGNATURE'

One of the earliest recognizable abnormalities implicated in serous carcinogenesis is the so called 'p53 signature'. 'p53 signatures' show a strong predilection for the distal fallopian tube. 'p53 signature' is defined as a cluster of morphologically normal fallopian tube cells that show aberrant staining by p53 immunohistochemistry, and requires a minimum of strong nuclear staining in greater than 12 consecutive cells of secretory type. TP53 mutation has been found in approximately half of the 'p53 signatures' by direct sequencing.[51]

'p53 signatures' are often small with less than 50 cells and multifocal in one-third of cases.[53] 'p53 signatures' are present in at least a third of the distal fallopian tubes of both BRCA1/2 mutation carriers and age matched controls.[51,53] Hence, 'p53 signatures' are common in normal appearing distal fallopian tubes. Multifocal 'p53 signatures' were also detected in women with Li-Fraumeni syndrome who underwent prophylactic salpingo-oophorectomy.[54] Li-Fraumeni syndrome is a multiple cancer syndrome caused by TP53 germline mutation, but this syndrome is not particularly associated with a high risk of high-grade serous carcinomas. 'p53 signatures' were found in continuity with STIC, suggesting a transition from one to the other.[51] Hence, loss of p53 function must be accompanied by at least one more event (see below) to initiate serous carcinogenesis.

SEROUS TUBAL INTRAEPITHELIAL CARCINOMA (STIC)

STICs show overlapping features with the 'p53 signature' but they are distinguished by morphologically recognizable nuclear atypia and increased proliferation. STICs are defined by three features:

1. Conspicuous nuclear atypia
2. Dramatically increased proliferation rate (usually greater than 75% ki67 labeling index or conspicuous increased compared with the background)
3. Evidence of TP53 mutation (usually indicated by over-expression but a minority may be completely negative, see below).[32]

STICs share the same TP53 mutation with coexisting metastatic high-grade serous carcinomas of the ovary or peritoneum[51,54–56] Approximately 75% of pelvic high-grade serous carcinomas show a coexisting STIC.[48]

The prevalence of STIC is 8 to 10% in BRCA1 and BRCA2 mutations carriers.[53] STICs are usually clinically occult, noninvasive and 2.7 mm in median size but may be as small as 1 mm.[47] Clearly the prevalence of STIC is dependent on the thoroughness of pathologic examination. It is currently recommended that the fallopian tubes should be sectioned according to the SEE-FIM protocol, after formalin fixation. Dissection of ovaries and fallopian tubes should result in sections less than 3 mm thick. The ovaries should be sectioned perpendicular to their long axis.[6] If such an approach is used, multistep deeper levels do not improve the detection of carcinoma.[47] STIC is not confined to BRCA1/BRCA2 mutation carriers. Shaw and colleagues reported two STICs in the control group of 64 women (3%) who underwent gynecologic surgery for reasons unrelated to malignancy. Larger studies are needed to establish the true prevalence of STIC in the general population.

TP53 MUTATION AND EXPRESSION

Diligent search for TP53 mutations in well-classified cohorts have revealed a near universal presence of TP53 mutations in high-grade serous carcinomas.[4] As for other tumor entities, TP53 mutation consists of approximately two thirds missense mutations and one third null mutations.[12,57] Null mutation refers to a mutation that results in a nonsense or premature stop codon that translates into a non-functional or truncated protein. Theoretically, such nonfunctional proteins should not be translated due to the nonsense-mediated mRNA decay pathway, which degrades mRNAs containing nonsense mutations. Hence, null mutations result in complete loss of p53 expression and disruption of p53 function. On the other hand, missense TP53 mutations are associated with nuclear protein accumulation, which results in moderate to strong nuclear staining, by immunohistochemistry, in more than 50% of nuclei (typically >80%). Therefore, a scoring system for p53 immunohistochemistry has been suggested that correlates with the underlying mutational status.[58,59] Complete loss of p53 expression correlates with null mutation, and over-expression in more than 50% of tumor cell nuclei correlates with missense mutation. Both staining patterns are examples of aberrant staining. Any staining between 0% and 50% indicates TP53 wild type. Using this approach, there is a considerable similarity in aberrant p53 expression (88%) with the overall TP53 mutation rate as well as correlation between the type of mutation and the staining pattern (two third over-expression/missense mutation, one third complete negativity/null mutation).[60] Still we are awaiting a large confirmatory study, which directly correlates immunohistochemistry with known mutational status.

p53 loss of function occurs in the majority of high-grade serous carcinomas and seems to be a defining feature (TP53 mutations have been detected only in rare cases of other types (see **Table 1**)). HGSCs that lack TP53 mutation may have other pathway alterations including upstream regulators such as MDM2/MDM4 resulting in the same net effect.[4] It remains to be clarified whether different types of TP53 mutations can delineate clinically relevant subsets of HGSC (see below molecular prognostic markers).

BRCA1/BRCA2 DEFICIENCY

FUNCTION

BRCA1/BRCA2 proteins are critical parts of the cellular machinery used to repair double-stranded DNA breaks though a process known as homologous ('error free') recombination. The effective repair of DNA damage requires damage-sensing mechanisms, and then transduction of damage signals to downstream effectors (including *p53*) that arrest the cell cycle at checkpoints, and effectors (including *BRCA1*) that repair the damage. ATM (ataxia telangiectasia mutated) and ATR (ataxia telangiectasia and Rad3 related) are central to the DNA-damage response. Double-stranded DNA breaks activate ATR and ATM kinases that phosphorylate *p53* and *BRCA1*. Chromatin is remodelled around double-stranded DNA breaks, presumably to facilitate repair processes including the phosphorylation of the C-terminal tail of the histone H2AX. *BRCA1* appears to have a central regulatory role in homologous recombination by operating as a scaffold protein. *BRCA1* recruits several interacting proteins such as *BRCA2* and RAD51 to the site of DNA damage. Loss of *BRCA1/BRCA2* function results in deficient double stranded DNA repair, followed by an attempt to a switch to non-homologous mechanism of DNA repair, which is error prone but may compensate for some of the function.[61] Nevertheless, *BRCA1/BRCA2* deficiency increases the chances of segmental chromosomal rearrangements, which ultimately may cause chromosomal instability.

RELATION TO HIGH-GRADE SEROUS CARCINOMAS

Among specimens from women undergoing prophylactic salpingo-oophorectomy with germline *BRCA1/BRCA2* mutations, the precursor lesion of HGSC, STIC, has been identified within the distal fallopian tube.[7,50] A comprehensive study on a small set of well-characterized ovarian carcinomas confirmed that *BRCA1/BRCA2* alterations of either germline or somatic origin are confined to HGSC and are not seen in other types.[15] This information will likely become of immediate importance due to the development of therapies targeting BRCA deficient cancers.

PREVALENCE OF SOMATIC *BRCA1/2* DEFICIENCIES

Approximately half of HGSCs show a loss of *BRCA1/BRCA2* function.[15] Causes of this loss include germline (hereditary) and somatic *BRCA1/BRCA2* mutations, and *BRCA*1 promoter hypermethylation.[15,62] The second allele in these cases may be lost due to loss of heterozygosity (LOH) or biallelic hypermethylation. Epigentic silencing of *BRCA2* occurs rarely if ever, yet sporadic cases with loss of *BRCA2* expression have been reported suggesting other mechanisms of transcriptional silencing for *BRCA2*.[63] Somatic mutations of *BRCA1/BRCA2* are uncommon,[15] indicating that the majority of these mutations are germline.

FAMILY AND EPIDEMIOLOGIC STUDIES

The genes that confer a high-penetrance susceptibility to breast and ovarian cancers were identified in the mid-1990s through the study of families with increased numbers of cases at young age.[64,65] It is now accepted that greater than 90% of hereditary breast and ovarian cancer cancers are due to germline mutations occurring in *BRCA1* or *BRCA2*. In contrast to sporadic cases, where two 'hits' are required to inactivate *BRCA1/BRCA2*, a single *BRCA* 'hit' is required in hereditary cases as one allele is already mutated. In two meta-analyses of 22 and 10 studies, the cumulative life-time risk of ovarian carcinomas was estimated to be 40% for *BRCA1* and 11% to 19% for *BRCA2* germline mutation carriers.[37,66] It is not known why *BRCA1* mutations confer an ovarian cancer risk 2-fold higher than *BRCA2* germline mutations. Furthermore, patients with *BRCA1* germline mutations are diagnosed about a decade earlier than *BRCA2* related and sporadic high-grade serous carcinomas (mean age at diagnosis is 60 years).[67] The prevalence of germline *BRCA1* and *BRCA2* mutations in serous carcinomas was 11% and 6% for *BRCA1* and *BRCA2*, respectively.[14] The prevalence of *BRCA* germline mutations in the general population of Ontario is estimated as 0.3% (*BRCA1*) and 0.7% (*BRCA2*), respectively (compared with 1.2 and 1.3% for Ashkenazi Jews, respectively).[68]

BRCA1/BRCA2 GERMLINE MUTATION AND SCREENING

The *BRCA1* (chromosome 17q21–24) gene contains 24 small exons spanning about 81 kb region of DNA or approximately 5500 nucleotides. *BRCA2* (chromosome 13q12.3) contains 26 exons spanning over 10,200 nucleotides, which is almost double the size of *BRCA1*. More than 10,000 mutations and unclassified variants have been cataloged at the Breast Cancer Information Core (BIC, http://research. nhgri.nih.gov/bic/). Although several screening methods have been developed for detecting hereditary risk, direct sequencing of the entire coding region remains the gold standard. Notably, three common deletions and two duplications that account for up to one third of *BRCA1* mutations are not detectable by direct sequencing. Multiplex ligation-dependent amplification (MLPA) has been suggested as an additional method to detect these large genomic rearrangements.[69]

Genetic testing for *BRCA1* and *BRCA2* mutations in patients with a family history of breast and/or ovarian cancer has become routine practice in genetic counseling. Women with documented germline *BRCA 1/BRCA2* mutation or a strong family history of breast/ovarian carcinoma may undergo bilateral prophylactic salpingo-oopherectomy after childbearing is complete to reduce the risk of developing pelvic high-grade serous carcinomas. A few patients will harbor occult carcinoma, most commonly located with the distal fallopian tube and chemotherapy might be offered to these women.[70] The appropriate management of women diagnosed with STIC is not clear at present.[44] However, not all carriers of *BRCA1/BRCA2* germline mutations have a family history. There is a need to further narrow down the pool of women diagnosed with ovarian carcinomas that should be offered genetic counseling. Given the prevalence of 15 to 20% in high-grade serous carcinomas, selection of morphologic type alone would mean that approximately every sixth case would be tested positive for *BRCA1/BRCA2* germline mutation.[14] Other histomorphological and clinical features may also be considered such as increased intraepithelial lymphocytes or age.[71,72] With respect to identification of hereditary risk and for triaging to targeted therapy (see below), it would be of outmost interest to develop a testing strategy for the molecular *BRCA* status for routine use in laboratory medicine in the future.

In summary, 15 to 20% of high-grade serous carcinomas are associated with *BRCA1/BRCA2* germline mutations and there is accumulating evidence that silencing of BRCA1 or deregulation of related genes in the BRCA1/BRCA2 pathway are involved in a significant proportion of sporadic high-grade serous carcinomas.[73] Outstanding questions are whether different mechanisms of BRCA1/BRCA2 deficiency are equivalent in function, (eg, are the consequences of germline mutations similar to epigenetic silencing or whether BRCA1 alterations are similar to that of BRCA2?) They may be not because mRNA expression profiles of BRCA1 related cases are distinct from BRCA2 related tumors.[74] The mechanism through which tumors without BRCA1/BRCA2 loss achieve chromosomal instability? It is likely that alternative alterations result in a net loss of BRCA function affecting interacting proteins such as upstream kinases ATR and ATM or BRCA1 interacting proteins, eg, BRAD1 or members of the Fanconi anemia complex. For example, the BRCA2 interacting protein EMSY, which is amplified in 17% of high-grade serous carcinomas, may interfere with BRCA2 function.[75] It is likely that the upcoming publication of the TCGA project will contain specific data relevant to this question.

CHROMOSOMAL INSTABILITY

HGSC display chromosomal instability with high numbers of DNA copy number alterations compared with other ovarian carcinoma types (**Fig. 2**). Loss of the *BRCA1/BRCA2* genes in the background of *TP53* mutation creates a genomic environment where DNA breaks are tolerated and not repaired with fidelity. This leads to a myriaid of copy number gains, microdeletions, amplifications and rearrangements. Global genome analysis of high-grade serous carcinomas has revealed recurrent regions of somatic copy number aberrations in genes known to be involved in oncogenesis. Frequent gains have been detected at 8q, 3q, 1q and 20q.[76] Candidate genes of these and other regions include oncogenes such as *MYC* (50%,[77]), *CCNE1* (36%,[78]), *NOTCH3* (32%,[78]), *CCND1* (15%,[79]), which are known to be involved in regulation of proliferation. Genes that directly affect genomic integrity have been reported to show chromosomal gains, such as *AURKA* (28%,[80]), *EMSY* (18%,[75]). Loci with homozygous deletions containing *RB1* have been detected in 10% of cases.[81,82]

Increased proliferation results in rapid accrual of additional genetic abnormalities with each cell cycle. Defects in mitotic spindles further result in rapid accrual of global chromosomal aberrations with each cell cycle, measurable as aneuploidy.[83]

The high level of chromosomal instability and the paucity of recurrent mutation other than *TP53* presents a tremendous challenge with respect to identifying novel treatment strategies that target specific molecular defects in high-grade serous carcinomas. Another consequence of chromosomal instability is the high degree of intratumoral heterogeneity.[84]

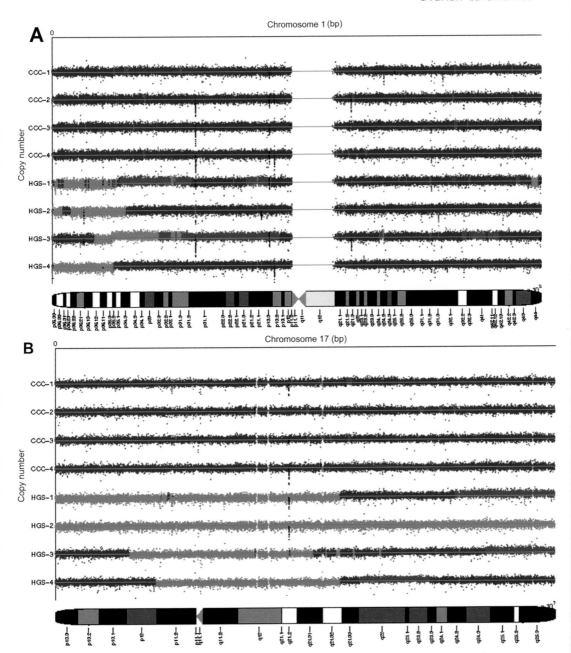

Fig. 2. Copy number changes of a high-grade serous and clear cell carcinomas by single nucleotide array.

MOLECULAR PROGNOSTIC MARKERS

Most of the potential molecular prognostic factors have been investigated in ovarian cancers. These biomarkers have not been independently validated, precluding clinical utility.

PROGNOSTIC SIGNIFICANCE OF p53 EXPRESSION

p53 is the most commonly studied biomarker. A recent metaanalysis pooling 53 immunohistochemistry studies on p53 expression in ovarian carcinoma reported a hazard ratio of 1.55 (95% confidence interval, 1.40 to 1.71) for p53 over-expression indicating a negative impact on prognosis, but remarkable heterogeneity between the studies was noted.[85] This is best illustrated by the range of reported frequency of p53 over-expression, from 14% to 82%.[85] Since DO7 has been established as the preferred antibody, and automated immunohistochemistry staining devices are now the norm, much of the analytical variation has been resolved. Now the differences among the studies are mainly related to heterogeneity of the study cohort, ie, frequency of non-serous types, which have ranged from 0% to 55%, and the interpretation of staining, in particular interpretation of no staining and the definition of cut-offs for over-expression, which have ranged from greater than 5% to greater than 90% of tumor cell nuclei staining positively.[85]

Most studies are confounded by the inclusion of cases of different histologic types. It has recently been shown that several biomarkers that seemed to be prognostic in a mixed cohort of all types of ovarian carcinoma were not informative when the analysis was restricted to a single type.[29] For instance, p53 over-expression is characteristic of HGSC, which is associated with a poor prognosis. However, in a series composed only of over 500 HGSCs, p53 over-expression was associated with a reduced risk of recurrence compared with cases completely negative for p53 (HR = 0.70, 95% CI 0.55 to 0.89) in multivariate analysis including age, stage, residual tumor and stratification by cohort.[60] The association of complete loss of p53 expression with unfavorable outcome suggests functional differences of *TP53* mutations underlying over-expression, compared with those underlying complete loss of expression.

IMMUNE RESPONSE AND *BRCA*1

The prognostic significance of the host immune response, as defined by the presence of tumor infiltrating lymphocytes (ie, intraepithelial lymphocytes), has been initially reported to be an independent factor associated with favorable prognosis in 186 advanced stage ovarian cancers.[86] This has been validated for high-grade serous carcinomas.[72,87] In contrast, tumors that downregulate class I HLA antigen processing proteins were associated with an unfavorable prognosis.[88] Based on a small number of cases a trend was observed that increased immune response may be associated with *BRCA* dysfunction.[72] This finding needs further validation in a larger, independent case series.[89] It also has long been noted that patients with *BRCA*-associated hereditary ovarian cancer, ie, *BRCA*1 or *BRCA*2 germline mutation, have a favorable outcome compared with sporadic ovarian carcinomas,[67,90] likely due to the excellent response to platinum based chemotherapy.

MICRO RNA

Decreased expression of miRNA processing proteins Dicer and Drosha has been recently reported to be associated with unfavorable outcome.[91] Reduced expression of Dicer or Drosha results in reduced generation of miRNA from its precursors, leading to a reduction in posttranscriptional gene silencing with global effects on gene expression.[92]

mRNA SIGNATURES

An unbiased approach to stratify high-grade serous carcinomas into prognostically relevant subgroups has been performed by gene expression profiling.[93–97] These studies show that gene expression profiling consistently revealed prognostically different subgroups. Three studies[95–97] used a second dataset for validation.[94] Yet with respect to individual genes used as prognostic classifier there is limited overlap between the studies. Limited reproducibility of prognostic classifiers between different microarray studies can be attributed to methodological issues or the cohort composition.

MOLECULAR THERAPEUTIC TARGETS

Conceptually, the logical approach would be to restore the functions of p53 and BRCA1/BRCA2 by retroviral transfer of wild-type genes with restoration of normal expression in cancer cells. The efficacy of such an approach is questionable because it seems unlikely that all cancer cells can be infected; secondly, cancer cells have accumulated additional chromosomal abnormalities impairing the success of restoration of one or a few genes; and thirdly, strategies to rescue p53/BRCA1/BRCA2 expression may counteract chemotherapy sensitivity. Standard chemotherapy of ovarian carcinomas consists of carboplatin and paclitaxel, both components acting via different cytotoxic mechanisms. Platinum containing agents crosslink DNA (similar to alkylating agents), inducing DNA damage. This is particularly efficient in the presence of double-stranded DNA repair deficiency such as with BRCA1/BRCA2 deficiency. The damage cannot be repaired and accumulating damage drives cancer cells into cellular crisis. Paclitaxel stabilizes microtubules and as a result, interferes with the normal breakdown of microtubules during cell division. This is effective in rapidly proliferating tumors such as high-grade serous carcinomas.

PARP INHIBITION

Until recently targeting abnormalities in tumor suppressor genes has been a challenge as replacing tumor suppressor function in cancer cells has not proven feasible. Since cells with loss of BRCA function have defective double strand break repair they are dependent on other secondary DNA repair mechanisms and unlike normal cells will perish if these alternative pathways are disrupted. This therapeutic approach is known as synthetic lethality.[98]

There is compelling evidence that cells harboring BRCA defects are more sensitive to agents targeting other DNA repair pathways. For example, inhibition of base excision repair (BER)

There are several phase I/II randomized, double blind, multicentre studies to assess the safety and efficacy of AZD2281 (Astra Zeneca) in the treatment of women with serous ovarian cancer (www.clinicaltrials.gov). If this class of drugs becomes mainstream therapy for women with HGSC then there will be a great need for improved assays to develop markers predictive of response to PARP inhibitors.

LOW-GRADE SEROUS CARCINOMAS

Low-grade Serous Carcinomas Key Molecular Features	
Molecular Pathology Features	1. *KRAS/BRAF* mutations mutually exclusive 2. Low proliferation
Key Molecular Prognostic Markers	None
Key Molecular Therapeutic Target	MAP Kinase inhibitors
Knowledge deficiencies	1. Given that LGSCs or borderline tumors are generally not seen in the fallopian tube, what is their histogenesis? 2. Could molecular features such as *KRAS* mutation be used to determine which borderline tumors are at greater risk to progress to LGSCs? 3. Will LGSCs respond to MEK inhibitors? If not what other therapeutic targets can be targeted?

is selectively lethal in BRCA deficient cells. Poly (ADP-ribose) polymerase 1 (PARP1) is a critical component of the BER pathway, which repairs DNA single strand breaks. Single stranded breaks occur commonly endogeneous but also may be induced by DNA-crosslinking agents, such as platinum. PARP1 inhibition leads to failure of the repair of single stranded breaks. If a persistent single-strand break, is encountered by the replication fork, mitosis will be arrested and these breaks eventually progress to double-stranded DNA breaks. In a BRCA-deficient state, these double-stranded DNA breaks cannot be repaired by homologous recombination leading to cellular crisis.[61] The PARP inhibitor Olaparib has been investigated in a phase I clinical trial and displayed promising antitumor activity with acceptable adverse effects.[99] Although it appears that BRCA1/2-deficient high-grade serous carcinomas are highly sensitive to PARP inhibitors, these changes can be reversible. Secondary mutations in the *BRCA1/2* genes that restore the wild-type reading frame and functional protein can give rise to acquired chemoresistance.[100–102] It remains to be seen how common this phenomenon is.

MOLECULAR PATHOLOGY FEATURES OF LOW-GRADE SEROUS CARCINOMAS

The separation of low-grade serous carcinomas from high-grade serous carcinomas is a relatively recent development, recognizing that these tumors are fundamentally different diseases with respect to underlying molecular alterations and clinical behavior.[31,103] Low-grade serous carcinomas (LGSCs) account for 3% of ovarian carcinomas and are relatively uncommon both when compared with serous borderline tumors (SBOTs) and high-grade serous carcinomas (HGSCs).[2] Unlike other low-grade subtypes, LGSCs are usually diagnosed at high stage,[2] at a median age of 43 years.[104] In general the outcome of LGSCs is somewhat favorable when compared with HGSCs.[104] However, when LGSCs are compared with optimally debulked (0 cm residual tumor) and adjuvantly treated HGSC, the outcome of LGSC is unfavorable with a 10-year disease specific survival rate of 51% compared with 56% for this specific HGSC subset.[105] This suggests that the long-term outcome of LGSC is not better than that of optimally treated HGSC. This poor prognosis may be due to a lack of response to platinum/paclitaxel chemotherapy,[103,104] a feature that is not surprising given the genomic stability of these cancers. Hence, LGSCs pose a therapeutic challenge, with cytoreductive surgery being the primary therapy and the only therapy of choice for the often multiple recurrences. Although initial studies are underway (see below) there is a need for more effective therapy for LGSC.

CELL LINEAGE

Low-grade serous carcinomas share molecular alterations with serous borderline tumors (SBOT) suggesting a common pathogenesis and continuum of disease from SBOT to LGSC.[19] This is in concordance with the clinicopathological observation that (60%) of LGSCs are associated with SBOT[106] and recurrences of SBOT can present as LGSC.[103] However, unlike other nonserous carcinomas, serous borderline tumors of conventional type are only rarely seen with associated invasive carcinoma in the ovary. Hence, an unresolved issue is what discriminates LGSC from serous borderline tumors on a molecular level and whether a progression model holds true for all SBOTs.

MAPK PATHWAY ALTERATIONS

A dualistic pathway for serous carcinogenesis is established based on distinct critical molecular

carcinomas.[109] These tumors contain *KRAS* mutation characteristic for low-grade serous carcinomas suggesting that low-grade and high-grade serous carcinomas are not related.[110] Activating *KRAS* mutations in codon 12 or 13 or *BRAF* mutations in codon 600 have been found in approximately 65% of low-grade serous carcinomas and are mutually exclusive events.[3,19] In addition, *ERBB2* mutations were identified in 6% of serous borderline tumors, lacking *KRAS* or *BRAF* mutations.[107] These MAPK pathway alterations are being currently targeted within a phase II study performed by the Gynecologic Oncology Group (GOG). Women with recurrent low-grade serous carcinoma are treated with the mitogen-activated protein kinase kinase (MAP2K1/2, MEK1/2) inhibitor AZD6244 (AstraZeneca).[111] MAPK inhibitors might interrupt the anti apoptotic cascade and induce cell senescence and would be a desirable treatment option especially in light of the low response rate to chemotherapy of low-grade serous carcinomas.[112] Although it is intuitive to target the MAPK pathway, potential challenges include the side effects on normal tissue given the central role of MAPK in homeostasis to stress response. As this is a rare cancer type it is unlikely that progress will be made on any front without broad based international collaboration.

ENDOMETRIOID CARCINOMAS

Endometrioid – Key Molecular Features	
Molecular Pathology Features	1. PTEN/PI3K pathway 2. Wnt/CTNNB1 pathway 3. ARID1A
Key Molecular Prognostic Markers	None
Key Molecular Therapeutic Target	PTEN/PI3K/mTOR pathway?
Knowledge deficiencies	1. What portion of endometrioid carcinomas are of uterine origin? 2. What is the cell of origin for non endometriosis associated endometrioid carcinomas? 3. What molecular feature defines true high-grade endometrioid carcinomas? 4. Will metastatic endometrioid carcinomas respond to therapies targeting known disrupted pathways?

abnormalities in LGSC and HGSC.[31] LGSCs show alterations of the MAP-kinase pathway (*KRAS, BRAF, ERBB2* mutation[3,107]) and an absence of *TP53* mutations.[108] Low-grade serous carcinomas can occasionally progress to higher grade

MOLECULAR PATHOLOGY FEATURES OF ENDOMETRIOID CARCINOMAS

Endometrioid carcinomas account for 12% ovarian carcinomas; greater than 80% are diagnosed at stage I or II.[2] Similar to their endometrial counterparts, more than 90% of endometrioid carcinomas are low-grade (grade 1 or grade 2). Because they are predominantly low grade and low stage at presentation, the burden of mortality associated with this type is relatively low.[105] While high stage endometrioid carcinomas may be associated with an adverse outcome compared with high-grade serous carcinomas,[113] reliable data are sparse given the rarity of high stage tumors of this type. mRNA expression profiling and principle component analysis showed that many grade 3 endometrioid carcinomas are molecularly indistinguishable from high-grade serous carcinomas.[11,27,114] Subsequently, morphologic criteria have been refined and many of the tumors diagnosed as grade 3 endometrioid carcinomas in the past would now be considered high-grade serous carcinomas,[1,115] an approach supported by biomarker expression.[113,115] As a consequence, reproducibility of histopathological typing has been improved.[116] Endometrioid carcinomas typically display low-grade nuclear atypia and are chromosomally stable compared with HGSC. The most common molecular alterations involve change of function mutation within the PTEN/PI3K and Wnt/CTNNB1 pathways. Changes in both of these two pathways were needed to produce a mouse model for endometrioid carcinomas supporting their interdependence.[11]

RISK FACTORS AND CELL LINEAGE

Associated endometrioisis has been identified in 37% of endometrioid carcinomas[117] compared with a 6% baseline incidence in a control population.[118] According to the theory of retrograde menstruation that accounts for endometrioisis, 'ovarian' endometrioid carcinomas may be derived from displaced endometrium.[44]

There is coexistence of endometrial and ovarian endometrioid carcinomas in a subset of cases, which also points to a potential role of hormonal environment in the genesis of endometrioid carcinoma of the ovary, given the well-characterized role of unopposed estrogenic stimulation as a risk factor for endometrial adenocarcinoma of endometrioid type. Virtually all endometrioid carcinomas of the ovary express estrogen receptor protein. Candidate gene approach showed that a SNP within the progesterone receptor is associated with a 17% risk increase of endometrioid carcinomas.[119]

The prevalence of Lynch syndrome with MMR deficiencies in patients with endometrioid ovarian carcinomas may be as high as 3%, similar the prevalence in endometrial endometrioid and colorectal carcinomas.[120]

PTEN/PI3K PATHWAY

Approximately one third of endometrioid carcinomas show mutation in either PTEN (19%,[11]) or in PIK3CA (12%,[11]). PIK3CA encodes the regulatory subunit p110alpha of class IA PI3K and mutations cluster in exon 9 and exon 20. In endometrioid carcinomas of the endometrium, mutations in PTEN and PIK3CA occur often concomitantly indicating that these mutations are not necessarily redundant but might have synergistic effects.[121] Mutations in PTEN or PIK3-CA result in an increased activity of the PI3K pathway (**Fig. 3**).

WNT SIGNALING PATHWAY

The most common mutation in endometrioid carcinomas is an activating CTNNB1 mutation present in up to 65% of cases.[122] Hotspots for mutations are phosphorylation sites of serine-threonine residues coded in exon 3 of the CTNNB1 targeted by GSK3 (see **Fig. 3**). CTNNB1 encodes β-catenin.

Since direct sequencing is cumbersome, immunohistochemistry has been suggested as a surrogate marker for assessment of the mutational status of CTNNB1. CTNNB1 (β-catenin) is also a submembrane component of the cadherin-mediated cell–cell adhesion system, strengthening the linkage of CDH1 and CTNNA1 to the actin cytoskeleton. Normal β-catenin is primarily in a submembrane location resulting in a membranous staining pattern by immunohistochemistry. CTNNB1 mutations correlate with increasing cytoplasmic and nuclear staining pattern with β-catenin antibodies, although the alteration is often seen only focally. Nuclear β-catenin accumulation is often found in areas of squamous differentiation, which are associated with CTNNB1 mutation. CTNNB1 mutations have been detected in up to 85% of endometrioid carcinomas with squamous morules.[123] Moreover, CTNNB1 mutations are generally identical to those in surrounding neoplastic glandular tissue. This suggests that CTNNB1 mutation may promote squamous differentiation and that squamous differentiation might serve as a surrogate

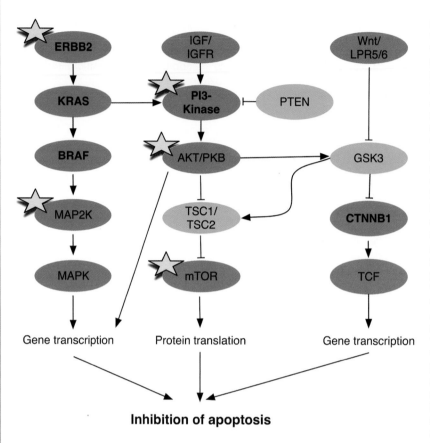

Fig. 3. Simplified overview of signaling pathways implemented in specific ovarian carcinoma types. *Left* MAP kinase pathway: upon activation of receptor tyrosin kinases from the epidermal growth factor family at the plasma membrane, downstream signals are transferred via KRAS/BRAF/MAP2K1/2(MEK1/2)/MAPK such as ERK1/p44MAPK (MAPK3) and ERK2/p42 MAPK (MAPK3). Constitutive activation of the MAPK signal transduction pathway by *ERBB2* amplification (mucinous) or activating mutation of *KRAS/BRAF* (low-grade serous) results in activation of the transcription factors JUN and FOS that results in increased cell survival by inhibiting apoptosis.[141,142] *Middle* PI3K/AKT pathway is also activated by certain receptor tyrosin kinases such as insulin growth factor receptor or KRAS. PI3K catalyzes the formation of phosphatidyl inositol-3,4,5-triphosphate (PIP3) from PIP2. PTEN is a dual specific phosphatase that is able to dephosphorylate both proteins and phospholipids. Its main substrate is PIP3; hence PTEN antagonizes PIK action on PIP3. PIP3 recruits AKT (PKB) to the membrane, its site of activation. Key substrates of AKT mediated phosphorylation include activation of the forkhead transcription factors such as FOXO and inhibition of TSC2 ("tuberin"), the latter leading to activation of rapamycin-sensitive TOR complex (mTORC1). The mTOR complex is a major regulator of ribosome and therefore protein synthesis. Activation of the PI3K/AKT pathway (clear cell and endometrioid) results in increased cell survival by inhibiting apoptosis. *Right* Wnt signaling pathway: Wnt activates GSK3, which tightly regulates CTNNB1 (β-catenin) levels. Phosphorylation of specific exon 3 residues by GSK3 requires a multiprotein complex including APC and axin among others and induces β-catenin degradation through a ubiquitin-proteasome process. Mutated *CTNNB1* (endometrioid) escapes this degradation resulting in increased cytoplasmic level of β-catenin, nuclear translocation, and enhanced participation in transcriptional regulation through the formation of bipartite complexes with the TCF transcription factor. Target genes of Wnt/CTNNB1 signaling include *MYC*, *CCNNB1* and *MMP7*. The Wnt signaling pathway is involved in pleiotropic cellular functions including differentiation. It also results in increased cell survival by inhibiting apoptosis. *Cross links*: for example, inhibition of GSK3 in will lead to inactivation of TSC1/2, followed by mTOR activation. This is one example of the complexity of cross talk between the Wnt and PI3K pathways. We are far from understanding how these pathways cooperate during oncogenesis. Bold indicates molecular alteration detected in a significant portion of tumors (see **Table 1**). Yellow star indicates targeted treatment intervention. Red indicates proteins with predominant oncogene function, while blue indicates predominant tumor suppressor functions.

marker for underlying *CTNNB1* mutation. Given the often-focal nuclear expression of β-catenin in endometrioid carcinomas, there is a need for more reliable test to infer the molecular status of CTNNB1.

KEY MOLECULAR PROGNOSTIC MARKERS

Prognostic marker studies on cohorts of endometrioid carcinomas are sparse and historically include a large portion of grade 3 endometrioid carcinomas; many of those now would be considered high-grade serous carcinomas.

KEY MOLECULAR THERAPEUTIC TARGET

Given that unopposed estrogen provides the hormonal effect that sets the background for endometrioid carcinogenesis, antiestrogenic treatment with either progestin or tamoxifen might influence endometrioid types of ovarian carcinomas preferentially. Selective estrogen receptor modulators are currently being investigated in clinical trials of recurrent endometrial cancer.[124]

PI3K PATHWAY

Given the high frequency of alterations in the PI3K/AKT pathway, it seems reasonable and rational to target this pathway in endometrioid carcinomas. The PI3K/AKT pathway, however, plays fundamental roles in homeostasis such as glucose metabolism. The downstream mTOR complex has pleiotropic and essential functions in protein translation. As is the case with targeting any pathway that is essential for normal cellular function avoiding side major effects remains a challenge. For example, PI3-K inhibition and resulting AKT inhibition causes toxicity such as hyperglycemia. XL765, as another example, is an oral dual PI3K and mTOR inhibitor with clinical phase I results in various solid tumors. In 26% of patients with advanced cancers treated with this drug, stable disease was achieved but adverse effects were dose limiting.[125]

Rapamycin inhibits the activity of mTOR and has been used as an immunosuppressant for years. Three rapamycin analogs have been tested in clinical phase II studies in women with recurrent or metastastic endometrial carcinomas. Of 91 patients, 56% had some clinical benefit, defined as partial response or stable disease.[126]

HISTONE DEACETYLASE INHIBITORS

Histone deacetylation and acetylation act as global epigenetic controls of gene expression in addition to actions as a promoter of hypermethylation. Altered histone acetylation patterns have been reported in several tumor entities. Class I histone deacytelases are expressed in the majority of endometrioid carcinomas and associated with outcome indicating biologic significance.[127] Preclinical studies using drugs that act as histone deacetylase inhibitors have shown increased induction of apoptosis in endometrial cancer cell lines and reduction of tumor size in nude mouse models.[128]

CLEAR CELL CARCINOMAS

Clear Cell Carcinomas Key Molecular Features	
Molecular Pathology Features	PTEN/PI3K pathway ARID1A
Key Molecular Prognostic Markers	IGF2BP3
Key Molecular Therapeutic Target	PI3K pathway
Knowledge deficiencies	1. Why does CCC have a stronger association with endometriosis than endometrioid carcinoma? 2. What mutations underpin the transformation of endometriosis to CCC? 3. What is the cell of origin of non endometriosis associated CCC? 4. How should CCC be treated?

MOLECULAR PATHOLOGY FEATURES OF CLEAR CELL CARCINOMAS

RISK FACTORS

The Müllerian nature of clear cell carcinomas is supported by the strong association with endometrioisis.[118] A diligent pathology review of 122 classic clear cell carcinomas showed association with endometriosis in 61% of cases.[10] The proportion of clear cell carcinomas is highest in Asians compared with other races.[129]

The frequency of microsatellite instability was reported to be 17% for clear cell carcinomas in women who were diagnosed at an age younger than 50.[130]

PI3K PATHWAY

Clear cell carcinomas are characterized by a relatively low proliferation rate; hence, defects in anti-apoptotic pathway have been suggested to play an important role in clear cell carcinogenesis. Until very recently the mutational landscape for clear cell carcinomas was not very well described because studies were hampered by insufficient sample sizes. A study of 97 clear cell carcinomas samples identified mutations in exon 9 and 20 of *PIK3CA* in 33% of cases.[18] Most recently, *ARID1A* mutations were detected in almost half of CCC. The *ARID1A* gene product (BAF250A) is a component of the SWI/SNF chromatin-remodelling complex keeping in line with the observation that CCC are not chromosomal unstable but rather may be characterized by changes of chromosomal configurations (**Fig. 2**).[26,131]

KEY MOLECULAR PROGNOSTIC MARKERS

Similar mRNA expression profiles of renal, endometrial and ovarian clear cell carcinomas raised the possibilities of potential crossovers of molecular marker expression, although characteristic molecular abnormalities of renal cell carcinomas are lacking.[28] IGF2BP3 has been reported and validated as independent prognostic marker for renal clear cell carcinomas and the same was shown for ovarian clear cell carcinomas. With respect to clear cell carcinomas, this marker could potentially help to identify patients with stage I/II disease who might not benefit from current inefficient chemotherapy, but needs further validation in powered prospective cohort or at least in large multi-institutional retrospective cohorts.[132] Key Molecular Therapeutic Target Clear cell carcinomas have the highest frequency of *PIK3CA* mutation among ovarian carcinomas and might be specifically vulnerable to inhibition of the PI3K pathway.

Another crossover from renal clear cell carcinomas is the use of multi-targeted kinase inhibitors such as sunitinib,[133] which target the microvasculature.[134] Anecdotally, spontaneous regression of a stage IV clear cell carcinoma of the endometrium was documented in women with essential thrombocytosis,[135] which suggests that the microvasculature may be the Achilles heal of clear cell carcinomas.

The recent discovery of frequent mutations in the chromatin remodelling gene *ARID1a* in clear cell and endometrioid carcinomas and the demonstration that these are early event in the pathogenesis of such cancers both further links these two cancer types of endometriosis precursors and may provide therapeutic opportunities.[26] However, since *ARID1a* may play a tumor supressor function this mutational event will not be targetable in a direct fashion yet could yield to a synthetic lethal approach as has been used to target cancers with *BRCA* loss.

MUCINOUS CARCINOMAS

Mucinous Carcinomas Key Molecular Features	
Molecular Pathology Features	1. *KRAS* 2. *ERBB2* amplication
Key Molecular Prognostic Markers	None
Key Molecular Therapeutic Target	Trastuzumab
Knowledge deficiencies	1. What is the histogenesis of this disease? 2. Can mucinous carcinomas with a more aggressive course be identified through biomarkers? 3. Other than *ERBB2* amplification, what targetable features do mucinous carcinomas express?

MOLECULAR PATHOLOGY FEATURES OF MUCINOUS CARCINOMAS

Mucinous carcinomas account for 3 to 4% ovarian carcinomas, with more than 80% diagnosed at stage I or II.[2] Similar to endometrioid counterparts, more than 90% of mucinous carcinomas are low-grade (grade 1 or grade 2).[105] The burden of mortality associated with this type is relatively low,[105] however, when diagnosed at advanced stage the outcome is poor compared with HGSC due to the poor response rate to standard chemotherapy (12 to 26%).[136,137]

The origin of mucinous tumors remains puzzling. Mucinous carcinomas may be associated with Brenner tumors or teratomas. Mucinous carcinomas are usually of intestinal-type rather than of endocervical-type. Expression profiles of mucinous carcinomas resemble normal colon.[30]

Mucinous carcinomas are usually chromosomally stable. A frequent homozygous deletion of *CDKN2A* has been reported in 6/16 (38%) of mucinous tumors.[82] Mucinous carcinomas share a recurrent molecular alteration with low-grade serous carcinomas; activating *KRAS* mutations at codon 12 and 13 are the most common mutation in mucinous carcinomas and are present in up to 50% of cases.[20] These mutations are also common in gastrointestinal carcinomas (>50% in colorectal and >90% of pancreatic carcinomas) so that the

Fig. 4. Massive *ERBB2/HER2* amplification in a mucinous carcinoma shown by single nucleotide polymorphism array. (*Data from* McAlpine JN, Wiegand KC, Vang R, et al. HER2 overexpression and amplification is present in a subset of ovarian mucinous carcinomas and can be targeted with trastuzumab therapy. BMC Cancer 2009;9:433.)

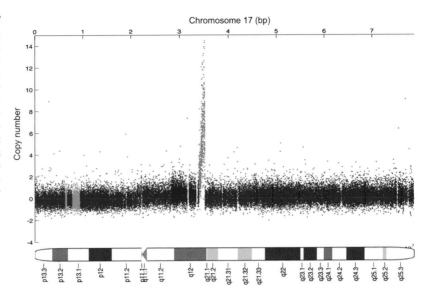

KRAS status cannot be used to distinguish primary ovarian mucinous tumor from metastatic carcinoma of gastrointestinal origin. In contrast to low-grade serous carcinomas, mucinous carcinomas carry no *BRAF* mutations. *KRAS* mutations have also been found in mucinous borderline tumors, which are more common that their carcinomatous counterparts.[138] Many mucinous tumors contain areas of carcinoma and borderline components, suggesting stepwise progression from borderline tumor to mucinous carcinomas. The molecular alterations that give rise to progression from borderline tumor to carcinoma remain enigmatic.

Activating *KRAS* mutations in codon 12 and 13 result in a constitutive activation of the MAPK pathway as mentioned previously. There is an alternative mechanism of MAPK pathway activation in 18% of mucinous tumors (borderline tumors and carcinomas), which is *ERBB2 (HER2)* amplification (**Fig. 4**).[22]

KEY MOLECULAR THERAPEUTIC TARGET

Given the fact that mucinous carcinomas respond poorly to chemotherapy, alternative treatment options are needed. *ERBB2* amplification is relatively common (18%). This is a higher frequency of *ERBB2* amplification than is seen in breast carcinomas, and it is similar to the frequency encountered in adenocarcinoma of the gastro-esophageal junction. Trastuzumab (Herceptin) therapy is an obvious treatment choice for these cases but there are few data on response of mucinous carcinomas of the ovary with *ERBB2* amplification.[22] There were large clinical trials of trastuzumab therapy in ovarian cancer with discouraging results,[139] but these trials included a majority of HGSCs that only rarely show *ERBB2* overexpression/amplification.[21,140] *ERBB2* and *KRAS* are members of the same pathway. It is likely that in case of downstream activating *KRAS* mutations, trastuzumab (Herceptin) would not be effective. Alternatively, mucinous carcinomas might be included together with low-grade serous carcinomas in trials of MAPK inhibitors.

SUMMARY

The five subtypes of ovarian carcinoma that are recognized in the current classification scheme are distinct diseases not only in terms of risk factors, morphologic appearance, clinical behavior and immunohistochemical profiles but also in terms of their underlying mutations. If we are to make progress in decreasing mortality from ovarian carcinoma then these distinctions need to be capitalized upon in the development of a new generation of subtype specific treatments.

REFERENCES

1. Gilks CB, Prat J. Ovarian carcinoma pathology and genetics: recent advances. Hum Pathol 2009;40: 1213–23.
2. Köbel M, Kalloger SE, Huntsman DG, et al. Differences in tumor type in low-stage versus

high-stage ovarian carcinomas. Int J Gynecol Pathol 2010;29:203–11.

3. Singer G, Oldt R, Cohen Y, et al. Mutations in BRAF and KRAS characterize the development of low-grade ovarian serous carcinoma. J Natl Cancer Inst 2003;95:484–6.

4. Ahmed AA, Etemadmoghadam D, Temple J, et al. Driver mutations in TP53 are ubiquitous in high grade serous carcinoma of the ovary. J Pathol 2010;221:49–56.

5. Shaw PA, McLaughlin JR, Zweemer RP, et al. Histo-pathologic features of genetically determined ovarian cancer. Int J Gynecol Pathol 2002;21:407–11.

6. Medeiros F, Muto MG, Lee Y, et al. The tubal fimbria is a preferred site for early adenocarcinoma in women with familial ovarian cancer syndrome. Am J Surg Pathol 2006;30:230–6.

7. Piek JM, van Diest PJ, Zweemer RP, et al. Dysplastic changes in prophylactically removed fallopian tubes of women predisposed to developing ovarian cancer. J Pathol 2001;195:451–6.

8. Flesken-Nikitin A, Choi KC, Eng JP, et al. Induction of carcinogenesis by concurrent inactivation of p53 and Rb1 in the mouse ovarian surface epithelium. Cancer Res 2003;63:3459–63.

9. Xing D, Orsulic S. A mouse model for the molecular characterization of brca1-associated ovarian carcinoma. Cancer Res 2006;66:8949–53.

10. Veras E, Mao TL, Ayhan A, et al. Cystic and adeno-fibromatous clear cell carcinomas of the ovary: distinctive tumors that differ in their pathogenesis and behavior: a clinicopathologic analysis of 122 cases. Am J Surg Pathol 2009;33:844–53.

11. Wu R, Hendrix-Lucas N, Kuick R, et al. Mouse model of human ovarian endometrioid adenocarci-noma based on somatic defects in the Wnt/beta-catenin and PI3K/Pten signaling pathways. Cancer Cell 2007;11:321–33.

12. Salani R, Kurman RJ, Giuntoli R, et al. Assessment of TP53 mutation using purified tissue samples of ovarian serous carcinomas reveals a higher muta-tion rate than previously reported and does not correlate with drug resistance. Int J Gynecol Cancer 2008;18:487–91.

13. Ho ES, Lai CR, Hsieh YT, et al. p53 mutation is infre-quent in clear cell carcinoma of the ovary. Gynecol Oncol 2001;80:189–93.

14. Risch HA, McLaughlin JR, Cole DE, et al. Preva-lence and penetrance of germline BRCA1 and BRCA2 mutations in a population series of 649 women with ovarian cancer. Am J Hum Genet 2001;68:700–10.

15. Press JZ, De Luca A, Boyd N, et al. Ovarian carci-nomas with genetic and epigenetic BRCA1 loss have distinct molecular abnormalities. BMC Cancer 2008;8:17.

16. Willner J, Wurz K, Allison KH, et al. Alternate molecular genetic pathways in ovarian carcinomas of common histological types. Hum Pathol 2007;38:607–13.

17. Catasús L, Bussaglia E, Rodrguez I, et al. Molecular genetic alterations in endometrioid carcinomas of the ovary: similar frequency of beta-catenin abnor-malities but lower rate of microsatellite instability and PTEN alterations than in uterine endometrioid carcinomas. Hum Pathol 2004;35:1360–8.

18. Kuo KT, Mao TL, Jones S, et al. Frequent activating mutations of PIK3CA in ovarian clear cell carci-noma. Am J Pathol 2009;174:1597–601.

19. Singer G, Kurman RJ, Chang HW, et al. Diverse tumorigenic pathways in ovarian serous carcinoma. Am J Pathol 2002;160:1223–8.

20. Gemignani ML, Schlaerth AC, Bogomolniy F, et al. Role of KRAS and BRAF gene mutations in mucinous ovarian carcinoma. Gynecol Oncol 2003;90:378–81.

21. Mayr D, Kanitz V, Amann G, et al. HER-2/neu gene amplification in ovarian tumours: a comprehensive immunohistochemical and FISH analysis on tissue microarrays. Histopathology 2006;48:149–56.

22. McAlpine JN, Wiegand KC, Vang R, et al. HER2 overexpression and amplification is present in a subset of ovarian mucinous carcinomas and can be targeted with trastuzumab therapy. BMC Cancer 2009;9:433.

23. Liu J, Albarracin CT, Chang KH, et al. Microsatellite instability and expression of hMLH1 and hMSH2 proteins in ovarian endometrioid cancer. Mod Path-ol 2004;17:75–80.

24. Cai KQ, Albarracin C, Rosen D, et al. Microsatellite instability and alteration of the expression of hMLH1 and hMSH2 in ovarian clear cell carcinoma. Hum Pathol 2004;35:552–9.

25. Pieretti M, Hopenhayn-Rich C, Khattar NH, et al. Heterogeneity of ovarian cancer: relationsships among histological group, stage of disease, tumor markers, patient characteristics, and survival. Cancer Invest 2002;20:11–23.

26. Wiegand KC, Shah SP, Al-Agha OM, et al. ARID1A mutations in endometrioisis-associated ovarian carcinomas. N Engl J Med 2010;363:1532–43.

27. Schwartz DR, Kardia SL, Shedden KA, et al. Gene expression in ovarian cancer reflects both morphology and biological behavior, distinguishing clear cell from other poor-prognosis ovarian carci-nomas. Cancer Res 2002;62:4722–9.

28. Zorn KK, Bonome T, Gangi L, et al. Gene expres-sion profiles of serous, endometrioid, and clear cell subtypes of ovarian and endometrial cancer. Clin Cancer Res 2005;11:6422–30.

29. Köbel M, Kalloger SE, Boyd N, et al. Ovarian carci-noma subtypes are different diseases: implications for biomarker studies. PLoS Med 2008;5:e232.

30. Marquez RT, Baggerly KA, Patterson AP, et al. Patterns of gene expression in different histotypes

of epithelial ovarian cancer correlate with those in normal fallopian tube, endometrium, and colon. Clin Cancer Res 2005;11:6116–26.

31. Shih Ie M, Kurman RJ. Ovarian tumorigenesis: a proposed model based on morphological and molecular genetic analysis. Am J Pathol 2004; 164:1511–8.

32. Jarboe E, Folkins A, Nucci MR, et al. Serous carcinogenesis in the fallopian tube: a descriptive classification. Int J Gynecol Pathol 2008;27:1–9.

33. Köbel M, Huntsman D, Gilks CB. Critical molecular abnormalities in high-grade serous carcinoma of the ovary. Expert Rev Mol Med 2008;10:e22.

34. Schildkraut JM, Calingaert B, Marchbanks PA, et al. Impact of progestin and estrogen potency in oral contraceptives on ovarian cancer risk. J Natl Cancer Inst 2002;94:32–8.

35. Whittemore AS, Harris R, Itnyre J. Characteristics relating to ovarian cancer risk: collaborative analysis of 12 US case-control studies. IV. The pathogenesis of epithelial ovarian cancer. Collaborative Ovarian Cancer Group. Am J Epidemiol 1992;136:1212–20.

36. Fathalla MF. Incessant ovulation–a factor in ovarian neoplasia? Lancet 1971;2:163.

37. Antoniou A, Pharoah PD, Narod S, et al. Average risks of breast and ovarian cancer associated with BRCA1 or BRCA2 mutations detected in case Series unselected for family history: a combined analysis of 22 studies. Am J Hum Genet 2003;72:1117–30.

38. Rebbeck TR, Mitra N, Domchek SM, et al. Modification of ovarian cancer risk by BRCA1/2-interacting genes in a multicenter cohort of BRCA1/2 mutation carriers. Cancer Res 2009;69:5801–10.

39. Fasching PA, Gayther S, Pearce L, et al. Role of genetic polymorphisms and ovarian cancer susceptibility. Mol Oncol 2009;3:171–81.

40. Schildkraut JM, Goode EL, Clyde MA, et al. Single nucleotide polymorphisms in the TP53 region and susceptibility to invasive epithelial ovarian cancer. Cancer Res 2009;69:2349–57.

41. Song H, Ramus SJ, Tyrer J, et al. A genome-wide association study identifies a new ovarian cancer susceptibility locus on 9p22.2. Nat Genet 2009; 41:996–1000.

42. Dubeau L. The cell of origin of ovarian epithelial tumors and the ovarian surface epithelium dogma: does the emperor have no clothes? Gynecol Oncol 1999;72:437–42.

43. Auersperg N, Wong AS, Choi KC, et al. Ovarian surface epithelium: biology, endocrinology, and pathology. Endocr Rev 2001;22:255–88.

44. Kurman RJ, Shih IeM. The origin and pathogenesis of epithelial ovarian cancer: a proposed unifying theory. Am J Surg Pathol 2010;34:433–43.

45. Crum CP, Drapkin R, Miron A, et al. The distal fallopian tube: a new model for pelvic serous carcinogenesis. Curr Opin Obstet Gynecol 2007;19:3–9.

46. Finch A, Beiner M, Lubinski J, et al. Salpingo-oophorectomy and the risk of ovarian, fallopian tube, and peritoneal cancers in women with a BRCA1 or BRCA2 Mutation. JAMA 2006;296:185–92.

47. Rabban JT, Krasik E, Chen LM, et al. Multistep level sections to detect occult fallopian tube carcinoma in risk-reducing salpingo-oophorectomies from women with BRCA mutations: implications for defining an optimal specimen dissection protocol. Am J Surg Pathol 2009;33:1878–85.

48. Kindelberger DW, Lee Y, Miron A, et al. Intraepithelial carcinoma of the fimbria and pelvic serous carcinoma: evidence for a causal relationship. Am J Surg Pathol 2007;31:161–9.

49. Salvador S, Gilks B, Köbel M, et al. The fallopian tube: primary site of most pelvic high-grade serous carcinomas. Int J Gynecol Cancer 2009;19:58–64.

50. Crum CP. Intercepting pelvic cancer in the distal fallopian tube: theories and realities. Mol Oncol 2009;3:165–70.

51. Lee Y, Miron A, Drapkin R, et al. A candidate precursor to serous carcinoma that originates in the distal fallopian tube. J Pathol 2007;211:26–35.

52. Tone AA, Begley H, Sharma M, et al. Gene expression profiles of luteal phase fallopian tube epithelium from BRCA mutation carriers resemble high-grade serous carcinoma. Clin Cancer Res 2008;14: 4067–78.

53. Shaw PA, Rouzbahman M, Pizer ES, et al. Candidate serous cancer precursors in fallopian tube epithelium of BRCA1/2 mutation carriers. Mod Pathol 2009;22:1133–8.

54. Xian W, Miron A, Roh M, et al. The Li-Fraumeni syndrome (LFS): a model for the initiation of p53 signatures in the distal fallopian tube. J Pathol 2010;220:17–23.

55. Carlson JW, Miron A, Jarboe EA, et al. Serous tubal intraepithelial carcinoma: its potential role in primary peritoneal serous carcinoma and serous cancer prevention. J Clin Oncol 2008;26:4160–5.

56. Salvador S, Rempel A, Soslow RA, et al. Chromosomal instability in fallopian tube precursor lesions of serous carcinoma and frequent monoclonality of synchronous ovarian and fallopian tube mucosal serous carcinoma. Gynecol Oncol 2008;110:408–17.

57. Havrilesky L, Darcy M, Hamdan H, et al. Prognostic significance of p53 mutation and p53 overexpression in advanced epithelial ovarian cancer: a Gynecologic Oncology Group Study. J Clin Oncol 2003; 21:3814–25.

58. Yemelyanova A, Vang R, Shih IM, et al. Correlation of immunohistochemical staining patterns of p53 with mutational analysis in ovarian carcinomas. Mod Pathol 2009;22:221A.

59. Lassus H, Leminen A, Lundin J, et al. Distinct subtypes of serous ovarian carcinoma identified by p53 determination. Gynecol Oncol 2003;91:504–12.

60. Köbel M, Reuss A, Bois AD, et al. The biological and clinical value of p53 expression in pelvic high-grade serous carcinomas. J Pathol 2010;222:191–8.

61. Tutt A, Ashworth A. The relationship between the roles of BRCA genes in DNA repair and cancer predisposition. Trends Mol Med 2002;8:571–6.

62. Baldwin RL, Nemeth E, Tran H, et al. BRCA1 promoter region hypermethylation in ovarian carcinoma: a population-based study. Cancer Res 2000;60:5329–33.

63. Hilton JL, Geisler JP, Rathe JA, et al. Inactivation of BRCA1 and BRCA2 in ovarian cancer. J Natl Cancer Inst 2002;94:1396–406.

64. Wooster R, Bignell G, Lancaster J, et al. Identification of the breast cancer susceptibility gene BRCA2. Nature 1995;378:789–92.

65. Miki Y, Swensen J, Shattuck-Eidens D, et al. A strong candidate for the breast and ovarian cancer susceptibility gene BRCA1. Science 1994; 266:66–71.

66. Chen S, Parmigiani G. Meta-analysis of BRCA1 and BRCA2 penetrance. J Clin Oncol 2007;25:1329–33.

67. Boyd J, Sonoda Y, Federici MG, et al. Clinicopathologic features of BRCA-linked and sporadic ovarian cancer. JAMA 2000;283:2260–5.

68. Risch HA, McLaughlin JR, Cole DE, et al. Population BRCA1 and BRCA2 mutation frequencies and cancer penetrances: a kin-cohort study in Ontario, Canada. J Natl Cancer Inst 2006;98:1694–706.

69. Montagna M, Dalla Palma M, Menin C, et al. Genomic rearrangements account for more than one-third of the BRCA1 mutations in northern Italian breast/ovarian cancer families. Hum Mol Genet 2003;12:1055–61.

70. Carcangiu ML, Peissel B, Pasini B, et al. Incidental carcinomas in prophylactic specimens in BRCA1 and BRCA2 germ-line mutation carriers, with emphasis on fallopian tube lesions: report of 6 cases and review of the literature. Am J Surg Pathol 2006;30:1222–30.

71. Soegaard M, Kjaer SK, Cox M, et al. BRCA1 and BRCA2 mutation prevalence and clinical characteristics of a population-based series of ovarian cancer cases from Denmark. Clin Cancer Res 2008;14:3761–7.

72. Clarke B, Tinker AV, Lee CH, et al. Intraepithelial T cells and prognosis in ovarian carcinoma: novel associations with stage, tumor type, and BRCA1 loss. Mod Pathol 2009;22:393–402.

73. Weberpals JI, Clark-Knowles KV, Vanderhyden BC. Sporadic epithelial ovarian cancer: clinical relevance of BRCA1 inhibition in the DNA damage and repair pathway. J Clin Oncol 2008;26:3259–67.

74. Jazaeri AA, Yee CJ, Sotiriou C, et al. Gene expression profiles of BRCA1-linked, BRCA2-linked, and sporadic ovarian cancers. J Natl Cancer Inst 2002;94:990–1000.

75. Brown LA, Irving J, Parker R, et al. Amplification of EMSY, a novel oncogene on 11q13, in high grade ovarian surface epithelial carcinomas. Gynecol Oncol 2006;100:264–70.

76. Gorringe KL, Jacobs S, Thompson ER, et al. High-resolution single nucleotide polymorphism array analysis of epithelial ovarian cancer reveals numerous microdeletions and amplifications. Clin Cancer Res 2007;13:4731–9.

77. Staebler A, Karberg B, Behm J, et al. Chromosomal losses of regions on 5q and lack of high-level amplifications at 8q24 are associated with favorable prognosis for ovarian serous carcinoma. Genes Chromosomes Cancer 2006;45:905–17.

78. Nakayama K, Nakayama N, Jinawath N, et al. Amplicon profiles in ovarian serous carcinomas. Int J Cancer 2007;120:2613–7.

79. Brown LA, Kalloger SE, Miller MA, et al. Amplification of 11q13 in ovarian carcinoma. Genes Chromosomes Cancer 2008;47:481–9.

80. Mendiola M, Barriuso J, Mariño-Enríquez A, et al. Aurora kinases as prognostic biomarkers in ovarian carcinoma. Hum Pathol 2009;40:631–8.

81. Kuo KT, Guan B, Feng Y, et al. Analysis of DNA copy number alterations in ovarian serous tumors identifies new molecular genetic changes in low-grade and high-grade carcinomas. Cancer Res 2009;69:4036–42.

82. Gorringe KL, Ramakrishna M, Williams LH, et al. Are there any more ovarian tumor suppressor genes? A new perspective using ultra high-resolution copy number and loss of heterozygosity analysis. Genes Chromosomes Cancer 2009;48:931–42.

83. Holland AJ, Cleveland DW. Boveri revisited: chromosomal instability, aneuploidy and tumorigenesis. Nat Rev Mol Cell Biol 2009;10:478–87.

84. Khalique L, Ayhan A, Weale ME, et al. Genetic intra-tumour heterogeneity in epithelial ovarian cancer and its implications for molecular diagnosis of tumours. J Pathol 2007;211:286–95.

85. de Graeff P, Crijns AP, de Jong S, et al. Modest effect of p53, EGFR and HER-2/neu on prognosis in epithelial ovarian cancer: a meta-analysis. Br J Cancer 2009;101:149–59.

86. Zhang L, Conejo-Garcia JR, Katsaros D, et al. Intratumoral T cells, recurrence, and survival in epithelial ovarian cancer. N Engl J Med 2003;348:203–13.

87. Sato E, Olson SH, Ahn J, et al. Intraepithelial CD8+ tumor-infiltrating lymphocytes and a high CD8+/regulatory T cell ratio are associated with favorable prognosis in ovarian cancer. Proc Natl Acad Sci U S A 2005;102:18538–43.

88. Han LY, Fletcher MS, Urbauer DL, et al. HLA class I antigen processing machinery component expression and intratumoral T-Cell infiltrate as independent prognostic markers in ovarian carcinoma. Clin Cancer Res 2008;14:3372–9.

89. Quinn JE, James CR, Stewart GE, et al. BRCA1 mRNA expression levels predict for overall survival in ovarian cancer after chemotherapy. Clin Cancer Res 2007;13:7413–20.

90. Tan DS, Rothermundt C, Thomas K, et al. "BRCA-ness" syndrome in ovarian cancer: a case-control study describing the clinical features and outcome of patients with epithelial ovarian cancer associated with BRCA1 and BRCA2 mutations. J Clin Oncol 2008;26:5530–6.

91. Merritt WM, Lin YG, Han LY, et al. Dicer, Drosha, and outcomes in patients with ovarian cancer. N Engl J Med 2008;359:2641–50 [Erratum in: N Engl J Med. 2010 Nov 4;363(19):1877].

92. Lee CH, Subramanian S, Beck AH, et al. MicroRNA profiling of BRCA1/2 mutation-carrying and non-mutation-carrying high-grade serous carcinomas of ovary. PLoS One 2009;4:e7314.

93. Berchuck A, Iversen ES, Lancaster JM, et al. Patterns of gene expression that characterize long-term survival in advanced stage serous ovarian cancers. Clin Cancer Res 2005;11:3686–96.

94. Dressman HK, Berchuck A, Chan G, et al. An integrated genomic-based approach to individualized treatment of patients with advanced-stage ovarian cancer. J Clin Oncol 2007;25:517–25.

95. Crijns AP, Fehrmann RS, de Jong S, et al. Survival-related profile, pathways, and transcription factors in ovarian cancer. PLoS Med 2009;6:e24.

96. Tothill RW, Tinker AV, George J, et al. Novel molecular subtypes of serous and endometrioid ovarian cancer linked to clinical outcome. Clin Cancer Res 2008;14:5198–208.

97. Denkert C, Budczies J, Darb-Esfahani S, et al. A prognostic gene expression index in ovarian cancer - validation across different independent data sets. J Pathol 2009;218:273–80.

98. Ashworth A. A synthetic lethal therapeutic approach: poly(ADP) ribose polymerase inhibitors for the treatment of cancers deficient in DNA double-strand break repair. J Clin Oncol 2008;26:3785–90.

99. Fong PC, Boss DS, Yap TA, et al. Inhibition of poly (ADP-ribose) polymerase in tumors from BRCA mutation carriers. N Engl J Med 2009;361:123–34.

100. Sakai W, Swisher EM, Karlan BY, et al. Secondary mutations as a mechanism of cisplatin resistance in BRCA2-mutated cancers. Nature 2008;451:1116–20.

101. Swisher EM, Sakai W, Karlan BY, et al. Secondary BRCA1 mutations in BRCA1-mutated ovarian carcinomas with platinum resistance. Cancer Res 2008; 68:2581–6.

102. Sakai W, Swisher EM, Jacquemont C, et al. Functional restoration of BRCA2 protein by secondary BRCA2 mutations in BRCA2-mutated ovarian carcinoma. Cancer Res 2009;69:6381–6.

103. Crispens MA, Bodurka D, Deavers M, et al. Response and survival in patients with progressive or recurrent serous ovarian tumors of low malignant potential. Obstet Gynecol 2002;99:3–10.

104. Gershenson DM, Sun CC, Lu KH, et al. Clinical behavior of stage II-IV low-grade serous carcinoma of the ovary. Obstet Gynecol 2006;108:361–8.

105. Köbel M, Kalloger SE, Santos JL, et al. Tumor type and substage predict survival in stage I and II ovarian carcinoma: insights and implications. Gynecol Oncol 2010;116:50–6.

106. Malpica A, Deavers MT, Lu K, et al. Grading ovarian serous carcinoma using a two-tier system. Am J Surg Pathol 2004;28:496–504.

107. Anglesio MS, Arnold JM, George J, et al. Mutation of ERBB2 provides a novel alternative mechanism for the ubiquitous activation of RAS-MAPK in ovarian serous low malignant potential tumors. Mol Cancer Res 2008;6:1678–90.

108. Singer G, Stöhr R, Cope L, et al. Patterns of p53 mutations separate ovarian serous borderline tumors and low- and high-grade carcinomas and provide support for a new model of ovarian carcinogenesis: a mutational analysis with immunohistochemical correlation. Am J Surg Pathol 2005;29:218–24.

109. Parker RL, Clement PB, Chercover DJ, et al. Early recurrence of ovarian serous borderline tumor as high-grade carcinoma: a report of two cases. Int J Gynecol Pathol 2004;23:265–72.

110. Dehari R, Kurman RJ, Logani S, et al. The development of high-grade serous carcinoma from atypical proliferative (borderline) serous tumors and low-grade micropapillary serous carcinoma: a morphologic and molecular genetic analysis. Am J Surg Pathol 2007;31:1007–12.

111. Schmeler KM, Gershenson DM. Low-grade serous ovarian cancer: a unique disease. Curr Oncol Rep 2008;10:519–23.

112. Pohl G, Ho CL, Kurman RJ, et al. Inactivation of the mitogen-activated protein kinase pathway as a potential target-based therapy in ovarian serous tumors with KRAS or BRAF mutations. Cancer Res 2005;65:1994–2000.

113. Gilks CB, Ionescu DN, Kalloger SE, et al. Tumor cell type can be reproducibly diagnosed and is of independent prognostic significance in patients with maximally debulked ovarian carcinoma. Hum Pathol 2008;39:1239–51.

114. Madore J, Ren F, Filali-Mouhim A, et al. Characterization of the molecular differences between ovarian endometrioid carcinoma and ovarian serous carcinoma. J Pathol 2010;220:392–400.

115. Soslow RA. Histologic subtypes of ovarian carcinoma: an overview. Int J Gynecol Pathol 2008;27: 161–74.

116. Köbel M, Kalloger SE, Baker PM, et al. Diagnosis of ovarian carcinoma cell type is highly reproducible: a transcanadian study. Am J Surg Pathol 2010;34: 984–93.

117. Lim MC, Chun KC, Shin SJ, et al. Clinical presentation of endometrioid epithelial ovarian cancer with concurrent endometriosis: a multicenter retrospective study. Cancer Epidemiol Biomarkers Prev 2010;19:398–404.

118. Nagle CM, Olsen CM, Webb PM, et al. Endometrioid and clear cell ovarian cancers: a comparative analysis of risk factors. Eur J Cancer 2008;44:2477–84.

119. Pearce CL, Wu AH, Gayther SA, et al. Progesterone receptor variation and risk of ovarian cancer is limited to the invasive endometrioid subtype: results from the Ovarian Cancer Association Consortium pooled analysis. Br J Cancer 2008;98:282–8.

120. Hampel H, Frankel WL, Martin E, et al. Screening for the Lynch syndrome (hereditary nonpolyposis colorectal cancer). N Engl J Med 2005;352:1851–60.

121. Oda K, Stokoe D, Taketani Y, et al. High frequency of coexistent mutations of PIK3CA and PTEN genes in endometrial carcinoma. Cancer Res 2005;65:10669–73.

122. Oliva E, Sarrió D, Brachtel EF, et al. High frequency of beta-catenin mutations in borderline endometrioid tumours of the ovary. J Pathol 2006;208:708–13.

123. Saegusa M, Machida BD, Okayasu I. Possible associations among expression of p14(ARF), p16(INK4a), p21(WAF1/CIP1), p27(KIP1), and p53 accumulation and the balance of apoptosis and cell proliferation in ovarian carcinomas. Cancer 2001;92:1177–89.

124. Engelsen IB, Akslen LA, Salvesen HB. Biologic markers in endometrial cancer treatment. APMIS 2009;117:693–707.

125. Molckovsky A, Siu LL. First-in-class, first-in-human phase I results of targeted agents: highlights of the 2008 American Society of Clinical Oncology meeting. J Hematol Oncol 2008;1:20.

126. Delmonte A, Sessa C. Molecule-targeted agents in endometrial cancer. Curr Opin Oncol 2008;20:554–9.

127. Weichert W, Denkert C, Noske A, et al. Expression of class I histone deacetylases indicates poor prognosis in endometrioid subtypes of ovarian and endometrial carcinomas. Neoplasia 2008;10:1021–7.

128. Takai N, Desmond JC, Kumagai T, et al. Histone deacetylase inhibitors have a profound antigrowth activity in endometrial cancer cells. Clin Cancer Res 2004;10:1141–9.

129. Chan J, Fuh K, Shin J, et al. The treatment and outcomes of early-stage epithelial ovarian cancer: have we made any progress? Br J Cancer 2008;98:1191–6.

130. Jensen KC, Mariappan MR, Putcha GV, et al. Microsatellite instability and mismatch repair protein defects in ovarian epithelial neoplasms in patients 50 years of age and younger. Am J Surg Pathol 2008;32:1029–37.

131. Jones S, Wang TL, Shih IeM, et al. Frequent mutations of chromatin remodeling gene ARID1A in ovarian clear cell carcinoma. Science 2010;330:228–31.

132. Köbel M, Xu H, Bourne PA, et al. IGF2BP3 (IMP3) expression is a marker of unfavorable prognosis in ovarian clear cell carcinoma. Mod Pathol 2009;22:469–75.

133. Motzer RJ, Hutson TE, Tomczak P, et al. Overall survival and updated results for sunitinib compared with interferon alfa in patients with metastatic renal cell carcinoma. J Clin Oncol 2009;27:3584–90.

134. Huang D, Ding Y, Li Y, et al. Sunitinib acts primarily on tumor endothelium rather than tumor cells to inhibit the growth of renal cell carcinoma. Cancer Res 2010;70:1053–62.

135. Parker R, Lanvin D, Gilks B, et al. Spontaneous regression of stage IV clear cell carcinoma of the endometrium in a patient with essential thrombocytosis. Gynecol Oncol 2001;82:395–9.

136. Hess V, A'Hern R, Nasiri N, et al. Mucinous epithelial ovarian cancer: a separate entity requiring specific treatment. J Clin Oncol 2004;22:1040–4.

137. Shimada M, Kigawa J, Ohishi Y, et al. Clinicopathological characteristics of mucinous adenocarcinoma of the ovary. Gynecol Oncol 2009;113:331–4.

138. Cuatrecasas M, Villanueva A, Matias-Guiu X, et al. K-ras mutations in mucinous ovarian tumors: a clinicopathologic and molecular study of 95 cases. Cancer 1997;79:1581–6.

139. Bookman MA, Darcy KM, Clarke-Pearson D, et al. Evaluation of monoclonal humanized anti-HER2 antibody, trastuzumab, in patients with recurrent or refractory ovarian or primary peritoneal carcinoma with overexpression of HER2: a phase II trial of the Gynecologic Oncology Group. J Clin Oncol 2003;21:283–90.

140. Lee CH, Huntsman DG, Cheang MC, et al. Assessment of Her-1, Her-2, and Her-3 expression and Her-2 amplification in advanced stage ovarian carcinoma. Int J Gynecol Pathol 2005;24:147–52.

141. Bonni A, Brunet A, West AE, et al. Cell survival promoted by the Ras-MAPK signaling pathway by transcription-dependent and -independent mechanisms. Science 1999;286:1358–62.

142. Michaloglou C, Vredeveld LC, Soengas MS, et al. BRAFE600-associated senescence-like cell cycle arrest of human naevi. Nature 2005;436:720–4.

143. Köbel M, Kalloger SE, Carrick J, et al. A limited panel of immunomarkers can reliably distinguish between clear cell and high-grade serous carcinoma of the ovary. Am J Surg Pathol 2009;33:14–21.

144. Phillips V, Kelly P, McCluggage WG. Increased p16 expression in high-grade serous and undifferentiated carcinoma compared with other morphologic types of ovarian carcinoma. Int J Gynecol Pathol 2009;28:179–86.

METASTATIC NEOPLASMS INVOLVING THE OVARY

W. Glenn McCluggage, FRCPath

KEYWORDS

• Ovary • Adenocarcinoma • Metastatic tumor • Immunohistochemistry

ABSTRACT

In this review, ovarian metastatic carcinomas from various sites, as well as other neoplasms secondarily involving the ovary are discussed. As well as describing the morphology, the value of immunohistochemistry in distinguishing between primary and metastatic neoplasms in the ovary is discussed. While immunohistochemistry has a valuable role to play and is paramount in some cases, the results should be interpreted with caution and with regard to the clinical picture and gross and microscopic pathologic findings.

OVARY

OVERVIEW

The ovary is a relatively common site of metastatic tumor.[1–4] Tumors may spread to this organ via a blood-borne or lymphatic route, transperitoneally or by direct extension. In many cases, there is a known history of a primary neoplasm but on occasions presentation is with symptoms related to an ovarian mass or an ovarian mass is discovered incidentally in a patient with no known history of malignancy. In such cases, the primary neoplasm may not manifest itself until some time later. In other cases, an ovarian mass is discovered in a patient with a history of a primary neoplasm elsewhere raising the possibility of a secondary within the ovary or a new independent primary. In these scenarios, it is the histopathologist who usually ultimately makes the diagnosis, although imaging and tumor markers may help. In this review, I discuss various metastatic tumors involving the ovary.

Microscopic and Clinical Features

In general, especially with mucinous carcinomas, but not exclusively so, features favoring a metastatic rather than a primary ovarian neoplasm, especially if present in constellation, include:

• Bilateral ovarian involvement (although metastatic carcinomas in the ovary may be unilateral and primary ovarian serous carcinomas are commonly bilateral)
• Relatively small size
• Nodular pattern of ovarian involvement
• Infiltrative pattern of stromal invasion
• Micoscopic surface deposits of tumor
• Marked lymphovascular invasion (especially in the ovarian hilum)
• Single cell infiltration and signet ring cells
• Cells floating in mucin
• Variation in growth pattern from one nodule to another
• Extraovarian spread.

However, none of these features is pathognomonic of a metastatic neoplasm. As an example, recently a small series of primary ovarian mucinous carcinomas with signet ring cells has been reported.[5] In a study of primary and metastatic ovarian mucinous carcinomas, features most in favor of a metastasis were bilateral ovarian involvement, microscopic surface implants and an infiltrative pattern of stromal invasion.[6] It should be borne in mind that many metastatic mucinous carcinomas involving the ovary contain morphologically bland foci resembling benign and borderline mucinous cystadenoma, a so-called maturation phenomenon. This is especially common with metastatic pancreatic and biliary

Department of Pathology, Royal Group of Hospitals Trust, Grosvenor Road, Belfast, BT12 6BA, Northern Ireland, UK
E-mail address: glenn.mccluggage@belfasttrust.hscni.net

Surgical Pathology 4 (2011) 297–330
doi:10.1016/j.path.2010.12.010
1875-9181/11/$ – see front matter © 2011 Elsevier Inc. All rights reserved.

tract adenocarcinomas but may occur with secondaries from various sites. Especially in the past, and to a lesser extent currently, there was a tendency for metastatic mucinous carcinomas involving the ovary to be misdiagnosed as a primary ovarian mucinous carcinoma or even occasionally as a borderline or benign mucinous cystadenoma (because of the maturation phenomenon).

A recent population based study has suggested that primary ovarian mucinous carcinomas are uncommon, representing less than 3% of primary ovarian carcinomas, a much lower percentage than that quoted in the older literature.[7] It is my opinion that, although relatively uncommon, they are more prevalent than this and part of the variation between institutions may be explained by variable diagnostic criteria amongst pathologists in the somewhat problematic distinction between a borderline mucinous tumor at the upper end of the spectrum with intraepithelial carcinoma and a mucinous carcinoma with expansile (non-destructive or non-infiltrative) invasion.[8] It is stressed that primary ovarian mucinous carcinomas with destructive (infiltrative) stromal invasion are rare, as are advanced stage primary ovarian mucinous carcinomas, although they do uncommonly occur.[7,8] Most primary ovarian mucinous carcinomas are unilateral and stage 1. A corollary to the aforementioned statement that metastatic mucinous carcinomas in the ovary may be misdiagnosed as a primary ovarian mucinous neoplasm is that, in my experience, there is now a tendency for pathologists to suggest that any mucinous carcinoma in the ovary is potentially metastatic. It is my opinion that, in the vast majority of cases, careful consideration of the gross and microscopic pathologic features allows a confident distinction between a primary and secondary ovarian mucinous neoplasm, although rarely there may be some doubt.

It has been suggested that the size of the neoplasm is a useful discriminator between a primary and secondary mucinous carcinoma, in that most primary ovarian mucinous carcinomas are large while most secondary mucinous carcinomas are relatively small.[9,10] A cut-off of 10 cm or 13 cm has been considered to be useful in this regard.[9,10] While this is true in most instances, there are obviously exceptions and size alone is not a reliable parameter in distinguishing between a primary and secondary mucinous carcinoma in the ovary. Another point worthy of note is that metastatic tumors in the ovary are often cystic or partially cystic, even when the primary neoplasm is not. Metastatic neoplasms in the ovary may also form follicle-like structures which bring to mind various primary ovarian neoplasms, including granulosa cell tumor and ovarian small cell carcinoma of hypercalcaemic type (OSCCHT). Metastatic neoplasms involving the ovary may be associated with a population of luteinised stromal cells. This phenomenon, which may occur with any mass lesion in the ovary, appears more common in metastatic adenocarcinomas than in other neoplasms and may result in androgenic or oestrogenic manifestations.

Krukenberg tumor

A few points regarding the term "Krukenberg tumor" are necessary here, and the reader is referred to a recent review of this.[1] The designation "Krukenberg tumor" is often loosely used for any metastatic carcinoma within the ovary and this is to be avoided. The term should be reserved for those metastatic adenocarcinomas with an appreciable (arbitrarily defined as >10%) component of signet ring cells and no evidence of another specific diagnosis, such as clear cell carcinoma or any other tumor type, which may contain signet ring cells. Some Krukenberg tumors have a morphologic picture which is dominated by other patterns, as discussed in the section on metastatic gastric carcinoma, the stomach being the most common primary site of a Krukenberg tumor. The classical description of a Krukenberg tumor included a cellular stromal reaction but, since this would exclude otherwise classical Krukenberg tumors, there seems little point in insisting on this criterion.

Markers for Ovarian Adenocarcinoma

In recent years, immunohistochemistry, including differential cytokeratin (CK 7 and 20) staining, has been widely used as an aid to distinguish between a primary and secondary ovarian adenocarcinoma and to ascertain the likely site of origin of a disseminated peritoneal adenocarcinoma.[11–14] These markers are also widely employed in cytologic preparations of ascitic fluid. While immunohistochemistry undoubtedly has a key role to play and is extremely important and even paramount in diagnosis in some cases, careful gross and microscopic pathologic examination usually results in a confident diagnosis. Moreover, the value of differential cytokeratin staining is not always understood by pathologists, some of whom equate a CK7 positive/CK20 negative immunophenotype in an adenocarcinoma as indicating an ovarian primary. However, a CK7 positive/CK20 negative immunophenotype is common in pancreatic, biliary, gastric, breast and pulmonary adenocarcinomas as well as in adenocarcinomas arising at other sites in the female genital tract.[15–18] Conversely, a CK20 positive/CK7 negative immunophenotype is characteristic of and is extremely suggestive of a primary colorectal adenocarcinoma, although this is not totally pathognomonic. A critical appraisal of the value of immunohistochemistry is presented with each metastatic tumor type discussed. Sometimes the procurement of additional sections provides more clues than immunohistochemistry, the results of which should always be interpreted in light of the clinical and gross and microscopic pathologic features. Having said that, there are undoubtedly cases where immunohistochemistry is diagnostic. **Table 1** details the characteristic immunophenotype of common adenocarcinomas and this is discussed at various places in this review.

COLORECTAL CARCINOMA INVOLVING OVARY

OVERVIEW

One of the most common metastatic tumors to involve the ovary is colorectal adenocarcinoma.[19] There may be a known history of colorectal adenocarcinoma or presentation may be with an ovarian mass in the absence of a known primary. In most cases, the primary tumor is in the rectum or sigmoid colon but it may be elsewhere. Patients with metastatic colorectal adenocarcinoma

involving the ovary not uncommonly have a mildly or moderately elevated serum CA125.[20] Metastatic colorectal adenocarcinoma in the ovary may morphologically closely mimic a primary ovarian endometrioid or mucinous adenocarcinoma. Metastatic colorectal adenocarcinoma in the ovary is statistically a more likely diagnosis than primary mucinous carcinoma or bilateral endometrioid carcinoma. In general, features which assist in distinguishing between a metastatic colorectal adenocarcinoma and a primary ovarian adenocarcinoma are similar to those which apply for other metastatic adenocarcinomas and which have already been discussed.[6] Most, but not all, metastatic colorectal adenocarcinomas involving the ovary are bilateral. However, primary ovarian endometrioid adenocarcinomas may also be bilateral (approximately 10 to 15% of cases). As discussed, primary ovarian mucinous adenocarcinomas are rarely bilateral and with bilateral ovarian mucinous neoplasms, a metastasis should always be considered.

Microscopic Features

Metastatic colorectal adenocarcinoma involving the ovary may be solid or partially or predominantly cystic. Most commonly, metastatic colorectal adenocarcinoma mimics a primary ovarian endometrioid adenocarcinoma since there is minimal intracytoplasmic mucin, a so-called pseudoendometrioid pattern.

Table 1
Typical immunophenotype of adenocarcinomas of various sites involving ovary

	CK7	CK20	CA125	CEA	ER	CDX2	CA19.9	WT1	TTF1	p16	GCDFP15
Ovarian Serous	D	N	D	N	N,F,D	N	N	D	N	D	N
Ovarian Endometrioid	D	N	D	N	D	N,F	N	N	N	N	N
Ovarian Clear Cell	D	N	D	N	N	N	N	N	N	N	N
ªOvarian Mucinous	D	N,F	N	N,F	N	N,F	N,F,D	N	N	N	N
Cervical	D	N	D	D	N,F	N	N	N	N	D	N
Colorectal	N	D	N	D	N	D	N,F,D	N	N	N	N
Appendiceal	N	D	N	D	N	D	N,F,D	N	N	N	N
Gastric	N,F,D	N,F,D	N,F,D	F,D	N	N,F,D	N,F,D	N	N	N	N
Pancreatic	N,F,D	N,F,D	N,F,D	F,D	N	F,D	F,D	N	N	N	N
Biliary	N,F,D	N,F,D	N	F,D	N	F,D	F,D	N	N	N	N
Breast	D	N	N,F	N	N,F,D	N	N	N	N	N	F,D
Pulmonary	D	N	N	N,F,D	N	N	N	N	D	N	N
Renal clear cell carcinoma	N	N	N	N	N	N	N	N	N	N	N

Although this table details the most common immunophenotypes, there are many exceptions.
Abbreviations: D, Diffuse; F, Focal; N, Negative.
ª Refers to more common intestinal or non-specific type.

Primary ovarian endometrioid adenocarcinoma

- Presence of squamous elements and endometriosis is suggestive of ovarian endometrioid adenocarcinoma
- "Dirty" and segmental necrosis and garland-like growth pattern is suggestive of a colorectal primary
- CK7 > CK20 with ER/PR expression favor endometrioid adenocarcinoma

Primary ovarian mucinous neoplasm

- Bilateral ovarian involvement is in favor of a metastasis
- CK7 > CK20 is characteristic of ovarian mucinous neoplasms, but metastases other than colorectal carcinoma can exhibit this phenotype

Primary ovarian clear cell carcinoma

- Bilateral ovarian involvement is in favor of a metastasis
- Presence of endometriosis is suggestive of ovarian clear cell carcinoma
- CK7 > CK20 favors clear cell carcinoma

The presence of significant dirty necrosis (necrotic materal containing nuclear debris), segmental necrosis and a "garland-like" growth pattern (glands, often with a cribriform architecture, arranged at the periphery of the necrotic material) are in .vor of a metastatic colorectal adenocarcinoma[19] (**Fig. 1**) but these features are also seen in some primary ovarian endometrioid and mucinous adenocarcinomas. One or more of the important triad of squamous elements, an adenofibromatous component, or coexisting endometriosis are strong pointers in favor of a primary ovarian endometrioid adenocarcinoma.[21] Metastatic colorectal adenocarcinomas are generally more atypical with pleomorphic hyperchromatic nuclei and are more mitotically active than ovarian endometrioid adenocarcinomas with a similar degree of glandular differentiation, although there is significant overlap.

Markers for Colorectal Carcinoma Involving Ovary

In the distinction between a primary ovarian endometrioid adenocarcinoma and a metastatic colorectal adenocarcinoma, immunohistochemistry is of paramount value and is almost totally discriminatory.[11–18] Although there are occasional

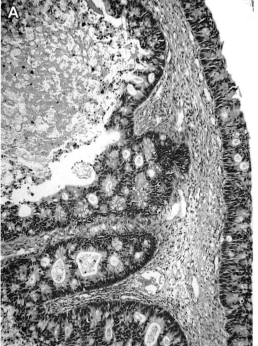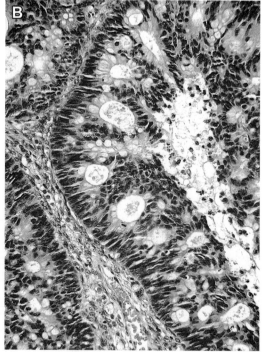

Fig. 1. Metastatic colorectal adenocarcinoma in ovary with extensive dirty necrosis (*A*). A garland-like growth pattern is seen (*B*).

exceptions, primary ovarian endometrioid adeno-carcinomas are:[22–25]

Endometrioid Adenocarcinoma Diffusely Positive with:

- CK7
- Estrogen receptor (ER)
- CA125.

Endometrioid Adenocarcinoma Negative or Focally Positive with:

- CK20
- CEA
- CDX2 (squamous morules in endometrioid adenocarcinomas of the ovary are commonly CDX2 positive[26]).

The converse immunophenotype is the rule in metastatic colorectal adenocarcinomas with a pseudoendometrioid appearance (**Fig. 2**).

More uncommonly, metastatic colorectal adenocarcinomas involving the ovary mimic an ovarian mucinous neoplasm. Those which are unilateral and cystic may closely mimic the gross appearance of a primary ovarian mucinous neoplasm. Histologically, there may also be a close resemblance to a primary ovarian mucinous neoplasm with areas resembling benign and borderline mucinous cystadenoma as well as obvious malignant foci with destructive stromal invasion; the latter may be revealed by the procurement of additional sections. Rare cases have abundant extracellular mucin, resulting in a colloid carcinoma-like picture. Analagous to the situation with other metastatic mucinous carcinomas, the morphologically bland foci (maturation phenomenon) can erroneously be in-terpreted as evidence of a primary ovarian neoplasm.

In distinguishing between a primary ovarian mucinous tumor and a metastatic colorectal adenocarcinoma, immunohistochemistry is less helpful than in the distinction between a primary ovarian endometrioid adenocarcinoma and a metastasis. This is because many primary ovarian mucinous neoplasms exhibit CK20 posi-tivity, which is usually focal but which may be widespread. They are also commonly positive, sometimes diffusely so, with CEA, CDX2, and CA19.9. The expression of these enteric markers is a reflection of intestinal differentiation in primary ovarian mucinous neoplasms. It is possible that some primary ovarian mucinous carcinomas which exhibit diffuse CK20 positivity represent intestinal type neoplasms arising within a teratoma, the other elements of which have been totally obliterated. A further confounding

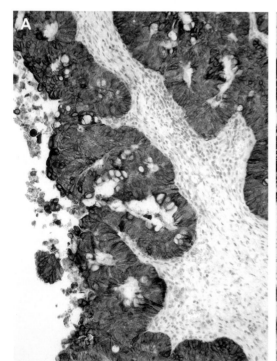
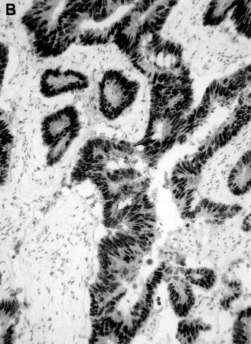

Fig. 2. Metastatic colorectal adenocarcinoma in ovary is positive with CK20 (*A*) and CDX2 (*B*).

factor is that colorectal adenocarcinomas with a mucinous appearance often exhibit focal CK7 positivity. In general, primary ovarian mucinous neoplasms are diffusely CK7 positive and negative or focally positive with CK20, although some cases exhibit widespread immunoreactivity. It is often the more "malignant" areas which are CK20 positive; for example, benign areas in a primary ovarian mucinous neoplasm are usually CK20 negative while borderline and malignant areas may be positive. Conversely, metastatic colorectal adenocarcinomas with a mucinous appearance are usually diffusely positive with CK20 and negative or focally immunoreactive with CK7. However, there is significant overlap and in an individual case differential cytokeratin staining may be of limited value.

Expression of the mucin gene MUC5AC may also be of value.[27] This is typically expressed in primary ovarian mucinous neoplasms but not in colorectal carcinomas; however, again there may be immunohistochemical marker overlap. It has been suggested that β-catenin is a useful immunohistochemical in the distinction between a primary ovarian mucinous tumor and a metastatic colorectal adenocarcinoma.[28] Many colorectal adenocarcinomas exhibit nuclear positivity but most primary ovarian mucinous neoplasms do not. In one study of primary ovarian mucinous and metastatic colorectal carcinomas, 83% of metastatic colorectal carcinomas exhibited nuclear positivity with β-catenin while only 9% of primary ovarian mucinous carcinomas did so.[28] It should be noted that ovarian endometrioid adenocarcinomas may exhibit nuclear β-catenin positivity, especially within the squamous morules (as discussed, these are also commonly CDX2 positive).[26]

Rare metastatic colorectal carcinoma: microscopic features and markers

Rare metastatic colorectal carcinomas involving the ovary have a clear cell appearance, mimicking either a primary ovarian clear cell carcinoma or a secretory variant of endometrioid carcinoma.[29] Thorough sampling may assist in revealing areas more diagnostic of metastatic colorectal adenocarcinoma. Primary ovarian clear cell and endometrioid carcinomas commonly arise in endometriosis and the presence of this is a strong pointer toward a primary ovarian neoplasm. Immunohistochemistry is also of value. Primary ovarian clear cell carcinoma is usually positive with CK7 and CA125 and negative with CK20, CEA and CDX2. The converse is true for metastatic colorectal adenocarcinomas with a clear cell appearance. Primary ovarian clear cell carcinomas

commonly exhibit immunoreactivity with hepatocyte nuclear factor 1 β.[30] They also have a characteristic morphologic appearance, often with an admixture of tubulocystic, solid and papillary growth patterns, as well as eosinophilic stromal hyaline material and hobnail cells.

APPENDICEAL TUMORS INVOLVING OVARY

OVERVIEW

The appendix is a not uncommon source of an ovarian metastasis and sometimes the pathologist does not think of the possibility of a primary neoplasm in that organ. Appendiceal metastasis within the ovary can have a varied morphologic appearance. One is an obvious mucinous adenocarcinoma with malignant glands, sometimes with abundant extracellular mucin, and signet ring cells (**Fig. 3**), and the appendix is one possible source of a classical Krukenberg tumor, as described later. In such cases, the ovarian disease may be unilateral or bilateral, with the right ovary

Differential Diagnosis
APPENDICEAL NEOPLASM INVOLVING OVARY

Primary ovarian mucinous neoplasm

- Bilateral ovarian involvement, surface involvement and extraovarian disease are in favor of a metastasis

- CK7 > CK20 is characteristic of ovarian mucinous neoplasms, but metastases other than colorectal carcinoma and appendiceal neoplasms can exhibit this phenotype

Other metastatic carcinomas, including gastric

- Signet ring carcinoma involving the ovary may be from a gastric or appendiceal primary; primary ovarian tumors with signet ring cells are very uncommon

- Immunohistochemistry may be useful (see text)

Goblet cell carcinoid (primary or metastatic)

- Goblet cell carcinoids in the ovary may appear similar to metastatic appendiceal carcinoma

- The presence of teratomatous elements is suggestive of a primary ovarian neoplasm

- Immunohistochemistry may be useful (see text)

Fig. 3. Metastatic appendiceal adenocarcinoma in ovary with signet ring cells and extracellular mucin.

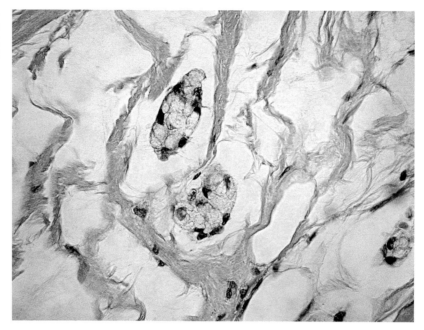

being more commonly involved than the left. Often, the appendix is firm or thickened but does not grossly harbour an obvious tumor mass. One clue to the appendix as a possible source of primary neoplasm in such cases is that the immunophenotype is often overtly "enteric" with diffuse positivity with CK20, CEA and CDX2 and negative staining with CK7. On morphology, the stomach is often considered the most likely site of primary but gastric adenocarcinomas usually have a different immunophenotype with positive staining with CK7 and typically more focal immunoreactivity with the enteric markers listed. A recent study has described a series of ovarian metastases from appendiceal tumors with goblet cell carcinoid-like and signet ring patterns.[31] In most cases, the ovarian metastases were bilateral. The ovarian and appendiceal tumors exhibited a variety of patterns, such as glandular formations and signet ring cells, and displayed goblet cell carcinoid-like patterns, including nests, cords or crypt-like tubules with goblet cells. Neuroendocrine markers were often positive. The overall prognosis was poor and it was concluded that these should be labeled as metastatic appendiceal adenocarcinomas rather than goblet cell carcinoid. Rare appendiceal metastases in the ovary result in a picture similar to colorectal adenocarcinoma with a pseudoendometrioid morphology.[32]

The coexistence of an appendiceal mucinous lesion, either adenoma or adenocarcinoma, and unilateral or bilateral ovarian mucinous tumors,

usually morphologically borderline or malignant, has been known for some time.[33–39] There is usually associated pseudomyxoma peritonei (PMP), a clinical term characterized by the presence of abundant mucinous material within the abdomen and peritoneal cavity. Previously it was considered than in women, PMP was most commonly due to rupture of an ovarian mucinous neoplasm. However, it is now clear that most cases of PMP are of appendicial (or much more rarely colorectal, gallbladder or pancreatic) origin and in such cases the ovarian mucinous tumors occur as a result of direct spread and implantation from the appendiceal neoplasm. Evidence for this (discussed following) comes from morphologic, immunohistochemical and molecular studies. It is stressed that PMP is a clinical term and, histologically, a number of different pictures may be seen.

Microscopic and Gross Features

The extracellular mucinous material may contain morphologically bland or low-grade adenomatous mucinous epithelium (**Fig. 4**A) (referred to as disseminated peritoneal adenomucinosis - DPAM) or the histologic features may be those of an overt mucinous adenocarcinoma, sometimes with signet ring cells and abundant extracellular mucin (referred to as peritoneal mucinous carcinomatosis-PMCA).[39] Occasional cases show overlap between these two morphologic pictures. In cases of PMP, the surgeon should always remove

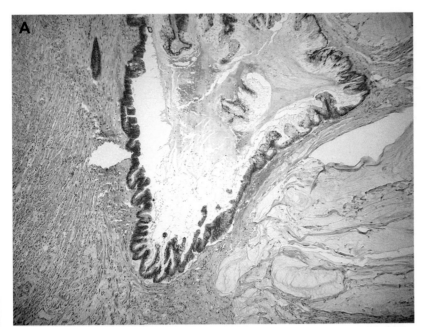

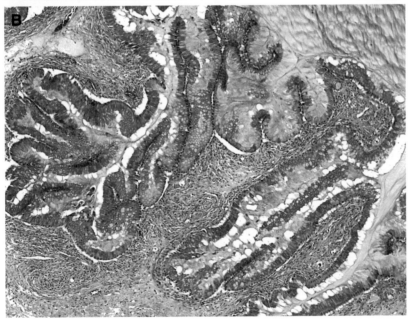

Fig. 4. Extraovarian mucinous material in PMP composed of low grade adenomatous epithelium embedded in abundant mucinous material (*A*). The ovarian tumor contains similar epithelium, mimicking a borderline mucinous tumor of intestinal type (*B*).

the appendix, even if a coexistent ovarian neoplasm is present. In some cases, the appendix is grossly normal but a small mucinous lesion is identified on histologic examination. In other cases, it may be difficult to identify the appendix because it is embedded in a mass of mucoid material. Pathologists should carefully section the appendix in cases of PMP and examine it in its entirety to look for a small lesion. Similarly, if a mass of mucoid material is removed from the

region of the appendix, this should be carefully examined to identify the appendix.

In cases of PMP, ovarian involvement is usually in the form of unilateral or bilateral multiloculated mucinous cystic neoplasms. Mucinous material is often seen on the surface of the masses and the locules contain thick mucin, which has been referred to as "bags of jelly." With unilateral involvement, the right ovary is more commonly affected, due to its proximity to the appendix.

Histologically, the picture most commonly resembles that of a borderline mucinous tumor of intestinal type (see **Fig. 4B**). There may also be benign appearing foci and sometimes overtly carcinomatous areas. There is often abundant extracellular mucin on the surface of the ovary and within the ovarian parenchyma (pseudomyxoma ovarii) containing strips of bland epithelium in the form of tall columnar cells with abundant intracellular mucin. In these cases, the primary appendiceal neoplasm is most often a low grade dysplastic mucinous cystadenoma. There may be histologic evidence of leakage of mucin and epithelium through the wall of the appendix or of prior appendiceal rupture. In cases where the appendiceal primary comprises an adenoma rather than an overt carcinoma, it is controversial as to whether the ovarian disease should be described as metastatic. My own preference is to regard this as representing direct spread and implantation from a ruptured appendiceal mucinous neoplasm rather than using the term metastasis. As stated, the ovarian involvement in such cases most often resembles a mucinous borderline tumor of intestinal type. However, the term borderline tumor should not be used since this propagates the now disproven belief that the ovary is the source of the primary neoplasm.

Much more uncommonly, the ovarian involvement comprises obvious high-grade mucinous adenocarcinoma with glandular and signet ring forms. It is beyond the scope of this review to describe in detail the pathologic features of the primary appendiceal lesion in cases of PMP and the reader is referred to several recent publications that discuss this and the terminology to be used in such cases.[40–42] The terminology used is varied and terms suggested include:

> Low grade appendiceal mucinous neoplasm (LAMN)
> Mucinous neoplasm of low malignant potential
> Peritoneal mucinous carcinomatosis, low grade or high grade depending on the exact morphologic appearances (**Fig. 5**).

Terms such as LAMN and low-grade peritoneal mucinous carcinomatosis are probably preferable to adenoma for the low grade end of the spectrum since there is an appreciable morbidity and mortality associated with PMP due to recurrent intestinal obstruction.

Markers for Appendiceal Neoplasms

Evidence that most cases of PMP are secondary to primary appendiceal (or colorectal) rather than ovarian neoplasms comes from immunohistochemical studies.[43,44] The epithelium of both the appendiceal and ovarian neoplasms and within the peritoneal mucinous material is diffusely positive with CK20, CEA and CDX2 and negative or focally immunoreactive with CK7, in keeping with an intestinal immunophenotype. Molecular studies have also provided evidence for a primary appendiceal neoplasm.[45,46] For example, identical K-ras mutations have been demonstrated in the appendiceal and ovarian neoplasms.[45,46] In a small number of cases, PMP is of ovarian origin since occasionally the appendix is removed and histologically examined in its entirety and no lesion is

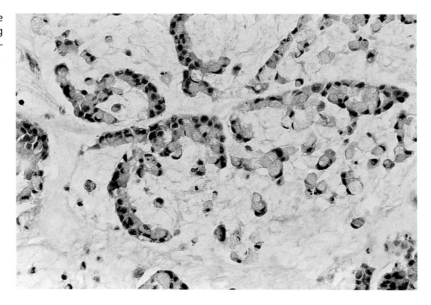

Fig. 5. PMP high grade containing signet ring tumor cells within abundant extracellular mucin.

found. Similarly, colonoscopy reveals no colo-rectal lesion and there is no possible alternative source of the PMP. In these cases, the ovarian mucinous neoplasm usually exhibits diffuse CK20, CEA and CDX2 positivity and is CK7 negative and it is probable that such cases represent intestinal type mucinous tumors arising from enteric elements within an ovarian teratoma.[47–49] In some cases, other teratomatous elements are present, supporting this hypothesis.

Metastatic Goblet Cell Carcinoid

Appendiceal goblet cell carcinoids rarely spread to the ovary and should be distinguished from the rare primary ovarian goblet cell carcinoid. As discussed earlier, the distinction between an appendiceal goblet cell carcinoid and an adenocarcinoma with goblet cell carcinoid-like features may be problematic and arbitrary. It has been suggested that in a primary appendiceal neoplasm, the term goblet cell carcinoid is inappropriate since these tumors often behave in an aggressive manner and the designation goblet cell carcinoid may inappropriately suggest a relatively benign lesion; the reader is referred to several recent publications which discuss this.[50,51] Features favoring a metastatic goblet cell carcinoid rather than a primary ovarian neoplasm are bilaterality and the other parameters described which help to distinguish primary from metastatic ovarian neoplasms in general. The presence of coexisting teratomatous elements is strong evidence of a primary ovarian tumor as most ovarian carcinoids arise in teratomatous neoplasms. Immunohistochemical markers are required to confirm neuroendocrine differentiation and help diagnose a goblet cell carcinoid. A potential point of diagnostic confusion is that some metastatic signet ring adenocarcinomas, for example of gastric or appendiceal origin, exhibit focal neuroendocrine differentiation.

GASTRIC CARCINOMA INVOLVING OVARY

Most gastric adenocarcinomas involving the ovary are bilateral and morphologically classical Krukenberg tumors with a component of signet ring cells in a sometimes reactive cellular stroma.

MICROSCOPIC AND GROSS FEATURES

Grossly, the ovaries are usually moderately enlarged, often with a bosselated external surface. On sectioning, the cut surface may be solid and firm, oedematous or gelatinous; small cysts may be present. Microscopic examination often reveals marked variation from area to area, often

Differential Diagnosis
GASTRIC CARCINOMA INVOLVING OVARY

Ovarian sex cord-stromal tumours, including signet ring-stromal tumour, fibroma, sclerosing stromal tumour

- These ovarian sex cord-stromal tumors may contain signet ring cells

- The presence of other epithelial arrangements, such as tubules, favors a metastasis

- Immunohistochemistry may be useful (see text)

Primary ovarian mucinous neoplasm

- The presence of signet ring cells, surface involvement, extraovarian spread and various other parameters associated with a secondary neoplasm assists in diagnosis

Other metastatic carcinomas, including appendiceal

- Signet ring carcinoma involving the ovary may be from a gastric or appendiceal primary

- Immunohistochemistry may be useful (see text)

with a nodular low power appearance. In some cases, the low power appearance may mimic a fibroma or some other spindle cell lesion. Signet ring cells are usually present but vary from the predominant pattern to a minor component of the neoplasm (**Fig. 6**).[52] Sometimes, the signet ring cells form nodular aggregates, resulting in a pseudotubular appearance (see **Fig. 6**). Tubules are commonly present and some tumors are predominantly composed of tubular formations, so called tubular Krukenberg tumors.[53] The stroma ranges from densely cellular to paucicellular and may be edematous or mucoid; extracellular mucin may be admixed with acellular fibrous stroma, resulting in an appearance referred to as "feathery degeneration." Sometimes, other morphologic features, such as cystic foci, squamous cells and clear cells are present (see **Fig. 6**). Glands may be lined by flattened cells, resulting in a microcystic appearance. There is often infiltration around and within pre-existing ovarian structures, such as corpora albicantia, and there may be easily recognisable lymphovascular invasion. Surface deposits are less commonly seen than with metastatic carcinomas from other intestinal sites, presumably because

Fig. 6. Metastatic gastric adenocarcinoma in ovary composed of signet ring cells (*A*) Sometimes, the signet ring cells form nodular aggregates (*B*).

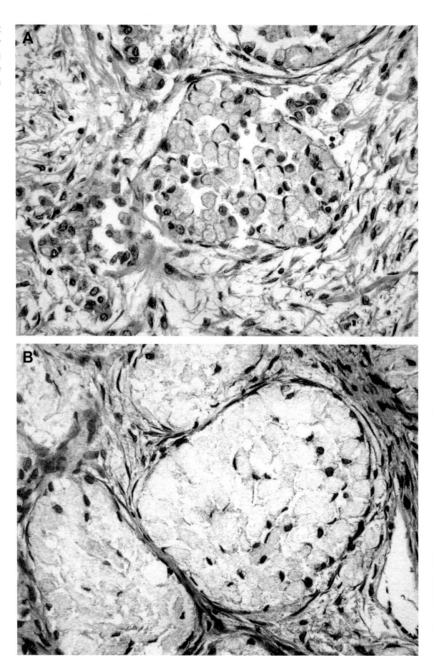

the latter involve the ovary by direct spread while gastric carcinomas spread to the ovary haematogenously. Mucin stains and immunohistochemistry with epithelial membrane antigen (EMA) and cytokeratins may be useful in highlighting the neoplastic population which is often more widespread than initially appreciated. The primary tumor within the stomach may be small or diffusely involve the wall resulting in a linitis plastica-like picture. The tumor may not be visible at endoscopy and in some cases the primary within the stomach may not manifest itself until some time later. There appears to be a peculiar tendency for metastatic gastric carcinomas to involve the ovary during pregnancy. Stromal luteinisation may occur, most commonly, but not exclusively, in pregnant patients and this can result in virilisation. Occasionally, an intestinal type gastric adenocarcinoma metastases to the ovary and results in a quite different histologic

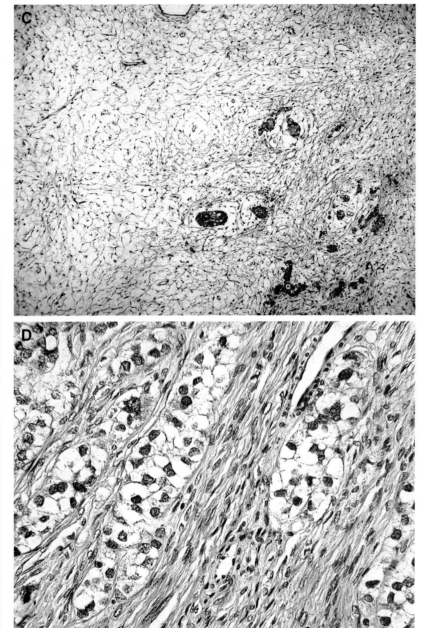

Fig. 6. Metastatic gastric adenocarcinoma in ovary. The stroma may be markedly edematous (*C*) and clear cells are present in some cases (*D*).

appearance to that of a typical Krukenberg tumor.[54] Intestinal type gastric adenocarcinomas metastatic to the ovary usually have a pseudoendometrioid or mucinous appearance, potentially mimicking a primary ovarian endometrioid or mucinous adenocarcinoma. Papillary, cribriform, trabecular and nested patterns may also be seen. A small number of these tumors have been examined by immunohistochemistry and most have been CK7 and CK20 positive.

PRIMARY KRUKENBERG TUMOR OF OVARY

Rare cases of so-called primary Krukenberg tumor of the ovary have been reported[55] but before making this diagnosis, extensive investigations should be undertaken to exclude a primary elsewhere. Furthermore, there should be a prolonged period of follow-up since, as stated, a primary gastric tumor may not manifest itself until some time later. It is also possible that some reports of primary Krukenberg tumor of the ovary represent signet ring-stromal tumor[56,57] or another ovarian sex cord-stromal tumor, such as fibroma or sclerosing stromal tumor, which may contain signet ring cells. Tubular Krukenberg tumors may mimic a Sertoli cell tumor or a Sertoli-Leydig cell tumor, the latter particularly if there is a component of non-neoplastic luteinised ovarian stromal cells. In the distinction between a Krukenberg tumor and a sex cord-stromal tumor, markers of ovarian sex cord - stromal neoplasms, such as inhibin and calretinin, may be useful in combination with mucin stains and EMA. Reactive non-neoplastic ovarian stromal cells in cases of Krukenberg tumor are often inhibin and calretinin positive, so close morphologic examination is necessary to ascertain which cells are immunoreactive. CK7 and CK20 staining is variable in metastatic gastric adenocarcinomas involving the ovary. Most, but not all, are CK7 positive while CK20 may be negative, focally positive or diffusely positive.

BREAST CARCINOMA INVOLVING OVARY

OVERVIEW

Patients with breast cancer are at increased risk of developing ovarian cancer and vice versa. This is especially, but not exclusively, so in the subset of patients with a hereditary predisposition to breast and ovarian cancer because of *BRCA1* or *BRCA2* mutation.[58] Usually, the breast carcinoma develops before the ovarian malignancy. In most patients with a history of breast carcinoma who are found to have a pelvic mass, this represents a new ovarian primary, usually of serous type.[59]

Breast carcinoma metastatic to the ovary may be of ductal or lobular type.[60,61] Although ductal carcinoma is the most common type of ovarian metastasis, lobular carcinoma is proportionally more likely to spread to the ovary. On occasions, metastatic breast cancer is identified in the ovary before a primary in the breast is discovered. The primary neoplasm may be small and detailed imaging may be necessary for detection. Rarely, the primary only manifests itself some time after the secondary in the ovary is discovered. Microscopic ovarian metastasis is occasionally discovered in therapeutic oophorectomy specimens in patients with breast cancer and in prophylactic risk reducing salpingo-oophorectomy specimens in patients with *BRCA1* or *BRCA2* mutation.

Microscopic and Gross Features

Ovarian metastasis from the breast is bilateral in most, but not all, cases.[60,61] The ovaries are

Differential Diagnosis
BREAST CARCINOMA INVOLVING OVARY

Primary ovarian serous or endometrioid adenocarcinoma

- These tumors express PAX8 and serous carcinoma frequently expresses WT1, unlike breast carcinoma

Granulosa cell tumor or other sex cord-stromal tumour

- The presence of various architectural arrangements characteristic of granulosa cell tumor assists

- These tumors express inhibin and calretinin and are negative for EMA, Ber EP4 and associated markers

Carcinoid tumor

- The presence of a "salt and pepper" chromatin assists in diagnosing a carcinoid tumor

- Chromogranin and synaptophysin expression favors carcinoid when breast carcinoma is not neuroendocrine-type

Lymphoma

- LCA and B- and T-cell markers are not expressed in breast carcinoma

usually enlarged, but often not markedly so, with a smooth or bosselated surface. Histology reveals the typical patterns associated with primary breast neoplasms. Ductal carcinomas may contain tubular glands, sometimes with a cribriform pattern, papillae, nests, trabeculae, diffuse sheets and small clusters of tumor cells (**Fig. 7A**). Signet ring cells are occasionally present. Ductal carcinoma metastatic to the ovary may mimic a primary ovarian endometrioid or serous carcinoma, the latter especially when there is a papillary architecture. Poorly differentiated metastatic breast carcinoma of ductal type may closely mimic a high grade serous or undifferentiated carcinoma. Lobular carcinoma within the ovary may be subtle and not obvious at scanning magnification. However, high power examination usually reveals the classical growth patterns, including single-file and insular arrangements, and the characteristic cytologic features including intracytoplasmic lumina (**Fig. 8**). Sometimes, a diffuse growth pattern is present. Signet-ring cells may be present. Those neoplasms with a diffuse pattern may mimic an adult granulosa cell tumor or

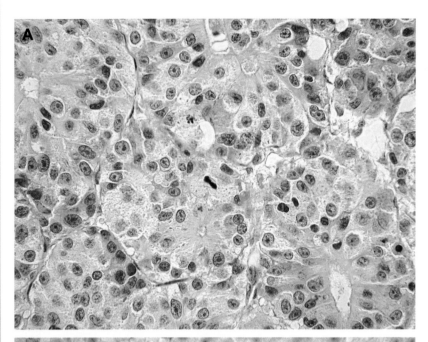

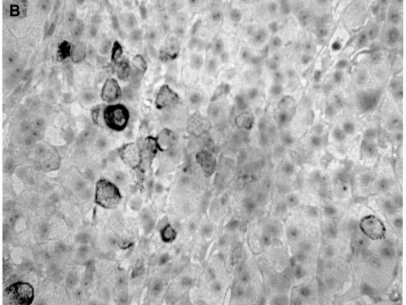

Fig. 7. Metastatic ductal breast carcinoma in ovary with a nested pattern (*A*). The tumor cells are focally positive with GCDFP15 (*B*).

a lymphoma while those with an insular pattern may mimic an adult granulosa cell tumor or a carcinoid tumor; in these situations, immunohistochemistry will be of value.

Markers for Breast Cancer Involving Ovary

Immunohistochemically, metastatic breast carcinoma is usually positive with CK7 and negative with CK20. ER and PR are often positive, as is HER2. Hormone receptor positivity may be useful both in diagnosis and in determining the likely response to adjuvant therapy. Hormone receptor positivity is, of course, not specific for a metastatic breast cancer since many primary ovarian and other gynecological malignancies are positive. Gross cystic disease fluid protein 15 (GCDFP15) (see **Fig. 7**B) and mammaglobin are commonly positive in breast carcinomas.[62] The former is a relatively specific marker of breast cancer but its sensitivity is low. Mammaglobin is a more sensitive marker of breast carcinoma than GCDFP15

Fig. 8. Metastatic breast lobular carcinoma involving ovary with a single-file pattern and intracytoplasmic lumina.

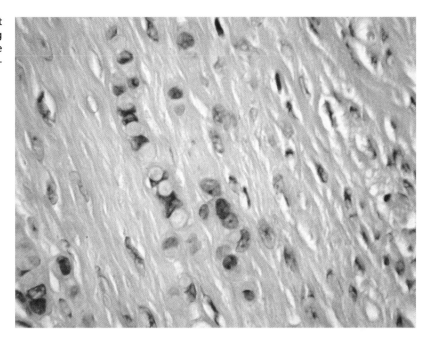

but is less specific since some gynaecological adenocarcinomas are positive,[63,64] although expression of this marker has not been extensively studied in primary ovarian adenocarcinomas. In the distinction between a metastatic breast carcinoma and an ovarian high grade serous carcinoma, WT1 and CA125 may be of value since these are commonly positive in serous carcinomas but usually negative in metastatic breast carcinoma, although a small percentage of the latter may be positive with both markers.[65] It has been shown recently that PAX8 is of value in the distinction between a metastatic breast carcinoma (PAX8 negative) and an ovarian serous or endometrioid adenocarcinoma (usually PAX8 positive).[66] In this distinction, PAX8 has been found to be more sensitive and more specific than WT1. Another recent study suggested PAX2 to be of value in the distinction between an ovarian serous carcinoma (PAX2 positive) and a breast carcinoma (PAX2 negative).[67]

PANCREATIC NEOPLASMS INVOLVING OVARY

OVERVIEW

Pancreatic adenocarcinomas may present with an ovarian metastasis in the absence of a known

 Differential Diagnosis
PANCREATIC AND BILIARY CARCINOMA INVOLVING OVARY

Primary ovarian mucinous neoplasm

- Bilateral ovarian involvement, surface involvement and extraovarian disease are in favor of a metastasis

- CK7 > CK20 is characteristic of ovarian mucinous neoplasms, but metastases from pancreas, biliary tract and stomach may display the same phenotype. Paradoxically, CA125 expression is more common in metastases than in primary ovarian mucinous neoplasms and DPC4 (SMAD4) expression is lost in about 50% of pancreatic ductal carcinomas

Primary ovarian endometrioid or serous adenocarcinoma

- These tumors express PAX8 and serous carcinoma frequently expresses WT1, unlike metastases from these organs

Carcinoid (metastatic pancreatic acinar cell carcinoma)

- Immunohistochemistry is useful (see text)

primary.[68] This is especially so with neoplasms located in the body or tail of the pancreas where symptoms related to the primary tumor may not be apparent until late in the course of the disease. Metastatic pancreatic adenocarcinomas involving the ovary may be solid neoplasms but not uncommonly they are large multiloculated cystic masses which may be unilateral or, more commonly, bilateral. Unilateral cystic metastasis from the pancreas is especially likely to be misdiagnosed as a primary ovarian neoplasm.

Microscopic Features

Microscopically, metastatic pancreatic adenocarcinoma usually resembles an ovarian mucinous neoplasm, often with morphologically bland areas, mimicking benign and borderline mucinous cystadenoma (**Fig. 9**).[68] As emphasized previously, this maturation phenomenon is not uncommon in metastatic mucinous carcinomas involving the ovary and may result in the pathologist erroneously diagnosing a primary ovarian mucinous tumor. However, with extensive sampling, obviously malignant areas, including foci of destructive stromal invasion, are usually identified, although this is not always the case. The presence of a nodular growth pattern, surface implants, and extensive lymphovascular permeation together with the other parameters described earlier are pointers toward a secondary neoplasm (see **Fig. 9**). In addition to often being bilateral,

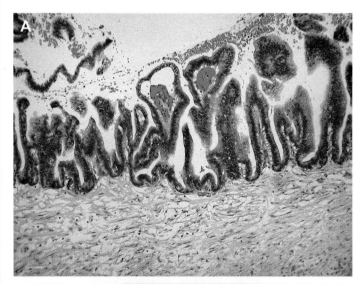

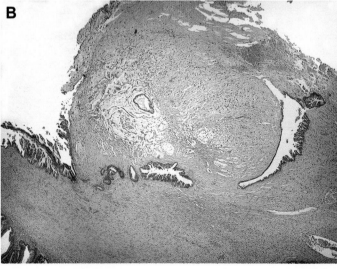

Fig. 9. Metastatic pancreatic adenocarcinoma in the ovary. In (*A*), the features mimic a primary ovarian mucinous borderline tumor. Tumor on the ovarian surface (*B*) is clue that one is dealing with a secondary neoplasm. See parts (*C*) and (*D*) on following page.

Fig. 9. Metastatic pancreatic adeno-carcinoma in the ovary. Tumor cells floating in mucin (*C*) and a nodular pattern of involvement (*D*) are clues that one is dealing with a secondary neoplasm.

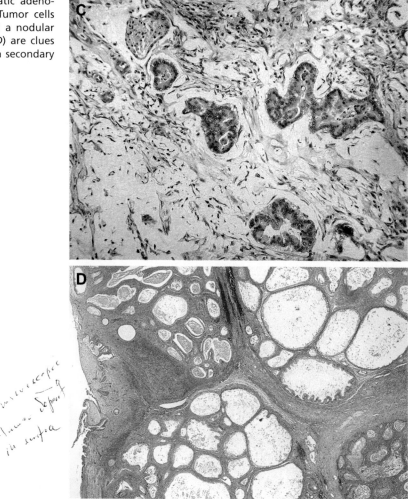

extraovarian disease involving the omentum or peritoneum may be present. It is once again emphasized that primary ovarian mucinous carcinomas are usually unilateral and stage 1. With a bilateral ovarian mucinous carcinoma or a mucinous carcinoma with extraovarian spread, a secondary should always be considered. Metastatic pancreatic carcinoma may also present with disseminated omental or peritoneal disease, mimicking a primary peritoneal tumor. While primary peritoneal serous carcinoma is a well recognized entity and is being diagnosed with increasing frequency (see below), primary perito-neal mucinous carcinomas are exceedingly rare if they occur at all.

Markers for Pancreatic Neoplasms Involving Ovary

Immunohistochemistry is of limited value in distin-guishing a primary ovarian mucinous neoplasm of intestinal type from a metastatic pancreatic carci-noma. Most commonly, both are diffusely positive with CK7 while CK20 is variable, being negative, focally or diffusely positive. CEA, CA19.9 and CDX2 may be positive in both tumor types. An absence of staining with DPC4 (DPC = deleted in pancreatic cancer) (SMAD4) may be a useful pointer toward a pancreatic adenocarcinoma since this nuclear transcription factor is inactivated in about 50% of pancreatic adenocarcinomas with the result that approximately half of these are negative.[69] Conversely, DPC4 is expressed in virtually all primary ovarian mucinous carcinomas. Rarely, especially in cases with extensive omental or peritoneal involvement, a pancreatic adenocarcinoma mimics an ovarian serous carcinoma or a primary peritoneal serous carcinoma. In this scenario, WT1 is of value since this is positive in almost all ovarian and peritoneal serous carcinomas but is negative in pancreatic carcinomas.[70] Pancreatic adenocarcinomas are not uncommonly positive with CA125 and some exhibit nuclear staining with PR (personal observations).

Metastatic Pancreatic Acinar Cell Carcinomas

Recently, a small series of metastatic pancreatic acinar cell carcinomas in the ovary has been reported.[71] Three of the four cases exhibited bilateral ovarian involvement and in 3 cases the ovarian neoplasm was discovered before the pancreatic tumor. Some of the neoplasms were characterized by a prominent acinar growth pattern with brightly eosinophilic granular cytoplasm. In other cases, the growth pattern was predominantly solid or cribriform. In all cases, prominent nucleoli were present. The main differential diagnosis was a carcinoid tumor. Positive staining with chymotrypsin and trypsin and negative staining with neuroendocrine markers assisted in diagnosis. There was focal inhibin staining in two cases, a potential diagnostic pitfall since a sex cord-stromal tumor might also enter into the differential diagnosis. Rarely, pancreatic islet cell tumors metastasize to the ovary.

GALLBLADDER AND BILIARY TRACT CARCINOMAS INVOLVING OVARY

OVERVIEW

Metastatic adenocarcinomas from the gallbladder and extrahepatic and intrahepatic bile ducts may involve the ovary.[72] This is uncommon in Western countries but there are geographic differences; for example, in Thailand, which has a high incidence of cholangiocarcinoma, metastatic biliary neoplasms in the ovary are much more common than in other parts of the world.[73] In general, the issues are similar to those encountered with metastatic pancreatic adenocarcinoma, although metastatic biliary carcinomas in the ovary more commonly result in solid than cystic masses. Two recent series have described in detail the clinicopathological features of these ovarian metastases.[73,74] Most mimic a primary ovarian mucinous neoplasm, usually adenocarcinoma, but occasionally a borderline or benign

neoplasm if the whole or much of the tumor exhibits a maturation phenomenon. The various features listed earlier which assist in the distinction between a primary ovarian mucinous neoplasm and a metastasis are of value and it is stressed that careful sampling with the examination of multiple sections is often contributory. Occasional cases mimic a primary ovarian high-grade endometrioid adenocarcinoma, a serous carcinoma, or an undifferentiated carcinoma. Uncommonly, metastatic biliary adenocarcinomas in the ovary are typical Krukenberg tumors with a component of signet ring cells. In general, immunohistochemistry is of limited value in the distinction between a primary ovarian mucinous neoplasm and a metastasis from these sites since both are usually diffusely positive with CK7 while CK20 may be negative, focally positive or occasionally diffusely positive. CEA, CA19.9 and CDX2 may be positive in both.

HEPATIC CARCINOMAS INVOLVING OVARY

OVERVIEW

As already discussed, carcinomas arising from the intrahepatic bile ducts may spread to the ovary. It is extremely rare for hepatocellular carcinoma (HCC) to metastasise to the ovary and there is usually a history of a primary liver tumor. However, rarely HCC presents with an ovarian metastasis in the absence of a known primary.[75] The morphologic features are similar to those seen within the liver with large polygonal tumor cells with abundant eosinophilic cytoplasm, arranged in insular, trabecular and pseudoglandular formations, sometimes containing bile pigment and hyaline globules.

THE MAIN DIFFERENTIAL DIAGNOSES ARE:

- Primary hepatoid carcinoma of the ovary
- Hepatoid variant of yolk sac tumor
- Metastatic hepatoid carcinoma from other organs
- Other primary ovarian epithelial neoplasms with an oxyphilic appearance, such as the eosinophilic variant of endometrioid and clear cell carcinoma
- Steroid cell tumors.

Extensive sampling may reveal more typical areas in yolk sac tumors (these usually occur in a young age group in contrast to the older age of most patients with metastatic HCC), clear cell carcinomas and endometrioid adenocarcinomas. Similarly, many primary hepatoid carcinomas of the ovary are associated with a component of a more usual surface epithelial carcinoma. However, in some cases imaging may be necessary to exclude a primary liver neoplasm. A single example of hepatoblastoma with ovarian metastasis has been documented.[76]

Markers for Hepatic Carcinoma Involving Ovary

Metastatic HCC in the ovary is often α fetoprotein and Hep PAR 1 positive. However, these are also commonly positive in the hepatoid variant of yolk sac tumor, primary hepatoid carcinoma of the ovary and metastatic hepatoid carcinomas from other organs and are consequently of no value in distinguishing these from a metastatic HCC.[77]

RENAL CARCINOMA INVOLVING OVARY

OVERVIEW

Renal cell carcinoma rarely metastasises to the ovary.[78] On occasion, there is no history of a primary renal neoplasm and the ovarian metastasis is the first presentation. The most common renal tumor to metastasise to the ovary is the typical clear cell carcinoma (CCC) and this may mimic a primary ovarian CCC. Morphologic differences exist between renal and ovarian CCC. A heterogenous appearance with an admixture of patterns, including tubulocystic, papillary and solid formations, and hobnail cells is much more common in primary ovarian neoplasms. Renal CCC usually has a characteristic sinusoidal vascular pattern. However, there may be morphologic overlap. The presence of endometriosis in the same or contralateral ovary is a pointer toward a primary ovarian neoplasm, as ovarian CCC commonly arises in endometriosis. With a CCC involving the ovary without the typical morphologic appearances of an ovarian primary, imaging may be necessary to exclude a renal tumor.

Markers for Renal Carcinoma Involving Ovary

A panel of markers assists in distinguishing ovarian from renal CCC.[79,80] Primary ovarian CCC is CK7 and CA125 positive while renal CCC is usually CK7 negative and positive with CD10 and renal cell carcinoma (RCC) marker. CK20 is negative in both. ER and PR are uncommonly positive in CCC of the ovary. In a study investigating ER and PR immunoreactivity in renal carcinomas, 2 of 182 cases (1.1%) exhibited positivity in less than 10% of tumor cell nuclei.[81] Hepatocyte nuclear factor 1β is a recently described useful

marker of primary ovarian CCC[30] and this might be anticipated to be of value in the distinction between an ovarian and a renal CCC. However, this marker has not been evaluated in primary renal CCC. Metastatic renal CCC in the ovary may also closely mimic an ovarian steroid cell tumor with clear cytoplasm. In this differential diagnosis, inhibin is useful (positive in steroid cell tumors), in addition to the markers already discussed which are positive in renal CCC.

URINARY TRACT CARCINOMAS INVOLVING OVARY

OVERVIEW

Metastatic transitional cell carcinoma from the urinary bladder or elsewhere within the urinary tract involving the ovary is rare.[82] These may mimic a primary ovarian transitional cell carcinoma or an undifferentiated carcinoma. The presence of a component of benign or borderline Brenner tumor confirms an ovarian primary which, given the benign or borderline areas, is termed a malignant Brenner tumor. Bilateral ovarian involvement is in favor of a metastatic neoplasm, although some primary ovarian transitional cell carcinomas are bilateral. Many primary ovarian transitional cell carcinomas contain a component of a more usual surface epithelial tumor, especially serous carcinoma,[83] and extensive sampling may assist in this regard. One transitional carcinoma of the renal pelvis metastatic to the ovary had a component of signet ring cells, in keeping with a Krukenberg tumor.[84]

Markers for Urinary Tract Carcinoma Involving Ovary

Immunohistochemistry can assist in distinguishing between a primary ovarian transitional cell carcinoma and a metastatic transitional cell carcinoma from the urinary tract. Primary ovarian transitional cell carcinomas have an immunophenotype that is much more in keeping with Mullerian than urothelial differentiation.[85] They are positive with CK7 and negative with CK20. Moreover, they commonly exhibit nuclear postivity with WT1, analagous to ovarian serous carcinoma.[86] In contrast, transitional cell carcinomas of the urinary tract are commonly positive with both CK7 and 20 and also with urothelial markers, such as uroplakin-III, p63 and thrombomodulin.[87] In contrast to primary ovarian transitional cell carcinomas, Brenner tumors of the ovary exhibit true urothelial differentiation and are often positive with markers such as uroplakin-III, p63 and thrombomodulin.[88,89]

PULMONARY CARCINOMAS INVOLVING OVARY

OVERVIEW

Metastatic pulmonary carcinomas within the ovary are uncommon and most are discovered in a patient with a known history of lung carcinoma; however, occasionally the metastatic neoplasm within the ovary is discovered synchronously with or before the primary neoplasm manifesting itself. In a recent large series of metastatic pulmonary carcinomas involving the ovary[90]:

  44% were small cell carcinomas
  34% adenocarcinomas
  16% large cell carcinomas
  3% squamous carcinomas.

Most of the metastases were unilateral. Common morphologic features were multinodular growth, widespread necrosis and extensive lymphovascular permeation. Occasional neoplasms contained areas mimicking a borderline tumor (**Fig. 10**).

MARKERS FOR PULMONARY CARCINOMAS INVOLVING OVARY

TTF1 is positive, usually with diffuse nuclear immunoreactivity, in most primary pulmonary adenocarcinomas and small cell carcinomas and may be useful in diagnosis. However, it has recently been demonstrated that adenocarcinomas arising in the ovary, endometrium, or cervix exhibit TTF1 immunoreactivity in a not insignificant percentage of cases.[91–93] TTF1 positivity in gynecologic adenocarcinomas is usually focal but is occasionally diffuse and this may result in obvious diagnostic problems. Furthermore, TTF1 immunoreactivity in a small cell carcinoma is not specific for a pulmonary primary since small cell and large cell neuroendocrine carcinomas arising at various sites may be positive.[94] Many pulmonary adenocarcinomas are CEA positive while most primary gynecological adenocarcinomas are negative.

ENDOMETRIAL CARCINOMAS INVOLVING OVARY AND SYNCHRONOUS ENDOMETRIAL AND OVARIAN CARCINOMAS

OVERVIEW

A not uncommon scenario is simultaneous involvement of the uterine corpus and one or both ovaries by an adenocarcinoma. Most commonly, these adenocarcinomas are endometrioid in type but sometimes they are serous.[95–102] With different morphologic tumor types, for example an endometrioid adenocarcinoma in the uterus and a serous adenocarcinoma in the ovary, it is clear that these represent independent primary neoplasms, although mixed endometrioid and serous carcinomas not uncommonly occur within the uterus and the serous element may preferentially metastasize even when this represents a minor component of the primary neoplasm.

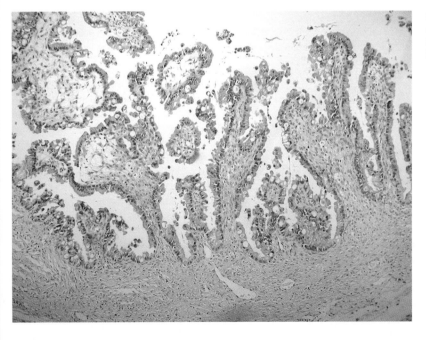

Fig. 10. Metastatic lung adenocarcinoma in ovary mimicking an ovarian borderline tumor.

The most common scenario is the presence of an endometrioid adenocarcinoma within the uterus and one or both ovaries. This association is found in approximately 5% of uterine endometrioid adenocarcinomas and 10 to 15% of ovarian endometrioid adenocarcinomas. In such cases, the neoplasms may represent synchronous independent primaries or metastasis from the uterus to the ovary or vice versa. Careful pathologic examination (discussed below) is the basis for deciding the relationship between the tumors. The question of whether these represent synchronous independent or metastatic carcinomas is of importance since adjuvant therapies may differ, as will the prognosis. For example, with an early stage, low-grade endometrioid adenocarcinoma of the uterine corpus and a separate independent stage IA or IB well differentiated endometrioid adenocarcinoma of the ovary, it is likely that no adjuvant therapy will be given. Conversely, adjuvant therapy is indicated with an ovarian tumor which has spread to the uterus (stage II) or with an endometrial carcinoma metastatic to the ovary (stage IIIA).

Endometrioid Adenocarcinoma

It is currently considered that early stage, low-grade endometrioid adenocarcinomas involving the uterus and one or both ovaries most likely represent synchronous independent primary neoplasms. The prognosis in such cases is usually good. Careful pathologic examination using "common sense" criteria is the basis for deciding the relationship between the uterine and ovarian neoplasms. Adjacent endometrial hyperplasia in the case of the uterine tumor and endometriosis (which may be subtle) or a component of benign or borderline adenofibroma in the case of the ovarian neoplasm are pointers toward an origin in these organs. With a deeply myoinvasive endometrial tumor exhibiting prominent lymphovascular invasion and tumor deposits in and on the surface of both ovaries, a uterine primary with ovarian metastasis is likely. The pattern of ovarian involvement may be a clue to a secondary neoplasm; for example, a nodular pattern of tumor growth, surface implants and prominent lymphovascular invasion within and surrounding an ovary which shows significant preservation of its parenchyma are clues to metastatic involvement. With endometrioid adenocarcinomas involving the uterus and one or both ovaries, immunohistochemistry is of no value in ascertaining the relationship between the tumors as the immunophenotype of a primary ovarian and uterine endometrioid adenocarcinoma is essentially identical.

Serous Carcinoma

With a serous carcinoma involving the uterus and one or both ovaries, the situation is different from endometrioid. Uterine serous carcinoma (USC) has a marked propensity for extrauterine spread which may occur even with a small primary tumor apparently confined to the endometrium. Similarly, the presumed precursor lesion of USC, serous endometrial intraepithelial carcinoma (serous EIC), may be associated with extrauterine involvement without demonstrable endometrial stromal or myometrial invasion.[103–107] USC and serous EIC may arise within endometrial polyps and in such cases may be associated with extrauterine involvement.[103–107] It is theoretically possible that, analogous to the situation with endometrioid carcinomas, the uterine and extrauterine (usually ovarian, peritoneal or omental) disease could represent independent primary neoplasms, indicative of a "field-change" effect. However, currently with serous neoplasia, it is considered much more likely that multifocal disease represents spread from one organ to another. The pattern of ovarian involvement described above may be a clue that one is dealing with a metastatic neoplasm in that organ. In problematic cases, WT1 staining may assist in distinguishing between a primary USC with metastasis to the ovary and independent synchronous neoplasms or metastasis from the ovary to the endometrium.[108–113] Most ovarian serous carcinomas (and primary tubal and peritoneal serous carcinomas) exhibit diffuse nuclear positivity with WT1. In contrast, USC is usually negative. However, the percentage of USCs exhibiting WT1 immunoreactivity has varied between studies and some cases are positive, occasionally with diffuse immunoreactivity.[108–113] It has been suggested that some WT1 positive USCs might have an origin in the fallopian tube.[114] It can be summarized that, although the published studies are somewhat contradictory and there is overlap, diffuse WT1 positivity in a serous neoplasm favors an ovarian, tubal or peritoneal origin. In contrast, negative staining is a pointer toward a primary uterine neoplasm. Uterine clear cell carcinoma and carcinosarcoma may also involve the ovary; this usually represents metastatic spread rather than synchronous independent uterine and ovarian primaries.

Markers to distinguish independent synchronous and metastatic adenocarcinomas

Several investigators have employed molecular techniques in an attempt to distinguish between independent synchronous and metastatic adenocarcinomas, especially of endometrioid type, involving the uterus and ovaries. However, there is no universal gold standard for the distinction between synchronous and metastatic neoplasms. Methods used include[115–121]:

> Comparative analysis between the separate neoplasms of loss of heterozygosity (LOH)
> Microsatellite instability (MI)
> Clonal X-inactivation
> β-catenin expression
> β-catenin, K-ras, PTEN and p53 mutations.

Theoretically, if two tumors exhibit the same molecular alterations they are likely to represent a primary neoplasm in one organ with metastasis to the other. However, it is stressed that although such techniques are of value, they are not performed routinely in most laboratories and the results should always be interpreted with caution. Careful pathologic examination remains the mainstay in diagnosis. Identical molecular alterations may be found in independent synchronous neoplasms involving the uterus and ovary. This can be explained by induction of the same genetic events by a common carcinogenic agent acting on the endometrium and on ectopic endometrial tissue within the ovary. Furthermore, a metastatic tumor may exhibit a different molecular profile to the primary neoplasm due to tumor progression.

It is clear that the best molecular approach to distinguish between independent synchronous and metastatic tumors is to combine several different techniques. In a small number of cases, identical p53 mutations have been demonstrated in the uterine and extrauterine lesions of patients with EIC or early USC and concurrent extrauterine disease.[122] Since USC exhibits a broad spectrum of p53 mutations, this is strong evidence in these cases that the extrauterine disease represents tumor metastasis and not an independent primary arising at an extrauterine site.

CERVICAL CARCINOMA INVOLVING OVARY

OVERVIEW

Cervical squamous carcinoma, adenocarcinoma and neuroendocrine carcinomas may metastasise to the ovary. Adenocarcinomas more commonly result in ovarian metastasis than squamous carcinomas. In most cases, there is little in the way of diagnostic difficulty, the ovarian metastasis being picked up at hysterectomy for cervical cancer or an ovarian mass being discovered in a patient with a known history of cervical cancer. However, occasionally presentation is with symptoms related to an ovarian mass, the cervical cancer being undetected. Before diagnosing a primary ovarian squamous carcinoma, a metastasis from the cervix or elsewhere should be excluded unless the tumor is associated with endometriosis, a dermoid cyst or some other ovarian lesion which potentially may give rise to a squamous carcinoma. Rarely, CIN3 spreads upwards to involve the endometrium, the tubal mucosa or the cortical surface of the ovary.[123] Ovarian cysts lined by dysplastic squamous epithelium resembling CIN3 have been described in association with CIN in the absence of endometrial or tubal involvement.[124,125]

Microscopic and Gross Features

Similar to other secondary adenocarcinomas, metastatic cervical adenocarcinoma involving the ovary may have a deceptively bland appearance and closely mimic a primary ovarian benign or borderline mucinous neoplasm. In such cases, the ovarian tumor may be unilateral or bilateral. As with other metastatic mucinous carcinomas in the ovary, extraovarian spread, a nodular pattern

> **Differential Diagnosis**
> CERVICAL CARCINOMA
> INVOLVING OVARY
>
> *Primary ovarian endometrioid adenocarcinoma*
>
> - The presence of surface involvement is in favor of metastatic carcinoma
>
> - The presence of significant mitotic and apoptotic activity in an architecturally low grade tumor is in favor of a metastasis
>
> - The presence of squamous elements and endometriosis is suggestive of ovarian endometrioid adenocarcinoma
>
> - Immunohistochemistry for p16 and HPV studies are useful
>
> *Primary ovarian mucinous neoplasm*
>
> - Bilateral ovarian involvement and surface involvement are in favor of a metastasis
>
> - Immunohistochemistry for p16 and HPV studies are useful
>
> *Primary ovarian squamous carcinoma*
>
> - Bilateral ovarian involvement is suggestive of a metastasis
>
> - Most primary ovarian squamous carcinomas arise in a teratoma
>
> - HPV studies are useful

of involvement, surface implants and prominent lymphovascular invasion, especially in tissues surrounding the ovary, are clues that one may be dealing with a metastatic lesion. Synchronous mucinous tumors of the cervix, including adenoma malignum, and ovaries have been described,[126–128] sometimes in association with Peutz-Jeghers syndrome. The presence of morphologically "benign" elements within the ovarian neoplasm has been interpreted as evidence of a primary here but it may be that, in some cases, these represent ovarian secondaries with bland areas mimicking benign or borderline mucinous cystadenoma. Other metastatic cervical adenocarcinomas within the ovary (perhaps the majority) closely mimic a primary ovarian endometrioid adenocarcinoma. A feature of some primary cervical adenocarcinomas and their ovarian metastases is that they exhibit a so-called hybrid morphology with features reminiscent of both mucinous and endometrioid differentiation. There is often prominent mitotic and apoptotic activity compared with the degree of glandular differentiation. With synchronous adenocarcinomas of the cervix and ovary, a metastasis from the cervix to the ovary should always be considered. A recent study has highlighted that in some cases with ovarian metastasis, the primary adenocarcinoma within the cervix may be extremely small with minimal, if any, recognizable invasive component.[129]

Markers for Metastatic Cervical Adenocarcinoma within Ovary

Immunohistochemical and molecular studies may assist in confirming a metastatic cervical adenocarcinoma within the ovary. In the distinction between a primary ovarian endometrioid adenocarcinoma and a metastasis from the cervix, ER may be of value since the former is usually positive and the latter negative. ER is of no value in the distinction between a primary ovarian mucinous neoplasm and a cervical metastasis since both are typically negative.[130] p16 may help in confirming a metastatic cervical adenocarcinoma since the majority of these are diffusely positive due to the presence of high-risk human papillomavirus (HPV), although some of the more unusual morphologic types, such as clear cell, mesonephric, gastric and minimal deviation, are negative.[131] Most primary ovarian endometrioid and mucinous carcinomas are p16 negative.[132] It should be noted that high grade ovarian serous carcinomas are often p16 positive, due to non-HPV related mechanisms.[133,134] However, these do not typically enter into the differential diagnosis of a metastatic cervical

adenocarcinoma. Molecular studies to demonstrate HPV also assist in confirming an ovarian metastasis from a cervical primary since HPV is demonstrable in the majority of cervical squamous and adenocarcinomas while primary ovarian carcinomas are negative.[129,130] The demonstration of identical HPV types in the cervical and ovarian neoplasms is strong evidence that the ovarian tumor is a metastasis from the cervix rather than a separate independent primary.

MALIGNANT MELANOMA INVOLVING OVARY

OVERVIEW

Most malignant melanomas involving the ovary are metastatic with young patients often being affected.[135,136] Primary ovarian melanoma is rare, most examples arising within a teratoma.[137,138] Unless shown to be associated with a teratoma, a malignant melanoma in the ovary should be considered most likely metastatic even with no history of a primary neoplasm elsewhere. In the absence of a known primary, a search should be

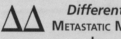

Differential Diagnosis
METASTATIC MALIGNANT MELANOMA INVOLVING OVARY

Primary ovarian undifferentiated carcinoma

- The presence of intranuclear inclusions and melanin pigment is suggestive of melanoma
- Absence of melanoma-associated immunophenotype and presence of epithelial differentiation are evidence again melanoma

Primary ovarian oxyphilic neoplasms

- Immunohistochemistry is useful (see text)

Primary ovarian clear cell neoplasms

- These typically lack melanoma-associated immunophenotype and display evidence of epithelial differentiation

Primary ovarian small round cell tumors

- Immunohistochemistry is useful (see text)

Sex cord-stromal tumors

- These tumors frequently express inhibin and calretinin, unlike melanomas, but markers such as Melan-A and S100 may be expressed in both sex cord-stromal tumors and melanomas

made for an extraovarian neoplasm and if not found it is possible that a cutaneous primary has regressed. However, malignant melanomas have been reported in the ovary without teratomatous elements and which have been considered most likely primary here.[138] Metastatic melanomas in the ovary may be bilateral but are more commonly unilateral.[135,136]

Diagnosis of a metastatic melanoma is straightforward if there is a history of melanoma which is known to the pathologist, there are bilateral black or brown ovarian masses and the characteristic morphologic features of melanoma are present, such as a nested pattern, epithelioid tumor cells with prominent nucleoli, nuclear inclusions, abundant eosinophilic cytoplasm, and melanin pigment (**Fig. 11**). However, malignant melanoma may have a variable histologic appearance and melanoma should always be considered with any unusual tumor morphology which does not conform to a typical primary ovarian neoplasm.

Metastatic melanoma in the ovary may have a diffuse growth pattern and mimic undifferentiated carcinoma or be composed of cells with

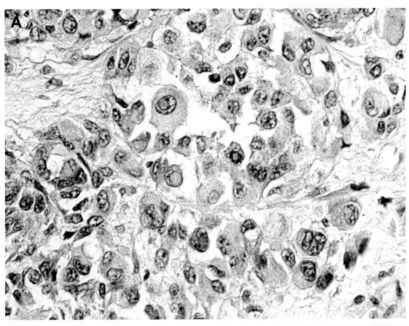

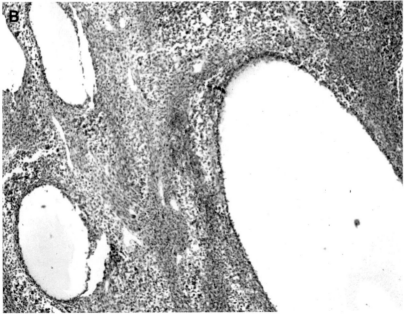

Fig. 11. Metastatic malignant melanoma in ovary composed of epithelioid cells with abundant eosinophilic cytoplasm and intranuclear inclusions (*A*). Another metastatic melanoma composed of cells with scant cytoplasm and forming follicles, closely mimicking ovarian small cell carcinoma of hypercalcemic type (*B*).

abundant eosinophilic or clear cytoplasm resulting in consideration of the broad range of neoplasms in the differentiated diagnosis of an oxyphilic or clear cell ovarian tumor.[139] Other metastatic melanomas are composed of cells with scant cytoplasm and enter into the differential diagnosis of an ovarian small round cell tumor (see **Fig. 11**).[140] Sometimes, follicle-like structures are present resulting in a close resemblance to juvenile granulosa cell tumor or ovarian small cell carcinoma of hypercalcaemic type. Other metastatic melanomas contain spindle cells, focally, predominantly or exclusively. Rhabdoid cells, nuclear grooves and a myxoid stroma have also been described. Sometimes, a mixture of morphologic appearances is present.

Markers for Malignant Melanoma Involving Ovary

Immunohistochemistry with S100, melan-A, micro-opthalmia transcription factor and HMB45 assists in confirming a diagnosis of malignant melanoma. However, ovarian sex cord-stromal tumors are commonly positive with S100 and melan-A.[141] Some neoplasms in this category, for example adult and juvenile granulosa cell tumor and steroid cell tumor (melanin pigment may be mistaken for the lipochrome pigment of a steroid cell tumor), may enter into the differential diagnosis of malignant melanoma. HMB45 is widely regarded as the most specific marker of malignant melanoma but some ovarian steroid cell tumors are positive.[142] Moreover, rarely malignant melanomas are positive with inhibin, resulting in obvious diagnostic difficulties.[136]

CARCINOID TUMORS INVOLVING OVARY

OVERVIEW

Carcinoid tumors involving the ovary may be primary or metastatic. Fewer than 1% of all carcinoids involve the ovary and primary ovarian carcinoids are more common in surgical pathology practice than metastatic neoplasms.[143] Most metastatic carcinoids involving the ovary are secondary from the small intestine. Apart from a history of an extraovarian carcinoid, features which help to distinguish a primary from a secondary carcinoid, in addition to those useful in the distinction between primary and metastatic ovarian neoplasms in general, are shown in **Table 2**.

Most primary ovarian carcinoids arise in a teratoma and rarely in association with another ovarian lesion, such as a Brenner tumor, a mucinous neoplasm or a Sertoli-Leydig cell tumor. However,

Table 2
Features useful in distinguishing primary from metastatic ovarian carcinoid

Primary Carcinoid	Secondary Carcinoid
Association with dermoid cyst or other neoplasm	No association with dermoid cyst
Usually unilateral	Often bilateral
Confined to ovary	May be extraovarian spread
Lymphovascular invasion rare	Lymphovascular invasion common

primary ovarian carcinoids may rarely occur in pure form. The histologic features of primary and metastatic ovarian carcinoids are similar with an insular (midgut) growth pattern being most common. It has been suggested that follicle-like spaces are more common in metastatic than primary ovarian carcinoids.[2] The differential diagnosis may be wide and positive staining with neuroendocrine markers assists in diagnosis.

Markers for Carcinoid Tumors Involving Ovary

Recent immunohistochemical studies of extraovarian carcinoids have suggested that CDX2 and TTF1 may help define the site of origin. CDX2 is expressed by enterochromaffin cells of the small intestine, the putative cell of origin of small intestinal carcinoids. This marker is selectively expressed by intestinal carcinoids, particularly of midgut origin, whereas TTF1 selectively marks bronchopulmonary carcinoids.[144–146] However, primary ovarian carcinoids of insular type are also CDX2 positive and this marker does not help to distinguish a primary ovarian carcinoid and a metastasis from the small intestine.[147] Primary ovarian goblet cell carcinoids are also CDX2 positive while trabecular carcinoids are negative.[147] This suggests that CDX2 is a marker of the morphologic phenotype of a carcinoid rather than of its site of origin. Metastatic goblet cell carcinoid from the appendix may rarely involve the ovary but, as discussed previously, most neoplasms diagnosed as such are best regarded as metastatic adenocarcinomas with goblet cell carcinoid-like features.

PRIMARY PERITONEAL TUMORS INVOLVING OVARY

OVERVIEW

Primary peritoneal serous carcinoma (PPSC), the most common primary peritoneal malignancy in

Table 3
Criteria for primary peritoneal serous carcinoma

Morphology is serous in type
Ovaries normal in size or enlarged by a benign process
Bulk of tumor is in peritoneum
No tumor in ovary or tumor confined to surface with no cortical invasion or <5 mm involvement of ovarian parenchyma
If prior oophorectomy, pathology report should be reviewed to document absence of carcinoma. If oophorectomy within 5 years, slides should be reviewed. Cervical, endometrial, ovarian and tubal primaries should be excluded

females, is morphologically identical to ovarian serous carcinoma. Both low grade and high grade variants occur. In many cases, it is arbitrary as to whether one is dealing with a PPSC with involvement of the ovaries or a small primary ovarian carcinoma which has metastasized widely. This is not a crucial distinction to make since management of both tumors is identical. The Gynecologic Oncology Group (GOG) has proposed criteria for PPSC, as opposed to primary ovarian serous carcinoma.[148] These criteria (**Table 3**), which are essentially arbitrary and which have been adopted by the World Health Organization, take account of the gross appearance of the ovaries and the impression of the surgeon. In cases of PPSC with involvement of the adnexa, the ovaries are small or enlarged by a benign process and microscopically tumor is confined to the capsular surface or invades minimally into the ovarian stroma (<5 mm). I would add that a primary neoplasm in the fallopian tube or uterus should also be excluded. The immunophenotype of PPSC and ovarian serous carcinoma does not differ.

Diffuse peritoneal malignant mesothelioma may involve the ovaries (**Fig. 12**).[149–151] Usually, there is widespread peritoneal disease with only minimal involvement of the surface of the ovaries. However, uncommonly there is prominent ovarian involvement, mimicking a primary ovarian neoplasm, and occasional cases of primary ovarian malignant mesothelioma have been described.[149] While a history of asbestos exposure does not necessarily precede a peritoneal mesothelioma, when this is present it can be helpful to diagnosis. Mesothelioma can morphologically mimic a serous carcinoma, both neoplasms exhibiting a prominent tubulopapillary architecture. Depending on the tumor distribution, this may result in a misdiagnosis of ovarian serous carcinoma or PPSC. Serous carcinomas are usually more atypical than mesotheliomas, which typically have more abundant columnar eosinophilic cytoplasm. Sarcomatoid and mixed mesotheliomas are uncommon in the peritoneum.

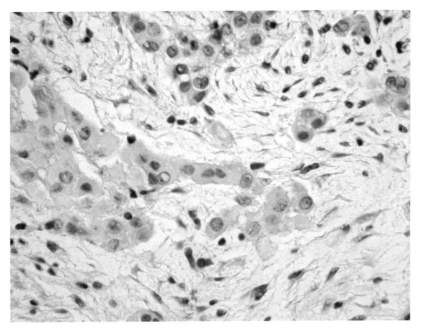

Fig. 12. Mesothelioma involving ovary with groups of epithelioid tumour cells with abundant eosinophilic cytoplasm. Refer to Figure 23 in Longacre: Benign and low-grade serous epithelial tumors: recent developments and diagnostic problems.

Markers to Distinguish Serous Carcinoma and Mesothelioma

Immunohistochemistry is useful in the distinction between a mesothelioma and a serous carcinoma and a panel of markers should be used. I find the two most useful markers to be BerEP4 (positive in serous carcinomas; negative in mesotheliomas) and calretinin (positive in mesotheliomas; negative in serous carcinomas).[152] Calretinin positivity should be nuclear (there may also be cytoplasmic immunoreactivity) to be of discriminatory value. Thrombomodulin, CK 5/6 and D2-40 may also be useful as mesothelial markers (although none of these markers is totally specific in the distinction between mesothelioma and serous carcinoma) while many serous carcinomas are ER positive. H-caldesmon may be of value since this is typically positive in mesotheliomas and negative in serous carcinomas.[153] Serous carcinomas and mesotheliomas both exhibit nuclear positivity with WT1.

DESMOPLASTIC SMALL ROUND CELL TUMOR (DSRCT) INVOLVING OVARY

OVERVIEW

Desmoplastic small round cell tumor (DSRCT) is a highly aggressive neoplasm most commonly involving the abdominal and pelvic cavity of young males.[154] In females, the clinical, radiological and operative findings may mimic bilateral ovarian neoplasms with omental and peritoneal secondaries.[155,156] The usual operative finding is of multiple large tumor deposits throughout the abdomen and pelvis.

Microscopic and Gross Features

Classically, the histologic picture is of cohesive sheets of small cells with hyperchromatic nuclei, scant cytoplasm and easily identifiable mitotic figures, set in an abundant fibrous stroma. There may be peripheral palisading. Variations to the classic histologic appearance exist; for example, the stroma may be scant, the cells may have abundant eosinophilic or clear cytoplasm and a variety of growth patterns may be present, such as corded and trabecular.[154] Glandular or tubular structures are rarely present, as are spindle cells. The differential diagnosis is wide and is that of an ovarian small round cell tumor.[140]

Markers for Desmoplastic Small Round Cell Tumor

Desmoplastic small round cell tumor has a characteristic immunophenotype, usually with coexpression of epithelial, mesenchymal and neural markers.[157] The tumor is usually positive with cytokeratins, EMA, vimentin and especially desmin, the latter with a punctate paranuclear pattern.[157] There is nuclear positivity with WT1 using antibodies against the C-terminal. The most widely used WT1 antibodies are those against the N-terminal which exhibit nuclear immunoreactivity in ovarian serous carcinomas, mesotheliomas and OSCCHT.[158] DSRCT often exhibits cytoplasmic staining with antibodies against the N-terminal of WT1.[159] Molecular studies have identified a translocation t(11;22) (p13;q12) as being unique to DSRCT.[160] Rare cases exhibit variant translocations.[161]

MISCELLANEOUS METASTATIC NEOPLASMS INVOLVING OVARY

OVERVIEW

A variety of other neoplasms rarely metastasise to the ovary. Occasional cases of metastatic thyroid carcinoma, usually of follicular type, have been reported.[162] Immunohistochemistry, using thyroglobulin and TTF1, may be useful in confirming a thyroid metastasis, although, as stated earlier, a not insignificant percentage of primary gynecologic adenocarcinomas are TTF1 positive. Primary thyroid neoplasms may obviously arise in the ovary within a teratoma which may be totally or extensively overgrown by the thyroid type tumor. In such cases, extensive sampling can assist in revealing other teratomatous elements. Hematopoietic neoplasms may involve the ovary, usually as part of a systemic process, as can the "small blue cell tumors of childhood."

Metastatic Gastrointestinal Stromal Tumors

A small series of metastatic gastrointestinal stromal tumors (GISTs) involving the ovary has been reported.[163] In three of five cases, the primary and metastatic neoplasms were discovered synchronously, in one case the ovarian metastasis was discovered before the primary neoplasm and in the other case the metastasis was removed 27 years after the intestinal primary. Morphologically, the tumors were either composed entirely of spindle cells or a mixture of spindle and epithelioid cells. The diagnosis was confirmed in all cases by positive c-kit (CD117) immunoreactivity. The main differential diagnosis was a smooth muscle neoplasm and negative desmin staining helped to exclude this. Of note, smooth muscle actin and h-caldesmon were positive in some cases. A correct diagnosis of GIST obviously has significant therapeutic implications given the specific therapy now available for these neoplasms.

Endometrial Stromal Sarcoma

A variety of other sarcomas rarely metastasize to the ovary. The most common sarcoma to result in ovarian metastasis is uterine endometrial stromal sarcoma (ESS).[164] Diagnosis is usually straightforward if there is a known history of ESS or if the ovarian metastasis is identified at the same time as the primary within the corpus. However, the history of a uterine primary may be remote or an ovary may be removed before the primary in the uterus is detected. The usual morphologic appearance is of a diffuse population of cells with ovoid to short spindle shaped nuclei and scant cytoplasm. In such cases, the chief differential diagnosis is likely to be some variant of sex cord-stromal tumor, particularly as the tongue-like growth pattern characteristic of uterine ESS is generally not seen in the ovarian metastasis. A rich network of arteriole-like vascular channels may be a clue to the diagnosis, as may cord-like hyalinisation. Other features sometimes present include sex cord-like differentiation and the formation of true endometrioid glands.[165] CD10 and hormone receptors may be useful in diagnosis since these are positive in most ESSs[166]; however, these are non-specific markers and a variety of other neoplasms may be positive. Inhibin is negative in ESSs, except in areas of sex cord-like differentiation. Distinction should also be made from the rare primary ovarian ESS which usually, but not always, arises in endometriosis.[167]

REFERENCES

1. Young RH. From krukenberg to today: the ever present problems posed by metastatic tumors in the ovary: part I. Historical perspective, general principles, mucinous tumors including the krukenberg tumor. Adv Anat Pathol 2006;13:205–27.
2. Young RH. From Krukenberg to today: the ever present problems posed by metastatic tumors in the ovary. Part II. Adv Anat Pathol 2007;14:149–77.
3. McCluggage WG, Wilkinson N. Metastatic neoplasms involving the ovary: a review with an emphasis on morphological and immunohistochemical features. Histopathology 2005;47:231–47.
4. Young RH, Scully RE. Metastatic tumors in the ovary: a problem – oriented approach and review of the recent literature. Semin Diagn Pathol 1991;8:250–76.
5. McCluggage WG, Young RH. Primary ovarian mucinous tumors with signet ring cells: report of 3 cases with discussion of so-called primary Krukenberg tumor. Am J Surg Pathol 2008;32:1373–9.
6. Lee KR, Young RH. The distinction between primary and metastatic mucinous carcinomas in the ovary. Gross and histologic findings in 50 cases. Am J Surg Pathol 2003;27:281–92.
7. Seidman JD, Horbayne-Szakaly I, Haiba M, et al. The histologic type and stage distribution of ovarian carcinomas of surface epithelial type. Int J Gynecol Pathol 2004;23:41–4.
8. McCluggage WG. My approach to and thoughts on the typing of ovarian carcinomas. J Clin Pathol 2008;61:152–63.
9. Seidman JD, Kurman RJ, Ronnett BM. Primary and metastatic mucinous adenocarcinomas in the ovaries: incidence in routine practice with a new approach to improve intraoperative diagnosis. Am J Surg Pathol 2003;27:985–93.
10. Yemelyanova AV, Vang R, Judson K, et al. Distinction of primary and metastatic mucinous tumors involving the ovary: analysis of size and laterality data by primary site with reevaluation of an algorithm for tumor classification. Am J Surg Pathol 2008;32:128–38.
11. McCluggage WG. Recent advances in immunohistochemistry in the diagnosis of ovarian neoplasms. J Clin Pathol 2000;53:558–60.
12. McCluggage WG. Recent advances in immunohistochemistry in gynaecological pathology. Histopathology 2002;46:309–26.
13. McCluggage WG, Young RH. Immunohistochemistry as a diagnostic aid in the evaluation of ovarian tumors. Semin Diagn Pathol 2005;22:3–32.
14. McCluggage WG. Immunohistochemical markers as a diagnostic aid in ovarian pathology. Diagn Histopathol 2008;14:335–51.
15. Berezowski K, Stasny JF, Kornstein MJ. Cytokeratins 7 and 20 and carcinoembryonic antigen in ovarian and colonic carcinoma. Mod Pathol 1996;9:1040–4.
16. Park SO, Kim HS, Hong EK, et al. Expression of cytokeratins 7 and 20 in primary carcinomas of the stomach and colorectum and their value in the differential diagnosis of metastatic carcinomas to the ovary. Hum Pathol 2002;33:1078–85.
17. Lagendijk JH, Mullink H, van Diest PJ, et al. Immunohistochemical differentiation between primary adenocarcinomas of the ovary and ovarian metastases of colon and breast origin. Comparison between a statistical and intuitive approach. J Clin Pathol 1999;52:283–90.
18. Uewa G, Sawada M, Ogawa H, et al. Immunohistochemical study of cytokeratin 7 for the differential diagnosis of adenocarcinoma in the ovary. Gynecol Oncol 1993;51:219–23.
19. Lash RH, Hart WR. Intestinal adenocarcinomas metastatic to the ovaries: a clinicopathologic

evaluation of 22 cases. Am J Surg Pathol 1989;11: 114–21.

20. Lewis MR, Euscher ED, Deavers MT, et al. Metastatic colorectal adenocarcinoma involving the ovary with elevated serum CA125: a potential diagnostic pitfall. Gynecol Oncol 2007;105:395–8.

21. Bell KA, Kurman RJ. A clinicopathologic analysis of atypical proliferative (borderline) tumours and well-differentiated endometrioid adenocarcinomas of the ovary. Am J Surg Pathol 2000;24:1465–79.

22. Raspollini MR, Amunni G, Villannucci A, et al. Utility of CDX-2 in distinguishing between primary and secondary (intestinal) mucinous ovarian carcinoma. Appl Immunohistochem Mol Morphol 2004; 12:127–31.

23. Werling RW, Yaziji H, Bacchi CE, et al. CDX2, a highly sensitive and specific marker of adenocarcinomas of intestinal origin: an immunhistochemical survey of 476 primary and metastatic carcinomas. Am J Surg Pathol 2003;27:303–10.

24. Groisman GM, Meir A, Sabo E. The value of cdx2 immunostaining in differentiating primary ovarian carcinomas from colonic carcinomas metastatic to the ovaries. Int J Gynecol Pathol 2003;23:52–7.

25. Tornillo L, Moch H, Diener PA, et al. CDX-2 immunostaining in primary and secondary ovarian carcinomas. J Clin Pathol 2004;57:641–3.

26. Houghton O, Connolly LE, McCluggage WG. Morules in endometrioid proliferations of the uterus and ovary consistently express the intestinal transcription factor CDX2. Histopathology 2008;53:156–65.

27. Albarracin CT, Jafri J, Montag AG, et al. Differential expression of MUC2 and MUC5AC mucin genes in primary ovarian and metastatic colonic carcinoma. Hum Pathol 2000;31:672–7.

28. Chou YY, Jeng YM, Kao HL, et al. Differentiation of ovarian mucinous carcinoma and metastatic colorectal adenocarcinoma by immunostaining with β-catenin. Histopathology 2003;43:151–6.

29. Young RH, Hart WR. Metastatic intestinal carcinomas simulating primary ovarian clear cell carcinoma and secretory endometrioid carcinoma: a clinicopathologic and immunohistochemical study of five cases. Am J Surg Pathol 1998;22:805–15.

30. Yamamoto S, Tsuda H, Aida S, et al. Immunohistochemical detection of hepatocyte nuclear factor 1beta in ovarian and endometrial clear-cell adenocarcinomas and nonneoplastic endometrium. Hum Pathol 2007;38:1074–80.

31. Hristov AC, Young RH, Vang R, et al. Ovarian metastases of appendiceal tumors with goblet cell carcinoidlike and signet ring cell patterns: a report of 30 cases. Am J Surg Pathol 2007;31: 1502–11.

32. Ronnett BM, Kurman RJ, Shmookler BM, et al. The morphologic spectrum of ovarian metastases of appendiceal adenocarcinomas: a clinicopathologic

and immunohistochemical analysis of tumors often misinterpreted as primary ovarian tumors or metastatic tumors from other gastrointestinal sites. Am J Surg Pathol 1997;21:1144–55.

33. Cuatrecasas M, Matias-Guiu X, Prat J. Synchronous mucinous tumors of the appendix and the ovary associated with pseudomyxoma peritonei: a clinicopathologic study of six cases with comparative analysis of c-Ki-ras mutations. Am J Surg Pathol 1996;20:739–46.

34. Prayson RA, Hart WR, Petras RE. Pseudomyxoma peritonei: a clinicopathologic study of 19 cases with emphasis on site of origin and nature of associated ovarian tumors. Am J Surg Pathol 1994;18: 591–603.

35. Young RH, Gilks CB, Scully RE. Mucinous tumors of the appendix associated with mucinous tumors of the ovary and pseudomyxoma peritonei: a clinicopathologic analysis of 22 cases supporting an origin in the appendix. Am J Surg Pathol 1991;15: 415–29.

36. Kahn MA, Demopoulos RI. Mucinous ovarian tumors with pseudomyxoma peritonei: a clinicopathologic study. Int J Gynecol Pathol 1992;11:15–23.

37. Ronnett BM, Kurman RJ, Zahn CM, et al. Pseudomyxoma peritonei in women: a clinicopathologic analysis of 30 cases with emphasis on site of origin, prognosis and relationship to ovarian mucinous tumors of low malignant potential. Hum Pathol 1995;56:509–24.

38. Ronnett BM, Yan H, Kurman RJ, et al. Patients with pseudomyxoma peritonei associated with disseminated peritoneal adenomucinosis have a significantly more favourable prognosis than patients with peritoneal mucinous carcinomatosis. Cancer 2001;92:85–91.

39. Ronnett BM, Zahn CM, Kurman RJ, et al. Disseminated peritoneal adenomucinosis and peritoneal mucinous carcinomatosis: a cliniocpathologic analysis of 109 cases with emphasis on distinguishing pathologic features, site of origin, prognosis and relationship to "pseudomyxoma peritonei". Am J Surg Pathol 1995;19:1390–408.

40. Pai RK, Longacre TA. Appendiceal mucinous tumors and pseudomyxoma peritonei: histologic features, diagnostic problems, and proposed classification. Adv Anat Pathol 2005;12:291–311.

41. Misdraji J, Young RH. Primary epithelial neoplasms and other epithelial lesions of the appendix (excluding carcinoid tumors). Semin Diagn Pathol 2004;21:120–33.

42. Misdraji J, Yantiss RK, Graeme-Cook FM, et al. Appendiceal mucinous neoplasms: a clinicopathologic analysis of 107 cases. Am J Surg Pathol 2003;27:1089–113.

43. Guerrieri C, Franlund B, Boeryd B. Expression of cytokeratin 7 in simultaneous mucinous tumors of

the ovary and appendix. Mod Pathol 1995;8:
573–6.

44. Ronnett BM, Shmookler BM, Diener-West M, et al. Immunohistochemical evidence supporting the appendiceal origin of pseudomyxoma peritonei in women. Int J Gynecol Pathol 1997;16:1–9.

45. Szych C, Staebler A, Connolly DC, et al. Molecular genetic evidence supporting the clonality and appendiceal origin of pseudomyxoma peritonei in women. Am J Pathol 1999;154:1849–55.

46. Chuaqui RF, Zhuang Z, Emmert-Buck MR, et al. Genetic analysis of synchronous mucinous tumors of the ovary and appendix. Hum Pathol 1996;27:165–71.

47. Ronnett BM, Seidman JD. Mucinous tumors arising in ovarian mature cystic teratomas. Relationship to the clinical syndrome of pseudomyxoma peritonei. Am J Surg Pathol 2003;27:650–7.

48. Pranesh N, Menasce LP, Wilson MS, et al. Pseudomyxoma peritonei: unusual origin from an ovarian mature cystic teratoma. J Clin Pathol 2005;58:1115–7.

49. Hwang JH, So KA, Modi G, et al. Borderline-like mucinous tumor arising in mature cystic teratoma of the ovary associated with pseudomyxoma peritonei. Int J Gynecol Pathol 2009;28:376–80.

50. Tang LH, Shia J, Soslow RA. Pathologic classification and clinical behavior of the spectrum of goblet cell carcinoid tumors of the appendix. Am J Surg Pathol 2008;32:1429–33.

51. Van Eeeden S, Offerhaus GJ, Hart AA, et al. Goblet cell carcinoid of the appendix: a specific type of carcinoma. Histopathology 2008;52:770–1.

52. Kiyokawa T, Young RH, Scully RE. Krukenberg tumors of the ovary: a clinicopathologic analysis of 120 cases with emphasis on their variable pathologic manifestations. Am J Surg Pathol 2006;30:277–99.

53. Bullon A, Arseneau J, Prat J, et al. Tubular Krukenberg tumor. A problem in histopathologic diagnosis. Am J Surg Pathol 1981;5:225–32.

54. Lerwill MF, Young RH. Ovarian metastases of intestinal-type gastric carcinoma: a clinicopathologic study of 4 cases with contrasting features to those of the Krukenberg tumor. Am J Surg Pathol 2006;30:1382–8.

55. Joshi VV. Primary Krukenberg tumor of ovary. Review of literature and case report. Cancer 1968;22:1199–207.

56. Vang R, Bague S, Tavassoli FA, et al. Signet-ring stromal tumor of the ovary: clinicopathologic analysis and comparison with Krukenberg tumor. Int J Gynecol Pathol 2004;23:45–51.

57. Dickersin GR, Young RH, Scully RE. Signet-ring stromal and related tumors of the ovary. Ultrastruct Pathol 1995;19:401–19.

58. Struewing JP, Hartge P, Wacholder S, et al. The risk of cancer associated with specific mutations of BRCA1 and BRCA2 among Ashkenazi Jews. N Engl J Med 1997;336:1401–8.

59. Curtin JP, Barakat RR, Hoskins WJ. Ovarian disease in women with breast cancer. Obstet Gynecol 1994;84:449–52.

60. Gagnon Y, Tetu B. Ovarian metastases of breast carcinoma. A clinico-pathologic study of 59 cases. Cancer 1989;64:892–8.

61. Young RH, Carey RW, Robboy SJ. Breast cancer masquerading as primary ovarian neoplasm. Cancer 1981;48:210–2.

62. Monteagudo C, Merino MJ, Laporte N, et al. Value of gross cystic disease fluid protein – 15 in distinguishing metastatic breast carcinomas among poorly differentiated neoplasms involving the ovary. Hum Pathol 1991;22:368–72.

63. Onuma K, Dabbs DJ, Bhargava R. Mammaglobin expression in the female genital tract: immunohistochemical analysis in benign and neoplastic endocervix and endometrium. Int J Gynecol Pathol 2008;27:418–25.

64. Bhargava R, Beriwal S, Dabbs DJ. Mammaglobin vs GCDFP-15: an immunohistochemical validation survey for sensitivity and specificity. Am J Clin Pathol 2007;127:103–13.

65. Tornos C, Soslow R, Chen S, et al. Expression of WT1, CA125, and GCDFP-15 as useful markers in the differential diagnosis of primary ovarian carcinomas versus metastatic breast cancer to the ovary. Am J Surg Pathol 2005;29:1482–9.

66. Nonaka D, Chiriboga L, Soslow RA. Expression of pax8 as a useful marker in distinguishing ovarian carcinomas from mammary carcinomas. Am J Surg Pathol 2008;32:1566–71.

67. Chivukula M, Dabbs DJ, O'Connor S, et al. PAX2: a novel Mullerian marker for serous papillary carcinomas to differentiate from micropapillary breast carcinoma. Int J Gynecol Pathol 2009;28:570–8.

68. Young RH, Hart WR. Metastases from carcinomas of the pancreas simulating primary mucinous tumors of the ovary: a report of seven cases. Am J Surg Pathol 1989;13:748–56.

69. Ji H, Isacson C, Seidman JD, et al. Cytokeratins 7 and 20, Dpc4 and MUC5AC in the distinction of metastatic mucinous carcinomas in the ovary from primary ovarian mucinous carcinomas: Dpc4 assists in identifying metastatic pancreatic carcinomas. Int J Gynecol Pathol 2002;21:391–400.

70. Goldstein NS, Bassi D, Uzieblo A. WT1 is an integral component of an antibody panel to distinguish pancreaticobiliary and some ovarian epithelial neoplasms. Am J Clin Pathol 2001;116:246–52.

71. Vakiani E, Young RH, Carcangiu ML, et al. Acinar cell carcinoma of the pancreas metastatic to the

ovary: a report of 4 cases. Am J Surg Pathol 2008; 32:1540–5.

72. Young RH, Scully RE. Ovarian metastases from carcinoma of the gallbladder and extrahepatic bile ducts simulating primary tumors of the ovary: a report of six cases. Int J Gynecol Pathol 1990;9: 60–72.

73. Khunamornpong S, Siriaunkgul S, Suprasert P, et al. Intrahepatic cholangiocarcinoma metastatic to the ovary: a report of 16 cases of an underemphasized form of secondary tumor in the ovary thatmaymimic primaryneoplasia.AmJSurgPathol2007;31:1788–99.

74. Khunamornpong S, Lerwill MF, Siriaunkgul S, et al. Carcinoma of extrahepatic bile ducts and gall-bladder metastatic to the ovary: a report of 16 cases. Int J Gynecol Pathol 2008;27:366–79.

75. Young RH, Gersell DJ, Clement PB, et al. Hepato-cellular carcinoma metastatic to the ovary: a report of three cases discovered during life with discus-sion of the differential diagnosis of hepatoid tumors of the ovary. Hum Pathol 1992;23:574–80.

76. Green LK, Silva EG. Hepatoblastoma in an adult with metastasis to the ovaries. Am J Clin Pathol 1989;92:110–5.

77. Pitman MB, Triratanachat S, Young RH, et al. Hepa-tocyte paraffin 1 antibody does not distinguish primary ovarian tumors with hepatoid differentiation from metastatic hepatocellular carcinoma. Int J Gy-necol Pathol 2004;23:58–64.

78. Young RH, Hart WR. Renal cell carcinoma meta-static to the ovary: a report of three cases empha-sizing possible confusion with ovarian clear cell adenocarcinoma. Int J Gynecol Pathol 1992;11: 96–104.

79. Cameron RI, Ashe P, O'Rourke DM, et al. A panel of immunohistochemical stains assists in the distinc-tion between ovarian and renal clear cell carci-noma. Int J Gynecol Pathol 2003;3:272–6.

80. Nolan LP, Heatley MK. The value of immunocyto-chemistry in distinguishing between clear cell carcinoma of the kidney and ovary. Int J Gynecol Pathol 2001;2(0):155–9.

81. Langer C, Ratschek M, Rehak P, et al. Steroid hormone receptor expression in renal cell carci-noma: immunohistochemical analysis of 182 tumours. J Urol 2004;171:611–4.

82. Young RH, Scully RE. Urothelial and ovarian carci-nomas of identical cell types: problems in interpre-tation. A report of three cases and review of the literature. Int J Gynecol Pathol 1988;7:197–211.

83. Eichhorn JH, Young RH. Transitional cell carcinoma of the ovary: a morphologic study of 100 cases with emphasis on differential diagnosis. Am J Surg Pathol 2004;28:453–63.

84. Irving JA, Vasques DR, McGuinness TB, et al. Kru-kenberg tumor of renal pelvic origin: report of a case with selected commentson ovarian tumors

metastatic from the urinary tract. Int J Gynecol Pathol 2006;25:147–50.

85. Soslow RA, Rouse RV, Hendrickson MR, et al. Tran-sitional cell neoplasms of the ovary and urinary bladder: a comparative immunohistochemical analysis. Int J Gynecol Pathol 1996;15:257–65.

86. Logani S, Oliva E, Amin MB, et al. Immunoprofile of ovarian tumors with putative transitional cell (uro-thelial) differentiation using novel urothelial markers: histogenetic and diagnostic implications. Am J Surg Pathol 2003;27:1434–41.

87. Ordonez NG. Transitional cell carcinoma of the ovary and bladder are immunophenotypically different. Histopathology 2000;36:433–8.

88. Riedel L, Czernobilsky B, Lifschitz-Mercer B, et al. Brenner tumors but not transitional cell carcinomas of the ovary show urothelial differentiation: immuno-histochemical staining of urothelial markers, including cytokeratins and uroplakins. Virchows Arch 2001;435:181–91.

89. Liao XY, Xue WC, Shen DH, et al. p63 expression in ovarian tumors: a marker for Brenner tumours but not transitional cell carcinomas. Histopathology 2007;51:477–83.

90. Irving JA, Young RH. Lung carcinoma metastatic to the ovary: a clinicopathologic study of 32 cases emphasizing their morphologic spectrum and problems in differential diagnosis. Am J Surg Pathol 2005;29:997–1006.

91. Kubba LA, McCluggage WG, Liu J, et al. Thyroid transcription factor-1 expression in ovarian epithe-lial neoplasms. Mod Pathol 2008;21:485–90.

92. Siami K, McCluggage WG, Ordonez NG, et al. Thyroid transcription factor-1 expression in endo-metrial and endocervical adenocarcinomas. Am J Surg Pathol 2007;31:1759–63.

93. Niu HL, Pasha TL, Pawel BR, et al. Thyroid tran-scription factor-1 expression in normal gynecologic tissues and its potential significance. Int J Gynecol Pathol 2009;28:301–7.

94. McCluggage WG, Sargent A, Bailey A, et al. Large cell neuroendocrine carcinoma of the uterine cervix exhibiting TTF1 immunoreactivity. Histopathology 2007;15:405–7.

95. Prat J, Matias-Guiu X, Barreto J. Simultaneous carcinoma involving the endometrium and the ovary. A clinicopathologic, immunohistochemical and DNA flow cytometric study of 18 cases. Cancer 1991;65:2455–9.

96. Zaino R, Whitney C, Brady MF, et al. Simultaneously detected endometrial and ovarian carcinoma: a prospective clinicopathologic study of 74 cases: a gynecologic oncology group study. Gynecol On-col 2001;83:355–62.

97. Sheu BC, Lin HH, Chen CK, et al. Synchronous primary carcinomas of the endometrium and ovary. Int J Gynaecol Obstet 1995;51:141–6.

98. Pearl ML, Johnston CM, Frank TS, et al. Synchronous dual primary ovarian and endometrioid carcinoma. Int J Gynaecol Obstet 1993;43:305–12.

99. Ayhan A, Yalcin OT, Tuncer ZS, et al. Synchronous primary malignancies of the female genital tract. Eur J Obstet Gynecol Reprod Biol 1992;45:63–6.

100. Montoya F, Martin M, Schneider J, et al. Simultaneous appearance of ovarian and endometrial carcinoma: a therapeutic challenge. Eur J Gynaecol Oncol 1989;10:135–9.

101. Ulbright TM, Roth LM. Metastatic and independent cancers of the endometrium and ovary: a clinicopathologic study of 34 cases. Hum Pathol 1985;16:28–34.

102. Zaino RJ, Unger ER, Whitney C. Synchronous carcinomas of the uterine corpus and ovary. Gynecol Oncol 1984;19:329–35.

103. Hendrickson M, Ross J, Eifel P, et al. Uterine papillary serous carcinoma. A highly malignant form of endometrial adenocarcinoma. Am J Surg Pathol 1982;6:93–108.

104. Ambros RA, Sherman ME, Zahn CM, et al. Endometrial intraepithelial carcinoma: distinctive lesion specifically associated with tumors displaying serous differentiation. Hum Pathol 1995;26:1260–7.

105. Wheeler DT, Bell KA, Kurman RJ, et al. Minimal uterine serous carcinoma: diagnosis and clinicopathologic correlation. Am J Surg Pathol 2000;24:797–806.

106. McCluggage WG, Sumathi VP, McManus DT. Uterine serous carcinoma and endometrial intraepithelial carcinoma arising in endometrial polyps: report of five cases including two associated with tamoxifen therapy. Hum Pathol 2003;34:939–43.

107. Silva EG, Jenkins R. Serous carcinoma in endometrial polyps. Mod Pathol 1990;3:120–8.

108. Goldstein NS, Uzieblo A. WT-1 immunoreactivity in uterine papillary serous carcinomas is different from ovarian serous carcinomas. Am J Clin Pathol 2002;117:541–5.

109. Al-Hussaini M, Stockman A, Foster H, et al. WT-1 assists in distinguishing ovarian from uterine serous carcinoma and in distinguishing between serous and endometrioid ovarian carcinoma. Histopathology 2004;44:109–15.

110. McCluggage WG. WT1 is of value in ascertaining the site of origin of serous carcinomas within the female genital tract. Int J Gynecol Pathol 2004;23:97–9.

111. Egan JA, Ionescu MC, Eapen E, et al. Can analysis of p53 and WT1 assist in distinguishing uterine serous carcinoma from uterine endometrioid carcinoma? Int J Gynecol Pathol 2004;23:119–22.

112. Euscher ED, Malpica A, Deavers MT, et al. Differential expression of WT-1 in serous carcinomas in the peritoneum with or without associated serous carcinoma in endometrial polyps. Am J Surg Pathol 2005;29:1074–8.

113. Hirschowitz L, Ganesan R, McCluggage WG. WT1, p53 and hormone receptor expression in uterine serous carcinoma. Histopathology 2009;55:478–82.

114. Jarboe EA, Miron A, Carlson JW, et al. Coexisting intraepithelial serous carcinomas of the endometrium and fallopian tube: frequency and potential significance. Int J Gynecol Pathol 2009;28:308–15.

115. Matias-Guiu X, Lagarda H, Catasus L, et al. Clonality analysis in synchronous or metachronous tumors of the female genital tract. Int J Gynecol Pathol 2002;21:205–11.

116. Shenson DL, Gallion HH, Powell DE, et al. Loss of heterozygosity and genomic instability in synchronous endometrioid tumors of the ovary and endometrium. Cancer 1995;4:650–7.

117. Moreno-Bueno G, Gamallo C, Perez-Gallego C, et al. beta-catenin expression pattern, beta-catenin gene mutations and microsatellite instability in endometrioid ovarian carcinomas and synchronous endometrial carcinomas. Diagn Mol Pathol 2001;10:116–22.

118. Fujita M, Enomoto T, Wada H, et al. Application of clonal analysis. Differential diagnosis for synchronous primary ovarian and endometrial cancers and metastatic cancer. Am J Clin Pathol 1996;105:350–9.

119. Emmert-Buck MR, Chuaqui R, Zhuang Z, et al. Molecular analysis of synchronous uterine and ovarian endometrioid tumors. Int J Gynecol Pathol 1997;16:143–8.

120. Lin WM, Forgacs E, Warshal DP, et al. Loss of heterozygosity and mutational analysis of the PTEN/MMAC1 gene in synchronous endometrial and ovarian carcinomas. Clin Cancer Res 1998;4:2577–83.

121. Brinkmann D, Ryan A, Ayhan A, et al. A molecular genetic and statistical approach for the diagnosis of dual-site cancers. J Natl Cancer Inst 2004;96:1441–6.

122. Baergen RN, Warren CP, Isacson C, et al. Early uterine serous carcinoma: clonal origin of extra-uterine disease. Int J Gynecol Pathol 2001;20:214–9.

123. Pins MR, Young RH, Crum CP, et al. Cervical squamous carcinoma in situ with intraepithelial extension to the upper genital tract and invasion of tubes and ovaries: report of a case with human papillomavirus analysis. Int J Gynecol Pathol 1997;16:272–8.

124. McGrady BJ, Sloan JM, Lamki H, et al. Bilateral ovarian cysts with squamous intraepithelial neoplasia. Int J Gynecol Pathol 1993;12:350–4.

125. Sworn MJ, Jones H, Letchworth AT, et al. Squamous intraepithelial neoplasia in an ovarian cyst, cervical intraepithelial neoplasia and human papillomavirus. Hum Pathol 1995;26:344–7.

126. LiVolsi VA, Merino MJ, Schwartz PE. Coexistent endocervical adenocarcinoma and mucinous adenocarcinoma of ovary: a clinicopathologic study of four cases. Int J Gynecol Pathol 1983;1:391–402.

127. Costa J. Peutz-Jeghers syndrome: case presentation. Obstet Gynecol 1977;50:15–7.

128. Young RH, Scully RE. Mucinous tumors of the ovary associated with mucinous adenocarcinomas of the cervix: a clinicopathologic analysis of 16 cases. Int J Gynecol Pathol 1988;7:99–111.

129. Ronnett BM, Yemelyanova AV, Vang R, et al. Endocervical adenocarcinomas with ovarian metastases: analysis of 29 cases with emphasis on minimally invasive cervical tumors and the ability of the metastases to simulate primary ovarian neoplasms. Am J Surg Pathol 2008;32:1835–53.

130. Elishaev E, Gilks CB, Miller D, et al. Synchronous and metachronous endocervical and ovarian neoplasms: evidence supporting interpretation of the ovarian neoplasms as metastatic endocervical adenocarcinomas simulating primary ovarian surface epithelial neoplasms. Am J Surg Pathol 2005;29:281–94.

131. Houghton O, Jamison J, Wilson R, et al. p16 immunoreactivity in unusual types of cervical adenocarcinoma does not reflect human papillomavirus infection. Histopathology 2010;57:342–50.

132. Vang R, Gown AM, Farinola M, et al. p16 expression in primary ovarian mucinous and endometrioid tumors and metastatic adenocarcinomas in the ovary: utility for identification of metastatic HPV-related endocervical adenocarcinomas. Am J Surg Pathol 2007;31:653–63.

133. Phillips V, Kelly P, McCluggage WG. Increased p16 expression in high grade serous and undifferentiated carcinoma compared with other morphologic types of ovarian carcinoma. Int J Gynecol Pathol 2009;28:179–86.

134. O'Neill CJ, McBride HA, Connolly LE, et al. High grade ovarian serous carcinoma exhibits significantly higher p16 expression than low grade serous carcinoma and serous borderline tumour. Histopathology 2007;50:773–9.

135. Young RH, Scully RE. Malignant melanoma metastatic to the ovary: a clinicopathologic analysis of 20 cases. Am J Surg Pathol 1991;15:849–60.

136. Gupta D, Deavers MT, Silva EG, et al. Malignant melanoma involving the ovary: a clinicopathologic and immunohistochemical study of 23 cases. Am J Surg Pathol 2004;28:771–80.

137. Davis GL. Malignant melanoma arising in mature ovarian cystic teratoma (dermoid cyst). Report of two cases and literature analysis. Int J Gynecol Pathol 1996;15:356–62.

138. McCluggage WG, Bissonnette JP, Young RH. Primary malignant melanoma of the ovary: a report of 9 definite or probable cases with emphasis on their morphologic diversity and mimicry of other primary and secondary ovarian neoplasms. Int J Gynecol Pathol 2006;25:321–9.

139. Young RH, Scully RE. Differential diagnosis of ovarian tumors based primarily on their patterns and cell types. Semin Diagn Pathol 2001;18:161–235.

140. McCluggage WG. Ovarian neoplasms composed of small round cells: a review. Adv Anat Pathol 2004;11:238–96.

141. Stewart CJ, Nandini CL, Richmond JA. Value of A103 (melan-A) immunostaining in the differential diagnosis of ovarian sex cord stromal tumours. J Clin Pathol 2000;53:206–11.

142. Deavers MT, Malpica A, Ordonez NG, et al. Ovarian steroid cell tumors: an immunohistochemical study including a comparison of calretinin with inhibin. Int J Gynecol Pathol 2003;22:162–7.

143. Robboy SJ, Scully RE, Norris HJ. Carcinoid metastatic to the ovary. A clinicopathologic analysis of 35 cases. Cancer 1974;33:798–811.

144. Erickson LA, Papouchado B, Dimashkieh H, et al. Cdx2 as a marker for neuroendocrine tumors of unknown primary sites. Endocr Pathol 2004;15:247–52.

145. Jaffee IM, Rahmani M, Singhal MG, et al. Expression of the intestinal transcription factor CDX2 in carcinoid tumors is a marker of midgut origin. Arch Pathol Lab Med 2006;130:1522–6.

146. Oliveira AM, Tazelaar HD, Myers JL, et al. Thyroid transcription factor-1 distinguishes metastatic pulmonary from well-differentiated neuroendocrine tumors of other sites. Am J Surg Pathol 2001;25:815–9.

147. Rabban JT, Lerwill MF, McCluggage WG, et al. Primary ovarian carcinoid tumors may express CDX-2: a potential pitfall in distinction from metastatic intestinal carcinoid tumors involving the ovary. Int J Gynecol Pathol 2009;28:41–8.

148. Bloss JD, Liao S, Buller RE, et al. Extraovarian peritoneal serous papillary carcinoma: a case-control retrospective comparison to papillary adenocarcinoma of the ovary. Gynecol Oncol 1993;50:347–51.

149. Clement PB, Young RH, Scully RE. Malignant mesotheliomas presenting as ovarian masses. A report of nine cases, including two primary ovarian mesotheliomas. Am J Surg Pathol 1996;20:1067–80.

150. Kerrigan SA, Tumnir RT, Clement PB, et al. Diffuse malignant epithelial mesotheliomas of the peritoneum in women: a clinicopathologic study of 25 cases. Cancer 2002;94:378–85.

151. Baker PM, Clement PB, Young RH. Malignant peritoneal mesotheliomas in women. A study of 75 cases with emphasis on their morphologic spectrum and differential diagnosis. Am J Clin Pathol 2005;123:724–37.

152. Attanoos RL, Webb R, Dojcinov SP, et al. Value of mesothelial and epithelial antibodies in distinguishing diffuse peritoneal mesothelioma in females from serous papillary carcinoma of the ovary and peritoneum. Histopathology 2002;40:237–44.

153. Comin CE, Saieva C, Messerini L. h-caldesmon, calretinin, estrogen receptor, and Ber-EP4: a useful combination of immunohistochemical markers for differentiating epithelioid peritoneal mesothelioma from serous papillary carcinoma of the ovary. Am J Surg Pathol 2007;31:1139–48.

154. Ordonez NG. Desmoplastic small round cell tumor I: a histopathologic study of 39 cases with emphasis on unusual histological patterns. Am J Surg Pathol 1998;22:1303–13.

155. Young RH, Eichhorn JH, Dickersin GR, et al. Ovarian involvement by the intra-abdominal desmoplastic small round cell tumor with divergent differentiation: a report of three cases. Hum Pathol 1992;23:454–64.

156. Elhajj M, Mazurka J, Daga D. Desmoplatic small round cell tumor presenting in the ovaries: report of a case and review of the literature. Int J Gynecol Cancer 2002;12:760–3.

157. Ordonez NG. Desmoplastic small round cell tumor II: an ultrastructural and immunohistochemical study with emphasis on new immunohistochemical markers. Am J Surg Pathol 1998;22:1314–27.

158. McCluggage WG, Oliva E, Connolly LE, et al. An immunohistochemical analysis of ovarian small cell carcinoma of hypercalcemic type. Int J Gynecol Pathol 2004;23:330–6.

159. McCluggage WG. WT-1 immunohistochemical expression in small round blue cell tumours. Histopathology 2008;52:631–2.

160. Gerald WL, Ladanyi M, Alava ED, et al. Clinical, pathologic and molecular spectrum of tumors associated with t(11;22) (p13; q12): desmoplastic small round cell tumor and its variants. J Clin Oncol 1998;16:3028–36.

161. Murphy AJ, Bishop K, Pereira C, et al. A new molecular variant of desmoplastic small round cell tumor: significance of WT1 staining in this entity. Hum Pathol 2008;12:1763–70.

162. Young RH, Jackson A, Wells M. Ovarian metastasis from thyroid carcinoma twelve years after partial thyroidectomy mimicking struma ovarii: report of a case. Int J Gynecol Pathol 1994;13:181–5.

163. Irving JA, Lerwill MF, Young RH. Gastrointestinal stromal tumors metastatic to the ovary: a report of five cases. Am J Surg Pathol 2005;29:920–6.

164. Young RH, Scully RE. Sarcomas metastatic to the ovary. A report of 21 cases. Int J Gynecol Pathol 1990;9:231–52.

165. McCluggage WG, Ganesan R, Herrington CS. Endometrial stromal sarcomas with extensive endometrioid glandular differentiation: report of a series with emphasis on the potential for misdiagnosis and discussion of the differential diagnosis. Histopathology 2009;54:365–73.

166. McCluggage WG, Sumathi VP, Maxwell P. CD10 is a sensitive and diagnostically useful immunohistochemical marker of normal endometrial stroma and of endometrial stromal neoplasms. Histopathology 2001;39:273–8.

167. Young RH, Prat J, Scully RE. Cancer. Endometrioid stromal sarcomas of the ovary. A clinicopathologic analysis of 23 cases. Cancer 1984;53:1143–55.

BENIGN AND LOW GRADE SEROUS EPITHELIAL TUMORS: RECENT DEVELOPMENTS AND DIAGNOSTIC PROBLEMS

Teri A. Longacre, MD

KEYWORDS

- Serous low malignant potential • Serous borderline • Serous low-grade carcinoma
- Serous micropapillary • Serous cribriform • Stromal microinvasion • Psammocarcinoma

ABSTRACT

Despite considerable controversy surrounding serous tumors of low malignant potential (S-LMP) or borderline tumors, there have been great strides in our understanding of the serous group of borderline and malignant pelvic epithelial neoplasms in the past decade. Most S-LMP have a favorable prognosis, but recurrences and progression to carcinoma occur, sometimes following a protracted clinical course. Pathologic risk factors covary, but the extraovarian implant status is the most important predictor for progressive disease. Progression of S-LMP usually takes the form of low-grade serous carcinoma, although transformation to high-grade carcinoma is occasionally seen. A pelvic S-LMP – low-grade serous carcinoma pathway has been proposed based on global gene expression profiling, shared mutations in KRAS or BRAF, and in most cases, the presence of S-LMP in low-grade serous carcinoma. Unlike high-grade serous carcinoma, low-grade serous carcinoma responds poorly to standard platinum-based chemotherapy. Development of more tailored therapy for S-LMP with invasive implants and low-grade serous carcinoma, ideally based on a relative risk model for disease progression is under active clinical investigation.

OVERVIEW

Tumors with serous differentiation are characterized by epithelial cells resembling the ciliated epithelial cells of the fallopian tube. These tumors encompass a group of three biologically distinct entities: serous adenoma; serous tumor of low malignant potential (S-LMP) or serous borderline tumor; and serous carcinoma (**Table 1**). The serous tumors at the benign and low grade malignant end of the spectrum recapitulate the typical tubal type histology more closely than those at the high grade malignant end of the spectrum. In addition, the low-grade tumors exhibit similar molecular features that are distinct from those seen in high-grade serous carcinomas. Mutations in BRAF and KRAS and activation of the MAP2 kinase pathway are common in S-LMP and low-grade serous carcinoma, whereas p53 mutations occur in the high-grade tumors. The overall degree of chromosomal instability is also much higher in

---

This discussion focuses on recent advances in the area of low-grade ovarian serous neoplasia with emphasis on key diagnostic criteria, differential diagnosis, and disease classification based on current understanding of low-grade serous carcinogenesis.

Department of Pathology, Stanford University School of Medicine, Stanford University, Room L235, 300 Pasteur Drive, Stanford, CA 94305, USA

E-mail address: longacre@stanford.edu

Surgical Pathology 4 (2011) 331–373
doi:10.1016/j.path.2010.12.011

Serous Adenoma: Key Points

1. Predominantly cystic (cystadenoma), solid and cystic (cystadenofibroma), or predominantly solid (adenofibroma). Must be greater than 1 cm

2. Polypoid excrescences, formed by collagenous or edematous stroma, may be prominent

3. Papillae, if present, are simple and nonbranching

4. Simple, nonstratified tubal-type epithelial lining composed of secretory and ciliated cells

5. Mitotic figures rare or absent

6. Nuclear atypia absent or mild at most

7. Psammoma bodies may be present

high-grade serous carcinomas than in the low-grade serous tumor group. Serous epithelial neoplasms commonly present in the ovaries, but primary presentation and/or involvement of fallopian tube and peritoneum also occurs.

SEROUS CYSTADENOMA (CYSTADENOFIBROMA, ADENOFIBROMA)

Overview

Benign serous tumors (cystadenoma, cystadenofibroma, adenofibroma) comprise 50% of all serous

Table 1
Classification of serous surface epithelial-stromal tumors (modified from World Health Organization)

Benign (cystadenoma, cystadenofibroma, adenofibroma) with focal proliferation	50%
Borderline (low malignant potential) with micropapillary features with stromal microinvasion with intraepithelial carcinoma with microinvasive carcinoma	15%
Malignant (adenocarcinoma, cystadenocarcinoma) low grade high grade	35%

Data from Lee KR, Tavassoli FA, Prat J, et al. Tumours of the ovary and peritoneum. In: Tavassoli FA, Devillee P, editors. Tumours of the breast and female genital organs. Lyon (France): IARC Press; 2003. p. 119–24.

ovarian neoplasms and almost 20% of all surface epithelial-stromal neoplasms of the ovary. They are confined to the ovary and occur in a wide age range, most commonly during the reproductive years.[1]

Gross Features

Serous cystadenomas range from 1 to 10 cm, and may occasionally attain the size of mucinous cystadenomas (15 to 30 cm). Most are unilocular, but multilocular tumors may be seen. The lining of the cysts are either entirely smooth or contain firm papillary, endophytic or exophytic projections. The cyst contents consist of clear fluid, but may be thick and slightly mucoid, resembling the contents of a mucinous tumor. Hemorrhage and necrosis are absent, unless torsion, secondary infection, or other complication has occurred. Serous cystadenofibromas are similar to cystadenomas, but contain foci of prominent fibromatous stroma. Adenofibromas are firm, white tumors containing small cysts or glands, with or without secondary firm papillary projections.

Microscopic Features

Benign serous tumors are composed of epithelium that recapitulates that seen in the fallopian tube. Ciliated cells are often prominent, but are not required. Cytologic atypia is absent. Psammoma bodies may be present in the adenofibromas, but are usually not seen in the predominantly cystic tumors. Mitotic figures are rare or absent. Papillary projections (**Fig. 1**), when present, are composed of dense fibrous stroma and lined by a simple layer of nonstratified epithelium (**Fig. 2**). Focal areas of serous epithelial proliferation similar to that seen in serous tumor of low malignant potential may be present, but should not exceed 10% of the tumor volume; these tumors are designated *serous tumor with focal proliferation*.

Diagnosis and Differential Diagnosis

Serous cystadenomas are lined by benign cuboidal or columnar ciliated epithelium resembling the epithelial lining of the fallopian tube. Polypoid excrescences, which may be quite prominent, are composed of fibrotic or edematous stroma with minimal epithelial stratification. Mitotic figures are sparse. Psammoma bodies may be present.

The only clinically significant differential diagnostic decision is between a benign serous tumor and a *serous tumor of low malignant potential (S-LMP)*. The distinction is based on extent of epithelial proliferation. S-LMP features more prominent branching papillary structures, epithelial stratification, and tufting with detached

Fig. 1. Serous cystadenofibroma. Broad, papillary projections are predominantly non-branching and lined by a simple layer of nonstratified epithelium overlying dense fibrous stroma.

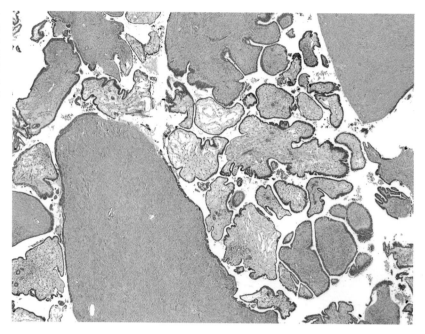

epithelial cell clusters. The cells in S-LMP often show mild cytologic atypia. In contrast to serous cystadenomas, occasional mitotic figures may be seen in S-LMP. This distinction is discussed more fully in the section on S-LMP below.

Rete ovarii and *serous epithelial inclusion cyst* may be mistaken for a benign serous tumor, but neither is of significant clinical consequence if misdiagnosed. Rete ovarii (**Fig. 3**) and rete cysts occur in the hilum (although extension into the medulla is not uncommon) and the latter is commonly associated with smooth muscle. Serous inclusion cysts are small (1 cm or smaller) and scattered within the ovarian cortical stroma (**Fig. 4**), whereas the

Fig. 2. Serous cystadenofibroma. Serous-type epithelium recapitulates the epithelium in the fallopian tube and is characterized by ciliated columnar cells with eosinophilic cytoplasm. The epithelium in benign serous cysts is nonstratified.

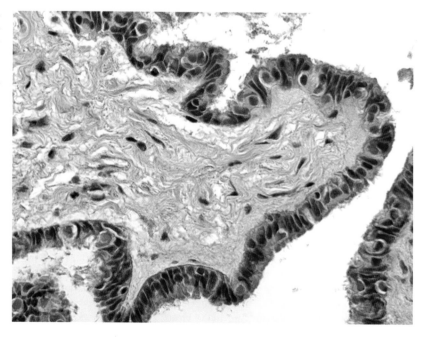

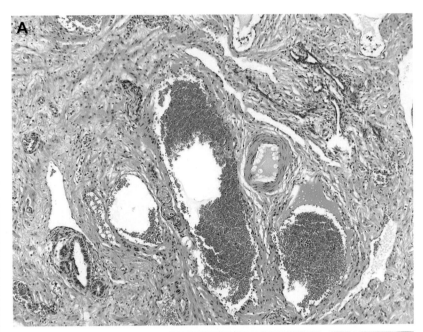

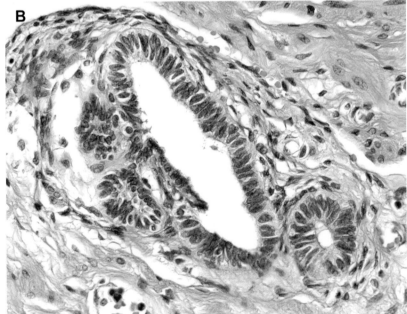

Fig. 3. (*A*) The rete ovarii is recognized by its characteristic hilar location, but extension into the medulla is not uncommon. (*B*) The ovarian homolog of the rete testis, the rete ovarii is formed by anastomosing clefts and tubules lined by columnar or low cuboidal epithelium.

small cystic and glandular structures in serous adenofibroma are embedded within dense fibromatous stroma.[1]

Struma ovarii may form a large cyst with small papillary projections, but colloid is usually present within the smaller follicular structures; immunostaining for TTF1 and thyroglobulin confirms thyroid differentiation (**Fig. 5**). Rare struma ovarii demonstrate recurrent behavior, but these would not be histologically confused with serous cystadenoma.

Occasionally, serous tumors can secrete material resembling that seen in a *mucinous epithelial neoplasm*, but the constituent cells of serous tumors do not contain intracytoplasmic mucin on mucin stains (PAS/diastase or mucicarmine). Stromal-poor *endometriosis* is distinguished by the presence of hemorrhage, hemosiderin, or the

Fig. 4. Ovarian glandular inclusions are commonly lined by tubal-type ciliated serous epithelium. They are typically scattered within the cortical region and distinguished from serous cystadenoma or cystadenofibroma on the basis of size (≤1 cm).

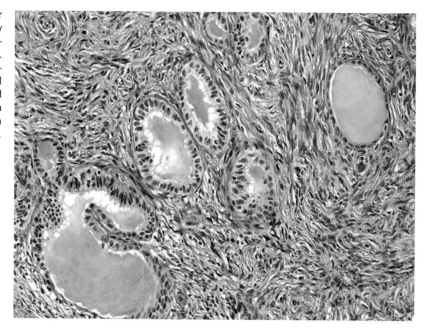

Serous Adenoma: Differential Diagnosis

Serous tumor of low malignant potential (S-LMP) (epithelial proliferation)

Struma ovarii (thyroglobulin and TTF1 positive)

Serous epithelial inclusion cyst (randomly distributed, not mass-forming)

Rete ovarii (hilar location)

Mucinous cystadenoma (intracytoplasmic mucin)

Endometriosis (endometrioid glands and stroma)

Serous Adenoma: Pitfalls

! Follicular cysts may mimic serous epithelial cysts when the lining granulosa cells assume a cuboidal appearance, but thecal cells are present in the outer cyst wall of follicular cysts.

---

demonstration of additional foci exhibiting characteristic endometrioid glands and stroma.

Prognosis

Serous cystadenoma is clinically benign and does not recur if completely excised.

SEROUS TUMOR OF LOW MALIGNANT POTENTIAL (BORDERLINE TUMOR)

Overview

S-LMP comprise approximately 15% of all ovarian serous neoplasms and account for the vast

---

S-LMP: Key Points

1. Hierarchical branching papillae

2. Clear or slightly eosinophilic granular cytoplasm

3. Mild to moderate nuclear atypia may be present

4. Mitotic figures sparse; no atypical mitotic figures

5. Psammoma bodies often present

6. Cellular tufting and stratification

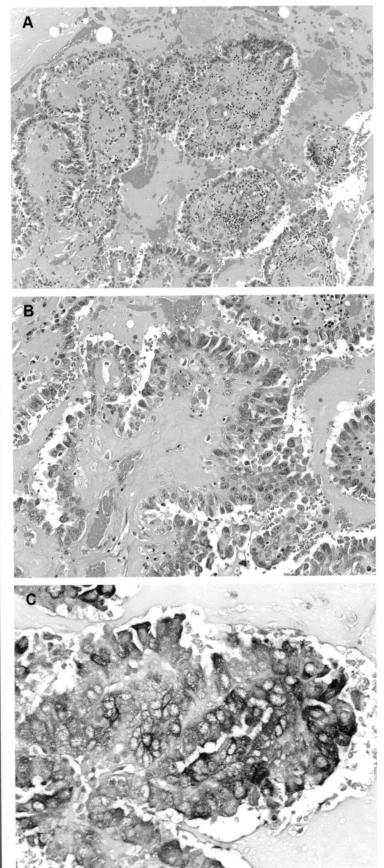

Fig. 5. Struma ovarii. (*A*) Papillary struma may be misdiagnosed as a serous epithelial tumor, either benign, borderline or carcinoma, depending on the degree of cytologic atypia that is present. (*B*) Mild cellular stratification with exfoliation into the cyst lumen further simulates a serous epithelial neoplasm in this example of papillary struma. However, ciliated cells are absent. (*C*) Immunstain for thyroglobulin confirms thyroid differentiation.

S-LMP: Differential Diagnosis

Serous cystadenoma (lacking epithelial proliferation, stratification, and tufting)

Low-grade serous carcinoma (stromal invasion present)

Papillary clear cell carcinoma (characteristic papillary architecture, associated endometriosis, round nuclei with nucleoli, cuboidal cell shape)

Localized, well differentiated papillary mesothelioma (calretinin positive)

Mucinous tumor of low malignant potential, endocervical-like (mixture of cell types)

Sertoli-Leydig cell tumor, retiform variant (inhibin and calretinin expression)

Granulosa cell tumor with pseudopapillary pattern (inhibin and calretinin expression)

S-LMP: Pitfalls

! Low-grade serous carcinoma is often associated with S-LMP; tumors with increased mitotic figures, increased cytologic atypia, or extensive cribriform and/or micropapllary architecture should be adequately sampling to exclude foci of carcinoma, especially if high stage.

! Stromal microinvasion in S-LMP may be multifocal, simulating low-grade serous carcinoma, but diffuse, widely invasive stromal involvement is absent.

Microscopic Features

S-LMP are composed of architecturally complex branching papillary and micropapillary structures not unlike that of low-grade serous carcinoma, but they do not feature destructive invasion of the ovarian stroma (**Fig. 7**). The nuclei are uniform or mildly atypical and mitotic activity is low. Atypical mitotic figures are absent. The constituent cells often exhibit a heterogeneous or polymorphous appearance due to the presence of columnar cells, pink cells, and ciliated cells with cellular stratification and tufting (detachment of pink cells into gland or cyst lumens) (**Fig. 8**). Psammoma bodies are often present, but are not diagnostic. Numerous psammoma bodies should prompt consideration for serous psammocarcinoma (see below).

MICROPAPILLARY ARCHITECTURE IN S-LMP: DEFINITION AND SIGNIFICANCE

Approximately 5 to 10% of all S-LMP contain foci of significant micropapillary architecture, defined

majority of all borderline surface epithelial-stromal neoplasms. S-LMP has the capacity for extra-ovarian spread, recurrence and progression to low-grade serous carcinoma, but even then the tempo of disease is significantly more indolent than high-grade serous carcinoma.

The molecular profile of mRNA gene expression patterns is significantly different for S-LMP and low-grade serous carcinoma versus high-grade serous carcinoma,[2,3] as is the pattern of genetic alterations, eg, the presence of point mutations in *BRAF* or *KRAS* is more frequently associated with S-LMP and low-grade serous carcinoma, while *p53* mutation and somatic or germline abnormalities in *BRCA1* and/or *BRCA2* are more frequently associated with high-grade serous carcinoma.[4–8] Low-grade serous carcinoma occurs at a slightly younger age than high-grade serous carcinoma (mean, 45 years vs 60 years), and often presents with disease beyond the confines of the ovary. Younger women may present with infertility.

Gross Features

S-LMP is more often bilateral and larger than benign serous tumors. These tumors are predominately cystic with variable amounts of papillary epithelial projections, or solid with surface papillary excrescences (or a combination thereof) (**Fig. 6**). Necrosis is not typically present, but may occur secondary to torsion and/or infarction.

Micropapillary S-LMP: Key Points

1. Non-hierarchical branching papillae

2. Papillae are x5 long as wide and at least 5 mm in continuous linear extent

3. Usually monomorphous cell population

4. Mild to moderate nuclear atypia

5. Often surface involvement and bilateral

6. Implants may be invasive (sample well)

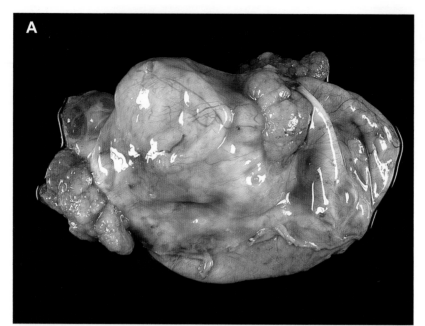

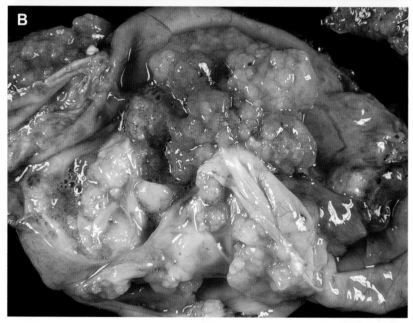

Fig. 6. S-LMP (serous borderline tumor). (*A*) The exterior surface of this partially deflated S-LMP cyst is punctuated by surface papillary excrescences. (*B*) Inner cyst lining contains similar excrescences, which may appear confluent. The cyst contents may be watery, frothy, or thick and mucoid in S-LMP.

as nonhierarchical branching of slender, elongated papillae that are at least five times as long as they are wide (**Fig. 9**).[9] A second, less common form of this variant consists of a sieve-like cribriform pattern (**Fig. 10**). In most cases, the constituent cells in this pattern of S-LMP exhibit a more uniform, hyperchromatic and monomorphous appearance than typical S-LMP. Pink cells, ciliated cells and tufting are not as frequent in tumors exhibiting a micropapillary growth pattern. Also, the degree of cytologic atypia may be slightly higher than that which is typically seen in S-LMP (see **Fig. 9**). The nuclei may be slightly irregular and usually contain small nucleoli. The degree of atypia

Fig. 7. Usual S-LMP with characteristic hierarchical, branching papillae.

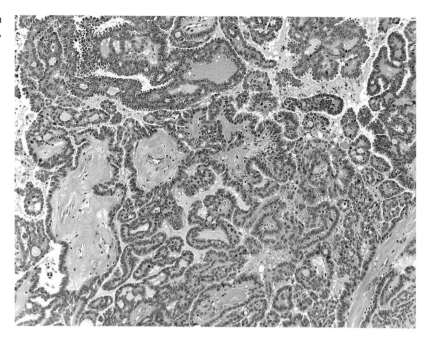

seen in many micropapillary S-LMP tumors is similar to that seen in low-grade serous carcinoma and psammocarcinoma (see below). Mitotic figures are present, but are not atypical and usually not significantly increased over that in the typical S-LMP. By definition, the micropapillary or cribriform elements must occupy a continuous 5-mm linear extent in the S-LMP to be designated as a micropapillary variant.[10]

The micropapillary variant of S-LMP is more frequently associated with bilateral ovarian involvement, the presence of exophytic ovarian

Fig. 8. S-LMP. Ciliated and eosinophilic cells line the papillae in a stratified fashion, often "falling off" into the cyst lumen. Atypia is minimal. Note paucity of mitotic figures.

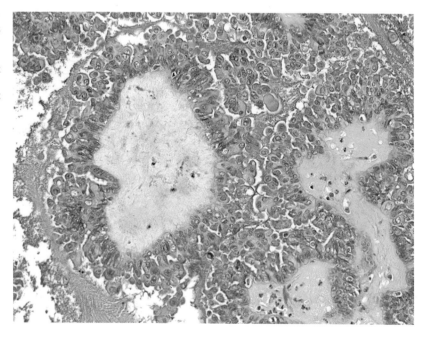

340

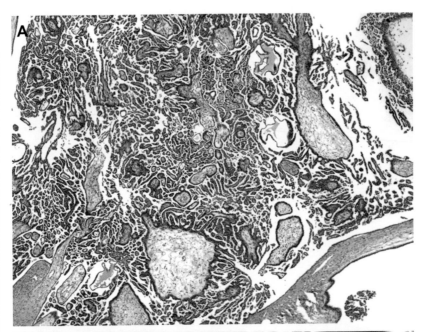

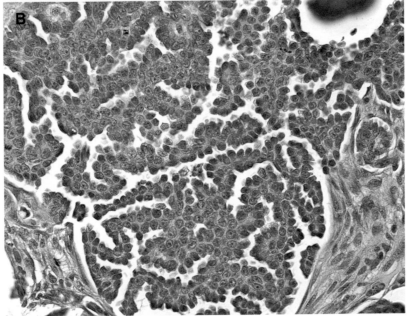

Fig. 9. Micropapillary S-LMP. (*A*) The papillae are elongated with uniform diameter from base to tip (so-called non-hierarchical branching). (*B*) The cells in micropapillary S-LMP tend to be more monomorphic and basophilic with more atypia than in the usual S-LMP.

△△ *Micropapillary S-LMP: Differential Diagnosis*
Low-grade serous carcinoma (stromal invasion present)
Serous tumor of low malignant potential (hierarchical branching present)
Clear cell carcinoma
Malignant mesothelioma (invasive; calretinin positive)

! *Micropapillary S-LMP: Pitfalls*
! The classification of micropapillary architecture is subjective; to achieve greater reproducibility for this diagnosis, a serous tumor should be designated as "micropapillary" only when the involved papillae are at least 5 times as long as they are wide *and* they encompass at least 5 mm in continuous linear extent.

Fig. 10. Cribriform S-LMP is characterized by broad papillae lined by serous-type epithelium arranged to form rounded spaces in a cribriform pattern. The constituent cells are often monomorphic and more basophilic than those in the usual S-LMP.

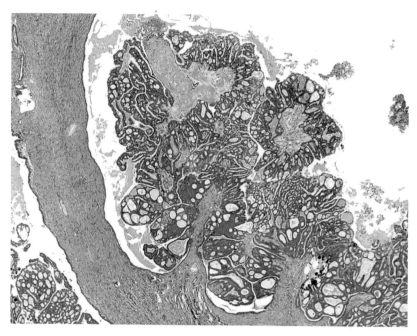

surface involvement and the presence of extra-ovarian implants. In some series, the micropapillary variant has also been more frequently associated with invasive implants; the poorer survival observed in earlier studies of micropapillary S-LMP has been attributed to the presence of invasive implants rather than to the micropapillary features in the ovarian neoplasm.[11–15] In 2004, a consensus workshop on serous tumors of the ovary concluded that micropapillary serous tumors should remain classified as S-LMP, but should be clearly distinguished from the typical type of S-LMP due to their distinctive clinicopathologic features at presentation.[16] In accordance with the WHO recommendations, serous tumors with micropapillary architecture but no stromal invasion should be designated as "S-LMP (or serous borderline tumor) with micropapillary features."[17] Although most such tumors exhibit diffuse micropapillary features, the extent of micropapillary architecture present in the ovarian tumor (eg, 15%, 40%, etc) should be specified in the comment section of the pathology report.[16]

STROMAL MICROINVASION IN S-LMP: DEFINITION AND SIGNIFICANCE

Approximately 10 to 15% of S-LMP feature stromal-epithelial patterns that resemble stromal invasion in other organ systems, but do not elicit a significant destructive stromal response.[18–20] Five patterns of stromal microinvasion have been described: individual eosinophilic cells and cell clusters (so-called "classic" microinvasion)[21] (**Figs. 11** and **12**); simple and non-complex branching papillae (**Fig. 13**); inverted macropapillae (**Fig. 14**); cribriform glands (**Fig. 15**); and micropapillae.[19] The classic pattern of microinvasion is the most common (but may be subtle and therefore often missed on initial microscopic examination, see **Fig. 12**), followed by simple papillary and inverted macropapillary patterns. Often, several patterns are present, particularly single cells, cell clusters and simple papillae. Cribriform and complex branching or micropapillary patterns of stromal microinvasion are very uncommon and their presence should warrant additional sectioning to exclude larger, definitive foci of invasive serous carcinoma (**Fig. 16**). Classic microinvasion occurs disproportionally in patients presenting with S-LMP during pregnancy, usually with low stage disease, and does not appear to be associated with any risk of progression in that setting. Unlike the classic pattern of stromal microinvasion, the presence of intrastromal elongated and/or complex branching micropapillae, with or without background micropapillary ovarian histology, may represent a comparatively higher risk lesion, particularly when multiple foci featuring this pattern of microinvasion are present in the primary ovarian tumor.[19]

The extent of the stromal invasion, in terms of number of discrete foci or presence of a diffuse

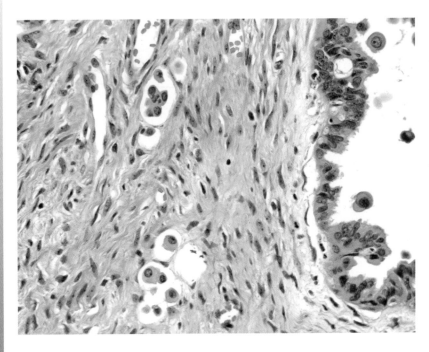

Fig. 11. Classic stromal microinvasion. Individual eosinophilic cells and small cell clusters are surrounded by a cleft-like space within the stroma of the papilla of this S-LMP. Similar appearing eosinophilic cells are seen detaching from the lining of the papilla at the right.

pattern is highly variable between S-LMP tumors. The WHO criteria for S-LMP require that individual foci of stromal microinvasion must not exceed 5 mm in linear extent or 10 mm² in area, but there is currently no published study with clinical follow-up to support a diagnosis of carcinoma in cases having histologic patterns acceptable for microinvasion, but measuring greater than 5 mm (or 10 mm²).[17] The foci may be diffusely scattered throughout the tumor and still qualify as microinvasion, provided they do not exceed the size limitations. Discrete foci are not summed. With the exception of the micropapillary and cribriform patterns, it is probably not important to separately

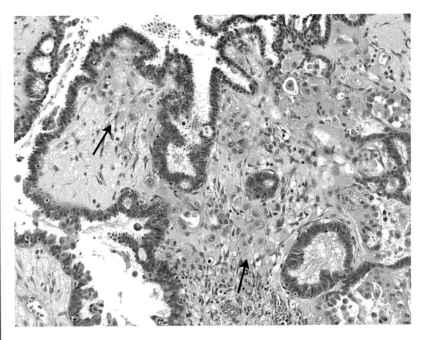

Fig. 12. Stromal microinvason can be subtle and easily overlooked in some cases due to the mergence of the pink cells with the surrounding pink, fibrous stroma (see *arrows*).

Fig. 13. Stromal microinvason may also feature simple, non-branching papillae within cleft-like spaces. Note admixed single cells and cell clusters (classic stromal microinvasion pattern).

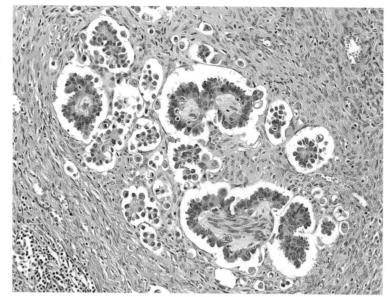

Fig. 14. A less common stromal microinvasion pattern features larger papillae surrounded by cleft-like spaces (so-called inverted macropapillae).

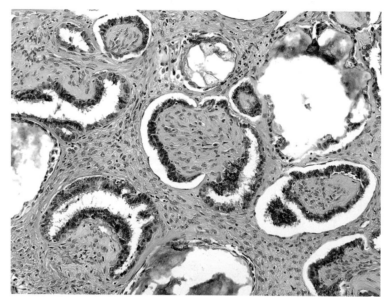

Fig. 15. Very rarely, stromal microinvasion may exhibit a cribriform pattern; tumors with this pattern should be carefully examined with additional sections to exclude larger foci of invasion, as this pattern is more commonly seen in invasive low-grade serous carcinoma.

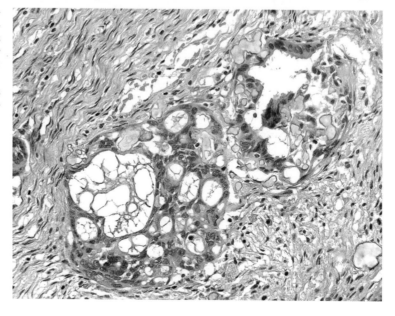

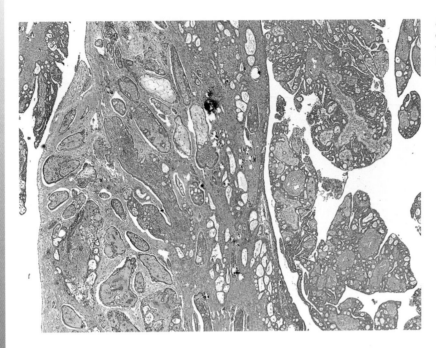

Fig. 16. Low-grade serous carcinoma with cribriform patten of stromal invasion.

identify individual patterns of stromal microinvasion in the pathology report.

Two patients with S-LMP in the Stanford series had foci of contiguous stromal invasion (classic pattern) measuring more than 5 mm in greatest linear dimension (7 and 12 mm) that would have precluded a diagnosis of S-LMP by WHO criteria, yet both were alive with no evidence of disease recurrence at last follow-up.[19] Although these data question the current quantitative criterion that would exclude a diagnosis of S-LMP based on size measurement alone, the presence of

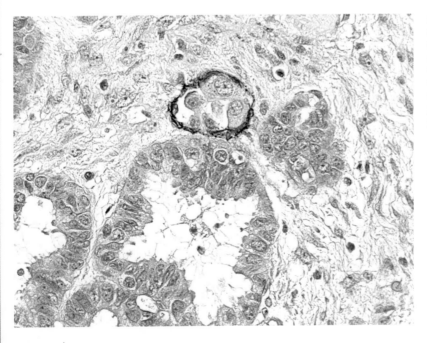

Fig. 17. D2–40 immunostain outlines lymphatic channel in this example of classic stromal microinvasion. Stromal microinvasion is associated with lymphatic invasion (LVSI) in up to two-thirds of S-LMP.

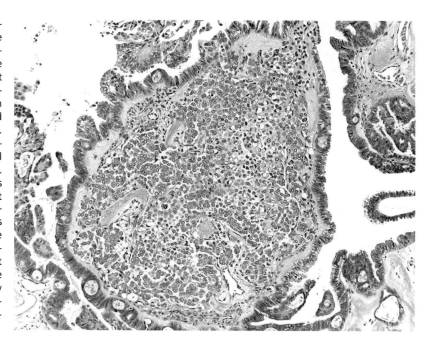

Fig. 18. Microinvasive serous carcinoma. The stroma in this papilla is extensively replaced by the presence of a confluent infiltration of monotonous epithelial cells with scanty cytoplasm and atypical, basophilic nuclei. The distinctive eosinophilia of classic stromal microinvasion is absent. When measuring less than 5 mm in linear extent (or 10 mm^2), the term "microinvasive carcinoma" is applied to such foci. The significance of this finding is unknown, but tumors harboring these foci should be carefully evaluated for the presence of invasive low-grade serous carcinoma.

discrete aggregates of stromal-epithelial patterns of microinvasion measuring more than 5 mm in an otherwise typical S-LMP is relatively uncommon. Until more data are available, caution should be exercised when small foci of cribriform, micropapillary, or inverted macropapillary patterns are encountered in an S-LMP. At the very least, the pathologist should ensure that the tumor has been well sampled and level sections of all suspicious areas featuring these architectural patterns of stromal micorinvasion should be performed to exclude an occult, larger focus of invasion. Because of the uncertainty regarding prognosis with these particular patterns, their presence should be separately identified in the pathology report with a specific comment concerning size and extent of involvement.

Although the literature has long held that patients with S-LMP containing foci of "stromal microinvasion" have a clinical outcome that is indistinguishable from patients with non-microinvasive S-LMP, it is likely that stromal microinvasion represents an early stage of destructive stromal invasion that has a very small, but statistically significant risk for disease progression. Therefore, the presence, extent, and type of microinvasion (eg, micropapillary, macropapillary, or cribriform) should be documented in the pathology report for all cases exhibiting non-standard forms of stromal microinvasion with a comment that this finding may place the patient

at a slightly increased risk for disease recurrence; long term follow up is warranted.

The presence of lymphatic vascular invasion (LVI) may be seen in up to 60% of S-LMP with microinvasion (**Fig. 17**). The presence of LVI in this setting is independent of age, stage, primary ovarian histology, and implant status and does not appear to confer a poorer prognosis.

Rarely, S-LMP contain foci of microinvasive carcinoma, which are distinguished from stromal microinvasion by the presence of destructive invasion of ovarian stroma by cytologically malignant cells (**Fig. 18**). The clinical significance of this finding is unknown. Like stromal microinvasion, such foci must not exceed 5 mm in linear extent or 10 mm^2 in area to qualify as microinvasive carcinoma.

"MINIMAL S-LMP": THE CONCEPT OF FOCAL PROLIFERATION

By definition, serous tumors with focal borderline change (<10% volume) in an otherwise benign tumor are designated serous cystadenoma (or cystadenofibroma) with focal proliferation.[17] Such tumors are considered to be benign with no risk for recurrence or disease progression; however, few studies have specifically examined serous tumors with focal proliferation. Since many patients with this finding do not undergo staging procedures, little is known about the incidence of serous disease elsewhere in the abdomen. In our experience, it is not altogether uncommon for patients with S-LMP in one ovary to have findings consistent with focal proliferation in the opposite ovary. Similarly, reproductive aged women with focal proliferation who have been treated by cystectomy have, on occasion subsequently developed an additional focal proliferative tumor or S-LMP in the ipsilateral or contralateral ovary. Therefore, while tumors with focal proliferation are distinguished from S-LMP, it is likely that serous cysts harboring these foci of proliferation represent a very low risk end of the spectrum of borderline proliferation.

Diagnosis and Differential Diagnosis

The chief differential diagnostic decisions are between benign serous tumor and S-LMP on the one hand and between S-LMP and low-grade serous carcinoma on the other. When the serous histology is ambiguous or other proliferations present histologic appearances that mimic S-LMP, the differential diagnosis is widened to include a variety of other surface epithelial, germ cell, sex cord-stromal, and non-ovarian lesions.

S-LMP is distinguished from *serous cystadenoma* on the basis of epithelial proliferation. In comparison to serous cystadenoma, S-LMP features more prominent papillary structures, epithelial stratification and tufting with detached epithelial cell clusters, mild cytologic atypia and occasional mitotic figures. By (arbitrary) definition, serous tumors featuring 10% or less proliferation of borderline-type are designated as serous tumors with focal proliferation.

The presence of prominent psammomatous calcifications in a low-grade serous epithelial neoplasm should prompt consideration for *serous psammocarcinoma*. Serous psammocarcinoma features cytologic atypia similar to that of low-grade serous carcinoma, but is distinguished from that entity by tumor cell nests containing at least 75% or more psammoma bodies (**Fig. 19**). Unlike S-LMP, stromal invasion is found and peritoneal disease is usually more prominent than ovarian disease in these patients; widespread lymphatic vessel involvement (in the ovary, endometrium, cervix, etc) is not uncommon.

Low-grade serous carcinoma is distinguished from S-LMP by the presence of destructive stromal invasion (>10 mm^2) or confluence of cytologically malignant cells in the stromal component of a predominately fibromatous tumor. This often takes one or more of several histologic patterns that are described in the section addressing low-grade serous carcinoma.

Mucinous borderline tumors endocervical-like (also referred to as seromucinous type) are distinguished from S-LMP by the presence of both serous and mucinous endocervical-like epithelial cells with abundant neutrophils (**Fig. 20**), and more frequent association with endometriosis.

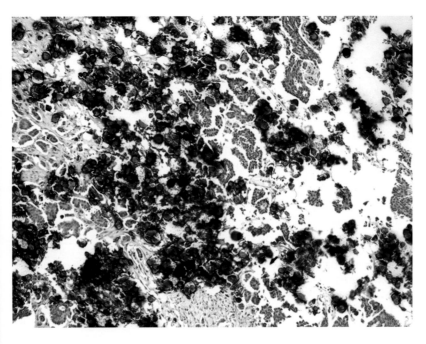

Fig. 19. Serous psammocarcinoma. Invasive nests of serous epithelium are associated with numerous psammoma bodies. Nuclear atypia is similar to that of low-grade serous carcinoma.

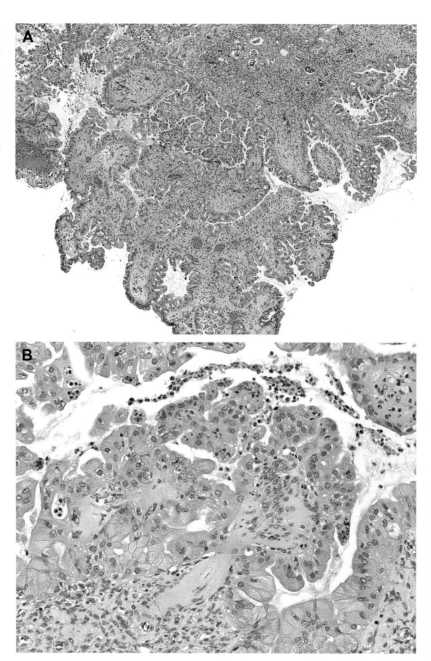

Fig. 20. Mucinous borderline tumor, endocervical-like. (*A*) Low power architecture is similar to S-LMP. (*B*) The papillae are lined by eosinophilic cells with cilia and endocervical-like mucinous epithelium. Note neutrophils within cyst lumen and papillae.

Although these tumors may also be associated with peritoneal implants, no tumor-associated deaths been reported and the prognosis is excellent.

Struma ovarii (thyroid differentiation) with cystic and papillary architecture may resemble S-LMP, but the constituent cells are more uniform in appearance, lack cilia and are immunoreactive for thyroglobulin and TTF1. Rarely, combined S-LMP and struma ovarii can be present.

Sertoli-Leydig cell tumors with retiform pattern exhibit a papillary architecture (**Fig. 21**), but typically

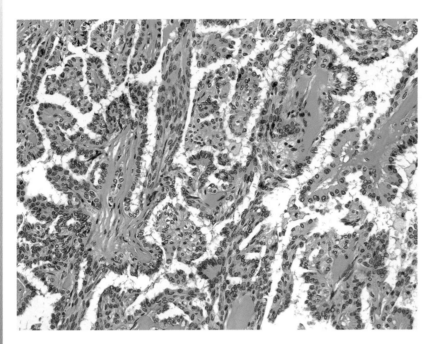

Fig. 21. Sertoli-Leydig cell tumor with retiform elements. The papillae in retiform Sertoli-Leydig cell tumors project into elongate, slitlike spaces and contain stromal cores. Cellular tufting and stratification are typically absent or if present, not nearly as well developed as in usual S-LMP.

also have distinctive features of sex cord-stromal differentiation provided there is adequate tumor sampling. Problematic cases can be resolved by immunohistochemical detection of inhibin and calretenin expression in the sex cord-stromal tumor.

Mesothelial proliferations may mimic a surface ovarian (or extra-ovarian) S-LMP, particularly when they occur in the adnexal region (**Fig. 22**). Most mimics occur within the well differentiated spectrum of papillary mesothelioma. *Localized, well differentiated papillary mesothelioma* presents most commonly in the peritoneum of young women (20 to 30 years of age) and is recognized by the characteristic well developed, minimally branching papillary or tubulopapillary architecture, fibrous connective tissue cores, and uniform, non-stratified cuboidal or low columnar epithelial cell lining (see **Fig 22**). The prognosis for this tumor is good, provided adequate sampling has excluded areas with cytologic atypia, increased mitotic index, or a more architecturally diffuse proliferation; each of which is a feature of diffuse papillary malignant mesothelioma (**Fig. 23**). Similarly, invasion into underlying tissues invalidates the diagnosis of well differentiated papillary mesothelioma. Problematic cases can usually be resolved by immunohistochemistry: strong, positive nuclear staining for calretinin with negative staining for the

epithelial marker Ber-EP4 in mesothelioma and a reversed staining pattern in S-LMP.

Clear cell carcinomas with prominent papillary architecture may be mistaken for S-LMP leading to delayed staging and treatment (**Fig. 24**). The diagnostic confusion arises in part due to occurrence in reproductive aged women and in part due to the low level of mitotic activity present in many clear cell carcinomas.[22] Features most helpful in recognizing papillary clear cell carcinoma are unilateral ovarian disease, non-hierarchical branching of the papillae, a monomorphous cell population, and the presence of more typical clear cell carcinoma patterns elsewhere in the tumor.[22] The presence of endometriosis, although not specific, should also prompt consideration for papillary clear cell carcinoma. In the problematic case, ER and WT1 may be useful adjunctive studies, since S-LMP expresses both markers and clear cell carcinomas often do not.[23,24]

Papillary clear cell cystadenoma may present in the broad ligament, over the ovarian surface, or along the fimbriated margin of the fallopian tube, simulating a primary tubal epithelial neoplasm (**Fig. 25**). This latter tumor occurs predominantly, although not always in patients in Von Hippel-Lindau syndrome and is distinguished from serous tumors by absence of stratification, bland cytology

Fig. 22. Localized well differentiated papillary mesothelioma. (*A*) The papillae are well developed and minimally branching, with papillary or tubulopapillary architecture. (*B*) The presence of uniform, nonstratified flattened or low cuboidal epithelium distinguishes low grade mesothelial proliferations from low grade serous proliferations.

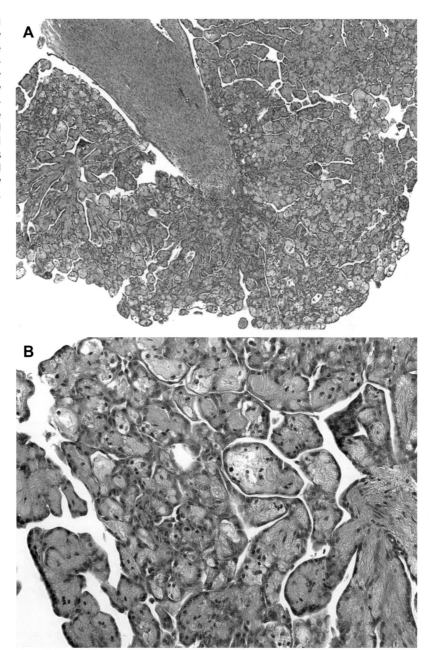

and often, a vacuolated clear cytoplasm in the constituent cells.[25]

Granulosa cell tumors with a prominent pseudo-papillary pattern may simulate epithelial tumors of the ovary with papillary architecture.[26] Although this pattern is a closer mimic of transitional or en-dometrioid differentiation, S-LMP may also enter into the differential diagnosis due to the bland, often monomorphic cytologic features seen in the adult variant (**Fig. 26**). Identification of areas that are more characteristic of granulosa cell tumor and judicious use of immunohistochemistry resolves most cases. It has been suggested that the pseudopapillary pattern in these tumors may

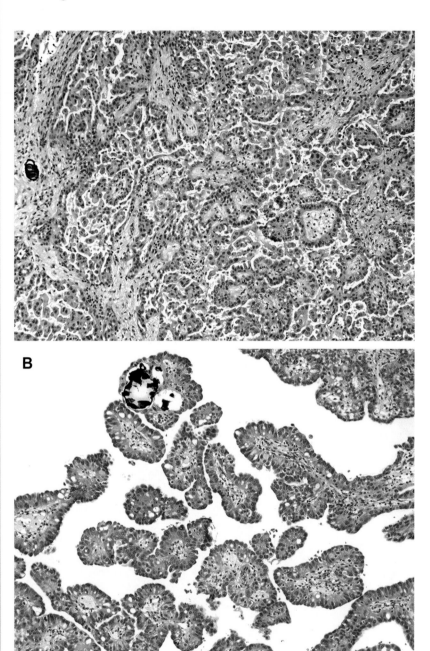

Fig. 23. (*A*) Invasive papillary malignant mesothelioma. Note psammoma body. (*B*) The mesothelial cells are cuboidal or low columnar and show scattered cytoplasmic vacuoles.

Fig. 24. (*A*) Clear cell carcinoma with prominent papillary architecture and relatively monomorphic cell population. (*B*) Scattered hobnail cells are present. Note nuclear hyperchromasia and atypia.

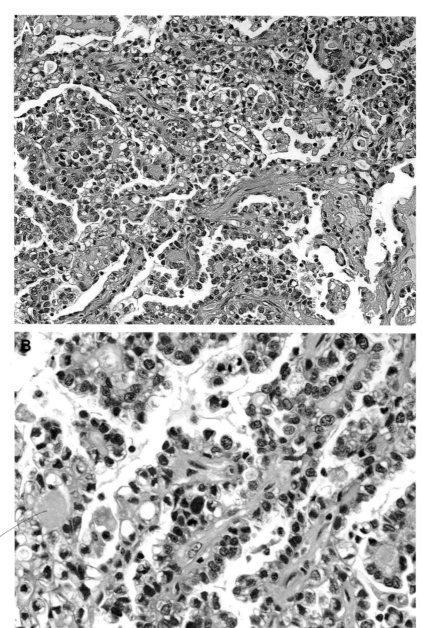

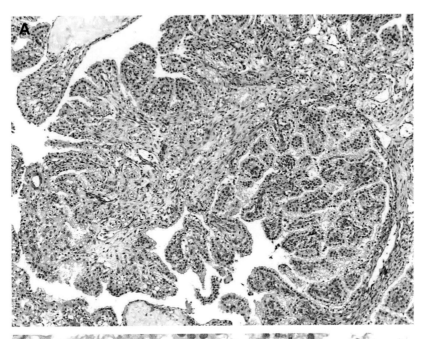

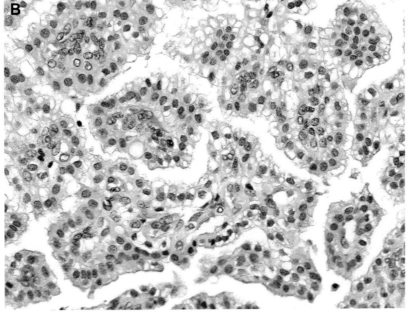

Fig. 25. (*A*) Papillary clear cell cystadenoma in Von Hippel-Lindau syndrome. (*B*) Tubules and papillae are lined by a single layer of low cuboidal cells with clear cytoplasm and uniform, bland nuclei.

Fig. 26. Adult granulosa cell tumor with pseudo-papillary pattern. Small and larger pseudopapillae are lined by a uniform cell population. The cells are stratified and appear to fall off into a cystic cavity similar to S-LMP, but the cytologic features differ (darker nuclear chromatin, grooved nuclei, and monomorphic cell population in granulosa cell tumor).

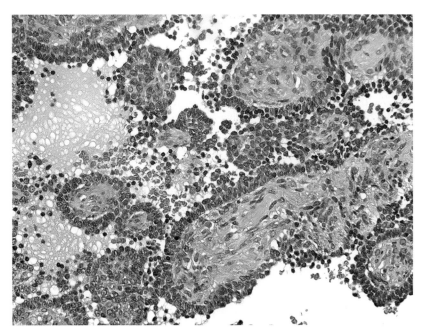

be related to the cystic change that is a feature of many granulosa cell tumors.[26]

PERITONEAL IMPLANTS IN S-LMP: DEFINITION AND SIGNIFICANCE

Approximately 30 to 40% of S-LMP are associated with similar-appearing lesions in the pelvis and intraabdominal sites, including lymph nodes (= high stage disease).[13] These lesions, termed implants, may be microscopic or macroscopic and are subclassified into noninvasive and invasive types, based on the presence of destructive infiltration into underlying normal tissue structures (**Table 2**).[12,13,15,27–31] The distinction is important because S-LMP with invasive implants is associated with significantly more aggressive disease than S-LMP with non-invasive implants. Although the numbers vary somewhat from study to study, approximately 50% of patients with ovarian S-LMP and invasive implants die of disease. In the Stanford series of 276 patients with S-LMP and 5 years or longer follow-up, 45% of patients with invasive implants succumbed to their disease within 10 years of diagnosis.[13]

Noninvasive implants may be primarily epithelial (**Fig. 27**), primarily desmoplastic (**Fig. 28**), or a mixture of epithelial and desmoplastic, depending on the degree of stromal reaction. Both epithelial-type and desmoplastic-type noninvasive implants may be seen over the surface or inner cystic lining of the ovarian tumor (when

desmoplastic, these are often referred to as "autoimplants"[32] (**Fig. 29**) as well as the peritoneum, omentum and lymph nodes. In the omentum, both types may coat the entire surface and/or extend along connective tissue septa, creating the impression of infiltration (both macroscopically and microscopically). However, in all of these cases, the neoplastic cells are confined to pre-existing tissue planes and do not breach the stromal-parenchymal interface (see **Figs. 27** and **28**). The stroma in desmoplastic implants resembles granulation tissue or nodular fasciitis and the gland-to-stroma ratio is low. The constituent epithelium consists of individual papillae, individual cells, and clusters of epithelial cells, as well as branching papillae, and glands with complex papillary infoldings. Often, the epithelial nuclei in desmoplastic implants may appear slightly more atypical than in the primary ovarian tumor, but marked nuclear atypia (marked nuclear hyperchromasia and prominent nucleoli) and numerous mitotic figures are absent.

Invasive implants are defined by the presence of unequivocal irregular, haphazard infiltration into subjacent normal tissue structures (**Fig. 30**); the infiltrating tumor is typically composed of glands with extensive bridging or papillary proliferations, but may be composed of small solid epithelial nests, single pink cells, cell clusters, and in some cases, widely separated, irregular or gaping glandular structures that simulate an invasive low-grade adenocarcinoma.[16] The constituent cells

Table 2
Extraovarian serous epithelial lesions (modified from World Health Organization)

	Diagnostic Features
Noninvasive implants[a]	
Epithelial implants	Smooth interface with underlying/surrounding normal tissue. Implant composed of branching papillae, glands with complex papillary infoldings, and single cell and small cell clusters. Mild to moderate atypia. Minimal or no reactive stroma.
Desmoplastic implants	Smooth interface with underlying/surrounding normal tissue. Implant composed of branching papillae, simple and complex glands with papillary infoldings, and single cell and small cell clusters. Mild to moderate atypia. Edematous, reactive nodular fasciitis-like stroma.
Indeterminate implants[b]	Implants with desmoplastic-type stromal response, but focal encroachment into underlying or adjacent parenchymal tissue, imparting a subtle irregular interface at low power magnification *or* Implants with focal micropapillary architecture but no evidence of infiltration into underlying parenchyma (ie, exhibit a smooth interface) *or* Implants with no evidence of infiltration into underlying parenchyma, but with cytologic atypia that exceeds that of the usual implant (ie, moderate atypia, insufficient to warrant a diagnosis of carcinoma)
Invasive implants[c]	Jagged and irregular interface with underlying/surrounding normal tissue, often entrapping fat lobules in omentum. Typically formed by branching papillae and simple and/or complex glands with papillary and micropapillary infoldings. Abundant epithelial component. Cytologic atypia sufficient to warrant a diagnosis of carcinoma.

[a] Implants should be distinguished from endosalpingiosis (which is a benign process and does not warrant up-staging of an accompanying ovarian S-LMP).
[b] Implants with no attached normal tissue (so-called detached implants) are classified as noninvasive (either epithelial or desmoplastic) provided the atypia is moderate at most (eg, no carcinomatous cytologic atypia) and the architecture is not overly complex (eg, cribriform or florid micropapillary). When *marked* cytologic and architectural atypia is present, the implant should probably be classified as invasive. Implants in which it is difficult to determine whether the interface is smooth and expansile or focally irregular and infiltrative should be classified as indeterminate.
[c] Less than 15% of extraovarian implants are invasive.
Data from Lee KR, Tavassoli FA, Prat J, et al. Tumours of the ovary and peritoneum. In: Tavassoli FA, Devillee P, editors. Tumours of the breast and female genital organs. Lyon (France): IARC Press; 2003. p. 119–24.

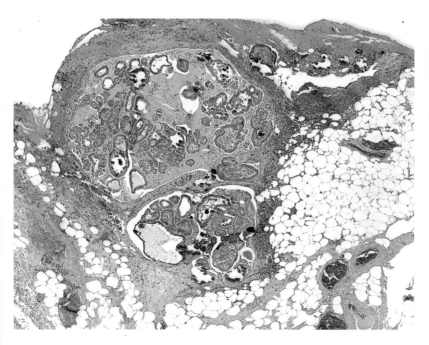

Fig. 27. Noninvasive. S-LMP implant, epithelial type. The epithelial component is similar to S-LMP arising in the ovary and the interface between the implant and underlying omentum is smoothly contoured with no invasion.

Fig. 28. (*A*) Noninvasive S-LMP implant, desmoplastic type is associated with a nodular fasciitis-like or granulation tissue stromal response, but the interface between the implant and underlying omentum is smoothly contoured with no invasion (*see arrows*). Unlike most invasive implants (see **Fig. 30**), the desmoplastic implant is predominantly composed of stroma. (*B*) The epithelial component is similar to S-LMP arising in the ovary.

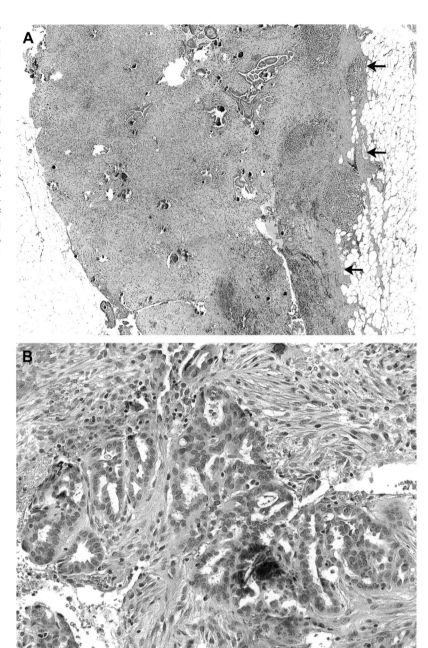

often exhibit a comparatively high nuclear to cytoplasm ratio, nuclear hyperchromasia and prominent nucleoli, resembling the epithelial cells in low-grade serous carcinoma, but the presence of such cells is not required for classification of an implant as invasive. The key criterion for diagnosing invasive implants in S-LMP is destructive *tissue invasion*, which is associated with varying degrees of stromal response.[16]

Sometimes, the surgeon plucks small biopsies from the peritoneal surface that consist entirely of implant tissue with no clear implant-parenchymal interface (**Fig. 31**). As long as these implants do not exhibit marked cytologic atypia (equal to at least the degree that is seen in low-grade serous carcinoma), such implants can be treated as if they were noninvasive implants, because they are not associated with any risk over and above that which is associated with the presence of S-LMP with high stage disease.[18,33]

Using this classification, most implants are noninvasive; only 10 to 15% of implants are

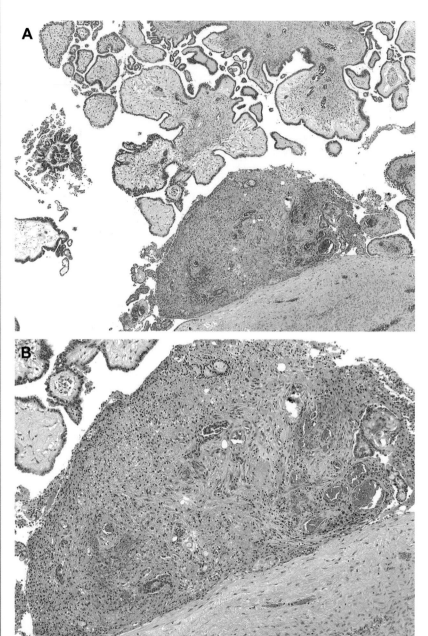

Fig. 29. (*A*) Autoimplant is essentially a desmoplastic implant in the ovary, typically deposited along the edge of a papilla or on the ovarian surface. (*B*) Higher magnification demonstrates predominance of granulation tissue-like stroma.

invasive.[13] Since both desmoplastic-type noninvasive and invasive implants may feature a prominent stromal response, occasional implants may be especially difficult to subclassify. The presence of marked epithelial prominence, often manifested by exuberant micropapillary architecture and significant cytologic atypia, manifested by nuclear hyperchromasia, high nuclear to cytoplasm ratio and increased mitotic figures may help resolve these problematic cases.[34] In absence of these findings,

implants can be classified as indeterminate, in analogy to the classification of dysplasia in the gastrointestinal tract.[13] The most common example of an indeterminate implant is a desmoplastic type implant with focal encroachment into underlying tissue, imparting a subtle irregular interface at low power magnification (**Fig. 32**). Not surprisingly, this indeterminate type of implant accounts for the majority of interobserver disagreement in the classification of S-LMP implants.[35]

Fig. 30. Invasive implant has irregular interface with surrounding omentum and invades underlying tissue. Note epithelial predominance, as opposed to stromal predominance in desmoplastic implant (see **Fig. 28**).

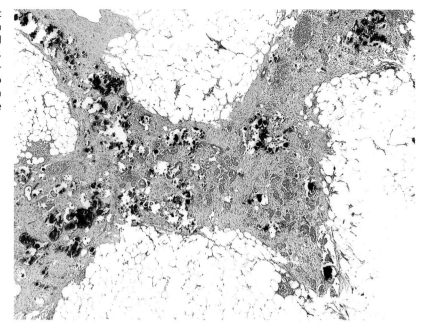

Diagnosis and Differential Diagnosis

Endosalpingiosis, defined as the presence of well-formed glands lined by serous (tubal-type) epithelium does not qualify as an implant, although it is a frequent finding in patients with S-LMP (**Fig. 33**). Endosalpingiosis can rarely contain simple, non-branching papillae protruding into the lumen of the glands (**Fig. 34**); in contrast,

S-LMP implants feature glandular structures with hierarchical branching and tufting of epithelium from papillary cores (see **Fig. 27**).[36]

Mesothelial hyperplasia may be quite prominent in patients with S-LMP, especially when there are extensive psammomatous calcifications distributed over the peritoneum (**Fig. 35**). A papillary architecture may also be present, but the papillae are

Fig. 31. Detached S-LMP implant. In this example, the implant is loosely attached to the uterine serosa. Ease of removal by the surgeon may result in a detached implant. Despite the absence of an interface with adjacent stroma, these implants are operationally similar to noninvasive implants unless they show architectural complexity or marked cytologic atypia.

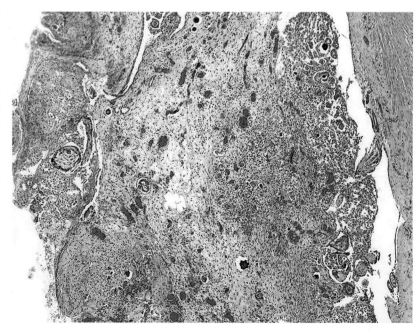

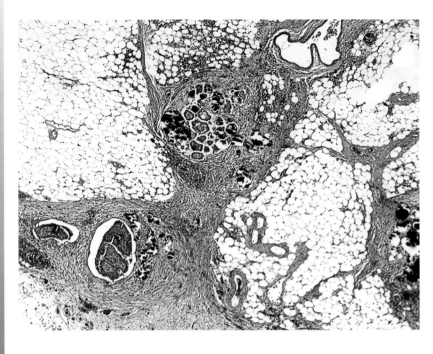

Fig. 32. S-LMP implant indeterminate for invasion. The interface with adjacent omental tissue is slightly irregular, but the implant is composed predominantly of stromal tissue.

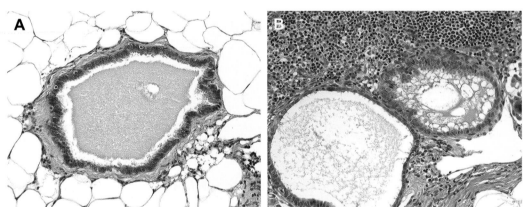

Fig. 33. (*A*) Endosalpingiosis in omentum and (*B*) in lymph node do not qualify as S-LMP implants and do not affect stage. The epithelium is ciliated, nonstratified, and cytologically bland.

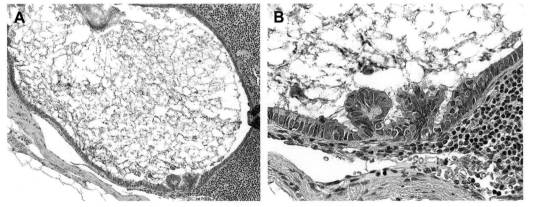

Fig. 34. (*A*) Endosalpingiosis with simple intraluminal projection. (*B*) The intraluminal papilla is insufficiently developed to warrant classification as S-LMP in this lymph node.

Fig. 35. Mesothelial hyperplasia with papillary architecture and psammoma bodies. Mesothelial hyperplasia often has fibroconnective tissue cores and/or tubulopapillary structures oriented in a linear fashion along the peritoneal surface. Psammoma bodies are often present, as are cellular aggregates (*left*).

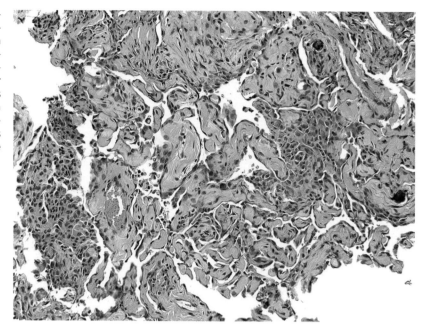

typically nonbranching and lined by a more uniform-appearing population of cuboidal epithelial cells.

LYMPH NODE INVOLVEMENT IN S-LMP: DEFINITION AND SIGNIFICANCE

Lymph node involvement (LNI) is not an independent prognostic factor for patient survival in patients with S-LMP, although approximately 15% of patients with S-LMP will be upstaged by LNI.[37,38] Lymph node involvement by S-LMP occurs in 20 to 30% of patients with S-LMP who undergo lymph node sampling. A variety of histologic patterns have been observed, but single cells, cell clusters, and papillae similar to that seen in typical S-LMP are most common

Fig. 36. Lymph node involvement by S-LMP is typically seen in subcapsular sinus of lymph node.

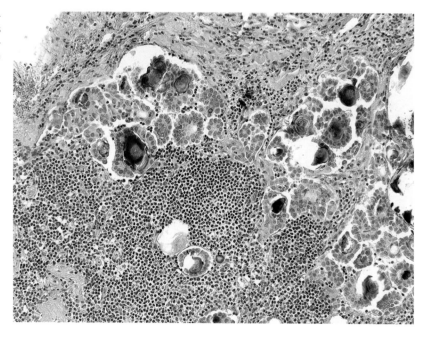

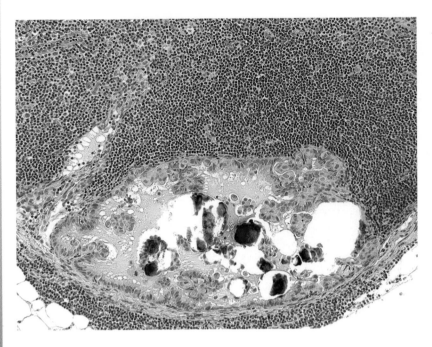

Fig. 37. Intraglandular pattern of lymph node involvement by S-LMP suggests possible development from pre-existing endosalpingiosis.

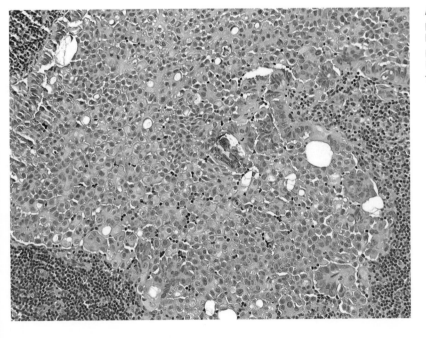

Fig. 38. Diffuse sinus and parenchymal expansion by individual eosinophilic cells in S-LMP. Note abortive papillary form at lower right.

(Fig. 36). Intraglandular (Fig. 37), micropapillary, and diffuse sinus and parenchymal expansion by eosinophilic cells (Fig. 38) also occur.[37] None of these histologic patterns of LNI is predictive of adverse outcome; however, the presence of a discrete, solid (eg, not an enlarged cyst) and confluent (ie, not interrupted by lymphoid cells), nodular aggregate of S-LMP greater than 1 mm within a lymph node is associated with decreased disease-free survival (Fig. 39). Most such cases are associated with a desmoplastic stromal response within the lymph node; often, invasive implants in the peritoneum are also present.[37] In problematic cases, examination of all remaining lymph nodes and peritoneal implants can help to determine whether or not a patient is at increased risk for recurrence.

Diagnosis and Differential Diagnosis

LNI should be distinguished from *endosalpingiosis*. Endosalpingiosis is defined by well-formed glands lined by a single layer of tubal-type epithelium (see

Fig. 33B) that may feature occasional simple, non-branching, and often blunted papillae protruding into the lumen of the gland without cytologic atypia (atypical endosalpingiosis). Any branching papillae or a mixture of papillae and cell clusters with the simple glands qualifies as nodal involvement by S-LMP and should be so classified.

Psammomatous calcifications may occur in pelvic and less commonly, periaortic lymph nodes in association with endosalpingiosis, S-LMP implants, serous carcinoma and mesothelial hyperplasia, as well as an isolated finding. In absence of an associated epithelial lesion, this finding is of no prognostic significance.

Nodal mesothelial cell hyperplasia, consisting of sinus collections of eosinophilic cells may mimic the pink cell pattern of LNI by S-LMP (Fig. 40).[39] Distinguishing features include the presence of other patterns of S-LMP (glands, papillae, etc), expression of BerEP4 in S-LMP, and expression of calretinen in mesothelial cell hyperplasia. Both processes express WT1 and so this marker is of limited utility in this distinction.

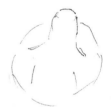

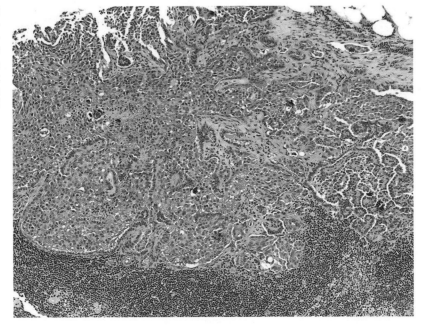

Fig. 39. Invasive implant within lymph node is composed of confluent epithelium uninterrupted by lymphoid tissue, measuring ≥1 mm. A fibroblastic stromal response is often present in invasive nodal implants.

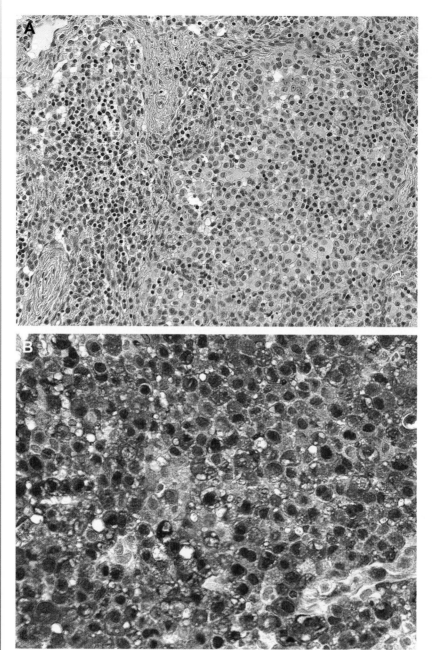

Fig. 40. (*A*) Mesothelial cells in lymph node may mimic lymph node involvement by S-LMP (see **Fig. 38**). (*B*) Calretinin expression confirms mesothelial differentiation in problematic cases.

PERITONEAL WASHINGS IN S-LMP

Positive findings on cytologic examination of ascitic fluid or abdominal/pelvic peritoneal washings may occur in S-LMP and this finding is incorporated in the formal staging. Positive peritoneal cytologic preparations are characterized by papillary aggregates and/or tight clusters of cells with minimal nuclear atypia (**Fig. 41**) and can be difficult to distinguish from benign serous epithelium (endosalpingiosis), reactive mesothelial proliferations, and low-grade serous carcinoma. S-LMP is distinguished from endosalpingiosis by the presence of a more complex papillary architecture, and from mesothelial proliferations on the basis of a heterogeneous mixture of ciliated and pink cells.

Fig. 41. S-LMP in cytologic preparations typically forms small papillary structures and is often associated with psammoma bodies. A definitive diagnosis of S-LMP, psammocarcinoma, or low-grade serous carcinoma requires tissue correlation in most cases.

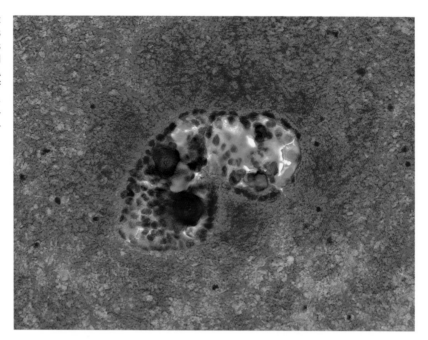

Psammoma bodies may be present, but are not diagnostic as they can be seen in all three lesions. Like mesothelial proliferations, S-LMP express WT1,[24] but unlike mesothelial proliferations, S-LMP also express Ber-EP4, MOC31, and CD15 (Leu-M1). In all cases, interpretation of the washings should be performed in concert with the rest of the surgical staging material and diagnosed accordingly – unless the washings exhibit significantly different cyto-architectural features, a diagnosis of serous carcinoma is misleading in the setting of S-LMP.

S-LMP WITH INTRAEPITHELIAL CARCINOMA

Very rarely, a serous neoplasm with the architecture of a borderline or low malignant potential tumor contains cells with cytologic atypia that is compatible with carcinoma, but no stromal invasion is identified.[1] The appropriate diagnosis for these tumors is S-LMP with intraepithelial carcinoma. However, when faced with such a tumor, additional sections almost always demonstrate marked cellular stratification (essentially sheets of cells) overlying the papillae or foci of destructive invasion, allowing the diagnosis of invasive serous carcinoma. S-LMP with intraepithelial carcinoma is very uncommon and other noninvasive epithelial lesions featuring high grade cytology, (ie, clear cell carcinoma with prominent papillary architecture) should be excluded.

Prognosis of S-LMP

Even in the presence of high stage disease, the disease tempo is characteristically indolent and protracted, often lasting years. Prolonged periods of dormancy and even spontaneous regression may occur. In a meta-analysis of studies S-LMP, disease-specific survival was >95% for patients with low stage (stage I) serous borderline disease and approximately 65% for patients with high stage (stage II–IV) disease.[30] Since late recurrences do occur in patients with S-LMP, and follow-up is limited in many of the studies analyzed, these are conservative estimates of risk of recurrence.[40]

Patients with invasive implants have an increased risk of disease recurrence and progression; survival is significantly worse than with uncomplicated S-LMP (approximately 50% at 10 years).[13] Given the poor survival rate, one could argue that all invasive implants should be regarded as early, low volume low-grade serous carcinoma.

S-LMP offers the potential for fertility sparing surgery, although initial staging surgery is often performed to accurately determine stage and exclude the presence of invasive implants.

Whether or not all patients with S-LMP need to undergo complete surgical staging is controversial. For reproductive aged women, cystectomy followed by oophorectomy on completion of child-bearing is often advised, since recurrences in the ipsilateral or contralateral ovary are high (>30%). Currently, there is no indication for adjuvant chemotherapy or radiation therapy for women with S-LMP who have disease confined to the ovary or non-invasive extraovarian implants. Patients with invasive implants have been treated with aggressive chemotherapy, but the efficacy of such treatment in this subset of patients has not been determined.

TRANSFORMATION TO SEROUS CARCINOMA

Overview

Transformation to low-grade serous carcinoma occurs in at least 7% of women with S-LMP, occasionally decades after initial diagnosis.[13,40] Transformation is associated with increased tempo of disease and a significantly more aggressive disease course with approximately 40%–50% overall survival. In some instances, transformation is preceded by several recurrences of S-LMP, which may or may not exhibit increasing degrees of atypical proliferation. In other cases, the transformation appears at the time of first recurrence.

Most transformations occur in the omentum, followed by intraabdominal or axillary lymph nodes.

Gross Features

Most transformations present as abdominal or pelvic masses. Occasionally, patients present with ascites.

Microscopic Features

Transformation in S-LMP is recognized histologically by the presence of florid epithelial proliferation with increased cytologic atypia in addition to destructive invasion; it is generally easily recognized on the basis of tumor volume and extent of tissue involvement (**Fig. 42**). It could be argued that invasive implants represent an early form of transformation and should also be classified as low-grade serous carcinoma. As currently defined, the distinction between invasive implants and invasive, low-grade serous carcinoma in this setting is admittedly subjective, but is used to convey a distinct, progressive change in the histology of the recurrent tumor compared with the original tumor.

Rarely, S-LMP transforms into high-grade serous carcinoma.[41] This transformation may occur early and is associated with a much more rapid course of disease. Limited studies indicate that in at least some cases, both tumors are derived from the same clone.[42]

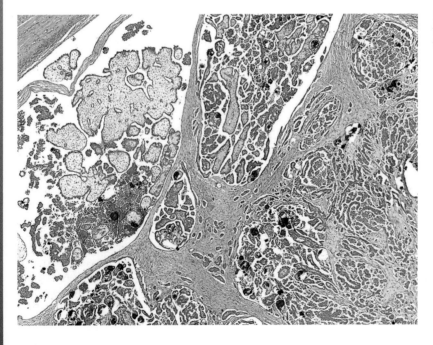

Fig. 42. S-LMP (*left*) transformation to low-grade serous carcinoma (*right*).

Diagnosis and Differential Diagnosis

Transformation to low-grade serous carcinoma is based on the presence of florid epithelial proliferation with increased cytologic atypia, often associated with a more pronounced branching papillary architecture, in addition to destructive invasion.

Recurrence of S-LMP may occur within lymph nodes and may form bulky masses within the peritoneum.[13,43] The diagnosis of transformation should only be made when microscopic examination reveals characteristic features of serous carcinoma, either low-grade or high-grade. Although transformation may initially present in a single site, it is often multifocal; therefore, evaluation of multiple sites may assist in confirming suspected transformation in problematic cases.

Prognosis

Patents with S-LMP who develop low-grade serous carcinoma have the same prognosis as those who initially present with low-grade serous carcinoma (so-called de novo low-grade serous carcinoma). The median survival is 82.8 months (vs 81.8 months for de novo low-grade serous carcinoma).[44] Although patients with low-grade serous carcinoma do not respond as well to platinum-based chemotherapy, the disease course is typically more protracted than with high-grade serous carcinoma.[45,46]

SEROUS PSAMMOCARCINOMA

Overview

Serous psammocarcinoma is a rare, very highly differentiated variant of low-grade serous carcinoma.[47] Almost all patients present with FIGO stage III disease. The ovaries are often not enlarged in serous psammocarcinoma. Due to the abundant psammomatous calcifications associated with this variant, patients may initially present with numerous psammoma bodies on multiple repeat Pap smears.

Gross Features

The ovaries are often minimally enlarged or if increased in size, exhibit minimal epithelial proliferation. Instead, the peritoneum is studded by psammomatous calcifications. Psammomatous calcifications may be visible as small granular opacities on plain films of the pelvis and abdomen.

Microscopic Features

Serous psammocarcinoma features solid nests of invasive serous epithelium (none of which contain >15 cells along the greatest dimension), exhibiting moderate nuclear atypia and extensive

Psammocarcinoma: Key Points

1. Often stage III at presentation; ovarian involvement may not be prominent

2. Nests of serous epithelial cells do not exceed 15 cells in greatest dimension

3. Psammomatous calcifications comprise at least 75% of the tumor cell nests

4. Cytologic atypia is that of low-grade serous carcinoma

5. Mitoses present, but not prominent

6. Lymphatic space invasion by tumor cells and psammoma bodies may be seen in peritoneum, fallopian tube, uterine cervix, and endometrium

psammomatous calcifications (see **Fig. 19**). The psammomatous calcifications involve at least 75% of the serous epithelium.[47] Mitotic figures are often present but should not be numerous. The main tumor may be extra-ovarian, with minimal true ovarian parenchymal involvement. Often, the ovaries exhibit features of a serous adenofibroma with numerous psammoma bodies, but no significant epithelial proliferation. Small papillae and psammoma bodies may be seen in lymphatic spaces of the peritoneum, fallopian tube, uterine cervix, and endometrium (**Fig. 43**). In addition, foci of psammomatous calcifications without associated serous epithelium may be seen throughout the pelvis and abdomen.

Diagnosis and Differential Diagnosis

The diagnosis of serous psammocarcinoma is strictly limited to serous tumors that exhibit cytologic features of low-grade serous carcinoma, but contain massive psammomatous calcifications, essentially blanketing 75% or more of the tumor cells. No single tumor cell nest should contain more than 15 cells in greatest linear dimension.

Serous tumor of low malignant potential (S-LMP) does not exhibit the degree of cytologic atypia associated with psammocarcinoma, although this can be quite subjective. The distinction is largely based on architectural features: S-LMP does not feature solid cell nests or an invasive pattern. Psammoma bodies are often present

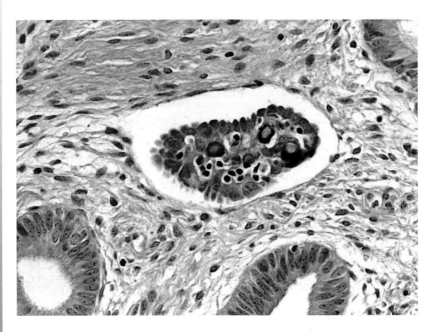

Fig. 43. Lymphovascular space invasion in endometrium of perimenopausal patient with psammocarcinoma.

in S-LMP, but rarely to the extent seen in serous psammocarcinoma. Lymphatic invasion is not a feature of S-LMP.

Low-grade serous carcinoma is characterized by more exuberant epithelial proliferation (see below). Small foci of prominent psammomatous calcification may be present in usual low-grade serous carcinoma, but additional sampling will always disclose areas of malignant serous epithelial proliferation without prominent psammomatous calcification. Lymphatic involvement is relatively uncommon in low-grade serous carcinoma, whereas it can be extensive in serous psammocarcinoma.

Psammomatous calcifications may stud the entire peritoneum in association with mesothelial hyperplasia, adhesions, and endosalpingiosis. *Mesothelial hyperplasia* is recognized on the basis of a more uniformly cuboidal epithelium, monomorphic cell population, and a single layer of epithelium lining papillae, when present.

Prognosis

Serous psammocarcinoma is rare and outcome data is limited, but the cases that have been reported behaved more like S-LMP than low-grade serous carcinoma.[47]

△△ **Psammocarcinoma: Differential Diagnosis**

Low-grade serous carcinoma (fewer psammoma bodies; more epithelial proliferation)

Serous tumor of low malignant potential (non-invasive)

Mesothelial hyperplasia (non-invasive; calretinin expression)

Peritoneal psammomatous calcifications with/without endosalpingiosis (associated epithelium, when present, is non-invasive)

 Psammocarcinoma: Pitfalls

! Prominent psammomatous calcifications may be focally present in a variety of other peritoneal lesions (eg, usual serous carcinoma, endosalpingiosis, peritoneal adhesions). Adequate sampling is required to establish the appropriate diagnosis.

LOW-GRADE SEROUS ADENOCARCINOMA

Overview

One of the more conceptually difficult and controversial areas in gynecologic pathology is the distinction between S-LMP (serous borderline tumor) and low-grade serous carcinoma. Because the cardinal distinguishing feature is the presence of destructive stromal invasion in serous carcinoma (and its absence in serous tumor of low malignant potential), the classification of various stromal-epithelial alterations that can occur in

these tumors conveys important diagnostic, prognostic, and therapeutic implications, particularly in the presence of high-stage disease. Low-grade serous carcinoma is less common than high-grade serous carcinoma. It occurs over a wide age range, but tends to be seen in younger women (median age 43 years vs 60 years for high-grade serous carcinoma).[46] Patients with low-grade serous carcinoma have a significantly poorer prognosis than patients with S-LMP, but experience a more prolonged survival than patients with high-grade serous carcinoma. The five year overall

Fig. 44. (*A*) Low-grade serous carcinoma may appear similar to S-LMP on macroscopic examination. (*B*) In this example of low-grade serous carcinoma, the papillary excrescences are more confluent than in the usual S-LMP.

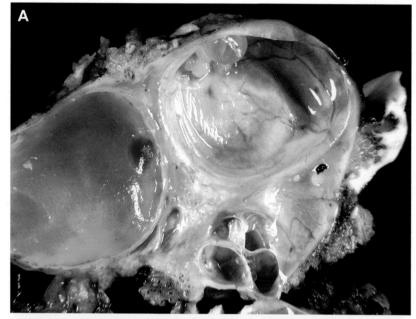

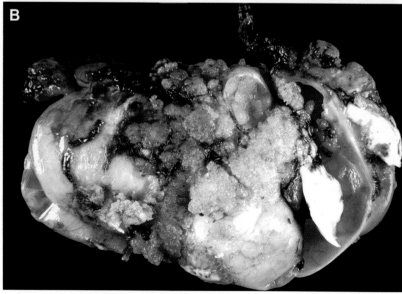

Low-Grade Serous Carcinoma: Key Points

1. Branching papillae, may be hierarchical or non-hierarchical *with* stromal invasion (must be >5 mm in greatest linear extent or >10 mm² in greatest diameter)

2. Stromal invasion patterns: small, nested papillary; solid spindle cell; inverted macropapillary; haphazard fused or cribriform glands

3. Moderate nuclear atypia

4. Mitotic figures increased, but usually <12MF/10HPF (rarely exceed 5–6MF/10HPF)

5. Psammoma bodies often present, but not required

6. Often high stage at presentation

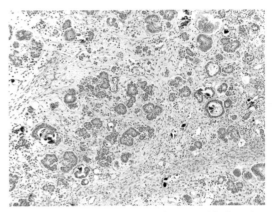

Fig. 45. Low-grade serous carcinoma with invasion into ovarian stroma. The pattern is reminiscent of the single cell and simple papillary-pattern of stromal microinvasion, but is widely invasive.

survival is approximately 70% for FIGO stage II–IV low-grade serous carcinoma (compared with 90% 5-year survival for FIGO stage II–IV S-LMP and 30 to 40% for FIGO stage II–IV high-grade serous carcinoma).[13,44]

Gross Features

The macroscopic features of low-grade serous carcinoma do not differ significantly from S-LMP (**Fig. 44**). The ovarian tumors typically exhibit exuberant papillary excrescences; surface involvement is often present. As in all ovarian tumors, solid nodules may be present and these should be well sampled.

Microscopic Features

Low-grade serous carcinoma is diagnosed on the basis of an exuberant epithelial proliferation and the presence of destructive stromal invasion, which typically takes one or more of the following forms:

1. *Extensive* stromal invasion (ie, involving a significant, contiguous volume of tumor, often in multiple tumor sections) featuring single cells and simple papillae admixed with branching micropapillae, cribriform glands, and inverted macropapillae. Unlike stromal microinvasion, this pattern is extensive (larger than 5 mm in linear extent or larger than 10 mm² in diameter) and typically evokes a stromal response (**Fig. 45**)

2. Small foci of severe epithelial stratification forming confluent nests of epithelial cells (confluent stromal invasion) (**Fig. 46**)

3. Dense aggregates of nested, small papillae with surrounding retraction resembling invasive micropapillary carcinoma of the breast (**Fig. 47**)

4. Haphazard and irregular infiltration of stroma by fused or cribriform glands, reminiscent of invasive ductal carcinoma of the breast (see **Fig. 16**)

5. Extensive inverted macropapillae (**Fig. 48**)

In addition, low-grade serous carcinomas may exhibit a higher mitotic rate and more severe degree of cytologic atypia than S-LMP, although this feature is admittedly subjective and a source of considerable interobserver disagreement. Most low-grade serous carcinomas contain additional foci of S-LMP, with or without micropapillary or cribriform features.[48,49]

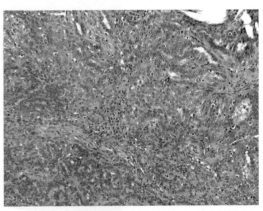

Fig. 46. Low-grade serous carcinoma with confluent pattern of invasion. The epithelial cells are atypical, but uniform in appearance and mitotic figures are inconspicuous, despite the solid appearance.

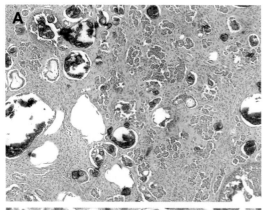

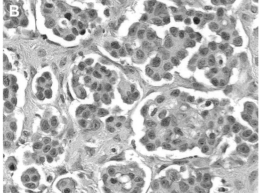

Fig. 47. (*A*) Low-grade serous carcinoma with micropapillary pattern similar to micropapillary carcinoma arising in the breast. (*B*) Moderate atypia is present (compare with degree of atypia typically seen in S-LMP, **Fig. 8**).

The occurrence of small foci of the above-described patterns of destructive stromal invasion in an otherwise typical S-LMP (eg, so-called "microinvasive carcinoma") is rare, as most have associated architectural and cytologic alterations. The optimal management for the patient whose diagnosis of low-grade serous carcinoma is based solely on this feature is unknown.

Diagnosis and Differential Diagnosis

The diagnosis of low-grade serous carcinoma requires the presence of destructive stromal invasion, measuring greater than 5 mm in linear extent or greater than 10 mm^2 in diameter. The malignant cells must exhibit low grade nuclear atypia. The presence of high-grade nuclear atypia warrants consideration for high-grade serous carcinoma. (Mitoses are present, but usually do not exceed 5 to 6 MF/10HPF). The differential diagnosis of low-grade serous carcinoma is similar to that for S-LMP and includes, papillary clear cell carcinoma, well differentiated papillary mesothelioma, high-grade serous carcinoma, endometrioid carcinoma, Sertoli Leydig cell tumor with retiform elements, and granulosa cell tumor with pseudopapillary pattern as well as S-LMP.

Diffuse malignant papillary mesothelioma[50] may be mistaken for a low-grade serous carcinoma; however, mesothelioma has a more prominent tubulopapillary architecture; moreover, the cells are more cuboidal and often have cytoplasmic vacuoles (see **Fig. 23**). Mesothelioma should show strong nuclear staining for calretenin with absent

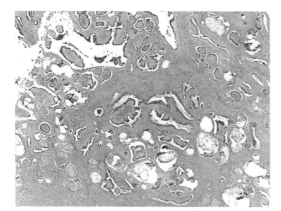

Fig. 48. Low-grade serous carcinoma with so-called "inverted macropapillary" pattern of stromal invasion is characterized by macropapillae surrounded by cleft-like spaces widely scattered throughout the ovarian stroma.

△△ *Low-Grade Serous Carcinoma: Differential Diagnosis*

Serous tumor of low malignant potential (S-LMP) (non-invasive)

Papillary clear cell carcinoma

Well differentiated papillary mesothelioma (non-invasive; cuboidal or flattened cells; calretinin positive)

Diffuse malignant papillary mesothelioma (surface peritoneal disease; cuboidal cells; calretinin expression)

High-grade serous carcinoma (nuclear pleomorphism and high mitotic index)

Endometrioid carcinoma (WT1 negative)

Sertoli Leydig cell tumor with retiform elements (inhibin and calretinin positive)

Granulosa cell tumor with pseudopapillary pattern (inhibin and calretinin positive)

staining for Ber-EP4, MOC31, or other carcinoma markers. CK5/6 and WT1 are less helpful in this differential diagnosis, since both can be expressed by well differentiated serous epithelial processes.[24] The distinction between malignant mesothelioma and serous carcinoma may also be suggested by the distribution of the two disease processes: massive tumor accumulation with diffuse encasement of abdominal organs in malignant mesothelioma versus discrete tumor aggregates studding the peritoneal surfaces in low-grade serous carcinoma.

The distinction between low-grade and *high-grade serous carcinoma* (see article by Al-Agha & Gilks in this publication) partly depends on the grading scheme being used (see grading below). Using the two-tiered MD Anderson criteria, low-grade carcinoma has mostly uniform oval to round nuclei with evenly distributed chromatin and mitotic index less than 12MF/10HPF, whereas high-grade carcinoma has more pleomorphic nuclei, irregular chromatin and high mitotic index (>12MF/10HPF). In our experience, the mitotic count is significantly lower than 12MF/10HPF in most low-grade serous carcinoma; and tumors exhibiting mitotic rates as high as 10 MF/10HPF should be carefully examined to exclude additional areas of high-grade carcinoma. The advantages of this two-tiered method are twofold: ease of use and prognostic value, since it appears to stratify patients with serous carcinoma into 2 distinct prognostic groups. Some tumors exhibit areas of unequivocal high grade histology amidst low grade, and in some instances, borderline histology. In these cases, the high grade designation is assigned with a note providing an assessment of the overall contribution of both grades, with the expectation that the higher grade component will drive prognosis.

Endometrioid carcinoma features more elongated villous papillary structures, glands with more rounded luminal contours and (often) foci of squamous (or morular) metaplasia (see article by Han & Soslow in this publication). Gland formation is not uncommon in serous carcinomas and should not be used as a sole criterion for endometrioid carcinoma. The diagnosis of endometrioid carcinoma should be reserved for those tumors resembling endometrial adenocarcinoma of endometrioid type.

Prognosis

The prognosis of low-grade serous carcinoma is dependent on stage of disease. Patients with stage IA disease who undergo complete excision and adequate staging have an extremely favorable prognosis. Patients with high stage disease are at significant risk for recurrence and death, although

Low-Grade Serous Carcinoma: Pitfalls

! Low-grade serous carcinoma may contain foci of spindle cells, simulating high-grade serous carcinoma, but marked nuclear pleomorphism is absent, and mitotic figures do not exceed 12MF/10HPF (and rarely exceed 5–6MF/10HPF).

! Areas of tumor infarction may mimic stromal invasion, but they are usually associated with a geographic zone of inflamed and edematous stroma, which may or may not contain disrupted and entrapped epithelial cells.

! Autoimplants (desmoplastic type implants in the primary ovarian tumor) may mimic stromal invasion, but they are distinguished from stromal invasion by their characteristic position along the tips and lateral borders of papillae and on the ovarian surface and their resemblance to noninvasive desmoplastic extraovarian implants elsewhere.

the course of disease tends to be more prolonged than with equivalent stage, high-grade serous carcinoma. The MD Anderson data indicates an overall survival of approximately 30% at 10 years, which decreases with more prolonged periods of follow up.[46] This reported survival for high stage, low-grade serous carcinoma is not significantly different from that of S-LMP with transformation to low-grade serous carcinoma. Patients with low-grade serous carcinoma are often treated with aggressive chemotherapy, but response is poor and alternative treatment regimens that are less toxic and more effective are needed.[51]

GRADING SEROUS CARCINOMA

There is no uniformly adopted grading scheme for (non-uterine) pelvic serous carcinoma. Most methods employ a combination of architectural and cytologic features. The GOG and Silverberg three-tiered schemes use architecture and cytology in the overall assessment of tumor grade, while the two-tiered system proposed by the MD Anderson group is based primarily on degree of nuclear atypia and secondarily on mitotic index. Still other systems employ a four-tiered grading scheme (eg, Broder's grade). The three major grading schemes currently in use are provided below:

1. The GOG grading system is essentially the same as that used for endometrial carcinoma; this

system is used for all histologic subtypes of ovarian cancer and is based primarily on architecture and secondarily, on cytologic atypia[52]:

> Grade 1: Less than 5% solid architecture. Nuclear atypia cannot reach the level seen in high-grade carcinoma (grade 3 nuclei are not allowed) (As in endometrial cancer, there are no guides as to the degree of cytologic atypia that is required to be scored as grade 3, although when grade 3 nuclei are present, they should constitute a significant proportion of the tumor (in other words, scattered grade 3 nuclei do not appear to qualify) before the tumor is upgraded to a grade 2 carcinoma.)
>
> Grade 2: Greater than 5% but less than 50% solid architecture
>
> Grade 3: Greater than 50% solid architecture

One problem with this method is the absence of guidelines in the overall assessment of architecture in ovarian carcinoma. Another problem is that it is not necessarily applicable to some histologic variants, such as clear cell carcinoma and mucinous carcinoma. On the other hand, a key advantage to this scheme is the use of the same system to grade ovarian cancer as endometrial cancer; this is useful comparative data when confronted with the problem of possible simultaneous primary tumors.

2. The Shimizu-Silverberg method uses a variation of the Nottingham system for grading breast cancer[53,54]:

> Architecture is assessed by primary pattern as follows: glandular = 1, papillary = 2, and solid = 3;
>
> Nuclear atypia is scored in the same way as the Nottingham method (mild = 1, moderate = 2, marked = 3);
>
> Mitotic activity is scored by the number of mitotic figures per 10 HPH [1HPF = 0.345 mm^2] in the most active region: 0–9 = 1, 10–24 = 2, 25 or more = 3.
>
> The total score is achieved by summing the individual scores and grade is assigned as in the Nottingham grade:
>
> Grade 1: Total score = 3, 4 or 5
>
> Grade 2: Total score = 6 or 7
>
> Grade 3: Total score = 8 or 9

The main advantages to this method are (1) familiarity of the system (since it is essentially a modification of a grading scheme that is widely used by pathologists), (2) incorporation of nuclear atypia and mitotic index, and (3) wider applicability to all histologic types (with the exception of clear cell carcinoma).

3. The M.D. Anderson group uses a two-tiered system based on assessment of nuclear atypia (primary criterion) and mitotic index (secondary criterion)[55]:

> Low Grade: Primary criterion: mostly uniform oval to round nuclei of uniform size with evenly distributed chromatin; nucleoli may be present. Secondary criterion: mitotic index ≤12MF/10HPF
>
> High Grade: Primary criterion: pleomorphic nuclei, irregular chromatin. Secondary criterion: mitotic index greater than 12MF/10HPF

Increasingly, this two-tiered grading scheme has been used for the following reasons:

1. There is considerable tumor heterogeneity in serous carcinoma, and in most cases of high-grade serous carcinoma, the assigned grade will vary by one grade depending on the extent of tumor sampling in a substantial proportion of cases.
2. The reproducibility in distinguishing grade 2 from grade 3 is poor.
3. The prognostic value in trying to make a distinction between grade 2 and grade 3 serous cancer varies amongst groups, but recent data suggest that the clinical and molecular genetic features of grade 2 serous carcinoma and grade 3 serous carcinoma are virtually identical.[56]
4. The cumulative clinical and molecular evidence suggests that the more biologically relevant distinction is between low-grade and high-grade serous tumors.

One of the potential drawbacks to the MD Anderson method is the incorporation of only 2 variables, with the key variable being that of nuclear atypia. One of the least reproducible assessments in the Nottingham grading method for breast carcinoma is the evaluation of nuclear atypia, but in that system the incorporation of 2 additional scores (architecture and mitotic index) blunts the potential for wide discrepancies in overall histologic grade due to variations in assignment of nuclear score. Whether a binary nuclear score in serous ovarian cancer is more reproducible than a ternary nuclear score in breast cancer is unknown.

REFERENCES

1. Scully RE, Young RH, Clement PB. Atlas of tumor pathology. Tumors of the ovary, maldeveloped gonads, fallopian tube, and broad ligament. Washington, DC: AFIP; 1998.
2. Gilks CB, Vanderhyden BC, Zhu S, et al. Distinction between serous tumors of low malignant potential

and serous carcinomas based on global mRNA expression profiling. Gynecol Oncol 2005;96:684–94.

3. Bonome T, Lee JY, Park DC, et al. Expression profiling of serous low malignant potential, low-grade, and high-grade tumors of the ovary. Cancer Res 2005;65:10602–12.

4. Caduff RF, Svoboda-Newman SM, Ferguson AW, et al. Comparison of mutations of Ki-RAS and p53 immunoreactivity in borderline and malignant epithelial ovarian tumors. Am J Surg Pathol 1999;23:323–8.

5. Shih Ie M, Kurman RJ. Ovarian tumorigenesis: a proposed model based on morphological and molecular genetic analysis. Am J Pathol 2004;164:1511–8.

6. Singer G, Oldt R 3rd, Cohen Y, et al. Shih Ie M. Mutations in BRAF and KRAS characterize the development of low-grade ovarian serous carcinoma. J Natl Cancer Inst 2003;95:484–6.

7. Singer G, Stohr R, Cope L, et al. Shih Ie M. Patterns of p53 mutations separate ovarian serous borderline tumors and low- and high-grade carcinomas and provide support for a new model of ovarian carcinogenesis: a mutational analysis with immunohistochemical correlation. Am J Surg Pathol 2005;29:218–24.

8. Werness BA, Ramus SJ, Whittemore AS, et al. Histopathology of familial ovarian tumors in women from families with and without germline BRCA1 mutations. Hum Pathol 2000;31:1420–4.

9. Eichhorn JH, Bell DA, Young RH, et al. Ovarian serous borderline tumors with micropapillary and cribriform patterns: a study of 40 cases and comparison with 44 cases without these patterns. Am J Surg Pathol 1999;23:397–409.

10. Burks RT, Sherman ME, Kurman RJ. Micropapillary serous carcinoma of the ovary. A distinctive low-grade carcinoma related to serous borderline tumors. Am J Surg Pathol 1996;20:1319–30.

11. Deavers MT, Gershenson DM, Tortolero-Luna G, et al. Micropapillary and cribriform patterns in ovarian serous tumors of low malignant potential: a study of 99 advanced stage cases. Am J Surg Pathol 2002;26:1129–41.

12. Gilks CB, Alkushi A, Yue JJ, et al. Advanced-stage serous borderline tumors of the ovary: a clinicopathological study of 49 cases. Int J Gynecol Pathol 2003;22:29–36.

13. Longacre TA, McKenney JK, Tazelaar HD, et al. Ovarian serous tumors of low malignant potential (borderline tumors): outcome-based study of 276 patients with long-term (> or =5-year) follow-up. Am J Surg Pathol 2005;29:707–23.

14. Prat J, De Nictolis M. Serous borderline tumors of the ovary: a long-term follow-up study of 137 cases, including 18 with a micropapillary pattern and 20 with microinvasion. Am J Surg Pathol 2002;26:1111–28.

15. Slomovitz BM, Caputo TA, Gretz HF 3rd, et al. A comparative analysis of 57 serous borderline tumors with and without a noninvasive micropapillary component. Am J Surg Pathol 2002;26:592–600.

16. Bell DA, Longacre TA, Prat J, et al. Serous borderline (low malignant potential, atypical proliferative) ovarian tumors: workshop perspectives. Hum Pathol 2004;35:934–48.

17. Lee KR, Tavassoli FA, Prat J, et al. Tumours of the ovary and peritoneum. In: Tavassoli FA, Devillee P, editors. Tumours of the breast and female genital organs. Lyon (France): IARC Press; 2003. p. 119–24.

18. Bell DA, Scully RE. Ovarian serous borderline tumors with stromal microinvasion: a report of 21 cases. Hum Pathol 1990;21:397–403.

19. McKenney JK, Balzer BL, Longacre TA. Patterns of stromal invasion in ovarian serous tumors of low malignant potential (borderline tumors): a reevaluation of the concept of stromal microinvasion. Am J Surg Pathol 2006;30:1209–21.

20. Tavassoli FA. Serous tumor of low malignant potential with early stromal invasion (serous LMP with microinvasion). Mod Pathol 1988;1:407–14.

21. Katzenstein AL, Mazur MT, Morgan TE, et al. Proliferative serous tumors of the ovary. Histologic features and prognosis. Am J Surg Pathol 1978;2:339–55.

22. Sangoi AR, Soslow RA, Teng NN, et al. Ovarian clear cell carcinoma with papillary features: a potential mimic of serous tumor of low malignant potential. Am J Surg Pathol 2008;32:269–74.

23. Han G, Gilks CB, Leung S, et al. Mixed ovarian epithelial carcinomas with clear cell and serous components are variants of high-grade serous carcinoma: an interobserver correlative and immunohistochemical study of 32 cases. Am J Surg Pathol 2008;32:955–64.

24. Acs G, Pasha T, Zhang PJ. WT1 is differentially expressed in serous, endometrioid, clear cell, and mucinous carcinomas of the peritoneum, fallopian tube, ovary, and endometrium. Int J Gynecol Pathol 2004;23:110–8.

25. Korn WT, Schatzki SC, DiSciullo AJ, et al. Papillary cystadenoma of the broad ligament in von Hippel-Lindau disease. Am J Obstet Gynecol 1990;163:596–8.

26. Irving JA, Young RH. Granulosa cell tumors of the ovary with a pseudopapillary pattern: a study of 14 cases of an unusual morphologic variant emphasizing their distinction from transitional cell neoplasms and other papillary ovarian tumors. Am J Surg Pathol 2008;32:581–6.

27. Bell DA, Weinstock MA, Scully RE. Peritoneal implants of ovarian serous borderline tumors. Histologic features and prognosis. Cancer 1988;62:2212–22.

28. Gershenson DM, Silva EG, Levy L, et al. Ovarian serous borderline tumors with invasive peritoneal implants. Cancer 1998;82:1096–103.

29. Gershenson DM, Silva EG, Tortolero-Luna G, et al. Serous borderline tumors of the ovary with noninvasive peritoneal implants. Cancer 1998;83:2157–63.

30. Seidman JD, Kurman RJ. Ovarian serous borderline tumors: a critical review of the literature with emphasis on prognostic indicators. Hum Pathol 2000;31:539–57.

31. Silva EG, Tornos C, Zhuang Z, et al. Tumor recurrence in stage I ovarian serous neoplasms of low malignant potential. Int J Gynecol Pathol 1998;17:1–6.

32. Rollins SE, Young RH, Bell DA. Autoimplants in serous borderline tumors of the ovary: a clinicopathologic study of 30 cases of a process to be distinguished from serous adenocarcinoma. Am J Surg Pathol 2006;30:457–62.

33. McKenney JK, Gilks CB, Longacre TA. Classification of extra-ovarian implants associated with ovarian serous tumors of low malignant potential (S-LMP). A clinicopathologic study of 181 cases. Mod Pathol 2005;18:195A.

34. Bell KA, Smith Sehdev AE, Kurman RJ. Refined diagnostic criteria for implants associated with ovarian atypical proliferative serous tumors (borderline) and micropapillary serous carcinomas. Am J Surg Pathol 2001;25:419–32.

35. Gilks CB, McKenney JK, Kalloger S, et al. Interobserver variation in the assessment of extra-ovarian implants of serous borderline tumors (serous tumors of low malignant potential). Mod Pathol 2005;18:184A.

36. Longacre TA, Kempson RL, Hendrickson MR. Well-differentiated serous neoplasms of the ovary. Pathology (Phila) 1993;1:255–306.

37. McKenney JK, Balzer BL, Longacre TA. Lymph node involvement in ovarian serous tumors of low malignant potential (borderline tumors): pathology, prognosis, and proposed classification. Am J Surg Pathol 2006;30:614–24.

38. Leake JF, Rader JS, Woodruff JD, et al. Retroperitoneal lymphatic involvement with epithelial ovarian tumors of low malignant potential. Gynecol Oncol 1991;42:124–30.

39. Clement PB, Young RH, Oliva E, et al. Hyperplastic mesothelial cells within abdominal lymph nodes: mimic of metastatic ovarian carcinoma and serous borderline tumor–a report of two cases associated with ovarian neoplasms. Mod Pathol 1996;9:879–86.

40. Silva EG, Gershenson DM, Malpica A, et al. The recurrence and the overall survival rates of ovarian serous borderline neoplasms with noninvasive implants is time dependent. Am J Surg Pathol 2006;30:1367–71.

41. Parker RL, Clement PB, Chercover DJ, et al. Early recurrence of ovarian serous borderline tumor as high-grade carcinoma: a report of two cases. Int J Gynecol Pathol 2004;23:265–72.

42. Dehari R, Kurman RJ, Logani S, et al. The development of high-grade serous carcinoma from atypical proliferative (borderline) serous tumors and low-grade micropapillary serous carcinoma: a morphologic and molecular genetic analysis. Am J Surg Pathol 2007;31:1007–12.

43. Chamberlin MD, Eltabbakh GH, Mount SL, et al. Metastatic serous borderline ovarian tumor in an internal mammary lymph node: a case report and review of the literature. Gynecol Oncol 2001;82:212–5.

44. Shvartsman HS, Sun CC, Bodurka DC, et al. Comparison of the clinical behavior of newly diagnosed stages II-IV low-grade serous carcinoma of the ovary with that of serous ovarian tumors of low malignant potential that recur as low-grade serous carcinoma. Gynecol Oncol 2007;105:625–9.

45. Gershenson DM, Sun CC, Bodurka D, et al. Recurrent low-grade serous ovarian carcinoma is relatively chemoresistant. Gynecol Oncol 2009;114:48–52.

46. Gershenson DM, Sun CC, Lu KH, et al. Clinical behavior of stage II-IV low-grade serous carcinoma of the ovary. Obstet Gynecol 2006;108:361–8.

47. Gilks CB, Bell DA, Scully RE. Serous psammocarcinoma of the ovary and peritoneum. Int J Gynecol Pathol 1990;9:110–21.

48. Silva EG, Tornos CS, Malpica A, et al. Ovarian serous neoplasms of low malignant potential associated with focal areas of serous carcinoma. Mod Pathol 1997;10:663–7.

49. Smith Sehdev AE, Sehdev PS, Kurman RJ. Noninvasive and invasive micropapillary (low-grade) serous carcinoma of the ovary: a clinicopathologic analysis of 135 cases. Am J Surg Pathol 2003;27:725–36.

50. Clement PB, Young RH, Scully RE. Malignant mesotheliomas presenting as ovarian masses. A report of nine cases, including two primary ovarian mesotheliomas. Am J Surg Pathol 1996;20:1067–80.

51. Schmeler KM, Sun CC, Bodurka DC, et al. Neoadjuvant chemotherapy for low-grade serous carcinoma of the ovary or peritoneum. Gynecol Oncol 2008;108:510–4.

52. Benda JA, Zaino R. GOG pathology manual. Buffalo (NY): Gynecologic Oncology Group; 1994.

53. Shimizu Y, Kamoi S, Amada S, et al. Toward the development of a universal grading system for ovarian epithelial carcinoma: testing of a proposed system in a series of 461 patients with uniform treatment and follow-up. Cancer 1998;82:893–901.

54. Silverberg SG. Histopathologic grading of ovarian carcinoma: a review and proposal. Int J Gynecol Pathol 2000;19:7–15.

55. Malpica A, Deavers MT, Tornos C, et al. Interobserver and intraobserver variability of a two-tier system for grading ovarian serous carcinoma. Am J Surg Pathol 2007;31:1168–74.

56. Ayhan A, Kurman RJ, Yemelyanova A, et al. Defining the cut point between low-grade and high-grade ovarian serous carcinomas: a clinicopathologic and molecular genetic analysis. Am J Surg Pathol 2009;33:1220–4.

HIGH-GRADE SEROUS CARCINOMA INVOLVING FALLOPIAN TUBE, OVARY AND PERITONEUM

Osama M. Al-Agha, MD, FRCPC, C. Blake Gilks, MD, FRCPC*

KEYWORDS

- Ovarian surface epithelial carcinoma • High-grade serous carcinoma
- Low-grade serous carcinoma • Ovary • Fallopian tube • Peritoneum • WT1
- p53 • p16 • BRCA • HNF1β • PAX8

ABSTRACT

The focus of this review is high-grade serous carcinoma (HGSC); for the purposes of this review, the term "pelvic SC" is used for HGSC that could be considered, based on historical definitions, to have arisen from ovary, fallopian tube, or peritoneum. These assignments of primary site are arbitrary and there is evidence that the distal fallopian tube is the site of origin of many pelvic HGSCs. The diagnosis of HGSC can be made readily based on routine histomorphologic examination in most cases; however, a variety of neoplasms can resemble HGSC. Thus, we review the key features of pelvic SC, current concepts of its pathogenesis, histopathological diagnostic criteria, discuss differential diagnosis, and review diagnostic ancillary studies that can be used in practice.

PELVIC HIGH-GRADE SEROUS CARCINOMA

OVERVIEW

The Concept of "Pelvic HGSC"

The World Health Organization's (WHO) classification of ovarian, tubal, and peritoneal tumors recognizes SC as one of the malignant epithelial neoplasms of these three organs,[1] and high-grade serous carcinoma (HGSC) is the most common epithelial malignancy arising at these sites.[2] However, the histogenesis of SC, specifically

Key Features
PELVIC HIGH-GRADE SEROUS CARCINOMA (HGSC)

High nuclear-to-cytoplasmic ratio, marked nuclear atypia, high mitotic index (>12 MF/10 HPF) with atypical mitotic figures, and marked pleomorphism with presence of wild-looking cells

Variety of patterns of growth including solid, papillary, glandular, microcystic and others

Tumor cells are highly stratified with a fenestrated appearance and irregular slit-like spaces

Papillae in HGSC are of complex architecture, lined by stratified cells, with cellular exfoliation

Tumor cells nests or micropapillae are commonly seen within clear spaces

Glandular HGSC predominantly shows tubular glands with serrated or slit-like lumens lined by round, large and highly atypical nuclei

Marked desmoplastic stromal reaction with necrosis and lymphovascular permeation

Psammoma bodies may be present, but are typically more numerous in LGSC

Expression of p53, WT1, ER, and PAX8

HGSC, in these organs has been the subject of recent debate. Pathologic criteria have been proposed to distinguish between tubal and ovarian HGSC,[3,4] and between peritoneal and ovarian

Department of Pathology and Laboratory Medicine, Vancouver General Hospital and University of British Columbia, Vancouver, BC, Canada
* Corresponding author.
E-mail address: Blake.Gilks@vch.ca

Surgical Pathology 4 (2011) 375–396
doi:10.1016/j.path.2010.12.004

HGSC.[5] These criteria are mainly based on the location of the dominant tumor mass (bulk of tumor). However, the criterion of the "dominant mass" is not necessarily valid as the location of the largest tumor does not necessarily identify the primary site. For example, small, inconspicuous low-grade mucinous tumors of the vermiform appendix, or adenocarcinomas of the uterine cervix can be associated with dominant ovarian masses.[6] In recent years, a significant number of studies have focused on the role of the distal fallopian tube in the histogenesis of cases of HGSC that would be described as primary ovarian or peritoneal tumors based on the "dominant mass" criteria. This evidence, discussed in detail later, has led to the widely held belief that most HGSCs arise from the tubal mucosa and spread to the ovary and/or the remainder of the abdominal cavity. As there are no morphologic or molecular differences between HGSC considered to be primary tubal, ovarian or peritoneal based on conventional criteria,[7] the concept and terminology of "pelvic HGSC" has been introduced to denote HGSC "arising" (based on dominant mass criterion) in these three sites: fallopian tube, ovary, and peritoneum.[8,9] It is important to note that pelvic HGSC should be separated from SC arising in the endometrium or cervix; the former differ from pelvic HGSC in typically lacking WT1 expression,[10] while the latter may be associated with HPV infection.[11] As well, endometrial and cervical SC do not show the strong association with germline *BRCA* mutations characteristic of pelvic HGSC. Thus, it is important to exclude a uterine primary in a case of HGSC involving ovary, fallopian tube and/or omentum, before diagnosing pelvic HGSC. Endometrial SC can spread beyond the uterus even in the absence of myometrial invasion. A study of HGSC comparing tumors with both ovarian and endometrial involvement to tumors with only ovarian involvement and tumors with only endometrial involvement, showed that the tumors with both endometrial and ovarian involvement were indistinguishable from the tumors with only endometrial involvement, and differed from tumors with only ovarian involvement.[12] Thus, if there is endometrial involvement in a case of HGSC, even in the presence of large ovarian masses and omental disease, in most cases it is appropriate to consider it to be a primary endometrial SC, acknowledging that in an individual case it is impossible to determine the primary site with certainty. An exception is shown in **Fig. 1**, where the endometrial involvement, in a patient with ovarian, peritoneal, and tubal serous carcinoma, is seen as tumor cells invading around benign endometrial glands, with prominent lymphovascular invasion, a pattern highly suggestive of metastasis to the endometrium. Hopefully immunohistochemical markers that will reliably distinguish between pelvic and endometrial HGSC will be identified but at the present time markers showing differential expression between pelvic and endometrial HGSC lack sufficient sensitivity and specificity for routine diagnostic use.[13]

The Theory of Tubal Origin

As indicated earlier (and for more information see the Shaw article in this publication on Familial

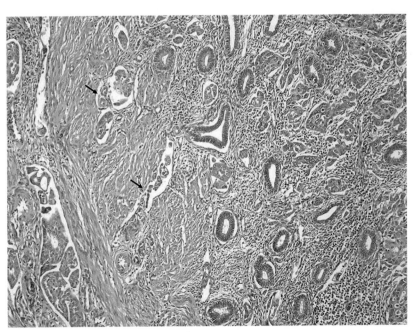

Fig. 1. Pelvic HGSC metastastatic to endometrium. The HGSC is seen infiltrating the endometrial stroma between benign endometrial glands. Extensive lymphovascular permeation is present (*arrows*). These findings support the metastatic nature of pelvic HGSC to the endometrium, a relatively uncommon occurrence (hematoxylin & eosin ×20).

Tumors), the fallopian tube has been implicated as the primary site of pelvic HGSC in many cases. Data in support of the tubal origin theory can be summarized as follows:

1. A small percentage of germline *BRCA1* or *BRCA2* mutation carriers have early SC of the distal, fimbriated end of the fallopian tube (tubal intraepithelial carcinoma; TIC) in risk reducing salpingo-oophorectomy specimens, without tumor in the ovary or peritoneum. This indicates that TIC is the precursor for most pelvic HGSCs in these patients.[14–17]

2. Sporadic pelvic HGSC, unassociated with a germline *BRCA* mutation, can also be linked to the distal fallopian tube, as approximately 50% of these patients have TIC on careful sectioning of the fallopian tubes.[7–9,18] These TICs are usually unilateral, in contrast to bilateral serosal fallopian tube involvement, suggesting that the former represents an initiating event and the latter a secondary, or metastatic event. In many cases, the fallopian tube cannot be identified, having presumably been obliterated by the tumor.

3. Analysis of tubal, ovarian, and peritoneal HGSCs from individual cases discloses identical *p53* mutations and identical cellular DNA content, indicating their monoclonality.[7,19]

4. Some studies have shown a decreased risk of HGSC development in ovaries after tubal ligation or hysterectomy,[15] the idea being that the source of HGSC (the distal, fimbriated end of the fallopian tube) either atrophies or is removed in these patients.

5. Most HGSCs involve the surface of the ovary and are advanced stage at presentation (in contrast to mucious, endometrioid, and clear cell carcinomas of ovary). An extraovarian source for HGSC can be explained if tumor cells exfoliated into the peritoneal cavity from the distal fimbriated end of the fallopian tube, with transcelomic spread and ovarian surface implantation.

Although it has been proposed that pelvic HGSC can originate from the ovarian surface epithelium (especially from the lining of cortical inclusion cysts)[20,21] the cysts are often lined by epithelium that shares immunophenotypic and molecular features with tubal epithelium.[22] PAX2 expression by pelvic HGSCs, which is characteristic of Müllerian tissues including both the distal fallopian tube and ciliated cortical inclusions cysts but not ovarian surface epithelium, suggests that these tumors arise from Müllerian-derived structures such as fallopian tube.[23] The paucity of reported cases of early/in-situ lesions in these cysts

suggests that it is less common than origination in the fallopian tube. Rarely, serous borderline tumors or LGSCs can evolve to HGSC, but this appears to be uncommon.[24–27] Overall, the tubal origin of pelvic HGSC is currently the most widely accepted hypothesis of origin for many/most pelvic HGSCs.

Risk Factors

Apart from hereditary HGSC that develops secondary to germline *BRCA1* or *BRCA2* mutations, risk factors for pelvic HGSC are relatively weak and incompletely understood. HGSC is not associated with estrogen stimulation (in contrast to endometrioid carcinoma)[28] but risk is reduced with increasing parity and oral contraceptive use,[29] while pelvic inflammatory disease is associated with increased risk.[30]

GROSS FEATURES

In the fallopian tubes, HGSC can be either exophytic, protruding into the lumen, or endophytic, infiltrating into the wall. The tumor can arise from any part of the tube but most commonly is in the outer or distal portion.[31] The tumor can be diffuse, occurring throughout the tubal lining, or localized, involving only a portion of the tube. In some cases, multifocal involvement can be present. The tube may appear enlarged, sometimes along its entire length, with closure of the fimbriated end and subsequent accumulation of fluid or blood in the tubal lumen, giving a fusiform or sausage-like external appearance resembling that of hydrosalpinx or pyosalpinx. Tumors arising from the fimbriated end of the tube can have a papillary appearance, protruding into the peritoneal cavity (**Fig. 2**). In some cases, the tube is not appreciably enlarged and the gross appearance is of slight irregularity in the tube thickness or thickened mucosa. In other cases, there is a tumor nodule attached to the fimbria by a thin stalk, occupying the potential space between fimbria and ovarian surface. In the ovaries, HGSC can be predominantly cystic, forming complex multiloculated cysts, (hence the nomenclature of serous cystadenocarcinoma), entirely solid, or both cystic and solid. Very often, the tumor contains papillae that can be seen grossly as papillary excrescences contained within the cysts or projecting from the ovarian surface.

Friability, necrosis and hemorrhage are very common gross features. Bilaterality is common, occurring in 84% of cases.[32] When HGSC involves the peritoneum it is usually diffuse but can take the form of localized masses. On documenting the

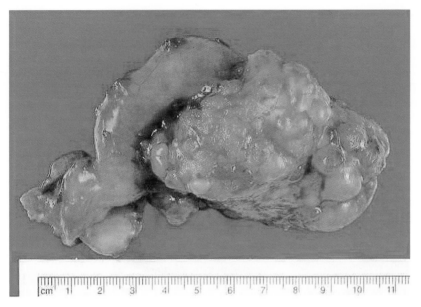

Fig. 2. Tubo-ovarian involvement by HGSC (pelvic HGSC). The tumor involves both the distal end of the fallopian tube and the ovary. The tumor is grossly solid with irregular surface and fuses both the ovary and fallopian tube, distorting normal anatomic landmarks.

findings on gross examination of specimens, attention should be given to the items listed in **Table 1**. Adequate tissue sampling is very important for accurate diagnosis, and cystic, solid and papillary areas should all be sampled, if present. Particular care should be taken on examining prophylactic salpingo-oophorectomy specimens from women with BRCA mutations or a family history of breast and/or ovarian carcinoma. Thorough and meticulous sampling and examination of fallopian tubes and ovarian tissue submitted is warranted as this might allow detection of occult HGSC or TIC. A protocol for systematic dissection and examination of the fallopian tubes and ovaries in such specimens has been described. This protocol is described in more detail by Shaw in Familial Tumors in this publication. The role of detailed examination of fallopian tubes routine (ie, other than in prophylactic specimens) is uncertain, but there is insufficient evidence at present to recommend its routine use.

MICROSCOPIC FEATURES

HGSC in the fallopian tube, ovary, and peritoneum show identical microscopic features. The cytologic features of HGSC are most characteristic, while the architectural features show considerable variability; accordingly, the cytologic changes will be described first. HGSC is characterized by

---

Table 1
Checklist of important features to note in the gross description of ovarian/tubal cancer specimens

Gross Description Items	Features to Note
Specimen integrity	Intact, ruptured, fragmented
Tumor site(s) and laterality	Right, left or both
Tumor size	Greatest dimension or overall dimensions
Ovarian/tubal serosal surface	Smooth, adhesions, tumor involvement (eg, nodularity or papillary excrescences), other lesions Check fimbriated end specifically
Gross appearance	Color, friability, hemorrhage and necrosis Solid or cystic. If cystic, areas of nodularity or papillary excrescences should be described The color and consistency of cystic fluid should be noted
Other organs or tissues (eg, omentum, segments of intestine)	Checked for tumor involvement

Fig. 3. HGSC is characterized by cytologic features of high-grade malignancy, including marked nuclear atypia (high nuclear-to-cytoplasmic ratio, prominent nucleoli, marked pleomorphism with the presence of bizarre nuclei), a high mitotic rate with atypical mitotic figures, and a high apoptotic rate (hematoxylin & eosin ×60).

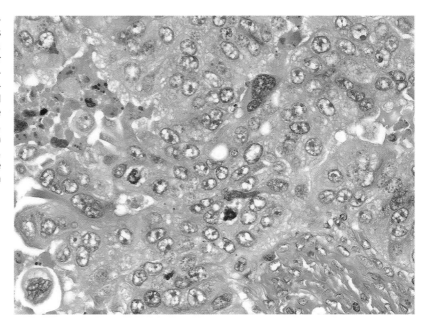

cytologic features of high-grade malignancy, including marked nuclear atypia (high nuclear-to-cytoplasmic ratio, prominent nucleoli, marked pleomorphism with the presence of bizarre nuclei), and a high mitotic rate with atypical mitotic figures (**Fig. 3**). While SC has traditionally been graded as 1, 2, or 3 (well, moderately, or poorly differentiated), this 3-tier system has been recently replaced by a 2-tier grading scheme proposed by Malpica and colleagues,[33] SC is divided into LGSC and HGSC based on nuclear grade as a primary criterion with mitotic index as a secondary criterion. In this 2-tier system, HGSC is defined as having marked nuclear atypia (tumor cells showing more than 3:1 variation in nuclear size and shape), and mitotic index of greater than 12 MF/10 HPF. In support of this 2-tier system, Vang and colleagues[34] found that

Fig. 4. Solid HGSC. The tumor cells are arranged in solid sheets with no glandular or papillary formations discerned. Some irregular slit-like spaces can be seen within the solid sheet (hematoxylin & eosin ×10).

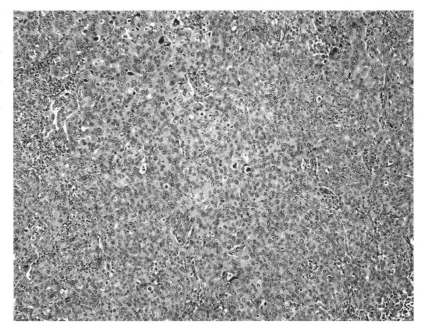

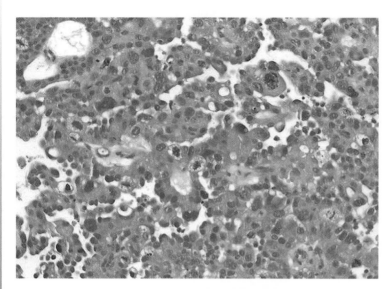

Fig. 5. Papillary HGSC. The papillae are covered by stratified, highly atypical epithelium with pronounced cellular budding or exfoliation (hematoxylin & eosin ×40).

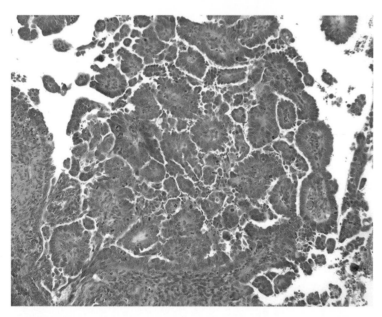

Fig. 6. Papillae of HGSC are of high architectural complexity and show non-hierarchical branching (hematoxylin & eosin ×20).

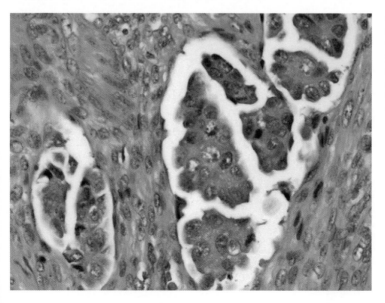

Fig. 7. Micropapillae of HGSC can be seen within clefted spaces in the stroma. These spaces may result from stromal retraction secondary to fixation or as a result of secretion of serous fluid by the tumor cells (hematoxylin & eosin ×40).

there were no significant biologic differences between grade 2 and grade 3 SC, graded using the 3-tier system, justifying combining them into a single category of HGSC.

HGSC can show different architectural patterns of growth including solid, papillary, glandular, and microcystic patterns. One tumor can show exclusively a single pattern of growth, but admixture of two or more patterns is usual.

The solid pattern is arguably the most common and consists of solid sheets of cells with occasional irregular slit-like spaces (**Fig. 4**). The designation of "undifferentiated" carcinoma should not be used for HGSC showing a predominantly solid component, but reserved for those tumors showing an undifferentiated pattern throughout.

In papillary HGSC, the papillae may be either large (macropapillae with broad fibrovascular cores or narrow fibrovascular cores lined by a thick, stratified epithelium) or small papillae (micropapillae lacking fibrovascular cores), but the latter are much more common. The papillae are covered by highly stratified epithelium showing exuberant cellular budding or exfoliation and non-hierarchical branching (**Figs. 5 and 6**). Micropapillae can be seen within clear clefted spaces in the stroma. These spaces do not have an endothelial lining and therefore care should be taken to not misinterpret them as tumor vascular invasion (these spaces may result from stromal retraction secondary to fixation or secretion of serous fluid by the tumor cells) (**Fig. 7**).

Glandular HGSC consists of glands that display irregular, serrated lumens (**Fig. 8**). Other patterns include transitional, microcystic, cribriform (**Fig. 9**) and multinucleated giant cell patterns. HGSC is very often associated with a marked desmoplastic stromal reaction. Necrosis and lymphovascular permeation is common. Although not specific for HGSC, and more commonly seen (and more numerous) in LGSC, psammoma bodies (concentrically lamellated calcifications) (**Fig. 10**) or larger calcific aggregates can occur in HGSC. Foci of clear cells can be seen in HGSC (**Fig. 11**). While this finding can suggest a component of clear cell carcinoma, Han and colleagues[35] found that these clear cells have the same immunoprofile as HGSC (distinctly different from clear cell carcinoma) indicating that such tumors are in fact HGSC with clear cell changes rather than mixed serous-clear cell carcinomas. Squamous differentiation is most unusual in HGSC and if present should prompt consideration of a diagnosis of endometrioid carcinoma.

While familiarity with the architectural patterns of HGSC is important for diagnostic purposes they do not serve to subclassify HGSC into clinically relevant subgroups and need not be mentioned in a diagnostic pathology report.

In the fallopian tube, close attention has recently been paid to the precursors of HGSC. The earliest precursor of HGSC in the fallopian tube is thought to be normal appearing epithelium that lacks atypia and proliferation but shows strong p53 expression (hence the term p53 signature). Tubal intraepithelial carcinoma (TIC) is an in situ malignancy that shows strong p53 positivity and neoplastic epithelium with nuclear stratification, loss of cell polarity, loss of

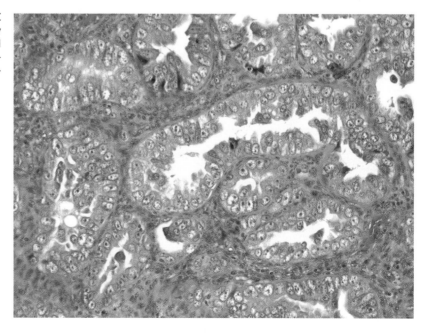

Fig. 8. Glandular HGSC showing glands lined by highly atypical luminal cells and irregular serrated lumens (hematoxylin & eosin ×40).

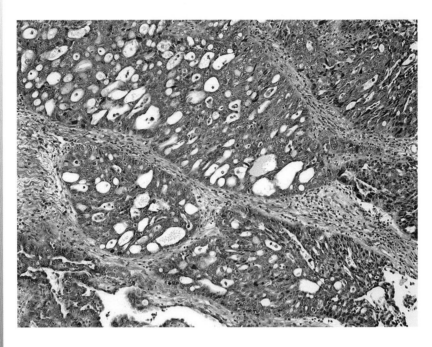

Fig. 9. Cribriform pattern of HGSC with small glandular spaces within sheets of tumor cells (hematoxylin & eosin ×40).

cilia, high-grade nuclear atypia (nuclear enlargement, prominent nucleoli, and coarse chromatin), abnormalities of cellular DNA content, and a high proliferative index. The lesion of TIC must span at least 10 to 12 consecutive tubal secretory cells. The lesional cells can undermine adjacent benign ciliated epithelial cells in a "pagetoid" pattern. Prominent papillae and detached cells floating in the lumen or off the surface of the fimbria also

characterize TIC (**Figs. 12** and **13**).[36] There are intermediate lesions falling between p53 signatures and TIC. These lesions show incomplete replacement of the ciliated cells, preserved cell polarity and cell-cell adhesion, and lower proliferative index relative to TIC. These lesions have been designated tubal intraepithelial lesions in transition (TILT) to distinguish them from both p53 signatures and TICs.[36] **Table 2** lists the diagnostic criteria of p53

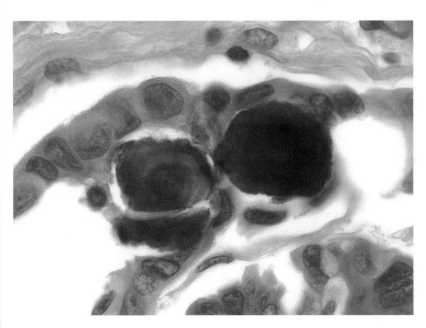

Fig. 10. Psmammoma bodies are concentrically lamellated calcifications that can occur in both HGSC and LGSC (hematoxylin & eosin ×60).

Fig. 11. Clear cell changes in HGSC. These changes can be misinterpreted as clear cell carcinoma (hematoxylin & eosin ×40).

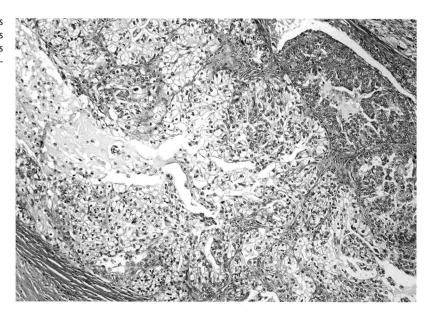

signatures, TILT, and TIC. At the present time, only TIC is a sufficiently validated and clinically relevant entity to merit diagnosis in practice. Note that TIC is diagnosed based on H&E features; in problematic cases a combination of p53 and Ki67 should be done and both should be strongly positive to support a diagnosis of TIC, but as some TIC are p53 negative (just as some HGSC are p53 negative), p53 immunostaining is not a prerequisite for a diagnosis of TIC. An algorithm depicting steps in tubal carcinogenesis of pelvic HGSC is presented in **Fig. 14**.

Fig. 12. Tubal intraepithelial carcinoma (TIC) with adjacent normal fallopian tube mucosa. TIC is an in-situ malignancy showing neoplastic epithelium with nuclear stratification, loss of cell polarity, loss of cilia, and high-grade nuclear atypia (hematoxylin & eosin ×40).

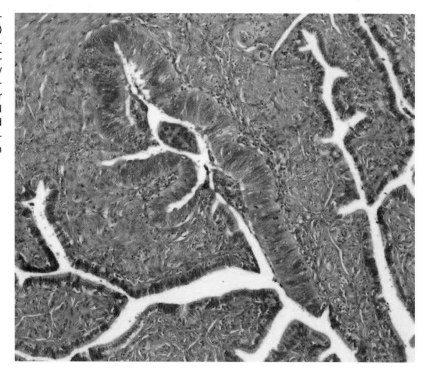

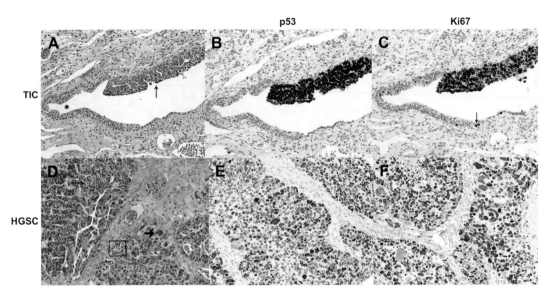

Fig. 13. Histologic and molecular features of in-situ and invasive high-grade serous carcinoma. (A) Tubal intra-epithelial carcinoma (TIC, *arrow*) and adjacent normal fallopian tube epithelium (hematoxylin & eosin). (B) Diffuse expression of p53 in nuclei of TIC and abrupt negativity of adjacent normal epithelium. (C) High prolif-eration rate of TIC with more than 50% of nuclei labeled with the proliferation marker Ki67. Normal epithelium shows occasional proliferating cells in the basal layer (*arrow*). (D) HGSC with marked nuclear pleomorphism and hyperchromatic enlarged nuclei (*short arrow*), high mitotic activity (*long arrow*) and high apoptotic activity (*framed*) (hematoxylin & eosin). (E) Diffuse expression of p53 in more than 80% of nuclei in HGSC, indicating an underlying *p53* missense mutation. (F) High proliferation rate with greater than 50% of HGSC nuclei labeled with the proliferation marker Ki67 (magnification in all figures ×200). (*From* Kobel M, Huntsman D, Gilks CB. Crit-ical molecular abnormalities in high-grade serous carcinoma of the ovary. Exp Rev Mol Med 2008;10:e22; with permission.)

Table 2
Diagnostic cytomorphological and immunocytochemical features of tubal precursors of pelvic HGSC

Tubal Lesion	Morphology and Immunocytochemistry
Latent precursor (p53 signature)	Normal appearing epithelium that lacks atypia and proliferation Strong p53 immunostaining (12 or more consecutive p53+ secretory cell nuclei) Low Ki67 index
Tubal intraepithelial lesion in transition (TILT)	Proliferation of atypical tubal secretory cells that have not completely replaced the normal epithelial cells Preservation of cell polarity Cohesive cell growth Incomplete loss of cilia (or intermixed with normal ciliated cells) Strong p53 immunostaining Increased Ki67 index (but lower than that of TIC)
Tubal intraepithelial carcinoma (TIC)	Disorganized growth and replacement of normal cells: Stratification (with variable thickness) Absence of cilia Loss of polarity Loss of cell to cell cohesion Strong p53 immunostaining Ki67 index higher than that of TILT

Fig. 14. Steps in tubal carcinogenesis, leading to pelvic HGSC.

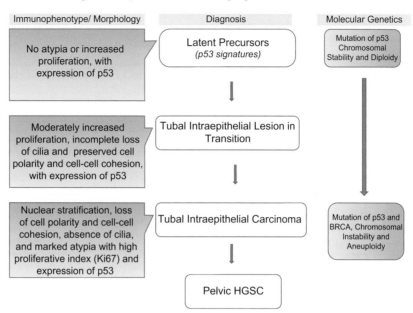

Carcinogenic Sequence of Pelvic High-grade Serous Carcinoma

Immunophenotype/ Morphology	Diagnosis	Molecular Genetics
No atypia or increased proliferation, with expression of p53	Latent Precursors *(p53 signatures)*	Mutation of p53 Chromosomal Stability and Diploidy
Moderately increased proliferation, incomplete loss of cilia and preserved cell polarity and cell-cell cohesion, with expression of p53	Tubal Intraepithelial Lesion in Transition	
Nuclear stratification, loss of cell polarity and cell-cell cohesion, absence of cilia, and marked atypia with high proliferative index (Ki67) and expression of p53	Tubal Intraepithelial Carcinoma	Mutation of p53 and BRCA, Chromosomal Instability and Aneuploidy
	Pelvic HGSC	

Although diagnosis of HGSC is primarily based on routine morphology, certain immunomarkers can aid in the cases whose histomorphology is not straightforward. The majority of pelvic HGSCs stain positively with antibodies directed against estrogen receptor (ER), p53, Wilms tumor gene product-1 (WT1), mesothelin,[37] CA-125,[38,39] epithelial membrane antigen (EMA), cytokeratin 7,[40] PAX8,[41,42] and PAX2.[23] Overexpression of p16 has also been observed in pelvic HGSC (but the molecular mechanism here is unrelated to human papilloma virus infection).[43–46] Several new markers including Rsf-1 (HBXAP)[47] and Nac1[48] have emerged. Ki67 labeling index of HGSC is very high and is usually higher than that of other ovarian carcinomas.[39] In one study,[46] the mean Ki67 (MIB1) proliferative index of 46 cases of HGSC was 55.4%. **Table 3** summarizes the ancillary studies of value in diagnosis of HGSC.

HGSC sampled after chemotherapy shows alterations that impact on morphologic assessment. These alterations occur in nuclei, cytoplasm and/or stroma. The nuclear alterations include bizarre appearance with hyperchromasia and chromatin smudging (**Fig. 15**). These are usually accompanied by alterations in the cytoplasm (intense eosinophilia, vacuolation, or foamy appearance), and stroma (fibrosis, inflammation, foamy histiocytes, cholesterol clefts, and dystrophic calcification).[49] Miller and colleagues[50] found that the immunoprofile of post-chemotherapy HGSC was very similar to that of untreated tumors and, thus, immunohistochemistry can be used when chemotherapy changes pose diagnostic challenges.

When the pathology report is generated, the report should convey data related to prognosis and guide treatment planning. In addition, it might be used for academic review in research and teaching. The report should therefore state the features listed in **Box 1**. Concerning the tumor primary site, in the light of the aforementioned speculations about the origin of pelvic HGSC, it is arguably better to avoid describing tumors with multifocal involvement as "ovarian," "peritoneal," or "tubal" in the final pathology report, and simply list the sites involved. We are in a period of transition and find that we frequently resort to a diagnostic comment in cases of pelvic HGSC to briefly discuss the possible primary site, frequently acknowledging some uncertainty in a given case. Fortunately, the treatment is the same for "ovarian," "peritoneal," and "tubal" HGSC. It is critically important that clinicians be familiar with new and changing diagnostic terminology; for example, the term "tubal intraepithelial carcinoma" is not necessarily an in situ carcinoma as it has risk of spread to the abdominal cavity, even in the absence of tubal wall invasion.[37]

Table 3
Ancillary studies of value in diagnosis of pelvic high-grade serous carcinoma (HGSC)

Ancillary Study	Utility
Immunohistochemistry	
p53	Distinguishes between HGSC (p53+ve) and p53−ve tumors such as clear cell carcinoma or LGSC
	Helps detect the tubal precursors of pelvic HGSC (strong p53 positivity relative to the normal tubal cells)
WT1	Distinguishes between pelvic HGSC (WT1+ve) and endometrioid adenocarcinoma, clear cell carcinoma or metastatic endometrial HGSC (WT−ve)
ER	Distinguishes between HGSC (ER+ve) and ER−ve tumors such as clear cell carcinoma and malignant mesothelioma
p16	Distinguishes between primary pelvic HGSC (p16+ve) and clear cell carcinoma or endometrioid carcinomas (p16−ve)
Cytokeratin 7 (CK7)	Distinguishes between primary pelvic HGSC (CK7+ve) and metastatic CK7−ve carcinomas, such as carcinomas of lower gastrointestinal tract
Ki67	Helps distinguish between HGSC and LGSC (moderately to highly elevated In HGSC)
	Distinguishes TIC from latent precursors (p53 signatures and TILT)
Genetic Mutations	
p53 mutation	Distinguishes between HGSC (+ve for *p53* mutation) and LGSC (−ve for *p53* mutation)
BRCA1/2 mutation	Germline mutations present in hereditary HGSC, somatic mutations present in some sporadic HGSC

DIFFERENTIAL DIAGNOSIS

Distinction Between HGSC and LGSC

LGSC and HGSC are now believed to be two distinct tumors which differ in genetic abnormalities, pathways of tumorigenesis and clinical behavior. Clinically, HGSCs are aggressive tumors affecting older women, whereas LGSCs are relatively indolent tumors affecting women of somewhat younger age.[51,52] LGSCs are more refractory to chemotherapy than HGSCs, probably because of the lower proliferative rate of the former.[53] It is thought that LGSCs arise by stepwise progression from benign through borderline to malignant tumors, while HGSCs are thought to arise de novo.[54] Molecular genetic studies have demonstrated that LGSC is more likely to have mutations in BRAF and KRAS[19,55] while HGSC

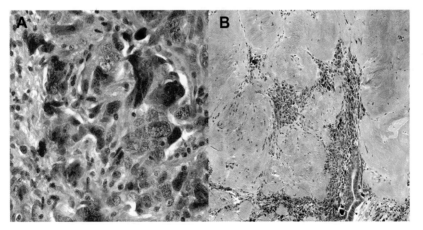

Fig. 15. Post-chemotherapy effects in HGSC. The nuclear alterations (*A*) consist of bizarre nuclear enlargement with hyperchromatism and chromatin smudging. The stromal alterations (*B*) include densely fibrotic stroma which contains inflammatory cells and hemosiderin pigment. These alterations may interfere with diagnosis of tumor subtype (hematoxylin & eosin A ×40, B ×10).

Box 1
Checklist of information to include in final diagnostic report for ovarian/tubal cancer specimens
Tumor histologic type and, if appropriate, grade
Tumor size
Tumor laterality
Status of ovarian surface
Status of tubal mucosa and serosa
Cytology (ascites or peritoneal washing)
Regional lymph node status
Metastasis
Other significant non-neoplastic features

△△ ***Differential Diagnosis***
PELVIC HIGH-GRADE SEROUS CARCINOMA

Primary Tumors

- High-grade endometrioid carcinoma - *WT1 is negative*
- Clear cell carcinoma - *WT1 is negative, HNF-1β is positive*
- Carcinosarcoma - *mesenchymal component*
- Epithelial malignant mesothelioma - *calretinin is positive*
- Low grade serous carcinoma/serous borderline tumor with micropapillary architecture - *more uniform nuclei and lower mitotic rate*
- Undifferentiated carcinoma - *absence of any papillary growth, WT1 is negative*
- Yolk sac tumor - *OCT3/4 is positive*

Metastatic Tumors

- Metastatic endometrial HGSC - *endometrial involvement*
- Metastatic carcinomas of non-Müllerian origin - *WT1 is negative, express non-gynecologic tissue-specific markers*

commonly shows mutations in *p53* and *BRCA1* or *BRCA2*.[56] Women with germline *BRCA* mutations are at increased risk of HGSC, but not of serous borderline tumor or LGSC, underscoring differences in pathogenesis between HGSC and LGSC.[17,57] The distinction between HGSC and LGSC is made primarily based on nuclear features, with less than threefold variation in nuclear size in LGSC (**Fig. 16**).[33,34] A secondary diagnostic criterion is mitotic activity, LGSC having less than 12 MF/10HPF. There are also differences in architectural features between LGSC and HGSC, with micropapillary architecture and psammoma bodies more common in the former, while HGSC frequently shows solid growth pattern, at least focally, an uncommon feature in LGSC. Immunohistochemistry is not particularly helpful (and is seldom required) to separate LGSC and HGSC; p53 and Ki67 may be of use but are not well validated. **Table 4** summarizes the major distinguishing features of HGSC and LGSC.

Distinction Between HGSC and Other High-grade Gynecologic Carcinomas

For more detail on the morphologic features of non-serous ovarian carcinomas, please also refer to article by Han and Soslow in this publication, *Non-Serous Ovarian Epithelial Tumors*. Because HGSC shows a wide spectrum of morphologic features, the differential diagnosis is broad. We can facilitate this discussion by examining the differential diagnoses of HGSC on the basis of pattern of growth; **Table 5** presents the differential diagnosis of HGSC based on growth pattern.

Solid HGSC has only a minor component with papillary or glandular differentiation, but these areas are critical in diagnosis. The morphologic features of the tumor overlap with high-grade endometrioid carcinoma. Features favoring HGSC rather than a poorly differentiated endometrioid adenocarcinoma include slit-like spaces and smaller, more complex papillae with a greater degree of cellular budding. Foci of squamous differentiation or the presence of a low-grade endometrioid component strongly support a diagnosis of endometrioid carcinoma. WT1 and vimentin immunostaining may also be of value in that most pelvic HGSCs are immunoreactive to WT1 (>80%) but not to vimentin, while the immunoreactivity pattern to these markers in endometrioid carcinoma is the opposite (almost all stain positively for vimentin while fewer than 5% stain for WT1).[58,59] Carcinosarcoma (or malignant Müllerian mixed tumor) enters the differential diagnosis of HGSC as a high-grade tumor that can harbor HGSC as its malignant epithelial component, however, the presence of malignant sarcomatous elements, either homologous (eg, smooth muscle, fibrosarcoma-like) or heterologous (eg, rhabdomyoblastic, chondrocytic) allows recognition. A variant of solid pattern of HGSC is "transitional" carcinoma. This pattern usually coexists with other more typical HGSC, and shows

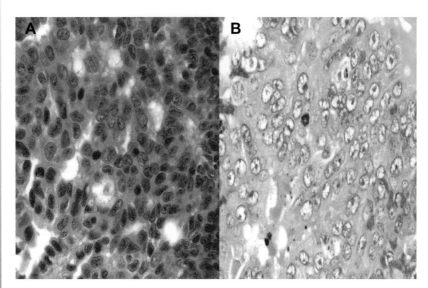

Fig. 16. The cytologic and nuclear features of LGSC (*A*) versus HGSC (*B*). In contrast to LGSC, HGSC shows much greater nuclear atypia (more than threefold variation in nuclear size and shape) and numerous mitoses with atypical mitotic figures (>12/10 HPF in HGSC and ≤12/10 in LGSC) (hematoxylin & eosin ×60).

the same immunophenotype as HGSC; it is best considered a variant of HGSC rather than a distinct subtype of ovarian carcinoma. Some high-grade carcinomas show no specific differentiation and such tumors are diagnosed as undifferentiated carcinoma.[1] Most such tumors do show focal recognizable serous differentiation, and have an immunoprofile indistinguishable from HGSC. It is our practice to only diagnose undifferentiated carcinoma when a tumor is undifferentiated throughout. If there is any morphologic evidence of HGSC we diagnose such a tumor as HGSC, even if this is a minor component. If there is doubt in such a case, it might be prudent to consider

classifying the tumor as HGSC, with the use of WT1 immunohistochemical staining for confirmation, before arriving at a diagnosis of undifferentiated carcinoma.[55]

Papillary HGSC may resemble villoglandular variant of endometrioid adenocarcinoma but the latter is usually of low grade and the cells have a uniform, columnar morphology with bland nuclei, and the papillary structures are generally simple and thin, without the broad fibrovascular cores and prominent exfoliation of HGSC. Clear cell carcinoma shares the high-grade nuclear atypia of HGSC, but hobnail and clear cells, with relatively low mitotic activity (compared with

Table 4
Features allowing distinction between low-grade and high-grade serous carcinomas

Feature	Low-Grade Serous Carcinoma	High-Grade Serous Carcinoma
Nuclei[a]	Uniform, with less than 3 fold variation in nuclear size, and small (low grade; grade 1)	Pleomorphic, with greater than 3 fold variation in nuclear size, and large (high grade; grade 2 or 3)
Mitotic Index[a]	Low (≤12 MF/10HPF)	High (>12 MF/10HPF) with atypical mitotic figures
Necrosis	Absent	Common
Immunohistochemistry		
p53	Negative, focal, or patchy	Diffuse and strong expression
p16	Negative, focal, or patchy	Diffuse and strong expression
Ki67	Low	Moderate to high
Genetic Mutations	KRAS, BRAF, with chromosomal stability	p53, BRCA1/2, with chromosomal instability
Chemosensitivity	Low	High

[a] Nuclear features and mitotic index are the major criteria for the distinction between HGSC and LGSC, with nuclear features being the primary criterion.

Table 5
Mimickers of high-grade serous carcinoma (classified based on growth pattern)

Growth Pattern	Mimickers	Major Discriminating Features
Solid	High-grade endometrioid carcinoma (either primary ovarian or metastatic uterine)	Squamous differentiation and WT1−ve immunophenotype
	Carcinosarcoma	Malignant sarcomatous elements
	Metastatic high-grade non-gynecologic carcinomas	Immunoreactivity with tissue-specific immunopanel
Papillary	Clear cell carcinoma	Hobnail appearance of the nuclei; and HNF1β+ve immunophenotype
	Malignant mesothelioma	Immunoreactivity with mesothelioma-restricted markers (eg, calretinin and D2-40)
	Low-grade serous carcinoma/serous borderline tumor with micropapillary architecture	Low-grade nuclei and low mitotic rate (≤12 MF/10HPF)
	Metastatic non-gynecologic carcinomas with papillary growth pattern	Immunoreactivity with tissue-specific immunopanel
Glandular	Low-grade endometrioid carcinoma	Squamous differentiation, absence of features of high-grade malignancy, and WT1−ve immunophenotype
	Embryonal carcinoma	Immunoreactivity to CD30 and OCT3/4
	Metastatic, non-gynecologic adenocarcinomas	Immunoreactivity with tissue-specific immunopanel

HGSC) characterize clear cell carcinoma. Moreover, the stromal cores of the papillae in clear cell carcinoma are characteristically hyalinized, and there is less cellular stratification than in HGSC (**Fig. 17**). In problematic cases, an immunopanel consisting of WT1, ER, and HNF1β can be helpful to separate the two (clear cell carcinoma typically demonstrates an immunophenotype of WT1−, ER−, and HNF1β+, which is opposite to that of HGSC) (see also in this publication, Han and Soslow: *Non-Serous Ovarian Epithelial Tumors*).[43]

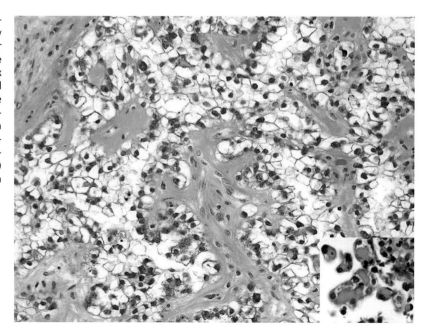

Fig. 17. Clear cell carcinoma of the ovary showing cells with clear cytoplasm. The papillae in CCC are less complex than those of HGSC and their stromal cores are characteristically hyalinised. Occasional cells in CCC can show cytoplasmic inclusions of hyalinized globules (*inset*) (hematoxylin & eosin ×20, insert ×60).

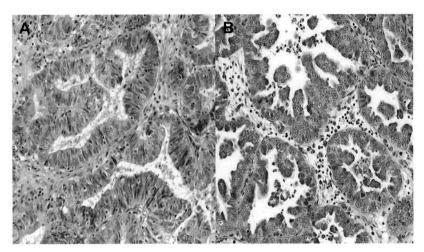

Fig. 18. Ovarian endometrioid adenocarcinoma (*A*) versus glandular HGSC (*B*). Endometrioid adenocarcinoma with glandular formation is low grade and the nuclei are columnar with basal polarity, and lacking high-grade atypia, as opposed to glandular HGSC with glands showing more irregular luminal outlines than those of endometrioid adenocarcinoma. The lining cells of HGSC glands are markedly atypical (hematoxylin & eosin ×40).

Glandular HGSC is easily confused with other adenocarcinomas, especially endometrioid adenocarcinoma. However, endometrioid adenocarcinomas with glandular formation are typically low grade and thus the nuclei are usually columnar, maintain basal polarity, and lack high-grade atypia, as opposed to glandular HGSC (**Fig. 18**).

Embryonal carcinoma, although rare, shares cytologic features of high-grade malignancy with HGSC. Tumor cells in embryonal carcinoma show solid sheets or nest arrangement, besides the glandular pattern of growth. The tumor cells are anaplastic with vacuolated cytoplasm, and hyperchromatic and vesicular nuclei with prominent nucleoli. Embryonal carcinoma is positive for OCT3/4 and CD30, and is seen in a younger age group than HGSC (median age at diagnosis is 12 years for embryonal carcinoma).

Microcystic HGSC can resemble yolk sac tumor. The presence of the characteristic features of yolk sac tumor such as Schiller-Duval bodies and hyaline globules and the lack of the aforementioned features of HGSC favors yolk sac tumor.

Immunohistochemistry may be helpful in that expression of WT1, ER, cytokeratin 7, and EMA are more frequent in HGSC, whereas expression of α-fetoprotein and absence of the above markers are more typical of yolk sac tumor. As for embryonal carcinoma, patients with yolk sac tumor are much younger than those with HGSC.

Pelvic Versus Endometrial HGSC

As endometrial and pelvic (tubal/ovarian/peritoneal) HGSC exhibit similar morphologic features, determining the site of the primary tumor may be difficult if there is concurrent involvement of endometrium and tube/ovary/peritoneum. As noted previously, most cases with endometrial involvement should be considered primary endometrial SC, while acknowledging that there is some uncertainty about primary site assignment; this may change in the future, as better diagnostic tools to establish primary site emerge.

Table 6 presents the immunohistochemical markers used in the distinction between the three most common gynecologic carcinomas involving

---

Table 6
Immunohistochemical markers useful in the distinction between the three common gynecologic carcinoma subtypes (serous, endometrioid and clear cell carcinoma)

				Marker	
Tumor	WT1	ER	p53	p16	Additional Markers
Endometrioid carcinoma	−	+	−	− or patchy+	Vimentin+ CEA−
Pelvic HGSC	+	+	+	+	Cytokeratin 7+
Clear cell carcinoma	−	−	−	−	HNF1β+

the ovary, serous carcinoma, endometrioid carcinoma and clear cell carcinoma.

Distinction Between Pelvic HGSC and Metastatic Carcinomas of Non-Müllerian Origin

Metastasis from non-Müllerian sites can mimic, clinically and pathologically, a primary pelvic HGSC. Familiarity with the patient's clinical history and comparison of the microscopic features of the primary tumor with those of the primary pelvic HGSC are critical in differential diagnosis. Immunohistochemistry may be helpful in problematic cases. Non-gynecologic tumors that display papillary pattern can be particularly challenging to separate from HGSC. Urinary bladder, breast, and lung carcinomas can show a papillary pattern and thus mimic HGSC. These tumors can be distinguished from HGSC with the HGSC markers (WT1, ER, and PAX8) combined with tissue-specific immunomarkers such as TTF-1 (for lung), uroplakin, cytokeratin 20, thrombomodulin (for urothelial carcinoma of the urinary bladder),[55] and GCDFP-15 (for breast carcinoma).[55,60] Note that TTF-1 can sometimes be expressed by primary ovarian carcinomas.

The specific scenario of a patient with a history of breast carcinoma who develops pelvic HGSC occurs not uncommonly, and may be a manifestation of a germline *BRCA* mutation. As patients with *BRCA1* mutations are more likely to have triple-negative, basal-like breast carcinomas with high-grade nuclear features, the differential diagnosis with HGSC can be difficult. Comparison of the previous breast carcinoma to the pelvic tumor will usually suffice to allow a diagnosis to be made; if immunostains are required, GCDFP-15, PAX8, and WT1 can be helpful. Epithelial malignant mesothelioma can exhibit a tubulopapillary pattern, resembling HGSC. Epithelial malignant mesothelioma cells are typically less pleomorphic, and show fewer and less atypical mitotic figures than HGSC. The papillae of malignant mesothelioma are less cellular and less complex than those of HGSC. The distinction between the two can be also facilitated by the use of immunohistochemistry (**Fig. 19**).

Adenocarcinoma-associated markers (eg, BerEP4, B72.3, and MOC31) combined with HGSC immunomarkers (eg, ER) and immunomarkers of mesothelial differentiation (eg, calretinin and D2-40) can be of value in the distinction. It is important to note that WT1 is co-expressed by both pelvic HGSC and malignant mesothelioma and, therefore, it is not helpful to separate the two.[61]

Distinction Between HGSC and its Mimics in Peritoneal Washing Specimens

Reactive atypical mesothelial cells and papillary mesothelial hyperplasia may mimic HGSC on peritoneal washings. The marked architectural and cytologic atypia in HGSC can, however, permit distinction. A panel of immunocytochemical stains on the cell block material (with the markers noted above) should help distinguish between

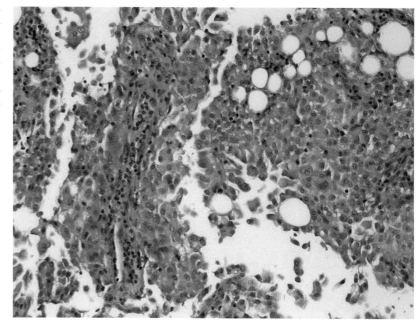

Fig. 19. Malignant mesothelioma of the peritoneum, epithelial type. Epithelial malignant mesothelioma cells are typically less pleomorphic, and show fewer and less atypical mitotic figures than HGSC (hematoxylin & eosin ×40).

mesothelial cells and HGSC tumor cells in difficult cases. Although psammoma bodies characterize SC, they can also be seen on the peritoneal washings of other conditions such as endosalpingiosis and borderline serous tumors. The presence of cilia, and the lack of single atypical cells, cytoplasmic vacuolation, marked nuclear atypia or two distinct cell populations are all features favoring a benign process (**Fig. 20**).[62]

Tubal Intraepithelial Carcinoma Versus Benign Hyperplasia of Tubal Mucosa

The fallopian tube epithelium commonly shows epithelial hyperplasia and mild atypia as reactive changes. Historically, the criteria for diagnosis of tubal intraepithelial carcinoma (TIC) were not well established, but there has been progress recently. TIC is characterized by cells with high-grade cytologic atypia, ie, large nuclei with prominent nucleoli and coarse chromatin, marked cellular proliferation, stratification with loss of cilia and basal polarity, and loss of cohesion with detached cells seen on luminal surface, while benign tubal hyperplasia shows stratification and mild atypia only. In problematic cases, immunostaining for p53 and Ki67 can be done. The cells of TIC typically show strong diffuse p53 positivity and a very high Ki67 labeling index relative to the background tubal cells.[37]

HGSC as a Component of Mixed Ovarian Carcinomas

According to the WHO diagnostic criteria, the diagnosis of mixed carcinoma can be made in tumors if the less prevalent type comprises 10% or more of the volume of the tumor.[1] We believe that this category has been overused in the past and recognition of the full spectrum of patterns of HGSC will dramatically reduce the number of cases of mixed carcinoma with a component of HGSC diagnosed. In particular, it is our experience that most tumors diagnosed as admixtures of HGSC and high-grade endometrioid, clear cell and/or undifferentiated carcinoma are best considered to be pure HGSC, as they show a uniform HGSC-specific immunophenotype throughout.

TREATMENT AND PROGNOSIS

The treatment of pelvic HGSC consists of full surgical staging (hysterectomy, salpingo-oophorectomy, omentectomy, peritoneal biopsies, and peritoneal washings, with or without lymph node biopsies or dissection). Two general therapeutic approaches are currently used: neoadjuvant chemotherapy with 3 or 4 cycles of chemotherapy before surgery and completion of chemotherapy thereafter (for patients with bulky,

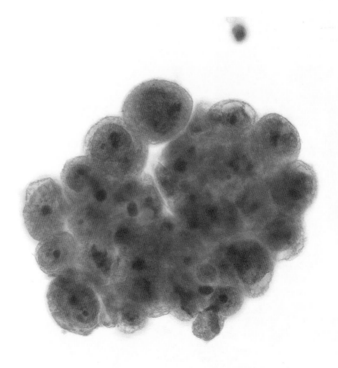

Fig. 20. HGSC Cytology: cluster of HGSC cells in a peritoneal washing specimen. The malignant cells of HGSC occur in a three-dimensional grouping and display marked cytologic and nuclear atypia (ThinPrep Papanicolaou stain ×60).

Pitfalls
PELVIC HIGH-GRADE SEROUS CARCINOMA

! Intracystic HGSC of the ovary without obvious stromal invasion can be misdiagnosed as serous borderline tumor (especially at frozen section). The presence of high-grade nuclei and high mitotic rate should establish the diagnosis of HGSC

! High-grade endometrioid carcinoma and clear cell carcinoma can have growth features similar to those of HGSC. Knowledge of the distinctive histopathological features and immunophenotype of these tumors should help in the distinction between them and HGSC

! HGSC can harbor areas with clear cell changes (HGSC with clear cell change) that can be misdiagnosed as clear cell carcinoma. The presence of typical HGSC and, in difficult cases immunostaining, should allow a correct diagnosis to be made

! In distinguishing between HGSC of the peritoneum and epithelial malignant mesothelioma of the peritoneum, the use of WT1 can be misleading as both tumors co-expresses the marker, and other markers such as MOC31, B72.3 and calretinin should be used instead

! Primary pelvic HGSC can be easily mistaken for metastatic non-gynecologic carcinomas, particularly metastatic breast carcinoma with micropapillary features. The use of GCDFP-15 (for breast carcinoma) and WT1 or PAX8 (for HGSC) can be helpful in the distinction

! Low-grade and high-grade serous carcinomas are two distinct tumor types rather than different grades of the same neoplasm. Therefore, accurate assessment and reporting of tumor grade is essential. Psammoma bodies are not specific to HGSC as they can be seen in benign serous tumors and endosalpingiosis, as well as low-grade serous carcinoma. Correlation with other histopathological and cytologic findings is critical for the correct diagnosis of HGSC

! Early tubal precursors of HGSC (p53 signatures) share p53 overexpression with TIC. However, TIC shows high-grade cytologic atypia with higher KI67 proliferative index. Depending on p53 expression as a sole diagnostic criterion for the distinction between these tubal lesions can lead to erroneous diagnoses

advanced stage, unresectable disease); or debulking surgery followed by adjuvant intraperitoneal and intravenous chemotherapy. Taxanes and platinum containing chemotherapeutic agents are standard for first-line therapy. The prognosis of pelvic HGSC depends on tumor stage. The large majority of cases of pelvic HGSC have spread beyond the pelvis at the time of presentation (stage III and IV) and these patients have five-year survival rates ranging from 10 to 50%, with disease resectability and chemosensitivity being the most important prognostic variables for placing patients within this range. Macroscopic residual disease after surgery is prognostically unfavorable, while surgeries that result in "optimal debulking" are associated with a relatively more favorable prognosis. Stage Ia or Ib HGSCs are very uncommon, and even these patients are at sufficiently high risk of recurrence that adjuvant chemotherapy is recommended. Despite the fact that HGSCs are typically sensitive to chemotherapy with response rates reaching 80%, the high frequency of subsequent tumor recurrence after surgery and progression to chemoresistance leads to the poor clinical outcome.[63–65] The natural history and clinical outcome of TIC has not yet been established in the literature. It has been suggested that TICs have a 5-year latent period before metastasizing transcelomically.[66] There is, at present, no consensus about whether adjuvant chemotherapy should be given when these lesions are detected as an incidental finding, and more information to guide detection and management of these lesions will undoubtedly be forthcoming over the years to come.

REFERENCES

1. Tavasolli FA, Devilee P. World Health Organization classification of tumors. Tumors of the breast and the female genital organs. Lyon (France): IARC Press-WHO; 2003.

2. Seidman JD, Horkayne-Szakaly I, Haiba M, et al. The histologic type and stage distribution of ovarian carcinomas of surface epithelial origin. Int J Gynecol Pathol 2004;23:41–4.

3. Hu CY, Taymor ML, Hertig AT. Primary carcinoma of the fallopian tube. Am J Obstet Gynecol 1950;59(1):58–67.

4. Sedlis A. Carcinoma of the fallopian tube. Surg Clin North Am 1978;58(1):121–9.

5. Young RH, Gilks CB, Scully RE. Mucinous tumors of the appendix associated with mucinous tumors of the ovary and pseudomyxoma peritonei. A clinicopathological analysis of 22 cases supporting an origin in the appendix. Am J Surg Pathol 1991;15(5):415–29.

6. Elishaev E, Gilks CB, Miller D, et al. Synchronous and metachronous endocervical and ovarian neoplasms: evidence supporting interpretation of the ovarian neoplasms as metastatic endocervical adenocarcinomas simulating primary ovarian surface epithelial neoplasms. Am J Surg Pathol 2005;29(3):281–94.

7. Carlson JW, Miron A, Jarboe EA, et al. Serous tubal intraepithelial carcinoma: its potential role in rimary peritoneal serous carcinoma and serous cancer prevention. J Clin Oncol 2008;26(25):4160.

8. Salvador S, Gilks B, Köbel M, et al. The fallopian tube: primary site of most pelvic high-grade serous carcinomas. Int J Gynecol Cancer 2009;19(1): 58–64.

9. Hashi A, Yuminamochi T, Murata S, et al. Wilms tumor gene immunoreactivity in primary serous carcinomas of the fallopian tube, ovary, endometrium, and peritoneum. Int J Gynecol Pathol 2003; 22(4):374–7.

10. Nofech-Mozes S, Khalifa MM, Ismiil N, et al. Detection of HPV-DNA by a PCR-based method in formalin-fixed, paraffin-embedded tissue from rare endocervical carcinoma types. Appl Immunohistochem Mol Morphol 2010;18(1):80–5.

11. Silva EG, Jenkins R. Serous carcinoma in endometrial polyps. Mod Pathol 1990;3(2):120–8.

12. Hirschowitz L, Ganesan R, McCluggage WG. WT1, p53 and hormone receptor expression in uterine serous carcinoma. Histopathology 2009; 55:478–82.

13. Piek JM, van Diest PJ, Zweemer RP, et al. Dysplastic changes in prophylactically removed fallopiantubes of women predisposed to developing ovarian cancer. J Pathol 2001;195:451–6.

14. Powell CB, Kenley E, Chen LM, et al. Risk-reducing salpingoooophorectomy in BRCA mutation carriers: role of serial sectioning in the detection of occult malignancy. J Clin Oncol 2005;1:127–32.

15. Finch A, Shaw P, Rosen B, et al. Clinical and pathologic findings of prophylactic salpingo-oophorectomies in 159 BRCA1 and BRCA2 carriers. Gynecol Oncol 2006;1:58–64.

16. Callahan MJ, Crum CP, Medeiros F, et al. Primary fallopian tube malignancies in BRCA-positive women undergoing surgery for ovarian cancer risk reduction. J Clin Oncol 2007;25:3985–90.

17. Vang R, Shih IeM, Kurman RJ. Ovarian low-grade and high-grade serous carcinoma: pathogenesis, clinicopathologic and molecular biologic features, and diagnostic problems. Adv Anat Pathol 2009;5: 267–82.

18. Salvador S, Rempel A, Soslow RA, et al. Chromosomal instability in fallopian tube precursor lesions of serous carcinoma and frequent monoclonality of synchronous ovarian and fallopian tube mucosal serous carcinoma. Gynecol Oncol 2008;3:408–17.

19. Singer G, Stöhr R, Cope L, et al. Patterns of p53 mutations separate ovarian serous borderline tumors and low- and high-grade carcinomas and provide support for a new model of ovarian carcinogenesis: a mutational analysis with immunohistochemical correlation. Am J Surg Pathol 2005;2:218–24.

20. Bell DA, Scully RE. Early de novo ovarian carcinoma. A study of fourteen cases. Cancer 1994; 73:1859–64.

21. Hutson R, Ramsdale J, Wells M. p53 protein expression in putative precursor lesions of epithelial ovarian cancer. Histopathology 1995;4:367–71.

22. Tong GX, Chiriboga L, Hamele-Bena D, et al. Expression of PAX2 in papillary serous carcinoma of the ovary: immunohistochemical evidence of fallopian tube or secondary Müllerian system origin? Mod Pathol 2007;8:856–63.

23. Parker RL, Clement PB, Chercover DJ, et al. Early recurrence of ovarian serous borderline tumor as high-grade carcinoma: a report of two cases. Int J Gynecol Pathol 2004;23:265–72.

24. Dehari R, Kurman RJ, Logani S, et al. The development of high-grade serous carcinoma from atypical proliferative (borderline) serous tumors and low-grade micropapillary serous carcinoma: a morphologic and molecular genetic analysis. Am J Surg Pathol 2007;7:1007–12.

25. Quddus MR, Rashid LB, Hansen K, et al. High-grade serous carcinoma arising in a low-grade serous carcinoma and micropapillary serous borderline tumor of the ovary in a 23-year-old woman. Histopathology 2009;54:771.

26. Silva EG, Tornos CS, Malpica A, et al. Ovarian serous neoplasms of low malignant potential associated with focal areas of serous carcinoma. Mod Pathol 1997;10:663–7.

27. Scully RE, Clement PB, Young RH. Ovarian surface epithelial-stromal tumors. In: Sternberg S, editor. Diagnostic surgical pathology. New York: Raven Press; 2004. p. 2552–3.

28. Risch HA, Marrett LD, Howe GR. Parity, contraception, infertility, and the risk of epithelial ovarian cancer. Am J Epidemiol 1994;7:585–97.

29. Parazzini F, La Vecchia C, Negri E, et al. Pelvic inflammatory disease and risk of ovarian cancer. Cancer Epidemiol Biomarkers Prev 1996;8:667–9.

30. Liapis A, Bakalianou K, Mpotsa E, et al. Fallopian tube malignancies: a retrospective clinical pathological study of 17 cases. J Obstet Gynaecol 2008;1:93–5.

31. Scully RE, Young RH, Clement PB. Tumors of the ovary, maldeveloped gonads, fallopian tube, and broad ligament. Atlas of tumor pathology. 3rd series, fascicle 23. Washington, DC: Armed Forces Institute of Pathology; 1992. p. 191.

32. Leitao MM, Boyd J, Hummer A, et al. Clinicopathologic analysis of early-stage sporadic ovarian carcinoma. Am J Surg Pathol 2004;28:147–59.

33. Malpica A, Deavers MT, Lu K, et al. Grading ovarian serous carcinoma using a two-tier system. Am J Surg Pathol 2004;4:496–504.

34. Vang R, Shih IeM, Salani R, et al. Subdividing ovarian and peritoneal serous carcinoma into moderately differentiated and poorly differentiated does not have biologic validity based on molecular genetic and in vitro drug resistance data. Am J Surg Pathol 2008;11:1667–74.

35. Han G, Gilks CB, Leung S, et al. Mixed ovarian epithelial carcinomas with clear cell and serous components are variants of high-grade serous carcinoma: an interobserver correlative and immunohistochemical study of 32 cases. Am J Surg Pathol 2008;7:955–64.

36. Crum CP. Intercepting pelvic cancer in the distal fallopian tube: theories and realities. Mol Oncol 2009;2:165–70.

37. Köbel M, Kalloger SE, Carrick J, et al. A limited panel of immunomarkers can reliably distinguish between clear cell and high-grade serous carcinoma of the ovary. Am J Surg Pathol 2009;1:14–21.

38. Lu KH, Patterson AP, Wang L, et al. Selection of potential markers for epithelial ovarian cancer with gene expression arrays and recursive descent partition analysis. Clin Cancer Res 2004;10:3291–300.

39. Lagendijk JH, Mullink H, van Diest PJ, et al. Immunohistochemical differentiation between primary adenocarcinomas of the ovary and ovarian metastases of colonic and breast origin: comparison between a statistical and an intuitive approach. J Clin Pathol 1999;52:283–90.

40. Nofech-Mozes S, Khalifa MA, Ismiil N, et al. Immunophenotyping of serous carcinoma of the female genital tract. Mod Pathol 2008;9:1147–55.

41. Nonaka D, Chiriboga L, Soslow RA. Expression of pax8 as a useful marker in distinguishing ovarian carcinomas from mammary carcinomas. Am J Surg Pathol 2008;32:1566–71.

42. Köbel M, Kalloger SE, Boyd N, et al. Ovarian carcinoma subtypes are different diseases: implications for biomarker studies. PLoS Med 2008;12:e232.

43. Armes JE, Lourie R, de Silva M, et al. Abnormalities of the RB1 pathway in ovarian serous papillary carcinoma as determined by overexpression of the p16 (INK4A) protein. Int J Gynecol Pathol 2005;24:363–8.

44. O'Neill CJ, McBride HA, Connolly LE, et al. High-grade ovarian serous carcinoma exhibits significantly higher p16 expression than low-grade serous carcinoma and serous borderline tumour. Histopathology 2007;50:773–9.

45. Deavers MT. Immunohistochemistry in gynecologic pathology. Arch Pathol Lab Med 2008;2:175–80.

46. Vang R, Gown AM, Farinola M, et al. p16 expression in primary ovarian mucinous and endometrioid tumors and metastatic adenocarcinomas in the ovary: utility for identification of metastatic HPV-related endocervical adenocarcinomas. Am J Surg Pathol 2007;31:653–63.

47. Shih I, Sheu JJ, Santillan A, et al. Amplification of a chromatin remodeling gene, Rsf-1/HBXAP, in ovarian carcinoma. Proc Natl Acad Sci U S A 2005;102:14004–9.

48. Nakayama K, Nakayama N, Davidson B, et al. A BTB/POZ protein, NAC-1, is related to tumor recurrence and is essential for tumor growth and survival. Proc Natl Acad Sci U S A 2006;103:18739–44.

49. McCluggage WG, Lyness RW, Atkinson RJ, et al. Morphological effects of chemotherapy on ovarian carcinoma. J Clin Pathol 2002;1:27–31.

50. Miller K, Price JH, Dobbs SP, et al. An immunohistochemical and morphological analysis of post-chemotherapy ovarian carcinoma. J Clin Pathol 2008;5:652–7.

51. Gershenson DM, Sun CC, Lu KH, et al. Clinical behavior of stage II–IV low-grade serous carcinoma of the ovary. Obstet Gynecol 2006;2:361–8.

52. Santillan A, Kim YW, Zahurak ML, et al. Differences of chemoresistance assay between invasive micropapillary/low-grade serous ovarian carcinoma and high-grade serous ovarian carcinoma. Int J Gynecol Cancer 2007;3:601–6.

53. Singer G, Kurman RJ, Chang HW, et al. Diverse tumorigenic pathways in ovarian serous carcinoma. Am J Pathol 2002;160:1223.

54. Soslow RA, Rouse RV, Hendrickson MR, et al. Transitional cell neoplasms of the ovary and urinary bladder: a comparative immunohistochemical analysis. Int J Gynecol Pathol 1996;15:257–65.

55. Lotan TL, Ye H, Melamed J, et al. Immunohistochemical panel to identify the primary site of invasive micropapillary carcinoma. Am J Surg Pathol 2009;33(7):1037–41.

56. Lancaster JM, Powell CB, Kauff ND, et al. Society of gynecologic oncologists education committee statement on risk assessment for inherited gynecologic cancer predispositions. Gynecol Oncol 2007;2:159–62.

57. Werness BA, Ramus SJ, Whittemore AS, et al. Histopathology of familial ovarian tumors in women from families with and without germline BRCA1 mutations. Hum Pathol 2000;31:1420.

58. McCluggage WG. My approach to and thoughts on the typing of ovarian carcinomas. J Clin Pathol 2008;2:152–63.

59. Al-Hussaini M, Stockman A, Foster H, et al. WT-1 assists in distinguishing ovarian from uterine serous carcinoma and in distinguishing between serous and endometrioid ovarian carcinoma. Histopathology 2004;2:109–15.

60. Tornos C, Soslow R, Chen S, et al. Expression of WT1, CA125, and GCDFP-15 as useful markers in

the differential diagnosis of primary ovarian carcinomas versus metastatic breast cancer to the ovary. Am J Surg Pathol 2005;29:1482–9.

61. McCaughey WT, Kirk ME, Lester W, et al. Peritoneal epithelial lesions associated with proliferative serous tumors of ovary. Histopathology 1984;8: 195–208.

62. Shield P. Peritoneal washing cytology. Cytopathology 2004;3:131–41.

63. International Collaborative Ovarian Neoplasm Group. Paclitaxel plus carboplatin versus standard chemotherapy with either single-agent carboplatin or cyclophosphamide, doxorubicin, and cisplatin in women with ovarian cancer: the ICON3 randomised trial. Lancet 2002;360(9332):505–15.

64. Soslow RA. Histologic subtypes of ovarian carcinoma: an overview. Int J Gynecol Pathol 2008;2: 161–74.

65. Lee Y, Medeiros F, Kindelberger D, et al. Advances in the recognition of tubal intraepithelial carcinoma: applications to cancer screening and the pathogenesis of ovarian cancer. Adv Anat Pathol 2006; 1:1–7.

66. Palmer C, Brown PO. The preclinical history of serous ovarian carcinoma: defining the target for early detection. PLoS Med 2009;6:e1000114.

NONSEROUS OVARIAN EPITHELIAL TUMORS

Guangming Han, MD[a,b], Robert A. Soslow, MD[a,*]

KEYWORDS

- Ovary • Intestinal mucinous borderline tumor • Intestinal mucinous carcinoma
- Clear cell carcinoma • Endometrioid borderline tumor • Endometrioid carcinoma
- Transitional cell carcinoma • Malignant Brenner tumor • Undifferentiated carcinoma ovary
- Mixed epithelial carcinoma

ABSTRACT

This review covers the group of relatively uncommon nonserous ovarian epithelial tumors. The authors focus on the group's distinctiveness from the much more common serous tumors and show the similarities across entities. Diagnostic criteria that separate the different entities are currently being debated. Particular problems include the reproducible diagnosis of high-grade endometrioid, transitional cell, mixed epithelial and undifferentiated carcinomas. Furthermore, despite recognition that most malignant mucinous tumors involving ovary represent metastases from extraovarian primary sites, many misdiagnoses still occur. The authors discuss the rationale behind the opinions about these problematic topics.

OVERVIEW

The nonserous ovarian epithelial tumors include intestinal mucinous, Mullerian mucinous, endometrioid, clear cell, transitional cell, squamous, undifferentiated and mixed epithelial varieties (**Table 1**). Benign, nonserous ovarian epithelial tumors, such as cystadenomas, are common worldwide, but nonserous ovarian carcinomas are relatively uncommon, particularly in North America and Europe. Assembling these fascinating tumors into one article emphasizes the group's distinctiveness from the much more common serous tumors and allows emphasis of similarities across entities. Mucinous, endometrioid and some clear cell carcinomas arise through stepwise progression from longstanding precursors such as cystadenomas and borderline tumors, and when transitional cell, undifferentiated and high stage clear cell carcinomas are excluded, the remaining tumors tend to display indolent clinical behavior.[1]

A discussion of these topics is contentious, as diagnostic criteria that separate the different entities are currently being debated. Particular problems include the reproducible diagnosis of high-grade endometrioid, transitional cell, mixed epithelial and undifferentiated carcinomas. Furthermore, despite recognition that most malignant mucinous tumors involving ovary represent metastases from extraovarian primary sites, many misdiagnoses still occur. The field is also plagued with arguments about nomenclature used to describe tumors that are proliferative, but neither highly atypical nor invasive: the "borderline tumors" (see **Table 1**). The term "borderline" tumor will be used in this review, mostly because of historical precedent and familiarity. Other terms used to describe borderline tumors are "tumors of low malignant potential," "tumors of borderline malignancy," and "atypical proliferative tumors." Aside from serous and Mullerian mucinous borderline tumors, borderline tumors are benign, do not present at high stage, do not recur, do not transform to carcinoma if completely resected and do not lead to disease specific morbidity or mortality. Since "atypical proliferative tumor" accurately describes these lesions' morphologic features without placing them in a malignant category, the term appears

[a] Department of Pathology, Memorial Sloan-Kettering Cancer Center, 1275 York Avenue New York, NY 10065, USA

[b] Department of Pathology & Laboratory Medicine, Foothills Medical Centre, University of Calgary, AB T2N 2T9, Canada

* Corresponding author.

E-mail address: soslowr@MSKCC.ORG

Surgical Pathology 4 (2011) 397–459
doi:10.1016/j.path.2010.12.012

Table 1
Nonserous ovarian epithelial tumors

Intestinal mucinous	
Mullerian mucinous[b]	Adenoma, borderline tumor[a] and carcinoma are recognized
Endometrioid	
Clear cell	
Brenner	
Transitional cell	
Squamous	
Undifferentiated	

[a] Synonyms include: tumor of low malignant potential and atypical proliferative tumor.
[b] Closely related tumors: endocervical-type mucinous; seromucinous.

most appropriate for borderline tumors lacking a serous component.

This article focuses on the most common non-serous ovarian epithelial tumors and discusses these authors' opinions about the problematic topics mentioned above and the rationale behind those opinions.

INTESTINAL MUCINOUS TUMORS

Primary ovarian mucinous carcinomas are very uncommon; a recent publication indicates that less than 3% of all ovarian carcinomas are mucinous.[2,3] A mucinous adenocarcinoma involving the ovary is statistically more likely to represent a metastasis from an extraovarian source than a primary ovarian tumor.

GROSS FEATURES

Intestinal Mucinous Cystadenoma and Cystadenofibroma

Mucinous cystadenomas constitute approximately 15% of benign ovarian epithelial

---

Key Features
PRIMARY OVARIAN MUCINOUS
CARCINOMA

- Large, unilateral tumor with intracytoplasmic mucin

- Background mucinous borderline tumor

- Expansile invasion>destructive stromal invasion

- CK7>CK20

- Metastatic carcinoma is excluded

---

neoplasms. Almost all are unilateral. They are unilocular or multilocular tumors of variable size with a mean of about 10 cm. The outer surface is smooth and lacks adherent mucin in almost all cases. Cut section reveals cysts containing thick gelatinous material. There may be Brenner tumor or teratomatous components in evidence. The amount of fibromatous stroma is variable.

Intestinal Mucinous Borderline Tumor

Mucinous borderline tumors are generally unilateral, large tumors, exceeding 10 to 12 cm in greatest dimension. Like the cystadenomas, these tumors lack tumor or adherent mucin on the ovarian surface. On cut section, they are multilocular, with cysts that contain mucinous material. Rare tumors contain solid nodules within them.

Intestinal Mucinous Carcinoma

Mucinous carcinomas and mucinous borderline tumors resemble one another to a substantial degree. In fact, it has been estimated that erroneous sampling of mucinous carcinomas at the time of frozen section leads to a mistaken diagnosis of borderline tumor in as many as 15% of cases.[4] The same generalities regarding unilaterality and large size apply. It is uncommon, but certainly not unheard of, to find tumor growth on the ovarian surface. Carcinomas usually contain more solid areas than borderline tumors and may feature necrosis (**Fig. 1**). Rare tumors also may contain solid, mural nodules.

MICROSCOPIC FEATURES

Intestinal mucinous tumors are composed of cells containing intracytoplasmic mucin and most feature goblet cells at least focally (**Fig. 2**). Extraovarian mucin by itself is not sufficient for classification as an intestinal mucinous neoplasm. A diagnosis of primary ovarian mucinous cystadenoma, borderline tumor or carcinoma should only be rendered with confidence when the tumor is unilateral and larger than 10 to 12 cm and the patient lacks a history of an extraovarian adenocarcinoma (**Box 1**).[3,5] Enhanced pathologic evaluation, including immunohistochemistry, is highly recommended when any uncharacteristic clinical, gross or microscopic feature is found.

Intestinal Mucinous Cystadenoma and Cystadenofibroma

These tumors feature one or more cysts separated by variable amounts of stroma (**Fig. 3**). The stroma may have a fibromatous appearance or resemble non-neoplastic ovarian stroma. The cysts are lined by columnar cells with obvious intracytoplasmic

Fig. 1. Gross appearance of a primary mucinous carcinoma of the ovary, intestinal type. Tumor has both cystic and solid areas.

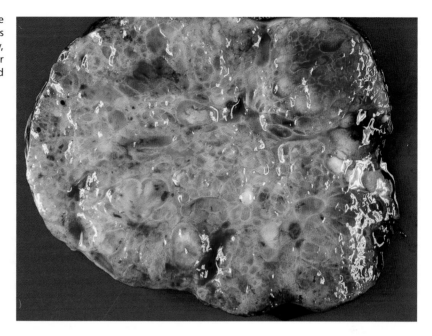

mucin (**Fig. 4**). Papillations and tufting are either not encountered or found in less than 10% of the tumor. Tumors with rare or focal papillations have been referred to as "mucinous cystadenomas with proliferative features,[6]" which is preferable terminology, or "mucinous cystadenomas with atypia."

Intestinal Mucinous Borderline Tumor

These tumors resemble cystadenomas with extensive papillations and tufting (**Fig. 5**). The precise degree of proliferation that separates the two entities has not been defined. As these tumors both feature benign clinical behavior, there is no compelling reason to err on the side of borderline tumor when tufting and papillations are not well developed. Some of the architectural and cytologic features of intestinal mucinous borderline tumors recapitulate non-neoplastic intestinal epithelium. In these areas, highly proliferative cells relatively lacking in cytoplasmic mucin, resembling intestinal

Fig. 2. The epithelial cells of intestinal mucinous tumors contain intracytoplasmic mucin and most feature goblet cells at least focally.

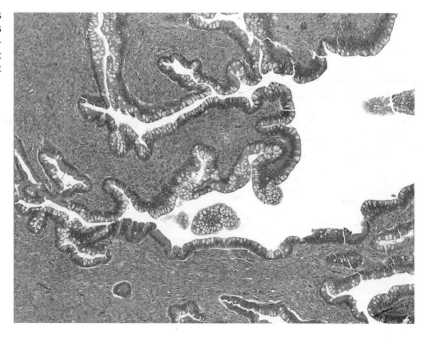

Box 1
Mucinous tumor algorithm[a]

Favor primary ovarian neoplasm[b]

Unilateral tumor > 10 to 12 cm

Favor metastatic carcinoma to ovary[c]

Unilateral tumor < 10 cm

Bilateral tumor

[a] May be used for endometrioid tumors as well
[b] History of extraovarian mucinous carcinoma is lacking and intraoperative examination fails to reveal another primary site
[c] Even when histologic appearance is benign or borderline
Data from Seidman JD, Kurman RJ, Ronnett BM. Primary and metastatic mucinous adenocarcinomas in the ovaries: incidence in routine practice with a new approach to improve intraoperative diagnosis. Am J Surg Pathol 2003;27(7):985–93; Yemelyanova AV, Vang R, Judson K, et al. Distinction of Primary and Metastatic mucinous tumors involving the ovary: analysis of size and laterality data by primary site with reevaluation of an algorithm for tumor classification. Am J Surg Pathol 2008;32(1):128–38.

evidence of expansile and destructive stromal invasion is lacking.[7,8] Cribriform architecture may be seen in intraepithelial carcinoma, but it fails to meet quantitative criteria for expansile-invasive adenocarcinoma. Widespread intraepithelial carcinoma is unusual and should suggest the possibility of full-fledged mucinous carcinoma or metastatic carcinoma from an extraovarian site, as discussed subsequently. Microinvasion in borderline tumors can also be encountered (**Fig. 7**). Small foci of destructive stromal invasion, defined subsequently, should be diagnosed as "microinvasion" if each focus measures less than 5 mm in greatest linear dimension or less than 10 mm² in greatest area in any one slide.[7,8] Microinvasive foci generally display cytoplasmic and nuclear features that differ from the background borderline tumor, similar to microinvasive squamous carcinoma of cervix with "paradoxical maturation." Microinvasion should be distinguished from ruptured glands with mucin extravasation (**Fig. 8**), as is frequently seen in inflammatory bowel disease.[9] When mucin extravasation is extensive, it is referred to as "pseudomyxoma ovarii." Although not a specific feature, pseudomyxoma ovarii (**Figs. 9** and **10**) should be considered a sign that the tumor may have originated in an extraovarian site, particularly the appendix. Very rare primary ovarian mucinous tumors may show limited amounts of mucin on the ovarian surface. These tumors can only be definitively classified as ovarian primaries when other features suggesting metastasis are lacking, and

crypts, are found at the base of papillary projections. The cells gradually assume increasing features of maturation, such that cells at the tips of the papillae have obvious intracytoplasmic mucin without mitotic activity. In some cases, a distinction between crypt-like and mature cells is not evident.

The term "intraepithelial carcinoma" (**Fig. 6**) has been applied when the nuclear grade is high and

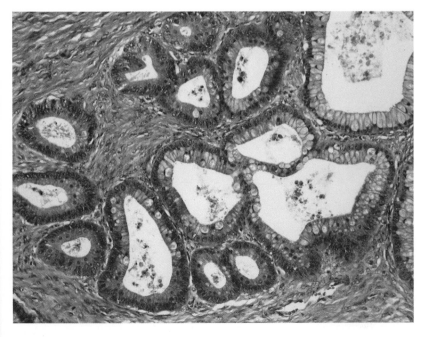

Fig. 3. Intestinal mucinous cystadenomas feature one or more glands and cysts separated by variable amounts of stroma.

Fig. 4. The cysts are lined by columnar cells with obvious intra-cytoplasmic mucin.

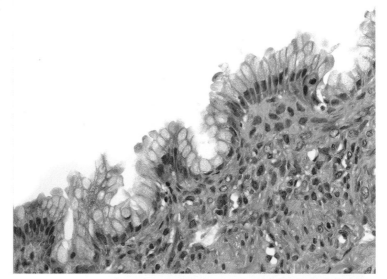

Fig. 5. (*A*) Intestinal mucinous borderline tumors typically demonstrate extensive papillation and tufting of the epithelium. (*B*) Cytologic features of intestinal mucinous borderline tumor.

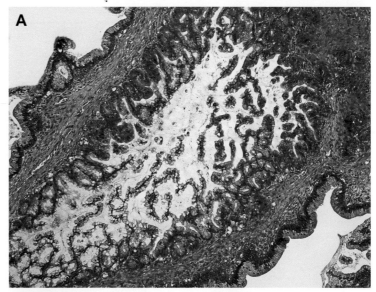

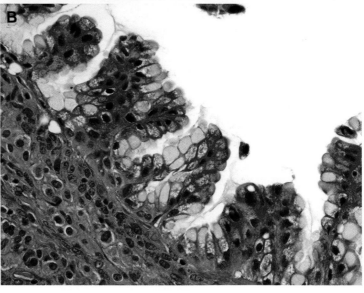

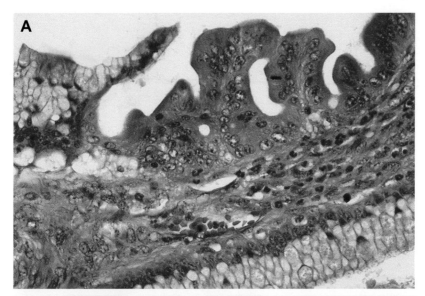

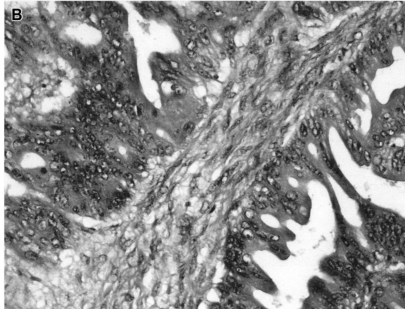

Fig. 6. (*A*) High grade nuclear features within an intestinal mucinous borderline tumor are in keeping with a diagnosis of intraepithelial carcinoma. (*B*) Foci of intraepithelial carcinoma may show architecturally complex growth patterns that fall short of those seen in expansile invasion.

a non-neoplastic appendix has been removed and has been examined in its entirety. Limited mucin deposition associated with primary ovarian tumors is thought to result from capsular disruption.

Intestinal Mucinous Carcinoma

Most intestinal mucinous carcinomas arise in a background of cystadenoma and borderline tumor. It is useful to imagine that these tumors

gradually enlarge in a symmetrical manner, with increasing proliferation and architectural complexity. The distinction between borderline tumor and carcinoma, then, is primarily based on architectural features. Growth patterns that resemble well differentiated endometrioid adenocarcinoma of the endometrium are considered evidence of expansile stromal invasion (**Fig. 11**).[7,8] These patterns include large cribriform glands, extensive gland fusion, maze-like patterns

Fig. 7. Focus of microinvasion in an intestinal mucinous borderline tumor. This focus measures less than 5 mm.

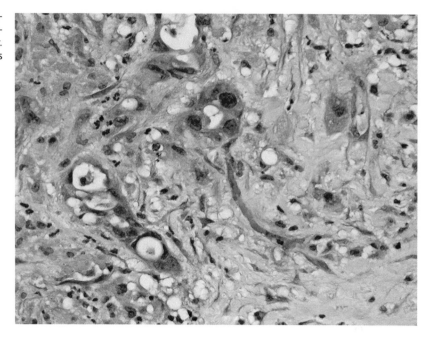

and extensive papillae (see **Fig. 11**).[10] When the diagnostic decisions involve consideration of borderline tumor and carcinoma, it is useful to apply Gleason grading rules; Gleason pattern 3 tumors are usually classified as borderline tumors whereas Gleason pattern 4 tumors are carcinomas. Foci of expansile invasion should measure at least 5 mm in greatest linear dimension in any one focus or more than 10 mm² in greatest area in any one slide.[7,8] Destructive stromal invasion is less frequently encountered (**Fig. 12**). This resembles the typical pattern of myometrial-invasive endometrial cancer, with irregularly shaped glands and small nests surrounded by reactive stroma. Extensive destructive stromal invasion is more typically seen in metastases to the ovary rather than in primary ovarian tumors, so this should prompt investigation for an extraovarian primary.

Fig. 8. Ruptured glands with extravasated mucin can sometimes mimic stromal invasion.

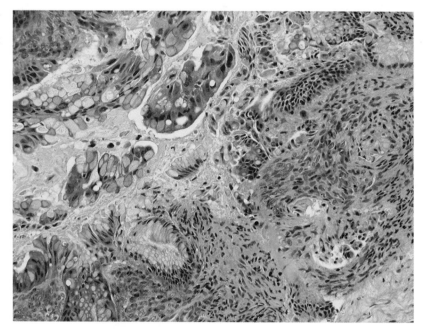

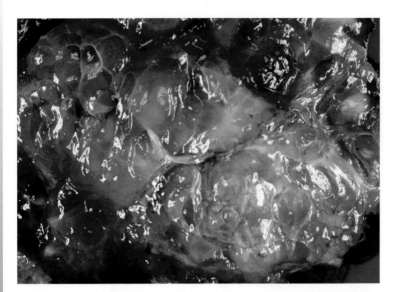

Fig. 9. Gross appearance of pseudomyxoma ovarii in a patient with a low grade appendiceal mucinous neoplasm.

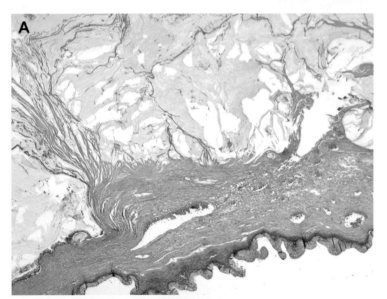

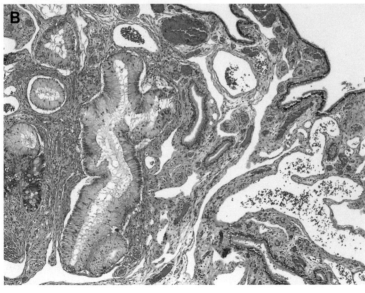

Fig. 10. Typically, ovarian involvement by low grade appendiceal mucinous neoplasm shows mucin-rich proliferations with only scant, benign, hyperplastic or low-grade dysplastic epithelium (*A*). Panel (*B*) shows hyperplastic-appearing mucinous epithelium from a low grade appendiceal mucinous neoplasm that colonizes and focally replaces fallopian tube epithelium.

Fig. 11. Mucinous carcinoma with expansile invasion has a growth pattern that resembles well differentiated endometrioid adenocarcinoma of the endometrium.

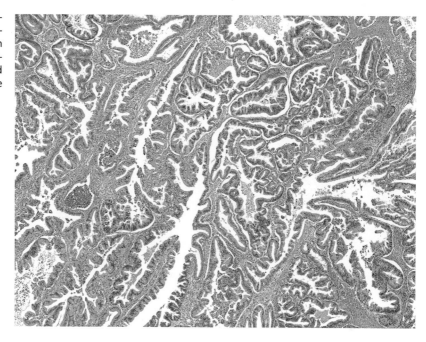

The cytoplasmic features of tumor cells vary from cells with eosinophilic cytoplasm and inapparent mucin to columnar cells with obvious apical mucin to goblet cells. Mucin should be demonstrable in at least 50% of tumor cells to qualify for mucinous carcinoma, and confirmatory endometrioid features, discussed subsequently, should be lacking. Most mucinous carcinomas display moderately atypical nuclei (**Fig. 13**), similar to that seen in moderately differentiated colorectal adenocarcinoma, as discussed subsequently.

Rare mucinous tumors contain unexpected components. The presence of mural nodules composed of spindle cells has received some attention in the literature.[11–14] Some have been classified as anaplastic carcinoma (**Fig. 14**), others as sarcoma and yet others as giant cell-rich tumors. Primary ovarian mucinous tumors may

Fig. 12. Destructive stromal invasion (right side of figure) in a primary mucinous carcinoma of the ovary is less frequent than expansile invasion (see **Fig. 11**).

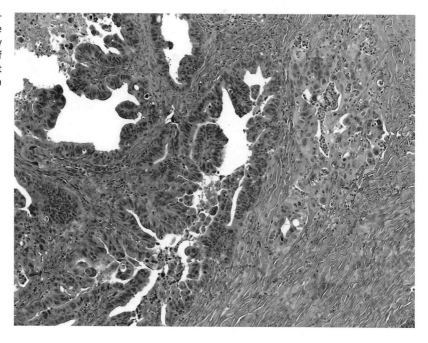

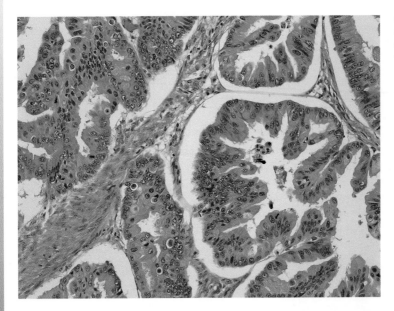

Fig. 13. Mucinous carcinoma with expansile invasion often shows concordance between architectural and nuclear grade.

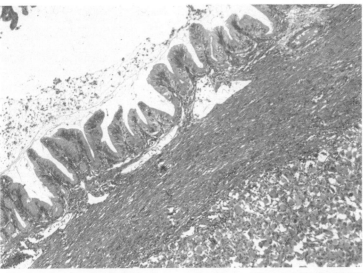

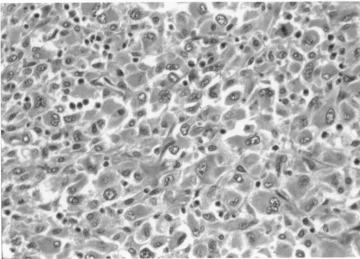

Fig. 14. Anaplastic carcinoma presenting as a mural nodule in a mucinous tumor. The epithelial lining of the cyst appears to be of borderline malignancy (*top*). The undifferentiated component is characterized by a diffuse arrangement of cells with abundant eosinophilic cytoplasm and grade 3 nuclei (*bottom*). The anaplastic carcinoma was strongly positive for cytokeratin (not shown). (*From* Prat J. Pathology of the Ovary. Philadelphia: Saunders; 2004; with permission.)

also contain foci of high-grade neuroendocrine carcinoma.[15]

There is no uniform approach to grading mucinous carcinomas of the ovary. Both 3-tiered grading schemes, FIGO (GOG) and Shimizu-Silverberg are currently the most commonly used in practice. The FIGO system, based primarily on architectural features, is identical to the FIGO grading system used for endometrioid carcinomas of the endometrium. Shimizu-Silverberg accounts for architecture, nuclear grade and mitotic activity.[16,17] With Shimizu-Silverberg, the typical ovarian mucinous carcinoma would score 1 point for glandular architecture, 2 or 3 points for nuclear atypia and 2 or 3 points for mitotic activity, which translates into either a grade 1 or grade 2 tumor. Grade 3 ovarian mucinous carcinomas are very rare.

Immunohistochemistry and Molecular Genetics

Primary intestinal mucinous carcinomas show co-expression of CK7 and CK20, with preferential expression of CK7 over CK20[18–21] in most cases (**Fig. 15**). This means that only CK20 staining with

Fig. 15. Primary intestinal mucinous carcinomas show co-expression of CK7 and CK20, with preferential expression of CK7 (*A*) over CK20 (*B*) in most cases.

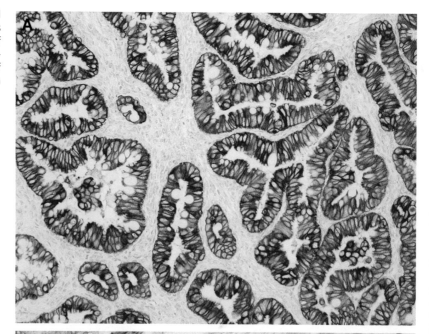

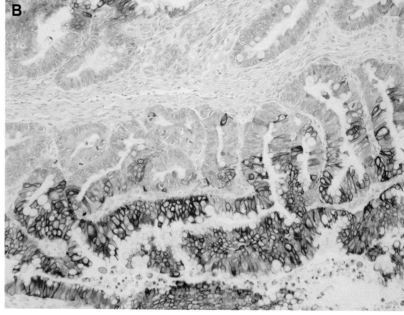

minimal or absent CK7 staining provides information about the presence of lower gastrointestinal differentiation (**Box 2**). Compared to colorectal carcinomas, primary intestinal mucinous carcinomas are negative for racemase and nuclear β-catenin.[22] The only primary ovarian tumor that demonstrates the CK7 negative/CK20 positive immunophenotype is an enteric-type neoplasm that arises in an ovarian teratoma.

When the differential diagnosis includes tumors other than colorectal and appendiceal tumors, the CK7/20 immunoprofile is not informative. Primary intestinal mucinous ovarian carcinomas are p16 negative, in contrast to endocervical adenocarcinomas,[23,24] and they lack expression of estrogen and progesterone receptors[25] and CA125, unlike endometrioid carcinomas. Compared to many pancreatic ductal carcinomas, about one-half of which lack SMAD4/DPC4 expression, SMAD4 expression is retained,[19] but primary ovarian intestinal mucinous carcinomas lack mesothelin and fascin.[26] Paradoxically, ductal adenocarcinoma of the pancreas is more likely to express CA125 than a primary ovarian intestinal mucinous neoplasm.

K-ras mutations are well described in ovarian mucinous neoplasms.[27,28] Mucinous neoplasms may rarely occur in the setting of Lynch syndrome/hereditary nonpolyposis colorectal carcinoma syndrome.[29]

Box 2
Mucinous tumor immunohistochemical algorithm

CK7 < CK20

- Metastatic colorectal, appendiceal or small intestinal neoplasm
- Primary ovarian mucinous neoplasm of enteric type, associated with teratoma

CK7 > CK20

- Primary ovarian mucinous neoplasm (provided unilateral tumor greater than 10 to 12 cm)
- Metastatic upper gastrointestinal, pancreatobiliary and gallbladder carcinomas (provided unilateral tumor <10 cm or bilateral tumor)

CK7 = CK20

- Metastatic colorectal and appendiceal neoplasm unlikely
- Consider primary and other metastatic tumors

DIFFERENTIAL DIAGNOSIS

The main differential diagnostic consideration is metastatic adenocarcinoma, including examples from the upper gastrointestinal and pancreatobiliary tracts, colon, and appendix. Other less commonly encountered problems involve the distinction of primary ovarian mucinous carcinoma and endometrioid carcinoma, low-grade serous carcinoma with intraluminal mucin, high-grade serous carcinoma with microcysts and signet ring cells and gynecologic tumors containing mucinous glandular elements. Unusual problems include the differentiation of metastatic endocervical carcinoma[23,24,30,31] and pulmonary carcinomas from primary mucinous ovarian carcinomas.[32]

Metastatic carcinoma **Box 3** should be considered when tumors are bilateral or unilateral and small (<10 to 12 cm), grossly multinodular, or display ovarian surface involvement. Microscopic features that are more commonly seen in metastases include extensive destructive stromal invasion, extensive pseudomyxoma ovarii, signet ring cell morphology and lymphovascular invasion (**Figs. 16–19**).[33] The presence of signet ring cells should raise consideration for Krukenberg tumor (**Fig. 20**),[34] a term generally used to describe signet ring cell carcinomas metastatic from the stomach, but signet ring cells do not predominate in some Krukenberg tumors and may be present in a variety of other primary and metastatic ovarian tumors, both benign[35] and malignant.[36,37] Not all mucinous carcinomas that metastasize to ovaries have a malignant appearance. Many biliary, gallbladder and pancreatic carcinomas display a deceptively benign or borderline appearance in the ovary[38–42] (see McCluggage Figure 9A, from

---

Box 3
Features favoring metastasis

- Bilateral disease
- Surface involvement
- Destructive stromal invasion
- Nodular growth pattern
- Single cells/signet ring cells
- Vascular invasion

Data from Lee KR, Young RH. The distinction between primary and metastatic mucinous carcinomas of the ovary: gross and histologic findings in 50 cases. Am J Surg Pathol 2003;27(3):281–92.

Differential Diagnosis
PRIMARY OVARIAN MUCINOUS CARCINOMA

Consider:	If this is Present:
Metastatic mucinous carcinoma	Bilateral, small and nodular tumors
Involvement by "pseudomyxoma peritonei"	Mucinous ascites
Mucinous borderline tumor	Lacking expansile and destructive stromal invasion
Endometroid carcinoma	ER/PR positive
Mucinous tumor associated with another primary ovarian neoplasm:	Teratoma Brenner tumor Carcinoid Small cell carcinoma of hypercalcemic type Heterologous Sertoli-Leydig cell tumor

the McCluggage article, Metastatic Carcinomas to Ovary, in this publication). Immunohistochemistry can be used in problematic cases, as outlined in the immunohistochemistry section, but it is acknowledged that, using commercially available antibodies, it may be difficult or impossible to target a primary extraovarian site, especially when the immunophenotype is CK7 positive with retained SMAD4/DPC 4 staining. As mentioned previously, CA125 is more likely to be positive in pancreatic ductal carcinoma using immunohistochemistry than is a primary ovarian intestinal mucinous tumor. The patient's history and distribution of disease still takes precedence in this circumstance. Clues to the presence of a metastatic pancreatobiliary carcinoma with misleadingly bland histologic features that suggest a benign primary ovarian mucinous tumor include bilateral tumor or a small unilateral tumor and a multinodular appearance.[38–40] Unless the tumor displays a negative SMAD4/DPC4 immunophenotype, immunohistochemistry would not be helpful for differential diagnosis. If there is any doubt about the location of the primary site, it is

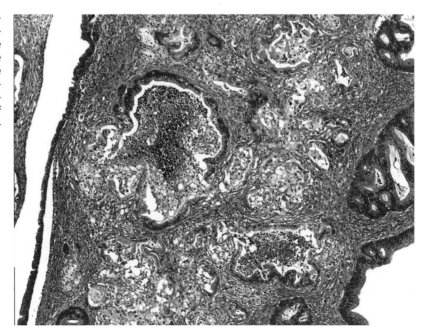

Fig. 16. Metastatic pancreatic ductal adenocarcinoma with extensive destructive invasion. Note that glands at the periphery have a low-grade, noninvasive appearance. This is typical of metastatic pancreatic ductal adenocarcinoma.

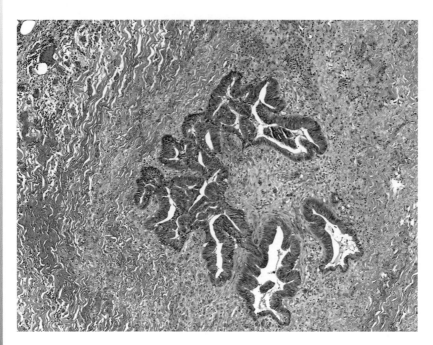

Fig. 17. Metastatic colonic adenocarcinoma demonstrates the nodular pattern and stromal reaction typically seen with metastasis.

reasonable to note in the surgical pathology report that the ovary can only be assigned as primary if all other possibilities are excluded.

Pseudomyxoma peritonei syndrome is treacherous because tumor in the ovary characteristically has a cytologically benign appearance. Occasional metastatic pancreatobiliary carcinomas may have a misleading appearance as well, with benign- and borderline-appearing deposits predominating over deposits that are easily recognized as adenocarcinoma. Correct diagnosis of these cases starts with an evaluation of the patient's clinical history and an appraisal of the disease distribution. Deposits of pseudomyxoma peritonei are found in patients with mucinous ascites and tumors showing ovarian surface involvement, extensive ovarian mucin dissection (pseudomyxoma ovarii) and the typical CK20 positive and CK7 negative immunophenotype. Tumors with these characteristics almost always derive from the appendix, with only rare exceptions,[43–45] discussed subsequently in this section.

Pseudomyxoma peritonei **Table 2**, the name used to describe copious mucinous ascites, exists in two distinct forms[43–46] with only occasional exceptions: mucin-rich proliferations with only scant, benign, hyperplastic or low-grade dysplastic epithelium (see **Fig. 10**) and mucin-rich tumors with copious, malignant appearing epithelium (**Fig. 21**). The former lesion is typical of ruptured mucinous cystic lesions of the appendix, while the second lesion may derive from any mucinous carcinoma. The former lesion is relatively indolent with low proliferative rates, while the latter is an aggressive, highly proliferative tumor. Pathologists agree that using the term "mucinous adenocarcinoma" to describe the latter lesions is appropriate, but there is no consensus regarding the best term for the former lesion (see **Table 2**). That is because the former lesion demonstrates extra-appendiceal spread, but neither arises from adenocarcinoma nor displays malignant cytologic features. Unlike typical forms of metastatic gastrointestinal adenocarcinoma, this lesion does not demonstrate omental adipose tissue invasion, lymph node metastasis or extra-abdominal dissemination. Tumor cells are also relatively chemoresistant. The current preferred terminology is therefore "low-grade (appendiceal) mucinous neoplasm" or "disseminated peritoneal adenomucinosis." It is not recommended to report these as "carcinomas" so that distinction with the highly proliferative and aggressive variants is maintained. It is also inappropriate to use terminology usually reserved for ovarian primary tumors, such as "borderline tumor" or "tumor of low malignant potential."

Fig. 18. Metastatic colonic adenocarcinoma with moderate cytologic atypia and frequent goblet cells, mimicking a primary ovarian mucinous tumor.

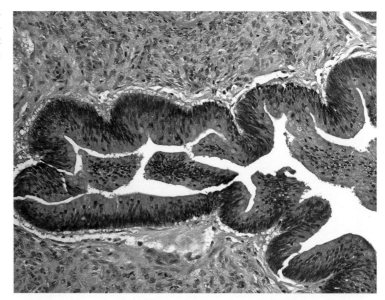

Fig. 19. Endocervical adenocarcinoma metastatic to ovary, mimicking primary ovarian mucinous tumor. Carcinoma exhibits frequent mitoses (A). Tumor cells are strongly and diffusely positive for p16 immunohistochemical staining (B).

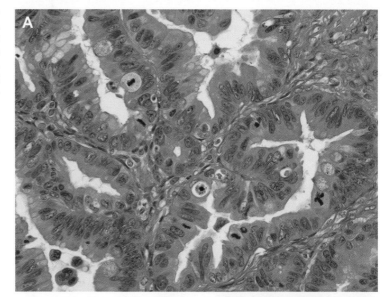

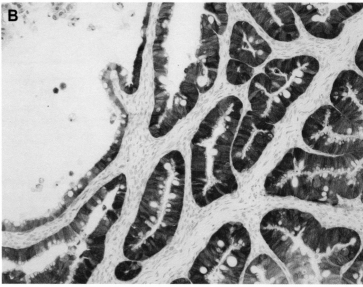

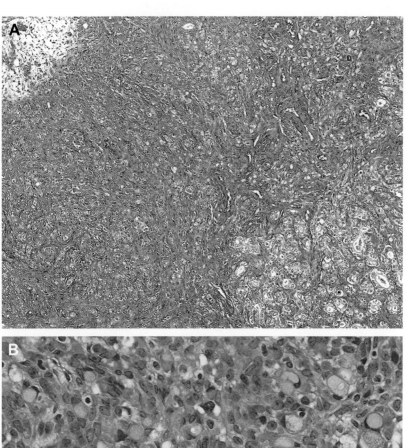

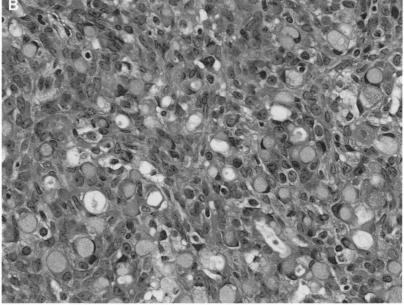

Fig. 20. The presence of signet ring cells in the ovary raises consideration of Krukenberg tumor (*A*). The cytologic details of the signet ring cells are shown in panel (*B*).

Coexisting mucinous borderline tumor and without endometriosis, an endometrioid adenofibromatous tumor, squamous metaplasia or ER/PR expression favor a mucinous neoplasm instead of an *endometrioid tumor*.[47] WT1 expression is typical of *serous carcinoma*. For metastases, p16 expression is typical of *endocervical carcinomas* of the usual type and TTF-1 expression is frequently encountered in *pulmonary adenocarcinomas* metastatic to ovaries,[32] although TTF-1 expression has recently been reported to be found in small percentages of primary gynecologic tumors.[48,49]

Table 2
"Pseudomyxoma peritonei" terminology

Cytologically low grade neoplasm with mucinous ascites	
Pseudomyxoma peritonei Mucinous borderline tumor Well differentiated mucinous adenocarcinoma	Terminology that should be *avoided* in pathology reports
Disseminated peritoneal adenomucinosis Disseminated or metastatic low grade appendiceal mucinous neoplasm	
Cytologically high grade neoplasm with mucinous ascites	
Pseudomyxoma peritonei	Terminology that should be *avoided* in pathology reports
Metastatic mucinous adenocarcinoma	

A number of ovarian tumors can contain mucinous epithelium that is usually histologically benign: *teratoma, Brenner tumor, carcinoid, small cell carcinoma of hypercalcemic type and heterologous Sertoli-Leydig cell tumor.* It has been hypothesized that some mucinous ovarian tumors represent overgrowth of a pre-existing Brenner tumor[50] or teratoma.[51] For practical purposes, then, it is reasonable to attempt to exclude the presence of these entities before making a diagnosis of pure intestinal mucinous ovarian tumor. Rare teratomas may harbor mucinous neoplasms, including carcinomas, with colorectal, gastric or appendiceal differentiation.[51] These malignancies can be histologically identical to eutopic examples and would be expected to display similar immunophenotypes. This means, for example, that colorectal-type adenocarcinoma can arise in the context of an ovarian teratoma (**Fig. 22**). The existence of tumors like this may account for the very rare primary ovarian mucinous carcinomas that have a lower gastrointestinal phenotype, as mentioned in the immunohistochemistry section. Correct diagnosis, therefore, would depend on documenting teratomatous components within the ovary and clinical exclusion of a colorectal primary. Appendix-like mucinous cystadenomas with pseudomyxoma peritonei have also been reported to arise in ovarian teratomas and very rare cases of pseudomyxoma peritonei have resulted.[51–53] Since this is exceptional, pseudomyxoma peritonei syndrome should continue to be considered almost exclusively a primary extraovarian, usually appendiceal process. An ovarian source should only be assigned when an ovarian teratoma is present and an entirely resected, sectioned and submitted appendix shows absolutely no gross or histologic abnormalities.

DIAGNOSIS

Ovarian intestinal mucinous neoplasms have a reputation for being morphologically heterogeneous. This means, in practical terms, that such a diagnosis cannot be established with certainty unless the entire tumor is resected, a very careful gross examination is undertaken and extensive sectioning takes place. Given the propensity of metastatic carcinomas to mimic primary ovarian mucinous tumors, it is crucial to be informed about the tumor's laterality, the status of the appendix, whether pseudomyxoma peritonei is present, the type of operation performed (ovarian cystectomy vs oophorectomy) and the patient's clinical history. Core biopsy of ovarian masses is discouraged as rupturing a malignant ovarian tumor automatically upstages the tumor and usually qualifies the patient for chemotherapy. Ovarian mucinous carcinomas are so rarely metastatic at presentation that almost nothing is known about the relevant diagnostic criteria that might be useful given a biopsy of tumor from a distant site.

The gross examination should include a meticulous evaluation of the ovarian surface to document the presence of any disruptions, implants or adherent mucin. If the tumor has a very simple architectural appearance on cut section (i.e. simple cysts without papillations, nodules or solid growth), it is reasonable to submit one section per centimeter. However, if the tumor is bilateral,

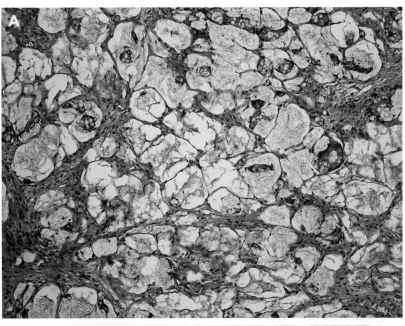

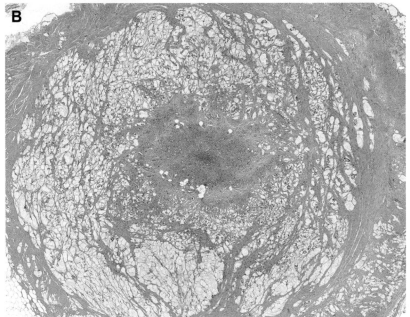

Fig. 21. Pseudomyxoma ovarii containing malignant appearing epithelium (*A*). This is a metastasis from a primary appendiceal adenocarcinoma (*B*).

shows ovarian surface abnormalities or intraoperative findings and clinical history that are uncharacteristic of an ovarian primary, submit additional sections, for a total of two per centimeter. If any macroscopic features suggest borderline tumor or carcinoma, it is reasonable to submit one section per centimeter initially. Additional sections are not needed if a diagnosis of primary ovarian mucinous carcinoma can be made without difficulty. In all other situations (i.e. borderline tumor, borderline tumor with microinvasion, borderline tumor with intraepithelial carcinoma, etc), two sections per centimeter should be submitted for microscopic examination.[54]

Fig. 22. Colorectal type adenocarcinoma can occasionally arise in an ovarian teratoma (the teratomatous component within the same ovary is shown in the inset).

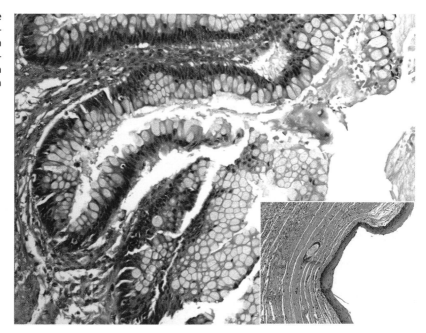

PROGNOSIS

Primary ovarian mucinous cystadenomas and borderline tumors[7,8] are benign if they are accurately diagnosed. Many metastatic pancreatobiliary adenocarcinomas display a paradoxically benign or borderline appearance in the ovary,[38–40] and it is well documented that ovarian deposits of low grade appendiceal mucinous neoplasm in the setting of pseudomyxoma peritonei resemble ovarian mucinous cystadenoma or borderline tumor.[43–45] Bone fide ovarian intestinal mucinous borderline tumors with intraepithelial carcinoma and/or microinvasion are generally considered benign tumors as well,[7,8] although there are rare reports of metastasis following such diagnoses.[8] As a general rule of thumb, mucinous tumors with severe, widespread nuclear atypia and a noninvasive profile should be treated very cautiously. It is statistically likely that such a tumor represented either a metastasis from a distant site or a full-fledged primary ovarian mucinous carcinoma.

Most reports about the dismal clinical outcomes of ovarian mucinous carcinoma are based upon review of metastases to the ovary that were misinterpreted as ovarian primary tumors. This is the subject of an upcoming publication from the Gynecologic Oncology Group in 2011. When metastases are excluded, it appears that a majority of patients with primary ovarian mucinous adenocarcinoma survive after complete staging surgery. The prognosis is driven principally by tumor stage; approximately one-half to two-thirds are FIGO stage I (confined to the ovary) in industrialized, Western countries.[2,3,7] Although they are rare, primary ovarian mucinous carcinomas are the third most common FIGO stage I ovarian carcinoma.[55] Extraovarian tumor deposition is rather uncommon, but it is highly unfavorable because, unlike high grade serous carcinomas, mucinous carcinomas are thought to be either relatively or absolutely resistant to taxanes and platinum-based

> ### *Pitfalls*
> #### PRIMARY OVARIAN MUCINOUS CARCINOMA
>
> ! Bilateral primary ovarian mucinous carcinomas cannot be diagnosed confidently
>
> ! Small (<10 to 12 cm), unilateral primary ovarian mucinous carcinomas cannot be diagnosed confidently
>
> ! Ovarian involvement by pseudomyxoma peritonei and metastatic pancreatobiliary carcinomas may resemble benign or borderline mucinous ovarian tumors
>
> ! Most examples express CK20 (although CK7 expression almost always exceeds CK20 in distribution and intensity)
>
> ! Many tumors, including primary ovarian mucinous carcinoma, co-express CK7 and 20

chemotherapeutic regimens.[56] The prognosis of FIGO stage I tumors is likely also affected by the presence of destructive stromal invasion, which is prognostically unfavorable.[7,9] Even tumors with expansile invasion only, however, have the potential to metastasize.[57] It has not been conclusively proven that tumor grade in stage I mucinous carcinomas is prognostically significant.[58] Recent work has shown that approximately 20% of ovarian mucinous carcinomas have *Her2* amplification and Her2 immunohistochemical overexpression, and anecdotal responses to trastuzumab are on record.[59]

ENDOMETRIOID TUMORS

The overall prevalence of ovarian endometrioid carcinoma has decreased owing to re-classification of many so-called "high-grade endometrioid carcinomas" as high-grade serous carcinoma. Nevertheless, ovarian endometrioid carcinoma is still the second most common ovarian carcinoma subtype in the West, accounting for approximately 10% of all ovarian carcinomas.[2] It is the most common FIGO stage I ovarian carcinoma and probably constitutes at least 50% of such cases.[55] Most ovarian endometrioid carcinomas are FIGO stage I or II.

GROSS FEATURES

Endometrioid Adenofibroma and Borderline Tumor

Pure endometrioid adenofibroma is very rare, but extensive sectioning of borderline tumors and carcinomas often discloses an adenofibromatous component. Endometrioid borderline tumor unassociated with carcinoma is very unusual as well. In their pure form, these tumors are unilateral and almost always predominantly solid. Small cysts may be present and an association with endometriosis apparent. Borderline tumors are not associated with extraovarian tumor implants involving peritoneum or the contralateral ovary unless they are synchronous tumors arising in endometriosis. Adenofibroma and borderline tumors can be associated with synchronous endometrial polyps, including polypoid adenomyoma, atypical polypoid adenomyoma, endometrial hyperplasia and even endometrioid adenocarcinoma of endometrium.

Endometrioid Carcinoma

Although it has been reported that endometrioid ovarian carcinomas are not infrequently bilateral, application of strict diagnostic criteria that exclude serous carcinoma makes bilateral endometrioid

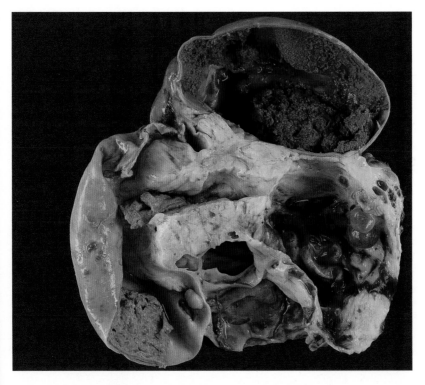

Fig. 23. Gross appearance of an endometrioid carcinoma presenting as a solid tumor nodule within an endometriotic cyst. (*Courtesy of* Dr Kay Park.)

ovarian carcinoma a rarity (Soslow RA, Park KJ, Murray MP, unpublished observations, 2010). Endometrioid ovarian carcinoma is frequently associated with endometriosis as well as endometrial neoplasms including atypical polypoid adenomyoma and endometrioid adenocarcinoma.[60,61] It has been estimated that 10 to 20% of endometrioid ovarian carcinomas are associated with synchronous endometrial carcinomas.[62,63] As noted previously, most endometrioid adenocarcinomas are confined to the ovary at presentation, although local extension to pelvic structures can sometimes be seen. Metastases to the abdomen and pelvic lymph nodes are rare. Adenocarcinomas may be solid, cystic, or solid and cystic. The solid tumors may resemble adenofibromatous tumors and the cystic tumors often display evidence of endometriosis. The presence of an endometriotic, chocolate-brown cyst containing a solid tumor nodule is a typical gross presentation of the entity (**Fig. 23**).

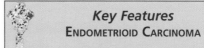

> ## *Key Features*
> ### ENDOMETRIOID CARCINOMA
>
> - Large, usually unilateral tumor
> - Resembles endometrioid adenocarcinoma of endometrium
> - Cytologic and architectural grades are concordant
> - Confirmatory endometrioid features are present (**Box 4**)
> - Expansile invasion>destructive stromal invasion
> - CK7 and ER positive; WT1 negative
> - Metastatic carcinoma is excluded

MICROSCOPIC FEATURES

Endometrioid Adenofibroma

This is a proliferation of benign appearing endometrioid glands set in fibromatous tissue (**Fig. 24**). The glands themselves and their distribution relative to the others resemble inactive, weakly proliferative or proliferative endometrium, or simple, non-atypical hyperplasia of the endometrium. Glands are well-formed and the nuclear grade is low. Endometrioid adenofibromas frequently have foci of squamous or morular metaplasia.

Endometrioid Borderline Tumor

The glandular components of endometrioid borderline tumors resemble complex hyperplasia of the endometrium,[60,61] with or without atypia

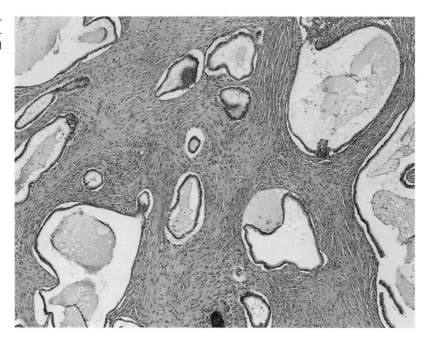

Fig. 24. Endometrioid cystadenofibroma with well-formed simple glands and fibromatous stroma.

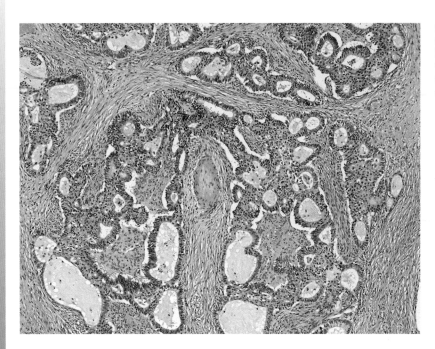

Fig. 25. Borderline endometrioid tumor resembles complex hyperplasia with or without atypia, often in a background cystadenofibroma.

(**Fig. 25**). The interglandular stroma is usually fibromatous. Diagnostic difficulties similar to those involving the distinction of complex atypical hyperplasia with morules versus endometrioid adenocarcinoma of the endometrium can sometimes be encountered when endometrioid borderline tumor has extensive morular metaplasia (**Fig. 26**). Microinvasion in borderline tumors can also be encountered.[60] The histologic features of microinvasion in endometrioid borderline tumors and

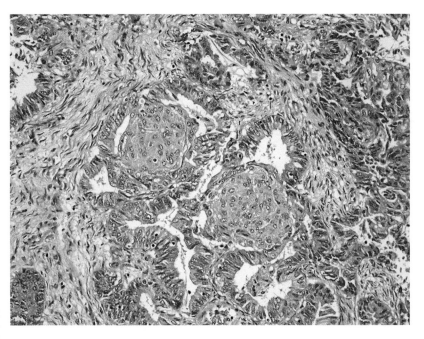

Fig. 26. A borderline endometrioid tumor with extensive morular metaplasia.

diagnostic criteria are the same as for intestinal mucinous borderline tumors. Please refer to the previous discussion on the topic.

Endometrioid Carcinoma

Endometrioid ovarian carcinomas should resemble endometrioid carcinomas of the endometrium (**Fig. 27**). Architectural patterns containing tubules with smooth luminal contours, cribriform structures, solid, sheet-like growth and papillae should be present in the context of an easily recognized endometrial-like background (**Fig. 28**).[47] In general, the cytologic features are concordant with the architectural features (**Fig. 29**) such that simple tubules or papillae are *not* lined by markedly atypical cells with extensive budding. Most endometrioid carcinomas contain either squamous or mucinous differentiation and many show secretory features. Instead of relying on tubular architecture and cribriform growth alone, a diagnosis of endometrioid ovarian carcinoma should only be established with confidence when "confirmatory endometrioid features" are present (see **Box 4**) Occasional examples demonstrate tubal metaplasia, sex cord-like features (**Fig. 30**)[64,65] or spindle cells (**Fig. 31**).[66]

Endometrioid carcinomas can arise in a background of a benign adenofibromatous tumor, usually borderline tumor. Endometrioid carcinoma is distinguished from endometrioid borderline tumor when stromal invasion is present. The most common pattern of stromal invasion is the expansile pattern (see **Fig. 4** in Mills and Longacre).[60,61] This pattern is thought to represent invasion because confluent growth of epithelium excludes stroma (see **Fig. 27**), although neither a stromal reaction nor jagged infiltration is seen. Criteria for distinguishing borderline tumor from carcinoma with expansile invasion are the same as those that permit distinction of complex atypical hyperplasia from endometrioid carcinoma of the endometrium[10] and mucinous borderline tumor from carcinoma; extensive gland fusion, large gland cribriforming, maze-like lumens, and extensive papillary architecture are considered evidence of invasion.[60,61] Destructive stromal invasion, a much less common pattern, is diagnosed when there are irregularly shaped groups of epithelial cells, glands, or nests within stroma displaying an edematous or desmoplastic reaction. This pattern resembles the typical pattern of myoinvasive endometrioid carcinoma of endometrium. Endometrioid carcinomas, like mucinous carcinomas, can be graded using the Shimizu-Silverberg system.[16,17] With Shimizu-Silverberg, the typical ovarian endometrioid carcinoma would score 1 point for glandular architecture, 1 or 2 points for nuclear atypia and 1 point for mitotic activity, which translates into a grade 1 tumor. As

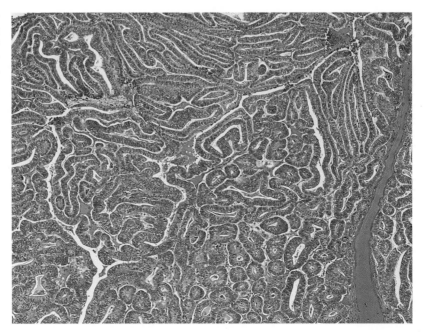

Fig. 27. Endometrioid carcinoma of the ovary with expansile invasion resembles endometrioid carcinoma in the endometrium.

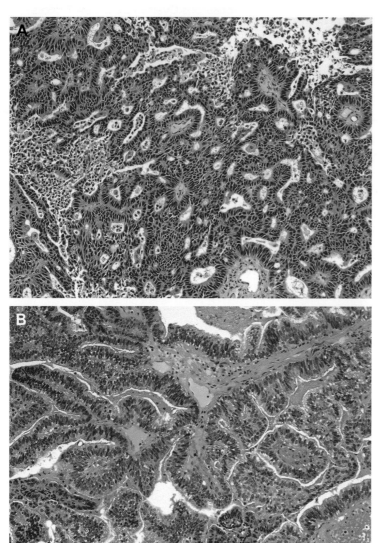

Fig. 28. Common patterns of endometrioid carcinoma include cribriform structures (*A*) and papillae (*B*).

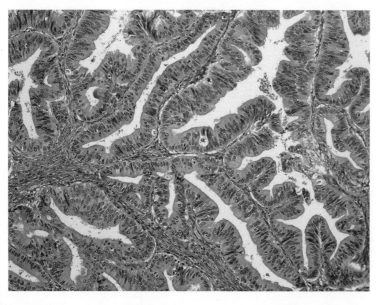

Fig. 29. In general, the cytologic and architectural features of endometrioid carcinoma are concordant.

Box 4
Confirmatory endometrioid features

Resemblance to endometrium and endometrioid neoplasms of the uterine corpus

- Tubules, cribriform structures, solid, sheet-like growth and papillae *with smooth luminal contours*, composed of columnar cells

- Cytologic features are concordant with the architectural features[a]

Squamous, morular, hobnail, eosinophilic and mucinous metaplasia, secretory change

Associated endometriosis, ovarian endometrioid adenofibroma, synchronous endometrioid neoplasm of endometrium

[a] ie, simple tubules or papillae are *not* lined by markedly atypical cells with extensive budding

---

Immunohistochemistry and Molecular Genetics

Endometrioid carcinomas express CK7, PAX8, EMA, B72.3, Ber EP4, estrogen receptor (ER) and progesterone receptor (PR) and vimentin in most cases and β-catenin[67–70] in a subset. In contrast to the usual serous carcinoma, endometrioid carcinomas lack WT1 expression[71,72] and p53 overexpression, although this has been described in purported poorly differentiated varieties.[73] They are negative or only weakly and focally positive for CK20, inhibin, calretinin, and mCEA.

Mutations in *CTNNB-1* (β-catenin),[67–70,74] *PIK3CA*[75] and *PTEN*[68,76] have been reported, as well as high levels of microsatellite instability. Some tumors may arise in the setting of Lynch syndrome/hereditary nonpolyposis colorectal carcinoma syndrome.[29]

DIFFERENTIAL DIAGNOSIS

is the case with endometrioid carcinoma of the endometrium, the presence of severe nuclear atypia in the presence of well formed glands and papillae should prompt consideration for serous or clear cell carcinoma. Such a tumor should not be diagnosed as endometrioid unless these possibilities are excluded. Grade 3 ovarian endometrioid carcinomas are very rare; they are discussed in more detail in the differential diagnosis section following.

Ovarian carcinomas that may be confused with endometrioid ovarian carcinoma include high-grade serous carcinoma when the nuclear features are highly atypical, low-grade serous carcinoma in examples with cytologically bland cribriform architecture, mucinous carcinoma (both primary and metastatic) when there is apparent intracytoplasmic mucin, clear cell carcinoma when there are numerous clear cells, and transitional carcinoma when there is extensive solid growth.[47]

Fig. 30. Endometrioid carcinoma with an area showing sex cord-like (Sertoliform) features.

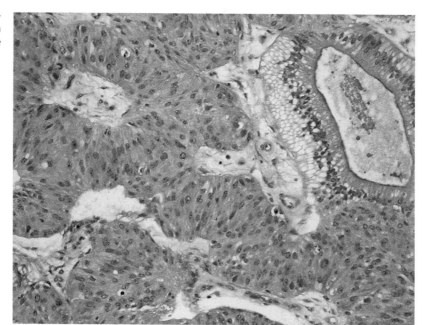

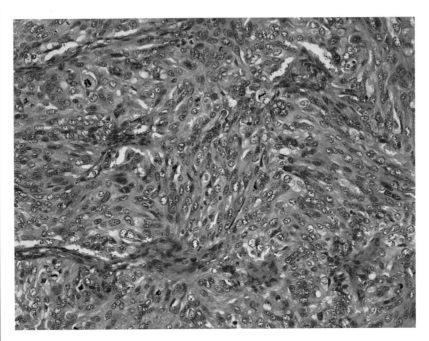

Fig. 31. Spindle cell features can sometimes be present in endometrioid carcinoma, particularly in examples with squamous differentiation and sex cord-like features.

A diagnosis of endometrioid carcinoma should be favored when a precursor lesion such as endometriosis or endometrioid borderline tumor is present, there is resemblance to eutopic endometrioid proliferations, metaplasias common to endometrioid tumors are identified, and the tumor displays ER and PR expression without WT1 expression or overexpression of p53. A cytologically bland, cribriform tumor unassociated with endometriosis, and showing WT1 expression along with ER and PR expression, for example, would likely be a low-grade serous carcinoma.

ΔΔ Differential Diagnosis
ENDOMETRIOID CARCINOMA

Consider:	If this is present:
High- and low-grade serous carcinoma	WT1 positive
Metastatic endometrioid carcinoma	Bilateral, multinodular, surface disease
Primary ovarian mucinous carcinoma	ER/PR negative
Metastatic mucinous adenocarcinoma (i.e. colorectal, endocervical)	Bilateral, multinodular, surface disease
Granulosa cell tumor	Inhibin positive; EMA negative
Sertoli and Sertoli-Leydig cell tumor	Inhibin positive; EMA negative
Yolk sac tumor	EMA negative, SALL4 positive
Wolffian tumor (FATWO)	Calretinin positive
Ependymoma	GFAP positive
Carcinoid	Chromogranin positive, ER/PR negative
Primitive neuroectodermal tumor (peripheral type)	CD99 diffusely positive
Carcinosarcoma	High-grade sarcomatous components
Transitional cell carcinoma	WT1 positive
Squamous cell carcinoma	No glandular differentiation

An endometriosis-associated tumor with columnar, moderately atypical clear cells lining simple, back-to-back tubules and retaining ER/PR expression would likely be an endometrioid carcinoma, not a clear cell carcinoma (see following).

Results from a gene expression analysis[74] support the idea that most ovarian carcinomas diagnosed as *high-grade or poorly differentiated endometrioid carcinomas* are not biologically related to low-grade endometrioid carcinomas. They lack *CTNNB1, PTEN, PIK3CA,* and *KRAS* mutations and microsatellite instability, which are considered typical of endometrioid neoplasms. Most have *p53* mutations instead. These and other related results have been interpreted in two ways. One is that low and high grade endometrioid carcinomas constitute the same histologic subtype of ovarian carcinoma, although they have disparate biological features. An alternate explanation, one that these authors favor, is that most high grade endometrioid carcinomas are not endometrioid at all; they are *high grade serous carcinomas with cribriform architecture* instead. (**Box 5** and **Fig. 32**). This conclusion can be supported by both clinical and immunohistochemical data. These contentious "high grade endometrioid carcinomas" frequently express WT1 and overexpress p53, unlike other endometrioid carcinomas, only extremely rarely demonstrate "confirmatory endometrioid features," are usually high stage at presentation and are frequently bilateral. Low-grade endometrioid carcinomas, in contrast, lack WT1 expression and p53 overexpression, almost always demonstrate "confirmatory endometrioid features," are low stage at presentation and unilateral. There exists a compelling reason to accurately diagnosis serous carcinoma and avoid misdiagnosis of "high grade endometrioid

carcinoma," particularly in young women. Missing a diagnosis of serous carcinoma may lead to insufficient screening for hereditary breast and ovarian cancer syndromes, since endometrioid carcinomas are currently not though to be part of the spectrum of tumors encountered in *BRCA-1* mutation carriers.

Of course, there are still rare high grade endometrioid carcinomas that display a WT1 negative immunophenotype and have confirmatory endometrioid features (**Fig. 33**), which usually include evolution from a pre-existing adenofibromatous tumor or endometriosis. So-called de-differentiated endometrioid carcinoma is another distinctive form of high grade tumor that is histogenetically related to other endometrioid carcinomas.[77,78]

When considering a diagnosis of ovarian endometrioid carcinoma, it is crucial to be sure that the tumor in question is not a *metastasis from an extraovarian source.* It is common to mistake a metastatic colorectal carcinoma for primary ovarian endometrioid carcinoma because both tumors display cribriform architecture and may be relatively lacking in cytoplasmic mucin (**Fig. 34**). The rules for distinguishing primary ovarian and metastatic mucinous carcinomas should be used for separating primary endometrioid and metastatic colorectal carcinoma as well (see **Box 3**). Histologically, endometrioid carcinomas should demonstrate the confirmatory endometrioid features enumerated previously (see **Box 4**), and both groups of tumors can be distinguished using immunohistochemistry. A carcinoma that expressed CK20 and CDX2 without CK7 or ER would support enteric differentiation and diffuse p16 expression would suggest the possibility of a metastatic endocervical carcinoma.

Unlike mucinous carcinomas, endometrioid carcinomas can be multifocal at presentation due to the synchronous development of similar-appearing tumors; they can also develop metachronously in different sites. These lesions should not be considered metastases from one site to another because their clinical evolution more closely resembles multiple stage I tumors rather than stage III tumors. The most common sites where one encounters *synchronous endometrioid tumors* are endometrium and ovary. The guidelines for evaluating such tumors are discussed separately (see *McCluggage: Metastatic Neoplasms Involving the Ovary* and *Mills & Longacre: Atypical Endometrial Hyperplasia and Well Differentiated Endometrioid Adenocarcinoma of the Uterine Corpus*). Be aware that some extragenital sites (ie, peritoneum, rectum, abdominal wall) might also harbor synchronous or

---

Box 5
Rationale behind reclassifying most "high-grade endometrioid carcinomas" as serous carcinoma

Focal presence of typical serous carcinoma patterns

High stage, bilateral ovarian presentation is typical

WT1 expression and *p53* overexpression

CTNNB1, PTEN, PIK3CA, and *KRAS* mutations and microsatellite instability are lacking; most have *p53* mutations instead

Some affected patients are *BRCA-1* mutation carriers

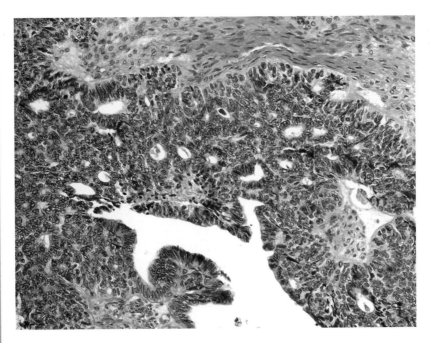

Fig. 32. Serous carcinoma with cribriform architecture, mimicking endometrioid carcinoma. The carcinoma is WT-1 positive.

metachronous endometrioid tumors with associated endometriosis. When confronted with an extragenital endometriosis-associated tumor, it is generally assumed that the extragenital lesion arose in that site. If a separate ovarian tumor also existed, the two tumors would be considered synchronous. Sometimes, the extraovarian synchronous lesion resembles endometrial hyperplasia, but not carcinoma. Criteria used for distinguishing endometriosis-associated complex atypical hyperplasia from adenocarcinoma are the same as those used for diagnosing adenocarcinoma in the endometrium itself. In general, endometriosis-associated complex atypical hyperplasia resembles endometrioid borderline tumor, except that the stroma in the endometriotic focus resembles endometrial stroma and is not obviously fibromatous as in borderline tumor.

Owing to the occasional presence of sex cord-like patterns in endometrioid carcinomas, the differential diagnosis would also include *sex cord stromal tumors* that contain granulosa or Sertoli cells or mixtures thereof (ie, adult and juvenile granulosa cell tumor, Sertoli and Sertoli-Leydig cell tumor, sex cord tumor with annular tubules, fibromas with minor sex cord elements, gynandroblastoma). *Yolk sac tumors* may rarely display endometrioid features,[79] while *Wolffian tumors*,[80]

ependymomas,[81,82] and *carcinoids* may all display architectural patterns that overlap with endometrioid tumors. Rare *primitive neuroectodermal tumors* (PNETs) can arise in the ovary.[82,83] The presence of rosettes may mimic the appearance of glands and nested growth patterns can suggest solid components of endometrioid adenocarcinoma. Clues to the correct diagnosis include primitive-appearing nuclei, exceedingly high mitotic rates and rosettes. The diagnosis can be suggested with immunohistochemical stains and confirmed with molecular testing in many cases. PNETs, particularly those of the peripheral variety (i.e. part of the spectrum of Ewing Sarcoma), express CD99 diffusely in a membrane pattern and are usually, but not always cytokeratin negative. Given this immunophenotype, it would be reasonable to also exclude the theoretical possibility of a primitive leukemia or lymphoma with a TdT immunostain. The vast majority of peripheral PNETs harbor t(11;22)(q24;q12), involving the *EWS* and *FLI1* genes. This can be evaluated by fluorescence in situ hybridization assays for the translocation or reverse transcription polymerase chain reaction for the translocation gene product. Rare PNETs are associated with malignant glandular epithelial and spindle cell components. The presence of these elements would suggest

Fig. 33. True high grade endometrioid carcinoma is uncommon. This tumor (*A*) is associated with endometrioid adenofibroma and squamous metaplasia (i.e. confirmatory endometrioid features). Panel (*B*) shows a cytologically high grade tumor with solid architecture. The tumor was unilateral and associated with endometrioid borderline tumor.

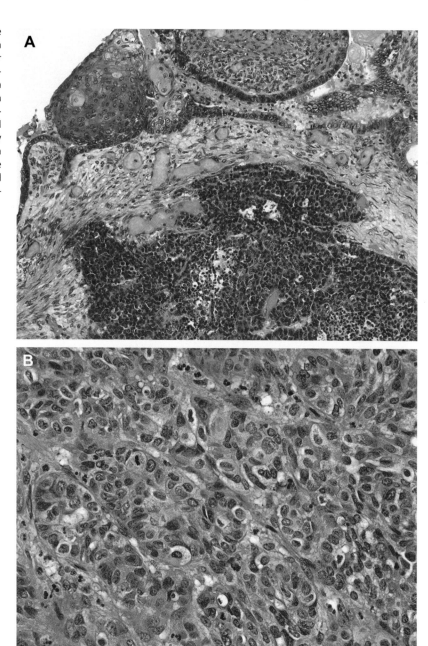

a diagnosis of carcinosarcoma, although in some cases the tumor overall bears a closer resemblance to immature teratoma of the ovary in which a central nervous system-type PNET (i.e. similar to medulloblastoma or ependymoblastoma) is present. The proper nomenclature and clinical evolution of such cases are unknown.

PROGNOSIS

Endometrioid cystadenofibromas and borderline tumors[60,61] are benign if they are accurately diagnosed. Occasional metastatic endocervical and colorectal carcinomas have been misdiagnosed as endometrioid borderline tumor, so caution is in order. Borderline tumors with microinvasion

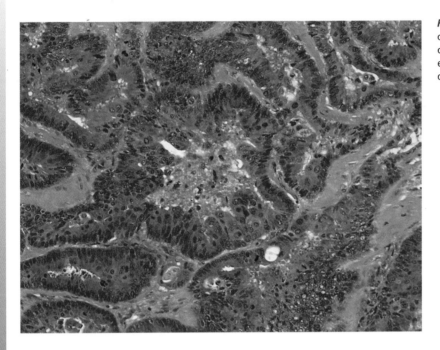

Fig. 34. Metastatic colonic carcinoma can mimic endometrioid carcinoma, especially when it is mucin depleted.

are generally considered to have a benign clinical profile.[60]

The prognosis of established endometrioid carcinoma is driven principally by tumor stage and accurate diagnosis. When the controversial high grade serous carcinomas with endometrioid features are excluded, it is extraordinary to find extrapelvic disease at presentation. Most examples are confined to the ovary, but extension to pelvic structures is sometimes found. Endometrioid ovarian carcinomas are the most common FIGO stage I ovarian carcinoma.[55] Clinical outcomes overall are therefore excellent, when accurately diagnosed, with 5-year survivals reported to be better than 85% or 90%. Stage I, typical endometrioid carcinoma (grade 1 or 2 of 3; low grade) has a 5-year survival that exceeds 95%.[58]

The general surgical approach is total abdominal hysterectomy and bilateral salpingo-oophorectomy with omentectomy, peritoneal biopsies and lymphadenectomy. However, in young patients desiring fertility sparing procedures, the hysterectomy and contralateral salpingo-oophorectomy can sometimes be avoided. Chemotherapy is usually reserved for tumors that are FIGO stage IC and higher and those that are poorly differentiated. It is therefore crucial to not mistake a synchronous tumor for a metastasis. Tumor involvement or disruption of the ovarian surface assigns a tumor to at least stage IC, but this can be very challenging to assess in practice. In contrast to what has been reported previously (much of which is based on extrapolations from suboptimally staged high grade serous carcinoma), ovarian surface involvement and tumor rupture are probably *not* adverse prognostic indicators in the setting of low-grade, stage I disease.[58] Sometimes, the portion of tumor

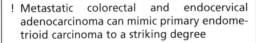

Pitfalls
ENDOMETRIOID CARCINOMA

! Metastatic colorectal and endocervical adenocarcinoma can mimic primary endometrioid carcinoma to a striking degree

! Metastatic endometrial carcinoma may mimic primary ovarian endometrioid carcinoma (see **Boxes 1** and **2** and McCluggage article)

! Tumors displaying primitive or high-grade nuclear features are unlikely to be endometrioid when solid architecture is lacking

! A cribriform tumor with high grade nuclei is statistically more likely to be high grade serous carcinoma than endometrioid carcinoma

! Mistaking serous carcinoma for endometrioid carcinoma may lead to insufficient screening for hereditary breast and ovarian cancer syndromes

on the ovarian surface is borderline tumor, adeno-fibroma or endometriosis, not carcinoma.

The clinical significance of accidental, intraoperative rupture as opposed to spontaneous, preoperative rupture has also not been studied in great depth, but a literature review seems to indicate that preoperative rupture is relatively prognostically unfavorable when compared with accidental, intraoperative rupture.[55,58] There is yet another problem with the distinction of stage I and II tumors–the problem posed by ovarian surface adhesions. Some gynecologists will assign any ovarian tumor adhesed to other pelvic structures to stage II, and treat the patient with chemotherapy regardless of whether the adhesion was a consequence of pre-existing endometriosis. Other gynecologists will reserve upstaging to stage II for tumors that demonstrate microscopic extension into the adhesion and surrounding structures and when sharp dissection is necessary for lysis. The latter seems reasonable.

CLEAR CELL TUMORS

OVERVIEW

Most ovarian clear cell tumors are carcinomas. They account for approximately 5% of all ovarian tumors[2] in North America, but ovarian clear cell carcinomas constitute a larger percentage of ovarian cancers in Japan.[84] Clear cell carcinoma represents approximately 25% of all stage I and II ovarian carcinomas.[55] Unlike serous carcinoma, less than one-third of clear cell carcinomas exhibit

Key Features
CLEAR CELL CARCINOMA

- Unilateral ovarian tumor, cystic and/or adenofibromatous
- Associated endometriosis common
- Low tumor stage > high tumor stage
- Papillary, tubulocystic and solid patterns
- Papillary examples lack extensive stratification and budding
- Cuboidal tumor cells with mostly uniform, but cytologically atypical nuclei
- Usually low mitotic rate
- HNF-1β positive and WT1 and ER/PR negative

extrapelvic spread at presentation.[85–87] As with other ovarian carcinoma types, presenting signs and symptoms are often nonspecific. Clear cell carcinomas, however, are known to be associated with paraneoplastic hypercalcemia and an increased risk of thromboembolic complications.

GROSS FEATURES

Clear Cell Adenofibroma and Borderline Tumor

These tumors are almost always associated with clear cell carcinoma. Most are unilateral. Grossly,

Fig. 35. Clear cell cysta-denofibroma showing areas resembling Swiss cheese.

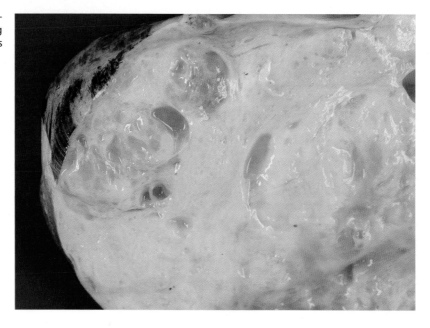

both tumors are typically described as fibromatous with innumerable, tiny cysts. This may impart a Swiss cheeselike or spongy appearance (**Fig. 35**).

Clear Cell Carcinoma

Ovarian clear cell carcinomas are almost always unilateral. One rarely encounters a surface metastasis from a contralateral, dominant ovarian tumor. Even rarer is a bilateral carcinoma that arises in the setting of clear cell adenofibroma. Surface adhesions are commonly present in ovarian clear cell carcinomas as a result of longstanding endometriosis. The typical gross appearance is a large, cystic and solid tumor, frequently associated with endometriosis (**Fig. 36**). When an endometriotic cyst is present, clear cell carcinoma manifests as clustered, round papillae protruding into the lumen or a solid tumor nodule. The appearance of an adenofibromatous tumor, as described above, is a less common presentation.

MICROSCOPIC FEATURES

Clear cell carcinomas can arise in a background of endometriosis, clear cell adenofibroma or both[88,89] Tumors that arise in these different backgrounds are believed to have distinct clinicopathologic and even biological characteristics.[90]

Clear Cell Carcinoma Precursors

More than half of clear cell carcinomas are associated with endometriosis. Some clear cell carcinomas also arise synchronously with other tumors known to be associated with endometriosis, such as ovarian endometrioid borderline tumor and adenocarcinoma (**Fig. 37**), ovarian seromucinous borderline tumor and endometrioid adenocarcinoma of the endometrium. "Atypical endometriosis" describes two types of lesions: complex atypical hyperplasia within endometriosis; and endometriosis with atypical hobnail metaplasia (**Fig. 38**). This is believed to be a possible precursor to clear cell carcinoma.[91-97] The absence of papillary, tubulocystic and solid growth patterns distinguishes the latter lesion from clear cell carcinoma, although it is acknowledged that some of these lesions may represent intraepithelial clear cell carcinoma (**Fig. 39**). Extensive sampling of atypical endometriotic lesions is therefore required to exclude microscopic foci of clear cell carcinoma.

Clear cell carcinomas arising in an adenofibromatous background are less common. Clear cell adenofibroma is composed of small, round, regularly distributed tubular glands with one layer of flat or low cuboidal cells lacking nuclear atypia, set in a fibromatous background (**Fig. 40**). Tumor cell cytoplasm can be scant, abundant and clear, or

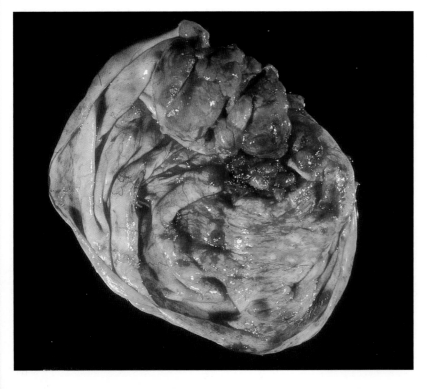

Fig. 36. Gross appearance of a clear cell carcinoma associated with a background endometriotic cyst. (*Courtesy of* Dr Esther Oliva.)

Fig. 37. Mixed endometrioid and clear cell carcinoma. Infiltrating clear cell carcinoma with a tubulocystic growth pattern (*at left*) is found adjacent to a low grade endometrioid adenocarcinoma. Mixed epithelial carcinomas such as this should show obvious morphological differences between components.

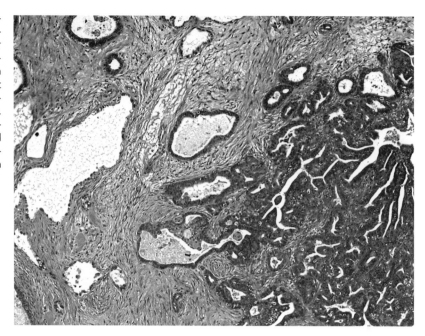

eosinophilic. Clear cell borderline tumor has a similar appearance, but has greater epithelial proliferation and the nuclei are cytologically atypical.[98,99] Like adenofibromas, borderline tumors retain the densely fibromatous stroma and the regular distribution of the tubules. Clear cell borderline tumor is distinguished from clear cell carcinoma by the lack of papillary projections into

Fig. 38. Atypical endometriosis. The epithelium shows atypical hobnail metaplasia.

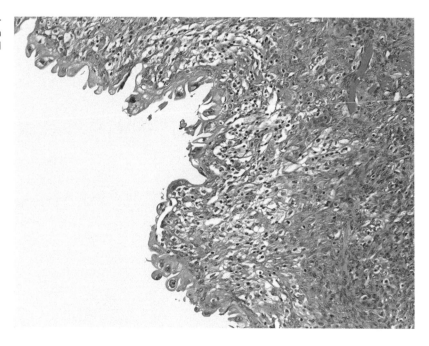

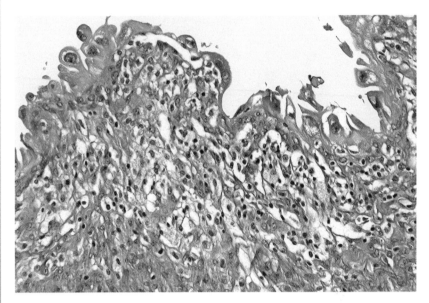

Fig. 39. Atypical endometri-osis can display cytologic features that raise concern for intraepithelial clear cell carcinoma.

the cysts and/or stromal invasion (**Fig. 41**). The stroma in carcinomas often demonstrates edema, myxoid change, or desmoplasia surrounding the tubules (**Fig. 42**), which are usually arranged haphazardly and irregularly clustered. Extensive sampling of tumors that resemble clear cell border-line tumor should be undertaken because clear cell carcinoma is almost always found within the same

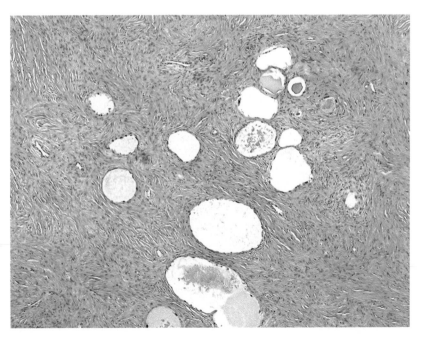

Fig. 40. Clear cell adeno-fibroma is composed of small, round tubular glands with one layer of flat or low cuboidal cells lacking nuclear atypia.

Fig. 41. Clear cell border-line tumor is an adenofibromatous tumor lacking both an invasive profile and intracystic papillae. The presence of cytologically atypical cells separates borderline tumor from clear cell adenofibroma. Clear cell borderline tumor is almost never found without carcinoma; extensive sectioning usually uncovers invasion and/or intracystic papillae.

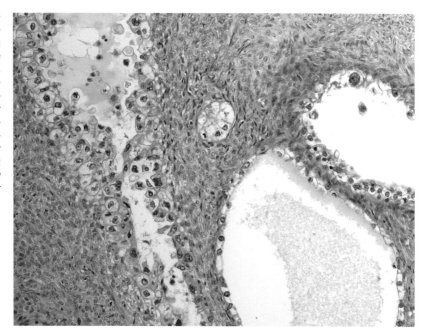

tumor. A diagnosis of clear cell adenofibroma or clear cell borderline tumor should therefore not be rendered at the time of frozen section. Indicating the likelihood of carcinoma, but deferring a final diagnosis until multiple permanent sections are reviewed is a prudent practice.

Clear Cell Carcinoma

Most clear cell carcinomas are at least partially composed of cells with clear cytoplasm (**Fig. 43**) due to accumulation of glycogen, but not mucin. Only a minority of these tumors contain

Fig. 42. Invasive clear cell carcinoma arising from clear cell adenofibroma. The stroma in the invasive areas demonstrates desmoplasia. The invasive tubules are irregularly arranged.

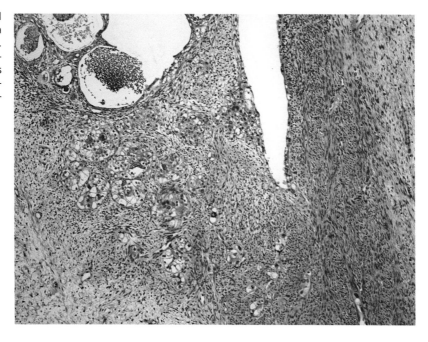

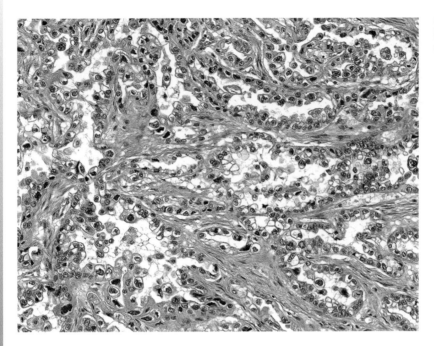

Fig. 43. Clear cytoplasm is seen in most clear cell carcinomas.

a population of uniformly clear cells, however.[100] Paradoxically, the presence of clear cytoplasm should not be used as the major diagnostic criterion since many other ovarian tumor types feature clear cells. Furthermore, rare ovarian clear cell carcinomas, referred to as "oxyphilic clear cell carcinomas," have eosinophilic cytoplasm (**Fig. 44**). Ovarian clear cell carcinoma should therefore be diagnosed primarily in the presence of typical architectural patterns and, secondarily,

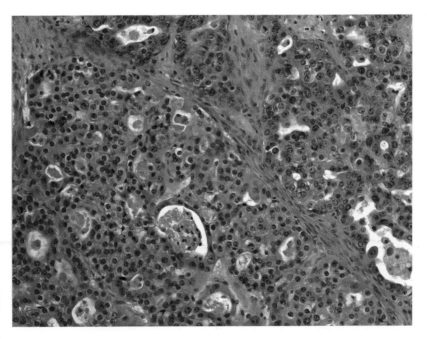

Fig. 44. Eosinophilic cytoplasm in an oxyphilic clear cell carcinoma.

Fig. 45. Flattened and cuboidal epithelium in a clear cell carcinoma with a tubulocystic growth pattern.

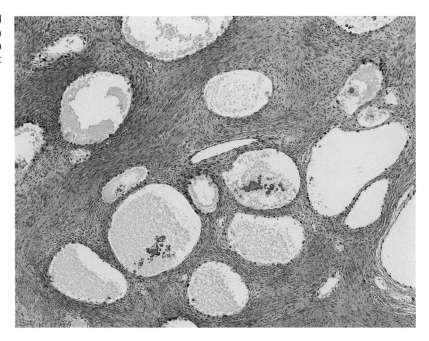

by the identification of cuboidal cell shape and characteristic nuclear features.[100]

The predominant tumor cell in ovarian clear cell carcinoma is cuboidal and, less frequently, flattened (**Fig. 45**). Columnar cells are much more frequently observed in mimics of clear cell

carcinoma such as serous and endometrioid carcinoma and serous borderline tumor. The nucleus-to-cytoplasm ratio of clear cell carcinoma cells is usually obviously lower than in serous carcinomas. "Hobnail" cells, with nuclei that protrude beyond the luminal border of a gland or

Fig. 46. Hobnail cells are frequently observed in clear cell carcinoma.

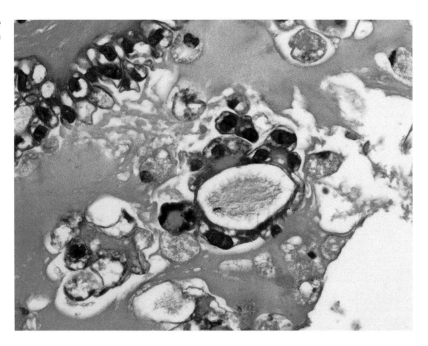

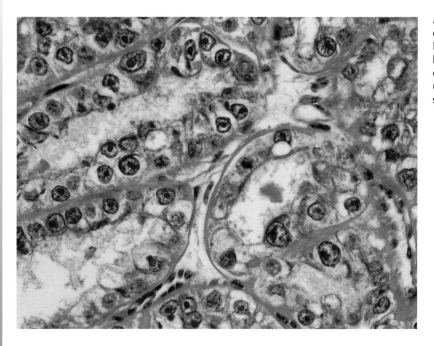

Fig. 47. The nuclei of clear cell carcinomas are large and round, may have a prominent nucleolus, and tend to be uniform in size and shape.

papilla, are observed in over 70% of clear cell carcinomas (**Fig. 46**),[100] but these may be focal and are not at all specific for clear cell carcinoma. The nuclei of most clear cell carcinomas are large and round, may have a prominent nucleolus, and tend to be of uniform shape (**Fig. 47**). Many examples have nuclei that are of uniform size as well. Cells containing large, oval-to-round, dark-staining nuclei are also encountered. Obvious variations in size and shape from one cell to the next occur, but bizarre cells tend to be scattered throughout the tumor or aggregated in small clusters (**Fig. 48**). Recurrent and high stage tumors composed of cells with an anaplastic appearance, in an inflammatory background, rarely occur. Occasional clear cell carcinomas with solid

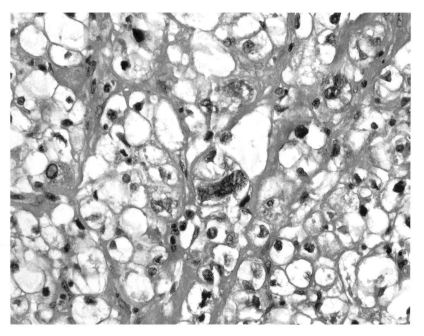

Fig. 48. Occasional bizarre cells can be seen within clear cell carcinoma.

Fig. 49. Clear cell carcinomas with solid architecture frequently contain cells with koilocyte-like nuclei.

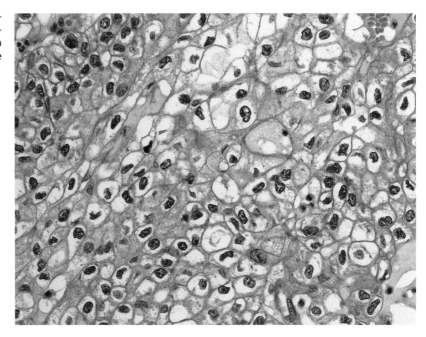

architecture contain cells with koilocyte-like nuclei (**Fig. 49**). The average mitotic rate is approximately 5 mitotic figures per 10 high power fields.[100,101] Bizarre and multipolar forms are unusual and mostly encountered in tumors with an anaplastic appearance.

Unlike serous carcinoma, the range of architectural patterns in ovarian clear cell carcinoma is limited. The common patterns include papillary, tubulocystic, and solid architectural varieties. Most clear cell carcinomas exhibit mixtures of these patterns, with the papillary patterns being by far the most common.[100] Tumors displaying purely tubulocystic or solid patterns are very unusual. The papillae of clear cell carcinomas differ from those of serous and endometrioid

Fig. 50. Clear cell carcinoma with papillary architecture and hyalinized stroma.

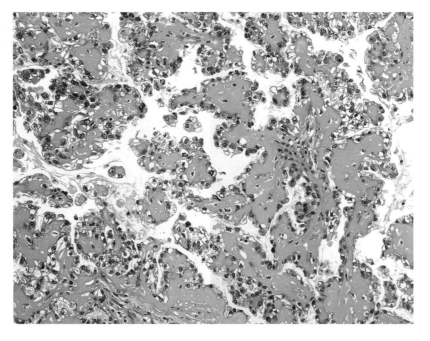

carcinomas. Clear cell carcinoma papillae are short and round and frequently have eosinophilic and hyalinized stroma (**Fig. 50**). Only one or two layers of cells line the papillae. Prominent epithelial tufting, a feature that is almost invariably seen in serous carcinomas, is usually lacking. Tubulocystic tumors are composed of infiltrating, tubular or cystically dilated glands lined by a flattened monolayer of tumor cells (**Fig. 51**). Recognition of the typical tubulocystic architecture remains the best way to identify this type of clear cell carcinoma since flattened tumor cells may resemble a benign tumor. The stroma surrounding the glands may show edema, myxoid changes, or desmoplasia. Solid ovarian clear cell carcinoma is almost always present together with papillary and/or tubulocystic patterns (see **Fig. 49**). Most solid clear cell carcinomas have a pavement or cobblestone-like appearance resulting from a flat sheet of square to rectangular tumor cells with sharp cytoplasmic boundaries.

Other morphologic features encountered in 10 to 30% of cases[100] are psammoma bodies, hyaline globules, basophilic secretions, open tumor rings, nuclear pseudoinclusions, targetoid bodies, intraluminal mucin, and an associated lymphoplasmacytic infiltrate. Some of these features, particularly the open tumor rings, targetoid bodies and lymphoplasmacytic infiltrate, are characteristic of clear cell carcinoma, but they are not specific (**Fig. 52**).

Mixed Epithelial Tumors Containing Clear Cells

Clear cell carcinoma can arise as part of a mixed epithelial carcinoma of the ovary, but mixed epithelial ovarian carcinoma with a clear cell carcinoma component should be diagnosed sparingly, only after confirmation that an absolutely typical and distinctive clear cell carcinoma component is present. A study of tumors diagnosed as mixed serous and clear cell carcinoma indicated only a low level of interobserver diagnostic agreement.[101] Using rigorous application of clear cell carcinoma diagnostic criteria, discussed above, and immunohistochemical staining, discussed subsequently, nearly all cases were reclassified as pure serous carcinomas without bona fide clear cell carcinoma components. Therefore, tumors containing cells with clear cytoplasm, but lacking typical clear cell carcinoma cytology and architecture, are not examples of clear cell carcinoma (**Fig. 53**).

Immunophenotype and Molecular Genetics

Clear cell carcinomas lack more than focal ER and WT1 expression.[101,102] p53 expression can be encountered, but diffuse and strong overexpression of the sort seen in most high-grade serous carcinomas is not characteristic.[101,103,104] Recently reported positive markers of clear cell differentiation include hypoxia-inducible factor

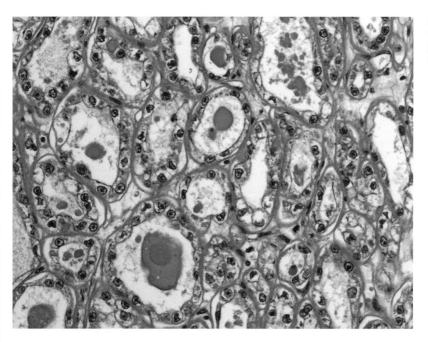

Fig. 51. Tubulocystic architecture is another common pattern seen with clear cell carcinoma.

Fig. 52. Examples of a number of morphologic features that are characteristic of clear cell carcinoma, but not specific. (*A*) Eosinophilic globules, which can be either intra or extra-cytoplasmic. (*B*) Psammoma bodies. (*C*) Open tumor rings.

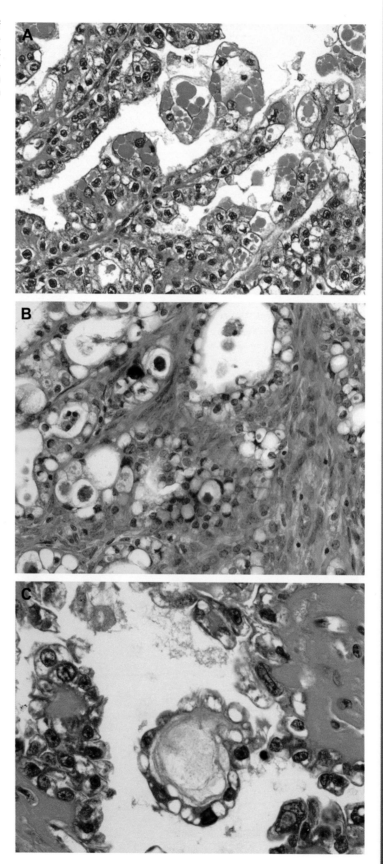

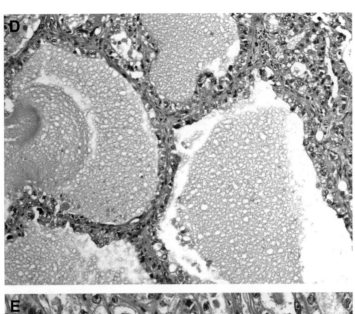

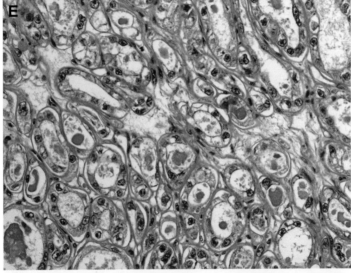

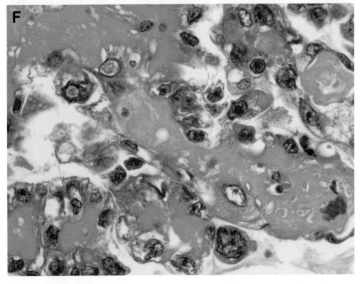

Fig. 52. (*D*) Basophilic secretions. (*E*) Targetoid bodies. (*F*) Nuclear pseudoinclusions.

Fig. 52. (*G*) Lymphoplasmacytic infiltrate.

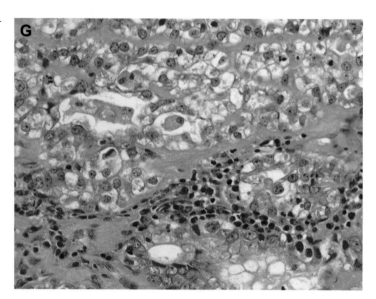

1 alpha (HIF-1α),[105,106] human kidney injury molecule-1,[107] hepatocyte nuclear factor-1 beta (HNF-1β),[102,108–110] vHL (von Hippel-Lindau)[111] and glypican-3.[112] HNF-1β is a transcription factor related to glycogen metabolism and is found in a number of normal tissues, including liver, pancreas, gastrointestinal tract, kidney and Arias-Stella change.[102,108–110] HNF-1β has recently emerged as a sensitive marker for ovarian clear cell carcinoma, with reported positive rate ranging from 82% to almost 100%.[100,102] The typical staining pattern is diffuse nuclear expression (**Fig. 54**). Only occasional focal positivity has been found in ovarian serous, endometrioid, and mucinous carcinomas.

Activating mutations of oncogene *PIK3CA* have been demonstrated in about one-third of ovarian clear cell carcinomas,[113] a higher frequency has been reported in other ovarian carcinoma subtypes. *PIK3CA* mutations lead to activation of the

Fig. 53. High-grade serous carcinoma with cytoplasmic clearing should not be diagnosed as mixed clear cell and serous carcinoma. Areas easily recognized as serous carcinoma were evident elsewhere. The tumor expressed WT1 and overexpressed p53.

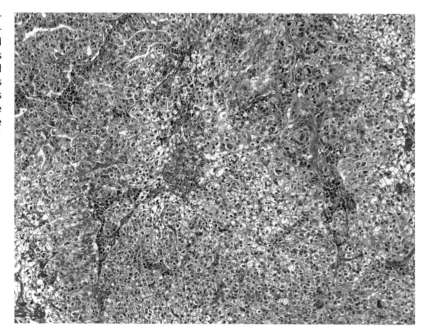

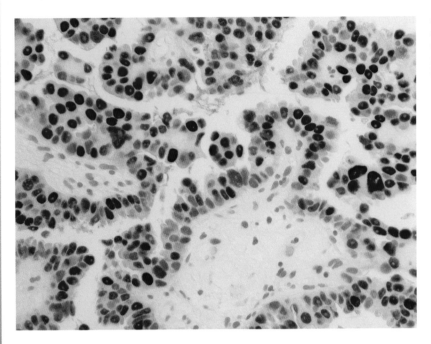

Fig. 54. Diffuse nuclear expression of HNF-1β is demonstrated by immunohistochemical staining in a clear cell carcinoma.

PI3 K/AKT pathway and may be used as a therapeutic target. Mutations in *K-ras*[114,115] and *PTEN*[76] have also been reported. Recent work indicates frequent *ARID1a* mutations in endometriosis-associated clear cell and endometrioid carcinomas.[116,117]

The incidence of certain gynecologic malignancies, including endometrial and ovarian carcinomas, are increased with Lynch Syndrome (hereditary nonpolyposis colorectal carcinoma [HNPCC]), a syndrome with defects in DNA mismatch repair (MMR) proteins due to germline mutations. This is discussed in more detail in *Familial Tumors of the Corpus by Garg & Soslow* in this publication. A recent study suggested that ovarian clear cell carcinoma was overrepresented among ovarian carcinomas with MMR defects in patients age 50 years or younger.[118] Synchronous ovarian clear cell carcinomas have also been reported in two patients with endometrial carcinoma and MMR abnormalities.[62,119] Several examples of microsatellite instability-high clear cell carcinoma[120–122] are also on record.

DIFFERENTIAL DIAGNOSIS

There are data that suggest that pure clear cell carcinomas of the ovary have been accurately and reproducibly diagnosed in the past,[1,101] but distinction from high grade serous carcinoma and endometrioid carcinoma remains a problem.

Difficulties separating mixed epithelial carcinomas with clear cell components from serous carcinoma have been emphasized recently[101] and were discussed previously in this article. The theoretical rationale for strict ovarian carcinoma subclassification is provided in *Kobel's and Huntsman's Molecular Overview of Ovarian Carcinogenesis,* in this publication. These matters will likely become increasingly more practically relevant as treatment protocols become tailored for different tumor types. Furthermore, because of the overrepresentation of clear cell carcinoma in young patients with Lynch syndrome, an accurate diagnosis may lead to an investigation that uncovers a germline genetic defect.

The differential diagnosis for a papillary ovarian carcinoma showing high nuclear grade is essentially restricted to *high-grade serous* and clear cell carcinomas when germ cell tumors and metastases are excluded. Round, hyalinized papillary cores, surrounded by one or two layers of cuboidal cells with uniform atypical nuclei, favor clear cell carcinoma. Extensive stratification and tufting of epithelium, columnar cell shape, diffuse severe nuclear pleomorphism, high nucleus-to-cytoplasmic ratios, mitotic rates in excess of 10 mitotic figures per 10 high power fields, and frequent atypical mitotic figures are findings associated with high grade serous carcinoma, even when tumor cells with cytoplasmic clearing are present. WT1 expression, especially along with ER expression, strongly favor a serous neoplasm

Differential Diagnosis
CLEAR CELL CARCINOMA

Consider:	If This is Present:
High-grade serous carcinoma	WT1 positive
Serous borderline tumor	WT1 positive
Low-grade serous carcinoma	WT1 positive
Endometrioid carcinomas	ER/PR positive with columnar cells
Endometrioid borderline tumor	ER/PR positive with columnar cells
Metastatic adenocarcinoma	Bilateral, multinodular tumors
Yolk sac tumor	EMA negative, SALL4 positive
Dysgerminoma	EMA negative; OCT4 positive
Juvenile granulosa cell tumor	Usually EMA negative; inhibin positive
Papillary mesothelioma	Calretinin and WT1 positive
Papillary cystadenoma	History of von Hippel Lindau
Endometriosis with Arias-Stella change	Hormonal stimulation
Tumors with oxyphilic and clear cells (Box 6)	

Box 6
Tumors with oxyphilic and clear cells

Clear cell carcinoma of ovary

Metastatic clear cell carcinoma

Endometrioid adenocarcinoma

Hepatoid carcinoma[123,124]

Hepatoid yolk sac tumor[125]

Metastatic hepatocellular carcinoma[126]

Steroid cell tumor and other sex cord-stromal tumors[127]

Epithelioid smooth muscle tumor[128]

Perivascular epithelioid cell tumor (PEComa)[129]

Undifferentiated carcinomas with rhabdoid morphology[130]

Gastrointestinal stromal tumors[131]

Intermediate trophoblastic tumors (placental site trophoblastic tumor; epithelioid trophoblastic tumor)[132]

Melanoma[133]

Clear cell sarcoma

Alveolar soft part sarcoma

Rhabdoid tumor

Epithelioid sarcoma

Epithelioid angiosarcoma

---

over clear cell carcinoma. HNF-1β expression without WT1, or ER expression is characteristic of clear cell carcinoma.

Occasional clear cell carcinomas with predominant papillary architecture can resemble *serous borderline tumor* or *low grade serous carcinoma*, especially at frozen section when only limited slides are available for review (**Fig. 55**). Clues to the correct diagnosis here include an adenofibromatous gross appearance, an associated endometriotic cyst and the identification of even occasional cells with significant nuclear atypia. Clinical features may also guide diagnosis, as bilateral tumors and those that are disseminated at presentation are more characteristic of serous neoplasia.[101,134] The immunohistochemical guidelines discussed in reference to serous carcinoma above would apply to this differential diagnosis as well.

Endometrioid carcinomas and borderline tumors may appear similar to clear cell carcinomas when they are papillary, display secretory changes in the cytoplasm, and when tumor cell cytoplasm is squamoid and contains abundant glycogen (**Fig. 56**).[135] Historical guidelines, all still absolutely relevant, restricted a diagnosis of clear cell carcinoma in this setting to tumors with high nuclear grade. However, occasional endometrioid carcinomas display moderate or severe nuclear atypia. Columnar cell shape, squamous metaplasia showing either keratinization or clearcut

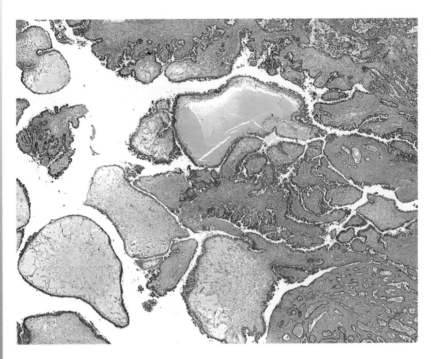

Fig. 55. Clear cell carcinoma can mimic serous borderline tumor or low grade serous carcinoma at low magnification.

intercellular bridges, subnuclear cytoplasmic clearing and cribriform architecture favor an endometrioid neoplasm. ER expression is typical of most endometrioid neoplasms as well. Endometrioid carcinomas with secretory changes may express HNF-1β, however. To diagnose a mixed endometrioid and clear cell ovarian carcinoma, look for typical clear cell architectural patterns, cuboidal cell shape, nuclear features that are distinct and easy to separate from the endometrioid component, and loss of ER expression within the clear cell component.

The typical *yolk sac tumor* patient is younger than age 20 years, while the typical clear cell carcinoma patient is at least four decades older;

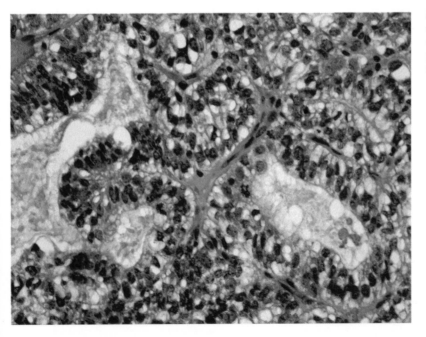

Fig. 56. Endometrioid carcinoma with secretory changes demonstrates cytoplasmic clearing, mimicking clear cell carcinoma.

Fig. 57. Yolk sac tumor, although having a wide range of appearances, can resemble clear cell carcinoma because of cytoplasmic clearing and tubulocystic architecture.

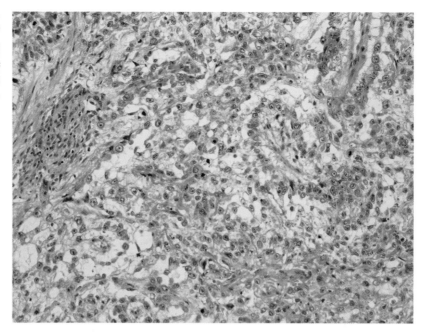

however, a small percentage of clear cell carcinoma patients presents at an age when a diagnosis of yolk sac tumor is considered. Yolk sac tumors, in general, have a much wider range of architectural appearances compared to clear cell carcinoma, more primitive appearing nuclei, a higher mitotic rate, elevated serum AFP levels, and can be associated with other germ cell tumors. Despite the wider range of architectural features in yolk sac tumor, patterns resembling papillary and tubulocystic clear cell carcinoma are frequently seen, and both yolk sac tumor and clear cell carcinoma typically contain clear cells and may display eosinophilic globules (**Fig. 57**). *Hepatoid yolk sac tumor*[125] may also resemble oxyphilic clear cell carcinoma. It has become almost the standard of care to use immunohistochemistry to distinguish between these two entities as they are treated differently and have disparate prognoses. Clear cell carcinomas in general express EMA and CK7, while yolk sac tumor expresses SALL4[136] and AFP without EMA or CK7 expression. The distribution of AFP positivity can be restricted in yolk sac tumor, while AFP can very rarely be positive in clear cell carcinoma.[137] Such cases may represent clear cell carcinomas with hepatoid differentiation. Immunohistochemistry does not aid in the distinction of primary ovarian tumors with hepatoid differentiation and metastatic hepatocellular carcinoma.[138]

Typical patients with *dysgerminoma* are substantially younger than those with clear cell carcinoma, but overlap exists. Morphologic features of a dysgerminoma that potentially mimic clear cell carcinoma are clear cytoplasm, prominent nucleoli, solid growth pattern and a chronic inflammatory infiltrate. Features suggesting dysgerminoma are tumor cells with central nuclei, a granulomatous reaction and, rarely, syncytiotrophoblastic giant cells. The presence of an other germ cell component would also favor dysgerminoma. As mentioned previously, solid clear cell carcinoma almost always has areas of papillary and/or tubulocystic growth patterns, which are not features typically seen in dysgerminoma. Several immunohistochemical markers may also be used to confirm the diagnosis. Cytokeratins are usually strongly and diffusely positive in clear cell carcinoma and are negative or focally positive in dysgerminomas. Similar to yolk sac tumor, the majority of dysgerminomas are diffusely positive for SALL4. OCT4 is another sensitive and specific marker for dysgerminoma and shows only focal immunoreactivity in clear cell carcinoma. EMA is usually positive in clear cell carcinoma and negative in dysgerminoma.

Juvenile granulosa cell tumor (JGCT) is another tumor that affects mainly children and young women, although it rarely occurs in older patients. Estrogenic manifestations are characteristic but not invariably present in JGCT, in contrast to clear cell carcinoma. While the presence of follicles lined by granulosa cells is a characteristic feature of JGCT, the cells lining these follicles can have a hobnail appearance and resemble tubulocystic clear cell carcinoma. Although the pseudopapillary growth pattern encountered in JGCT may resemble true papillae, they lack true fibrovascular cores. Inhibin and calretinin are usually positive in JGCT and negative in clear cell carcinoma, while EMA expression is more typical of clear cell carcinoma.

Similar to clear cell carcinoma, *papillary mesothelioma* is composed of flattened or cuboidal cells without extensive hierarchical branching, stratification, or tufting (**Fig. 58**). Unlike clear cell carcinoma, mesothelioma tends to present with diffuse or multifocal peritoneal disease, although rare cases with preferential ovarian involvement have been reported.[139] Exceptions occur and diagnosis can be difficult when confronted with only a core biopsy or a frozen section. Both tumors have small, round papillae, but papillary mesotheliomas tend to have myxoid stroma in fibrovascular cores. Both clear cell carcinoma and mesothelioma can have tumor cells with uniform nuclei, but mesothelioma nuclei are smaller, have more regularly distributed chromatin and usually lack prominent nucleoli. Most mesotheliomas have cells with eosinophilic cytoplasm, but some may be clear. Mesothelioma cells can have perinuclear, circumferential accumulations of intermediate filaments recognizable on hematoxylin and eosin stains and, in some cases, fuzzy apical membrane projections can be appreciated. These tumors have different immunophenotypes. Mesotheliomas express WT1, calretinin, or podoplanin, all lacking in clear cell carcinoma. EMA and CK7 expression would be expected in both tumor types, but only clear cell carcinoma expresses at least one of the glycoprotein markers, BerEP4 or B72.3.

Papillary cystadenoma (see **Fig. 25** in Longacre Benign and Low Grade Serous Epithelial Tumors: Recent Developments and Diagnostic Problems review elsewhere in this issue) is a rare tumor that is associated with von Hippel-Lindau (VHL) disease. It usually occurs in the broad ligament or mesosalpinx in women, while the epididymis is the most common site in men. It is characterized by papillae lined by a single layer of cuboidal clear cells and hyalinized stroma, just like ovarian clear cell carcinoma. In addition, both tumors are positive for CK7 and EMA. Features that favor a papillary cystadenoma include other VHL manifestations and an extraovarian presentation. Papillary cystadenomas lack mitotic activity, nuclear atypia and prominent nucleoli.[140]

Tumors metastatic to the ovaries can resemble ovarian clear cell carcinoma due to the presence of clear or eosinophilic cytoplasm and signet ring cells. Examples include Krukenberg tumor, which may demonstrate tubulocystic patterns and clear cells, and occasionally, renal cell carcinoma and malignant melanoma. Features favoring metastasis include small tumor size, predominant surface involvement, a multi-nodular growth pattern, bilaterality, and prominent lymphovascular invasion. Immunohistochemistry may also contribute especially when the differential diagnosis includes a carcinoma of lower gastrointestinal origin, which is typically strongly CK20 positive and CK7 negative. Positive PAX8 and HNF-1β would support the

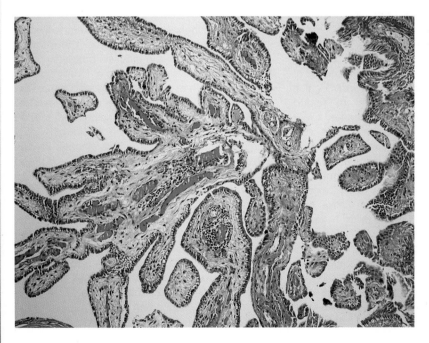

Fig. 58. Papillary mesothelioma is another tumor that potentially mimics clear cell carcinoma with its papillary architecture and low cuboidal epithelium.

Fig. 59. A number of different types of sex cord-stromal tumors frequently contain cells with clear cytoplasm. One example shownhere is a sex cord tumor with annular tubules.

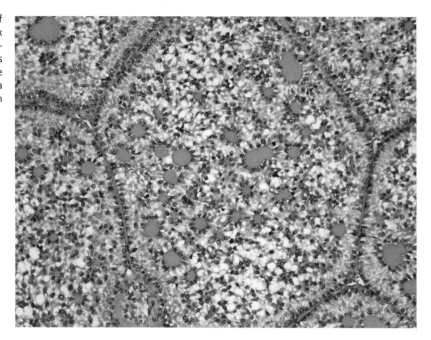

diagnosis of an ovarian clear cell carcinoma. These issues are discussed in more detail in the McCluggage article, Metastatic Neoplasms Involving the Ovary, in this publication.

Endometriosis with *Arias-Stella change* can appear very similar to clear cell carcinoma.[141] They both feature clear cells, hobnail forms and nuclear atypia, and can even have rare mitotic figures.[142] HNF-1β is expressed in both.[109] Clear cell carcinoma associated with endometriosis, in contrast to Arias-Stella change, usually presents as a mass lesion within an endometriotic cyst, a microscopic, infiltrative tubulocystic tumor in the wall of the cyst, or a mixed papillary and tubulocystic neoplasm arising in clear cell adenofibroma. Arias-Stella change, on the other hand, is present within the context of non-neoplastic and metaplastic changes in ectopic endometrium, including endometrioid stroma, lacks an invasive profile and does not, by itself, form a mass lesion. Physiologic or iatrogenic exposures to progestins as well as histologic manifestations of progestational effect (ie, pseudodecidua) are frequently present.

Tumors with oxyphilic and clear cells enter into the differential diagnosis with clear cell carcinoma (see **Box 6; Fig. 59**).

PROGNOSIS

Clear cell adenofibroma and borderline tumors are clinically benign, but it is emphasized that the presence of carcinoma should be excluded using every means necessary, as discussed previously. The survival of patients with clear cell carcinoma is stage dependent. The prognosis of stage I and II clear cell carcinoma is worse than that of ovarian

Pitfalls
CLEAR CELL CARCINOMA

! Assumptions about biological and clinical similarities to serous carcinoma are mistaken

! Although clear cell, serous and endometrioid carcinomas demonstrate many histologic similarities, immunophenotypes differ as do prognosis and response to chemotherapy

! Serous borderline tumor and papillary mesothelioma can resemble clear cell carcinoma, especially at frozen section

! Clear cell carcinoma can be diagnosed *without* evident stromal invasion, provided the cytologic features support the diagnosis and papillary architecture is present

! Tumor cells lining the tubules and cysts of clear cell carcinoma may appear attenuated and give the impression of a benign tumor

! Young patients may develop ovarian clear cell carcinoma. This should prompt consideration for:

  ! The differential diagnosis with yolk sac tumor

  ! The possibility of Lynch Syndrome

endometrioid and mucinous carcinomas, but better than high grade serous carcinomas.[58]

For stage I clear cell carcinoma, the five year survival is reported to range from 70% to almost 90%.[55,88,143] Stage Ia and Ib clear cell carcinoma has a very favorable 10 year disease-specific survival of 87%.[58,143] Other prognostic indicators have been reported. IGF2BP3 (IMP3) expression in low stage clear cell carcinoma reportedly identifies prognostically unfavorable subgroups.[135]

Tumors arising in an adenofibromatous background have been suggested to be less clinically aggressive than others in one study,[89] although this has not been confirmed by other groups.[88]

High stage clear cell carcinoma has a very poor prognosis, likely due to its relative chemoresistance to platinum and taxane-based chemotherapy. Radiation has recently been proposed as an effective therapy for clear cell carcinoma[144] and targeted therapy against components of the PIK3CA pathway and the tyrosine kinase receptors VEGF-R and PDGF-R are being studied.

TRANSITIONAL CELL TUMORS, INCLUDING BRENNER TUMORS

Two types of ovarian transitional cell tumors are recognized: Brenner tumors and tumors with a transitional cell-like appearance that lack a Brenner tumor component. The latter type displays substantial morphologic[145] and immunohistochemical[146] overlap with high-grade serous carcinomas (**Fig. 60**); therefore, they are discussed in *Al-Agha and Gilks topic on High-Grade Serous Carcinoma* in this publication. Like other primary ovarian epithelial stromal tumors, Brenner tumors are divided into benign, borderline and malignant varieties. As a group, these tumors bear more significant similarities to urothelial neoplasms than do transitional cell tumors unassociated with a Brenner component.

GROSS FEATURES

Benign Brenner tumors are not uncommon. When oophorectomy is performed for a clinically detectable Brenner tumor, it usually appears unilateral; however, microscopic, incidental, bilateral Brenner tumors are commonly found in practice. The tumors are typically solid and resemble ovarian fibromas, but small cysts may be present. Stromal calcification is frequently seen. Borderline and malignant Brenner tumors usually display more prominent cysts as compared to benign Brenner tumors.

MICROSCOPIC FEATURES

Brenner tumors are, in essence, transitional cell adenofibromas. Most also display mucinous differentiation, such that "mixed transitional cell and mucinous adenofibroma" is an even more accurate description (**Fig. 61**). Accordingly, Brenner tumors exhibit nests of bland transitional cells with longitudinal nuclear grooves, sometimes with admixed mucinous cells, in a fibromatous stroma. Nests with a large complement of mucinous cells

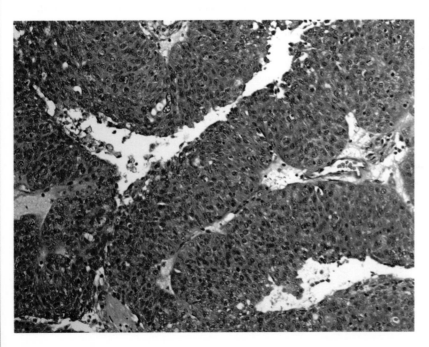

Fig. 60. Transitional cell carcinoma morphologically and immunohistochemically overlaps with high grade serous carcinoma.

Fig. 61. Brenner tumor nests frequently contain central cysts lined by mucinous epithelium and may be associated with mucinous adenofibroma.

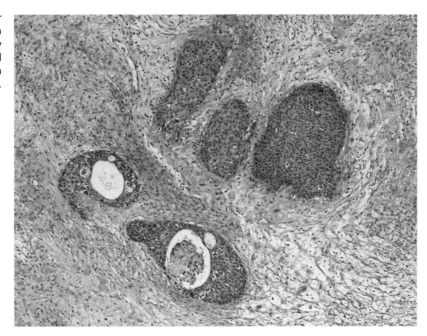

are usually cystically dilated and may contain mucinous secretions. As noted previously, the fibromatous stroma frequently contains coarse calcifications. Brenner tumors may also be associated with ovarian teratomas and related tumors, including struma ovarii and carcinoid.

The earliest detectable difference between benign Brenner tumor and borderline Brenner tumor is enlargement and fusion of epithelial cell nests with central cyst formation. The classic borderline Brenner tumor resembles noninvasive low grade papillary urothelial carcinoma, usually in a background of benign Brenner tumor—that is, these tumors are cystic, display papillary projections into the cyst lumen, and have a noninvasive contour at the periphery (**Fig. 62**).[147–151] Historically, the term "proliferating Brenner tumor" was used for neoplasms at the cytologically bland end of the spectrum whereas "borderline Brenner tumor" was used for tumors with more cytologic atypia.[149] Regardless, these lesions are benign when they lack stromal invasion. Borderline Brenner tumors that resemble noninvasive high grade papillary urothelial carcinoma tend to be diagnosed as "borderline Brenner tumor with intraepithelial carcinoma." Foci of microinvasion, as defined in the context of other types borderline tumors, can be found; any one focus should not exceed 5 mm in one dimension or 10 mm² in area.

Malignant Brenner tumors are extremely uncommon. The best examples of the entity display transitions from benign and borderline Brenner tumor to an obviously invasive carcinoma exceeding the dimensions of microinvasion (**Fig. 63**).[146–151] Irregularly shaped nests of neoplastic cells, frequently displaying squamous differentiation, are seen invading through fibromatous stroma with a desmoplastic reaction.

Brenner tumors, including malignant Brenner tumors, are immunohistochemical distinct from ovarian transitional cell carcinomas.[152–156] Brenner tumors coexpress CK7 and CK20, express p63 and uroplakin, while they lack WT1 expression and p53 overexpression.

DIFFERENTIAL DIAGNOSIS

The differential diagnosis of malignant Brenner tumor primarily includes *endometrioid carcinoma* and, to a lesser extent, *squamous carcinoma*, when metastasis from the urinary tract has been excluded. Extensive sectioning of an ovarian tumor is necessary when a lesion resembling keratinizing or nonkeratinizing squamous cell carcinoma is encountered. Gross examination should focus on the search for a precursor lesion. The presence of endometrioid adenofibroma or endometriosis favors classification as endometrioid carcinoma; the presence of teratoma favors

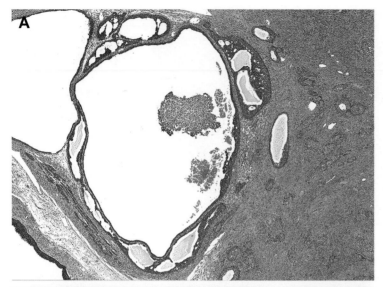

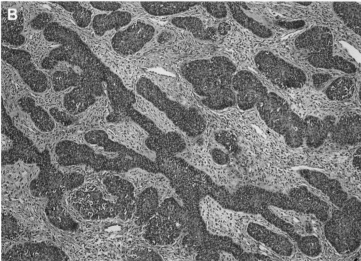

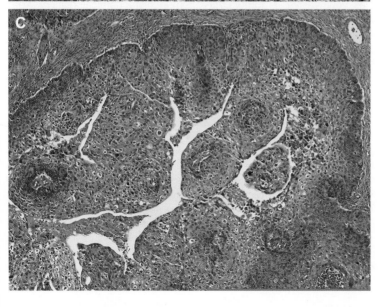

Fig. 62. Borderline Brenner tumor (*A*) is usually cystic and has recognizable benign Brenner components (*present at right*). Occasional borderline Brenner tumors display enlargement and fusion of epithelial nests, resembling inverted papilloma (*B*). Cytologically malignant epithelium, frequently papillary, may be found within borderline Brenner tumor (*C*). This is diagnosed as intraepithelial carcinoma as long as no invasion is identified.

Fig. 63. Malignant Brenner tumor is composed of invasive carcinoma that is present within the context of benign and/or borderline Brenner tumor. Panel (*A*) shows invasive carcinoma that originates in a borderline Brenner tumor with intraepithelial carcinoma (*shown at top*). Cytologic detail of the squamoid invasive component is shown in panel (*B*).

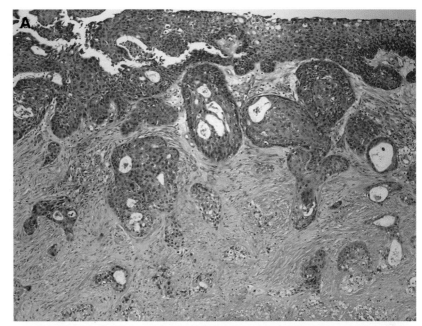

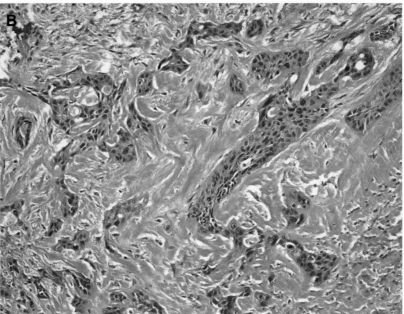

squamous carcinoma arising in that context; and the presence of a benign or borderline Brenner tumor supports a diagnosis of malignant Brenner tumor. If one of these precursor lesions is not found, it is advisable to consider a diagnosis of metastatic urothelial, squamous or endometrioid carcinoma. A discussion of transitional cell carcinomas (tumors unassociated with benign and borderline Brenner components) and their

relationship to serous carcinoma is provided in *Al-Agha and Gilks review on High-Grade Serous Carcinoma,* in this publication.

UNDIFFERENTIATED CARCINOMAS

Undifferentiated carcinoma should be regarded a diagnosis of exclusion. Currently, the absence of histological differentiating features is

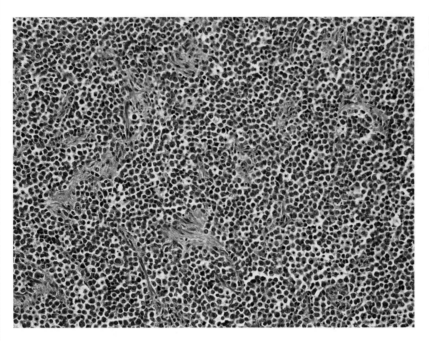

Fig. 64. Undifferentiated carcinoma is composed of relatively uniform, dyshesive tumor cells, resembling lymphoma.

considered sufficient to make this diagnosis. This means that a solid, high grade epithelial neoplasm present in the context of a tumor that can be diagnosed confidently as serous carcinoma, for example, should not be diagnosed as undifferentiated carcinoma. Some pathologists would also argue that WT1 expression in an apparently undifferentiated epithelial neoplasm should encourage

classification as serous carcinoma.[47] It is essential to exclude metastatic carcinomas and non-epithelial neoplasms as well.

As currently defined, undifferentiated carcinomas are a heterogeneous group of tumors. One specific type of undifferentiated carcinoma has been described recently.[130,157] The tumors are formed of sheets of small, dyshesive, uniform cells without

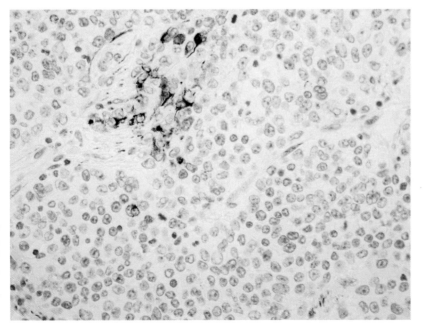

Fig. 65. Rare cells within an undifferentiated carcinoma stain positive for CK18.

glands, nests or trabeculae, and usually resemble lymphoma or "high-grade endometrioid stromal sarcoma" microscopically (**Fig. 64**). Many cases arise in a background of a differentiated endometrioid adenocarcinoma; these tumors have been termed "de-differentiated" carcinomas.[77,157] Support for epithelial differentiation should be sought before establishing a diagnosis of undifferentiated carcinoma, but usually only rare cells with EMA and/or CK18 expression are found (**Fig. 65**). These tumors may show focal expression of chromogranin and/or synaptophysin, but diffuse expression of neuroendocrine-associated markers should be lacking.

MIXED EPITHELIAL OVARIAN TUMORS

Mixed epithelial tumors such as mixed endometrioid and serous carcinomas can be diagnosed when at least two histologically distinctive elements are present and each constitutes at least 10% of the tumor. The elements should be obvious, separable, and characteristic for this designation to retain biologic relevance (see **Fig. 37**). Preferably, the immunophenotype of each component should be distinctive as well.[47] Mixed epithelial tumors should *not* be diagnosed when the overall morphology is a hybrid of features generally encountered in different ovarian cancer subtypes. The overall tumor grade should be based upon the highest grade component.

Three types of mixed epithelial carcinomas occur commonly enough in routine practice: [77,157]

1. Mixed endometrioid and clear cell carcinoma
2. Seromucinous borderline tumor
3. Dedifferentiated carcinoma.

Mixed endometrioid/serous carcinomas and *mixed clear cell/serous carcinomas,*[101] however, are statistically more likely to represent high grade serous carcinomas with morphologic heterogeneity than true mixtures of disparate types of ovarian carcinoma.

Seromucinous borderline tumor, also referred to as Mullerian mucinous borderline tumor, demonstrates an admixture of serous, endocervical mucinous and, frequently, endometrioid cells arranged in hierarchically branched papillae. The appearance overlaps significantly with papillary endometrioid borderline tumor showing tubal and mucinous metaplasia. The low power architecture resembles typical serous borderline tumor (**Fig. 66**), but the cellular constituents and the presence of neutrophilic infiltrates are distinctive (**Fig. 67** and, in Longacre's article in this publication, *Benign And Low Grade Serous Epithelial Tumors: Recent Developments And Diagnostic Problems*, see Fig. 20). Similar tumors that exhibit a predominance of endocervical mucinous cells (or endometrioid cells with extensive mucinous metaplasia) carry the term, "endocervical mucinous borderline tumor." Like serous

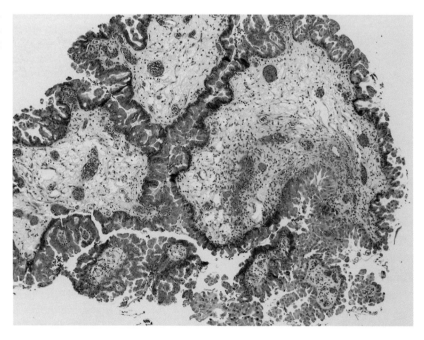

Fig. 66. Seromucinous borderline tumor resembles serous borderline tumor at low magnification.

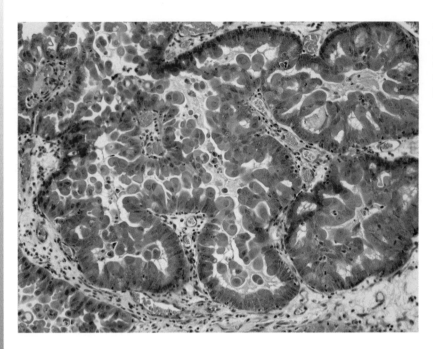

Fig. 67. The epithelium of seromucinous borderline tumor contains mucinous and polygonal cells with eosinophilic cytoplasm.

borderline tumor, seromucinous tumors may present with peritoneal implants and rarely recur and/or progress to carcinoma. This stands in contrast to intestinal mucinous borderline tumor,

as discussed earlier. Like endometrioid tumors, they are frequently associated with endometriosis[158,159] and sometime contain foci of low grade endometrioid,[160] mixed epithelial[160] or clear cell carcinoma.[161] The immunophenotype most closely resembles that of an endometrioid neoplasm and differs from typical serous and intestinal mucinous tumors.[25,162] Seromucinous borderline tumors express CK7, ER, PR and CA125, and they lack expression of CK20 and WT1. Although extraovarian implants, especially invasive implants, are thought to be prognostically unfavorable,[160] recurrence rates and progression to full fledged carcinoma are significantly less common as compared to serous borderline tumor.

RARE, NONSEROUS OVARIAN NEOPLASMS WITH EPITHELIAL DIFFERENTIATION

These tumors are listed in **Box 7**.

Box 7
Rare, nonserous ovarian neoplasms with epithelial differentiation

Monodermal teratoma

- Struma ovarii
- Carcinoid
- Neuroectodermal tumor[82]
- Adenocarcinoma and squamous cell carcinoma
- Sebaceous neoplasm

Tumors of rete ovary[163]
Small cell carcinoma of hypercalcemic type[164]
Small cell carcinoma of pulmonary type[165]
Large cell neuroendocrine carcinoma[15,123]
Hepatoid carcinoma[123]
Wilms tumor[166]
Gestational choriocarcinoma[167]
Adenoid cystic carcinoma[168]
Wolffian tumor[169]

REFERENCES

1. Gilks CB, Ionescu DN, Kalloger SE, et al. Tumor cell type can be reproducibly diagnosed and is of independent prognostic significance in patients with maximally debulked ovarian carcinoma. Hum Pathol 2008;39(8):1239–51.
2. Seidman JD, Horkayne-Szakaly I, Haiba M, et al. The histologic type and stage distribution of ovarian carcinomas of surface epithelial origin. Int J Gynecol Pathol 2004;23(1):41–4.

3. Seidman JD, Kurman RJ, Ronnett BM. Primary and metastatic mucinous adenocarcinomas in the ovaries: incidence in routine practice with a new approach to improve intraoperative diagnosis. Am J Surg Pathol 2003;27(7):985–93.

4. Kim JH, Kim TJ, Park YG, et al. Clinical analysis of intra-operative frozen section proven borderline tumors of the ovary. J Gynecol Oncol 2009;20(3): 176–80.

5. Yemelyanova AV, Vang R, Judson K, et al. Distinction of primary and metastatic mucinous tumors involving the ovary: analysis of size and laterality data by primary site with reevaluation of an algorithm for tumor classification. Am J Surg Pathol 2008;32(1):128–38.

6. Seidman JD, Soslow RA, Vang R, et al. Borderline ovarian tumors: diverse contemporary viewpoints on terminology and diagnostic criteria with illustrative images. Hum Pathol 2004;35(8):918–33.

7. Riopel MA, Ronnett BM, Kurman RJ. Evaluation of diagnostic criteria and behavior of ovarian intestinal- type mucinous tumors: atypical proliferative (borderline) tumors and intraepithelial, microinvasive, invasive, and metastatic carcinomas. Am J Surg Pathol 1999;23(6):617–35.

8. Lee KR, Scully RE. Mucinous tumors of the ovary: a clinicopathologic study of 196 borderline tumors (of intestinal type) and carcinomas, including an evaluation of 11 cases with 'pseudomyxoma peritonei'. Am J Surg Pathol 2000;24(11):1447–64.

9. Chen S, Leitao MM, Tornos C, et al. Invasion patterns in stage I endometrioid and mucinous ovarian carcinomas: a clinicopathologic analysis emphasizing favorable outcomes in carcinomas without destructive stromal invasion and the occasional malignant course of carcinomas with limited destructive stromal invasion. Mod Pathol 2005; 18(7):903–11.

10. Longacre TA, Chung MH, Jensen DN, et al. Proposed criteria for the diagnosis of well-differentiated endometrial carcinoma: A diagnostic test for myoinvasion. Am J Surg Pathol 1995;19:371–406.

11. Provenza C, Young RH, Prat J. Anaplastic carcinoma in mucinous ovarian tumors: a clinicopathologic study of 34 cases emphasizing the crucial impact of stage on prognosis, their histologic spectrum, and overlap with sarcomalike mural nodules. Am J Surg Pathol 2008;32(3):383–9.

12. Bague S, Rodriguez IM, Prat J. Sarcoma-like mural nodules in mucinous cystic tumors of the ovary revisited - A clinicopathologic analysis of 10 additional cases. Am J Surg Pathol 2002;26(11): 1467–76.

13. Rodriguez IM, Prat J. Mucinous tumors of the ovary: a clinicopathologic analysis of 75 borderline tumors (of intestinal type) and carcinomas. Am J Surg Pathol 2002;26(2):139–52.

14. Baergen RN, Rutgers JL. Mural nodules in common epithelial tumors of the ovary. Int J Gynecol Pathol 1994;13:62–71.

15. Veras E, Deavers MT, Silva EG, et al. Ovarian non-small cell neuroendocrine carcinoma: a clinicopathologic and immunohistochemical study of 11 cases. Am J Surg Pathol 2007;31(5):774–82.

16. Shimizu Y, Kamoi S, Amada S, et al. Toward the development of a universal grading system for ovarian epithelial carcinoma - Testing of a proposed system in a series of 461 patients with uniform treatment and follow-up. Cancer 1998;82(5):893–901.

17. Shimizu Y, Kamoi S, Amada S, et al. Toward the development of a universal grading system for ovarian epithelial carcinoma. I. Prognostic significance of histopathologic features–problems involved in the architectural grading system. Gynecol Oncol 1998;70:2–12 [see comments].

18. Vang R, Gown AM, Barry TS, et al. Cytokeratins 7 and 20 in primary and secondary mucinous tumors of the ovary: analysis of coordinate immunohistochemical expression profiles and staining distribution in 179 cases. Am J Surg Pathol 2006;30(9): 1130–9.

19. Ji H, Isacson C, Seidman JD, et al. Cytokeratins 7 and 20, Dpc4, and MUC5AC in the distinction of metastatic mucinous carcinomas in the ovary from primary ovarian mucinous tumors: Dpc4 assists in identifying metastatic pancreatic carcinomas. Int J Gynecol Pathol 2002;21(4):391–400.

20. Ronnett BM, Kurman RJ, Shmookler BM, et al. The morphologic spectrum of ovarian metastases of appendiceal adenocarcinomas - A clinicopathologic and immunohistochemical analysis of tumors often misinterpreted as primary ovarian tumors or metastatic tumors from other gastrointestinal sites. Am J Surg Pathol 1997;21(10):1144–55.

21. Ronnett BM, Shmookler BM, Diener-West M, et al. Immunohistochemical evidence supporting the appendiceal origin of pseudomyxoma peritonei in women. Int J Gynecol Pathol 1997;16:1–9.

22. Logani S, Oliva E, Arnell PM, et al. Use of novel immunohistochemical markers expressed in colonic adenocarcinoma to distinguish primary ovarian tumors from metastatic colorectal carcinoma. Mod Pathol 2005;18(1):19–25.

23. Elishaev E, Gilks CB, Miller D, et al. Synchronous and metachronous endocervical and ovarian neoplasms: evidence supporting interpretation of the ovarian neoplasms as metastatic endocervical adenocarcinomas simulating primary ovarian surface epithelial neoplasms. Am J Surg Pathol 2005;29(3):281–94.

24. Vang R, Gown AM, Farinola M, et al. p16 expression in primary ovarian mucinous and endometrioid tumors and metastatic adenocarcinomas in the ovary: utility for identification of metastatic HPV-

related endocervical adenocarcinomas. Am J Surg Pathol 2007;31(5):653–63.

25. Vang R, Gown AM, Barry TS, et al. Immunohistochemistry for estrogen and progesterone receptors in the distinction of primary and metastatic mucinous tumors in the ovary: an analysis of 124 cases. Mod Pathol 2006;19(1):97–105.

26. Cao D, Ji H, Ronnett BM. Expression of mesothelin, fascin, and prostate stem cell antigen in primary ovarian mucinous tumors and their utility in differentiating primary ovarian mucinous tumors from metastatic pancreatic mucinous carcinomas in the ovary. Int J Gynecol Pathol 2005;24(1):67–72.

27. Gemignani ML, Schlaerth AC, Bogomolniy F, et al. Role of KRAS and BRAF gene mutations in mucinous ovarian carcinoma. Gynecol Oncol 2003;90(2):378–81.

28. Enomoto T, Weghorst CM, Inoue M, et al. K-ras activation occurs frequently in mucinous adenocarcinomas and rarely in other common epithelial tumors of the human ovary. Am J Pathol 1991; 139(4):777–85.

29. Lynch HT, Lynch PM, Lanspa SJ, et al. Review of the Lynch syndrome: history, molecular genetics, screening, differential diagnosis, and medicolegal ramifications. Clin Genet 2009;76(1):1–18.

30. Yemelyanova A, Vang R, Seidman JD, et al. Endocervical adenocarcinomas with prominent endometrial or endomyometrial involvement simulating primary endometrial carcinomas: utility of HPV DNA detection and immunohistochemical expression of p16 and hormone receptors to confirm the cervical origin of the corpus tumor. Am J Surg Pathol 2009;33(6):914–24.

31. Ronnett BM, Yemelyanova AV, Vang R, et al. Endocervical adenocarcinomas with ovarian metastases: analysis of 29 cases with emphasis on minimally invasive cervical tumors and the ability of the metastases to simulate primary ovarian neoplasms. Am J Surg Pathol 2008;32(12): 1835–53.

32. Irving JA, Young RH. Lung carcinoma metastatic to the ovary: a clinicopathologic study of 32 cases emphasizing their morphologic spectrum and problems in differential diagnosis. Am J Surg Pathol 2005;29(8):997–1006.

33. Lee KR, Young RH. The distinction between primary and metastatic mucinous carcinomas of the ovary: gross and histologic findings in 50 cases. Am J Surg Pathol 2003;27(3):281–92.

34. Kiyokawa T, Young RH, Scully RE. Krukenberg tumors of the ovary: a clinicopathologic analysis of 120 cases with emphasis on their variable pathologic manifestations. Am J Surg Pathol 2006; 30(3):277–99.

35. Vang R, Bague S, Tavassoli FA, et al. Signet-ring stromal tumor of the ovary: clinicopathologic analysis and comparison with Krukenberg tumor. Int J Gynecol Pathol 2004;23(1):45–51.

36. Che M, Tornos C, Deavers MT, et al. Ovarian mixed-epithelial carcinomas with a microcystic pattern and signet-ring cells. Int J Gynecol Pathol 2001;20(4):323–8.

37. Baker PM, Oliva E, Young RH, et al. Ovarian mucinous carcinoids including some with a carcinomatous component - A report of 17 cases. Am J Surg Pathol 2001;25(5):557–68.

38. Khunamornpong S, Siriaunkgul S, Suprasert P, et al. Intrahepatic cholangiocarcinoma metastatic to the ovary: a report of 16 cases of an underemphasized form of secondary tumor in the ovary that may mimic primary neoplasia. Am J Surg Pathol 2007;31(12):1788–99.

39. Khunamornpong S, Suprasert P, Chiangmai WN, et al. Metastatic tumors to the ovaries: a study of 170 cases in northern Thailand. Int J Gynecol Cancer 2006;16(Suppl 1):132–8.

40. Khunamornpong S, Suprasert P, Pojchamarnwiputh S, et al. Primary and metastatic mucinous adenocarcinomas of the ovary: Evaluation of the diagnostic approach using tumor size and laterality. Gynecol Oncol 2006;101(1):152–7.

41. Young RH, Hart WR. Metastases from carcinomas of the pancreas simulating primary mucinous tumors of the ovary. A report of seven cases. Am J Surg Pathol 1989;13(9):748–56.

42. Young RH, Scully RE. Ovarian metastases from carcinoma of the gallbladder and extrahepatic bile ducts simulating primary tumors of the ovary. A report of six cases. Int J Gynecol Pathol 1990; 9:60–72.

43. Ronnett BM, Kurman RJ, Zahn CM, et al. Pseudomyxoma peritonei in women: A clinicopathologic analysis of 30 cases with emphasis on site of origin, prognosis, and relationship to ovarian mucinous tumors of low malignant potential. Hum Pathol 1995;26:509–24.

44. Ronnett BM, Zahn CM, Kurman RJ, et al. Disseminated peritoneal adenomucinosis and peritoneal mucinous carcinomatosis - A clinicopathologic analysis of 109 cases with emphasis on distinguishing pathologic features, site of origin, prognosis, and relationship to "Pseudomyxoma peritonei". Am J Surg Pathol 1995;19:1390–408.

45. Szych C, Staebler A, Connolly DC, et al. Molecular genetic evidence supporting the clonality and appendiceal origin of Pseudomyxoma peritonei in women. Am J Pathol 1999;154(6):1849–55.

46. Ronnett BM, Yan H, Kurman RJ, et al. Patients with pseudomyxoma peritonei associated with disseminated peritoneal adenomucinosis have a significantly more favorable prognosis than patients with peritoneal mucinous carcinomatosis. Cancer 2001;92(1):85–91.

47. Soslow RA. Histologic subtypes of ovarian carcinoma: an overview. Int J Gynecol Pathol 2008; 27(2):161–74.

48. Zhang PJ, Gao HG, Pasha TL, et al. TTF-1 expression in ovarian and uterine epithelial neoplasia and its potential significance, an immunohistochemical assessment with multiple monoclonal antibodies and different secondary detection systems. Int J Gynecol Pathol 2009;28(1):10–8.

49. Kubba LA, McCluggage WG, Liu J, et al. Thyroid transcription factor-1 expression in ovarian epithelial neoplasms. Mod Pathol 2008;21(4):485–90.

50. Seidman JD, Khedmati F. Exploring the histogenesis of ovarian mucinous and transitional cell (Brenner) neoplasms and their relationship with Walthard cell nests: a study of 120 tumors. Arch Pathol Lab Med 2008;132(11):1753–60.

51. McKenney JK, Soslow RA, Longacre TA. Ovarian mature teratomas with mucinous epithelial neoplasms: morphologic heterogeneity and association with pseudomyxoma peritonei. Am J Surg Pathol 2008;32(5):645–55.

52. Ronnett BM, Seidman JD. Mucinous tumors arising in ovarian mature cystic teratomas: relationship to the clinical syndrome of pseudomyxoma peritonei. Am J Surg Pathol 2003;27(5):650–7.

53. Vang R, Gown AM, Zhao C, et al. Ovarian mucinous tumors associated with mature cystic teratomas: morphologic and immunohistochemical analysis identifies a subset of potential teratomatous origin that shares features of lower gastrointestinal tract mucinous tumors more commonly encountered as secondary tumors in the ovary. Am J Surg Pathol 2007;31(6):854–69.

54. Ronnett BM, Kajdacsy-Balla A, Gilks CB, et al. Mucinous borderline ovarian tumors: points of general agreement and persistent controversies regarding nomenclature, diagnostic criteria, and behavior. Hum Pathol 2004;35(8):949–60.

55. Leitao MM Jr, Boyd J, Hummer A, et al. Clinicopathologic analysis of early-stage sporadic ovarian carcinoma. Am J Surg Pathol 2004;28(2):147–59.

56. Cloven NG, Kyshtoobayeva A, Burger RA, et al. In vitro chemoresistance and biomarker profiles are unique for histologic subtypes of epithelial ovarian cancer. Gynecol Oncol 2004;92(1):160–6.

57. Tabrizi AD, Kalloger SE, Kobel M, et al. Primary ovarian mucinous carcinoma of intestinal type: significance of pattern of invasion and immunohistochemical expression profile in a series of 31 cases. Int J Gynecol Pathol 2010;29(2):99–107.

58. Kobel M, Kalloger SE, Santos JL, et al. Tumor type and substage predict survival in stage I and II ovarian carcinoma: insights and implications. Gynecol Oncol 2010;116(1):50–6.

59. McAlpine JN, Wiegand KC, Vang R, et al. HER2 overexpression and amplification is present in a subset of ovarian mucinous carcinomas and can be targeted with trastuzumab therapy. BMC Cancer 2009;9:433.

60. Bell KA, Kurman RJ. A clinicopathologic analysis of atypical proliferative (borderline) tumors and well-differentiated endometrioid adenocarcinomas of the ovary. Am J Surg Pathol 2000;24(11):1465–79.

61. Roth LM, Emerson RE, Ulbright TM. Ovarian endometrioid tumors of low malignant potential: a clinicopathologic study of 30 cases with comparison to well-differentiated endometrioid adenocarcinoma. Am J Surg Pathol 2003;27(9):1253–9.

62. Garg K, Shih K, Barakat RR, et al. Endometrial carcinomas in women aged 40 years and younger: tumors associated with loss of DNA mismatch repair proteins comprise a distinct clinicopathologic subset. Am J Surg Pathol 2009;33(12):1869–77.

63. Soliman PT, Slomovitz BM, Broaddus RR, et al. Synchronous primary cancers of the endometrium and ovary: a single institution review of 84 cases. Gynecol Oncol 2004;94(2):456–62.

64. Young RH, Prat J, Scully RE. Ovarian endometrioid carcinomas resembling sex cord-stromal tumors. A clinicopathologic analysis of 13 cases. Am J Surg Pathol 1982;6:513–22.

65. Roth LM, Liban E, Czernobilsky B. Ovarian endometrioid tumors mimicking Sertoli and Sertoli-Leydig cell tumors: Sertoliform variant of endometrioid carcinoma. Cancer 1982;50(7):1322–31.

66. Tornos C, Silva EG, Ordonez NG, et al. Endometrioid carcinoma of the ovary with a prominent spindle-cell component, a source of diagnostic confusion - a report of 14 cases. Am J Surg Pathol 1995;19:1343–53.

67. Moreno-Bueno G, Gamallo C, Perez-Gallego L, et al. Beta-catenin expression pattern, beta-catenin gene mutations, and microsatellite instability in endometrioid ovarian carcinomas and synchronous endometrial carcinomas. Diagn Mol Pathol 2001;10(2):116–22.

68. Catasus L, Bussaglia E, Rodrguez I, et al. Molecular genetic alterations in endometrioid carcinomas of the ovary: similar frequency of beta-catenin abnormalities but lower rate of microsatellite instability and PTEN alterations than in uterine endometrioid carcinomas. Hum Pathol 2004;35(11):1360–8.

69. Irving JA, Catasus L, Gallardo A, et al. Synchronous endometrioid carcinomas of the uterine corpus and ovary: alterations in the beta-catenin (CTNNB1) pathway are associated with independent primary tumors and favorable prognosis. Hum Pathol 2005;36(6):605–19.

70. Oliva E, Sarrio D, Brachtel EF, et al. High frequency of beta-catenin mutations in borderline endometrioid tumours of the ovary. J Pathol 2006;208(5):708–13.

71. Acs G, Pasha T, Zhang PJ. WT1 is differentially expressed in serous, endometrioid, clear cell, and mucinous carcinomas of the peritoneum, fallopian tube, ovary, and endometrium. Int J Gynecol Pathol 2004;23(2):110–8.

72. Shimizu M, Toki T, Takagi Y, et al. Immunohistochemical detection of the Wilms' tumor gene (WT1) in epithelial ovarian tumors. Int J Gynecol Pathol 2000;19(2):158–63.

73. Caduff RF, Svoboda-Newman SM, Bartos RE, et al. Comparative analysis of histologic homologues of endometrial and ovarian carcinoma. Am J Surg Pathol 1998;22(3):319–26.

74. Wu R, Hendrix-Lucas N, Kuick R, et al. Mouse model of human ovarian endometrioid adenocarcinoma based on somatic defects in the Wnt/beta-catenin and PI3K/Pten signaling pathways. Cancer Cell 2007;11(4):321–33.

75. Wu R, Zhai Y, Fearon ER, et al. Diverse mechanisms of beta-catenin deregulation in ovarian endometrioid adenocarcinomas. Cancer Res 2001; 61(22):8247–55.

76. Sato N, Tsunoda H, Nishida M, et al. Loss of heterozygosity on 10q23.3 and mutation of the tumor suppressor gene PTEN in benign endometrial cyst of the ovary: possible sequence progression from benign endometrial cyst to endometrioid carcinoma and clear cell carcinoma of the ovary. Cancer Res 2000;60(24):7052–6.

77. Silva EG, Deavers MT, Bodurka DC, et al. Association of low-grade endometrioid carcinoma of the uterus and ovary with undifferentiated carcinoma: a new type of dedifferentiated carcinoma? Int J Gynecol Pathol 2006;25(1):52–8.

78. Tafe LJ, Garg K, Chew I, et al. Endometrial and ovarian carcinomas with undifferentiated components: clinically aggressive and frequently underrecognized neoplasms. Mod Pathol 2010;23(6):781–9.

79. Clement PB, Young RH, Scully RE. Endometrioid-like variant of ovarian yolk sac tumor. A clinicopathological analysis of eight cases. Am J Surg Pathol 1987;11:767–78.

80. Kariminejad MH, Scully RE. Female adnexal tumor of probable Wolffian origin: a distinctive pathologic entity. Cancer 1973;31:671–7.

81. Idowu MO, Rosenblum MK, Wei XJ, et al. Ependymomas of the central nervous system and adult extra-axial ependymomas are morphologically and immunohistochemically distinct–a comparative study with assessment of ovarian carcinomas for expression of glial fibrillary acidic protein. Am J Surg Pathol 2008;32(5):710–8.

82. Kleinman GM, Young RH, Scully RE. Primary neuroectodermal tumors of the ovary: a report of 25 cases. Am J Surg Pathol 1993;17:764–78.

83. Kawauchi S, Fukuda T, Miyamoto S, et al. Peripheral primitive neuroectodermal tumor of the ovary confirmed by CD99 immunostaining, karyotypic analysis, and RT-PCR for EWS/FLI-1 chimeric mRNA. Am J Surg Pathol 1998;22:1417–22.

84. Sugiyama T, Kamura T, Kigawa J, et al. Clinical characteristics of clear cell carcinoma of the ovary: a distinct histologic type with poor prognosis and resistance to platinum-based chemotherapy. Cancer 2000;88(11):2584–9.

85. Mizuno M, Kikkawa F, Shibata K, et al. Long-term follow-up and prognostic factor analysis in clear cell adenocarcinoma of the ovary. J Surg Oncol 2006;94(2):138–43.

86. Takano M, Kikuchi Y, Yaegashi N, et al. Clear cell carcinoma of the ovary: a retrospective multicentre experience of 254 patients with complete surgical staging. Br J Cancer 2006;94(10): 1369–74.

87. Behbakht K, Randall TC, Benjamin I, et al. Clinical characteristics of clear cell carcinoma of the ovary. Gynecol Oncol 1998;70:255–8.

88. Veras E, Mao TL, Ayhan A, et al. Cystic and adenofibromatous clear cell carcinomas of the ovary: distinctive tumors that differ in their pathogenesis and behavior: a clinicopathologic analysis of 122 cases. Am J Surg Pathol 2009;33(6):844–53.

89. Yamamoto S, Tsuda H, Yoshikawa T, et al. Clear cell adenocarcinoma associated with clear cell adenofibromatous components: a subgroup of ovarian clear cell adenocarcinoma with distinct clinicopathologic characteristics. Am J Surg Pathol 2007; 31(7):999–1006.

90. Yamamoto S, Tsuda H, Takano M, et al. Expression of platelet-derived growth factors and their receptors in ovarian clear-cell carcinoma and its putative precursors. Mod Pathol 2008;21(2):115–24.

91. Fukunaga M, Nomura K, Ishikawa E, et al. Ovarian atypical endometriosis: Its close association with malignant epithelial tumours. Histopathology 1997;30(3):249–55.

92. Seidman JD. Prognostic importance of hyperplasia and atypia in endometriosis. Int J Gynecol Pathol 1996;15(1):1–9.

93. Moll UM, Chumas JC, Chalas E, et al. Ovarian carcinoma arising in atypical endometriosis. Obstet Gynecol 1990;75:537–9.

94. Mandai M, Yamaguchi K, Matsumura N, et al. Ovarian cancer in endometriosis: molecular biology, pathology, and clinical management. Int J Clin Oncol 2009;14(5):383–91.

95. Kobayashi H. Ovarian cancer in endometriosis: epidemiology, natural history, and clinical diagnosis. Int J Clin Oncol 2009;14(5):378–82.

96. LaGrenade A, Silverberg SG. Ovarian tumors associated with atypical endometriosis. Hum Pathol 1988;19:1080–4.

97. Czernobilsky B, Morris WJ. A histologic study of ovarian endometriosis with emphasis on

hyperplastic and atypical changes. Obstet Gyne-col 1979;53(3):318–23.

98. Roth LM, Langley FA, Fox H, et al. Ovarian clear cell adenofibromatous tumors: benign, low malignant potential, and associated with invasive clear cell carcinoma. Cancer 1984;53:1156–63.

99. Bell DA, Scully RE. Benign and borderline clear cell adenofibromas of the ovary. Cancer 1985;56: 2922–31.

100. DeLair D, Soslow R, Gilks B, et al. The morphologic spectrum of immunohistochemically characterized clear cell carcinoma of the ovary: a study of 83 cases [abstract 961]. Mod Pathol 2009;22(Suppl 1):211A.

101. Han G, Gilks CB, Leung S, et al. Mixed ovarian epithelial carcinomas with clear cell and serous components are variants of high-grade serous carcinoma: an interobserver correlative and immunohistochemical study of 32 cases. Am J Surg Pathol 2008;32(7):955–64.

102. Kobel M, Kalloger SE, Carrick J, et al. A limited panel of immunomarkers can reliably distinguish between clear cell and high-grade serous carcinoma of the ovary. Am J Surg Pathol 2009;33(1):14–21.

103. Shimizu M, Nikaido T, Toki T, et al. Clear cell carcinoma has an expression pattern of cell cycle regulatory molecules that is unique among ovarian adenocarcinomas. Cancer 1999;85(3):669–77.

104. Otis CN, Krebs PA, Quezado MM, et al. Loss of heterozygosity in P53, BRCA1, and estrogen receptor genes and correlation to expression of p53 protein in ovarian epithelial tumors of different cell types and biological behavior. Hum Pathol 2000;31(2):233–8.

105. Lee S, Garner EI, Welch WR, et al. Over-expression of hypoxia-inducible factor 1 alpha in ovarian clear cell carcinoma. Gynecol Oncol 2007;106(2):311–7.

106. Miyazawa M, Yasuda M, Fujita M, et al. Therapeutic strategy targeting the mTOR-HIF-1alpha-VEGF pathway in ovarian clear cell adenocarcinoma. Pathol Int 2009;59(1):19–27.

107. Lin F, Zhang PL, Yang XJ, et al. Human kidney injury molecule-1 (hKIM-1): a useful immunohistochemical marker for diagnosing renal cell carcinoma and ovarian clear cell carcinoma. Am J Surg Pathol 2007;31(3):371–81.

108. Kato N, Sasou S, Motoyama T. Expression of hepatocyte nuclear factor-1beta (HNF-1beta) in clear cell tumors and endometriosis of the ovary. Mod Pathol 2006;19(1):83–9.

109. Yamamoto S, Tsuda H, Aida S, et al. Immunohistochemical detection of hepatocyte nuclear factor 1beta in ovarian and endometrial clear-cell adenocarcinomas and nonneoplastic endometrium. Hum Pathol 2007;38(7):1074–80.

110. Tsuchiya A, Sakamoto M, Yasuda J, et al. Expression profiling in ovarian clear cell carcinoma: identification of hepatocyte nuclear factor-1 beta as a molecular marker and a possible molecular target for therapy of ovarian clear cell carcinoma. Am J Pathol 2003;163(6):2503–12.

111. Lin F, Shi J, Liu H, et al. Immunohistochemical detection of the von Hippel-Lindau gene product (pVHL) in human tissues and tumors: a useful marker for metastatic renal cell carcinoma and clear cell carcinoma of the ovary and uterus. Am J Clin Pathol 2008;129(4):592–605.

112. Stadlmann S, Gueth U, Baumhoer D, et al. Glypican-3 expression in primary and recurrent ovarian carcinomas. Int J Gynecol Pathol 2007;26(3):341–4.

113. Kuo KT, Mao TL, Jones S, et al. Frequent activating mutations of PIK3CA in ovarian clear cell carcinoma. Am J Pathol 2009;174(5):1597–601.

114. Otsuka J, Okuda T, Sekizawa A, et al. K-ras mutation may promote carcinogenesis of endometriosis leading to ovarian clear cell carcinoma. Med Electron Microsc 2004;37(3):188–92.

115. Amemiya S, Sekizawa A, Otsuka J, et al. Malignant transformation of endometriosis and genetic alterations of K-ras and microsatellite instability. Int J Gynaecol Obstet 2004;86(3):371–6.

116. Wiegand KC, Shah SP, Al-Agha OM, et al. ARID1A mutations in endometrioisis-associated ovarian carcinomas. N Engl J Med 2010;363:1532–43.

117. Jones S, Wang TL, Shih IeM, et al. Frequent mutations of chromatin remodeling gene ARID1A in ovarian clear cell carcinoma. Science 2010;330: 228–31.

118. Jensen KC, Mariappan MR, Putcha GV, et al. Microsatellite instability and mismatch repair protein defects in ovarian epithelial neoplasms in patients 50 years of age and younger. Am J Surg Pathol Jul 2008;32(7):1029–37.

119. Garg K, Leitao MM Jr, Kauff ND, et al. Selection of endometrial carcinomas for DNA mismatch repair protein immunohistochemistry using patient age and tumor morphology enhances detection of mismatch repair abnormalities. Am J Surg Pathol 2009;33(6):925–33.

120. Ueda H, Watanabe Y, Nakai H, et al. Microsatellite status and immunohistochemical features of ovarian clear-cell carcinoma. Anticancer Res 2005;25(4):2785–8.

121. Cai KQ, Albarracin C, Rosen D, et al. Microsatellite instability and alteration of the expression of hMLH1 and hMSH2 in ovarian clear cell carcinoma. Hum Pathol 2004;35(5):552–9.

122. Gras E, Catasus L, Argueelles R, et al. Microsatellite instability, MLH-1 promoter hypermethylation, and frameshift mutations at coding mononucleotide repeat microsatellites in ovarian tumors. Cancer 2001;92(11):2829–36.

123. Ishikura H, Scully RE. Hepatoid carcinoma of the ovary. A newly described tumor. Cancer 1987;60: 2775–84.

124. Matsuta M, Ishikura H, Murakami K, et al. Hepatoid carcinoma of the ovary: a case report. Int J Gynecol Pathol 1991;10(3):302–10.

125. Prat J, Bhan AK, Dickersin GR, et al. Hepatoid yolk sac tumor of the ovary (endodermal sinus tumor with hepatoid differentiation): a light microscopic, ultrastructural and immunohistochemical study of seven cases. Cancer 1982;50:2355–68.

126. Young RH, Gersell DJ, Clement PB, et al. Hepatocellular carcinoma metastatic to the ovary: a report of three cases discovered during life with discussion of the differential diagnosis of hepatoid tumors of the ovary. Hum Pathol 1992;23:574–80.

127. Hayes MC, Scully RE. Ovarian steroid cell tumors (not otherwise specified). A clinicopathological analysis of 63 cases. Am J Surg Pathol 1987;11: 835–45.

128. Kurman RJ, Norris HJ. Mesenchymal tumors of the uterus. VI. Epithelioid smooth muscle tumors including leiomyoblastoma and clear cell leiomyoma: a clinical and pathological analysis of 26 cases. Cancer 1976;37:1853–65.

129. Vang R, Kempson RL. Perivascular epithelioid cell tumor ('PEComa') of the uterus: a subset of HMB-45-positive epithelioid mesenchymal neoplasms with an uncertain relationship to pure smooth muscle tumors. Am J Surg Pathol 2002;26(1):1–13.

130. Altrabulsi B, Malpica A, Deavers MT, et al. Undifferentiated Carcinoma of the Endometrium. Am J Surg Pathol 2005;29(10):1316–21.

131. Irving JA, Lerwill MF, Young RH. Gastrointestinal stromal tumors metastatic to the ovary: a report of five cases. Am J Surg Pathol 2005;29(7):920–6.

132. Shih IM, Kurman RJ. Epithelioid trophoblastic tumor - a neoplasm distinct from choriocarcinoma and placental site trophoblastic tumor simulating carcinoma. Am J Surg Pathol 1998;22:1393–403.

133. Young RH, Scully RE. Malignant melanoma metastatic to the ovary: a clinicopathologic analysis of 20 cases. Am J Surg Pathol 1991;15:849–60.

134. Sangoi AR, Soslow RA, Teng NN, et al. Ovarian clear cell carcinoma with papillary features: a potential mimic of serous tumor of low malignant potential. Am J Surg Pathol 2008;32(2):269–74.

135. Silva EG, Young RH. Endometrioid neoplasms with clear cells: a report of 21 cases in which the alteration is not of typical secretory type. Am J Surg Pathol 2007;31(8):1203–8.

136. Cao D, Guo S, Allan RW, et al. SALL4 is a novel sensitive and specific marker of ovarian primitive germ cell tumors and is particularly useful in distinguishing yolk sac tumor from clear cell carcinoma. Am J Surg Pathol 2009;33(6):894–904.

137. Cetin A, Bahat Z, Cilesiz P, et al. Ovarian clear cell adenocarcinoma producing alpha-fetoprotein: case report. Eur J Gynaecol Oncol 2007;28(3): 241–4.

138. Pitman MB, Triratanachat S, Young RH, et al. Hepatocyte paraffin 1 antibody does not distinguish primary ovarian tumors with hepatoid differentiation from metastatic hepatocellular carcinoma. Int J Gynecol Pathol 2004;23(1):58–64.

139. Clement PB, Young RH, Scully RE. Malignant mesotheliomas presenting as ovarian masses. A report of nine cases, including two primary ovarian mesotheliomas. Am J Surg Pathol 1996;20:1067–80.

140. Gersell DJ, King TC. Papillary cystadenoma of the mesosalpinx in von Hippel-Lindau disease. Am J Surg Pathol 1988;12:145–9.

141. Felix A, Nogales FF, Arias-Stella J. Polypoid endometriosis of the uterine cervix with arias-stella reaction in a patient taking phytoestrogens. Int J Gynecol Pathol 2010;29(2):185–8.

142. Arias-Stella J Jr, Arias-Velasquez A, Arias-Stella J. Normal and abnormal mitoses in the atypical endometrial change associated with chronic tissue effect. Am J Surg Pathol 1994;18:694–701.

143. Kobel M, Xu H, Bourne PA, et al. IGF2BP3 (IMP3) expression is a marker of unfavorable prognosis in ovarian carcinoma of clear cell subtype. Mod Pathol 2009;22(3):469–75.

144. Nagai Y, Inamine M, Hirakawa M, et al. Postoperative whole abdominal radiotherapy in clear cell adenocarcinoma of the ovary. Gynecol Oncol 2007;107(3):469–73.

145. Eichhorn JH, Young RH. Transitional cell carcinoma of the ovary: a morphologic study of 100 cases with emphasis on differential diagnosis. Am J Surg Pathol 2004;28(4):453–63.

146. Logani S, Oliva E, Amin MB, et al. Immunoprofile of ovarian tumors with putative transitional cell (urothelial) differentiation using novel urothelial markers: histogenetic and diagnostic implications. Am J Surg Pathol 2003;27(11):1434–41.

147. Ehrlich CE, Roth LM. The Brenner tumor. A clinicopathologic study of 57 cases. Cancer 1971;27: 332–42.

148. Fox H, Agrawal K, Langley FA. The Brenner tumour of the ovary. A clinicopathological study of 54 cases. J Obstet Gynaecol Br Commonw 1972;79: 661–5.

149. Miles PA, Norris HJ. Proliferative and malignant Brenner tumors of the ovary. Cancer 1972;30: 174–86.

150. Roth LM, Czernobilsky B. Ovarian Brenner tumors. II. Malignant. Cancer 1985;56:592–601.

151. Roth LM, Dallenbach-Hellweg G, Czernobilsky B. Ovarian Brenner tumors: I. Metaplastic, proliferating, and low malignant potential. Cancer 1985; 562:582–91.

152. Soslow RA, Rouse RV, Hendrickson MR, et al. Transitional cell neoplasms of the ovary and urinary bladder: a comparative immunohistochemical analysis. Int J Gynecol Pathol 1996;15:257–65.

153. Cuatrecasas M, Catasus L, Palacios J, et al. Transitional cell tumors of the ovary: a comparative clinicopathologic, immunohistochemical, and molecular genetic analysis of Brenner tumors and transitional cell carcinomas. Am J Surg Pathol 2009;33(4):556–67.

154. Liao XY, Xue WC, Shen DH, et al. p63 expression in ovarian tumours: a marker for Brenner tumours but not transitional cell carcinomas. Histopathology 2007;51(4):477–83.

155. Ordonez NG. Transitional cell carcinomas of the ovary and bladder are immunophenotypically different. Histopathology 2000;36(5):433–8.

156. Riedel I, Czernobilsky B, Lifschitz-Mercer B, et al. Brenner tumors but not transitional cell carcinomas of the ovary show urothelial differentiation: immunohistochemical staining of urothelial markers, including cytokeratins and uroplakins. Virchows Arch Int J Pathol 2001;438(2):181–91.

157. Tafe L, Garg K, Tornos C, et al. Undifferentiated carcinoma of the endometrium and ovary: a clinicopathologic correlation. Mod Pathol 2009;22(1): 238A.

158. Rutgers JL, Scully RE. Ovarian mullerian mucinous papillary cystadenomas of borderline malignancy. A clinicopathologic analysis. Cancer 1988;61: 340–8.

159. Rutgers JL, Scully RE. Ovarian mixed-epithelial papillary cystadenomas of borderline malignancy of mullerian type. A clinicopathologic analysis. Cancer 1988;61:546–54.

160. Shappell HW, Riopel MA, Smith Sehdev AE, et al. Diagnostic criteria and behavior of ovarian seromucinous (endocervical-type mucinous and mixed cell-type) tumors: atypical proliferative (borderline) tumors, intraepithelial, microinvasive, and invasive carcinomas. Am J Surg Pathol 2002;26(12): 1529–41.

161. Asad H, Soslow RA. Clinicopathologic and immunohistochemical analysis of mixed epithelial ovarian tumors with a clear cell carcinoma component [abstract 894]. Mod Pathol 2008;21(Suppl 1):195A.

162. Vang R, Gown AM, Barry TS, et al. Ovarian atypical proliferative (borderline) mucinous tumors: gastrointestinal and seromucinous (endocervical-like) types are immunophenotypically distinctive. Int J Gynecol Pathol 2006;25(1):83–9.

163. Rutgers JL, Scully RE. Cysts (cystadenomas) and tumors of the rete ovarii. Int J Gynecol Pathol 1988;7:330–42.

164. Young RH, Oliva E, Scully RE. Small cell carcinoma of the ovary, hypercalcemic type: A clinicopathological analysis of 150 cases. Am J Surg Pathol 1994;18:1102–16.

165. Eichhorn JH, Young RH, Scully RE. Primary ovarian small cell carcinoma of pulmonary type: A clinicopathologic, immunohistologic, and flow cytometric analysis of 11 cases. Am J Surg Pathol 1992;16: 926–38.

166. Isaac MA, Vijayalakshmi S, Madhu CS, et al. Pure cystic nephroblastoma of the ovary with a review of extrarenal Wilms' tumors. Hum Pathol 2000; 31(6):761–4.

167. Axe SR, Klein VR, Woodruff JD. Choriocarcinoma of the ovary. Obstet Gynecol 1985;66:111–4.

168. Eichhorn JH, Scully RE. "Adenoid cystic" and basaloid carcinomas of the ovary: evidence for a surface epithelial lineage. A report of 12 cases. Mod Pathol 1995;8:731–40.

169. Young RH, Scully RE. Ovarian tumors of probable Wolffian origin: a report of 11 cases. Am J Surg Pathol 1983;7:125–36.

HEREDITARY CARCINOMAS OF THE OVARY, FALLOPIAN TUBE, AND PERITONEUM

Patricia A. Shaw, MD[a,b],*

KEYWORDS

- BRCA1 • BRCA2 • Serous carcinoma • Hereditary nonpolyposis colon cancer
- Lynch syndrome • Prophylactic salpingo-oophorectomy • Tubal intraepithelial carcinoma
- Occult cancer

ABSTRACT

Approximately 10% of ovarian cancers are associated with inherited germline mutations, most commonly of the *BRCA1* or *BRCA2* genes. The majority of BRCA1 and BRCA2 cancers are high-grade serous carcinomas diagnosed at an advanced stage, and there are as yet no histologic features that distinguish these tumors from sporadic serous cancers. Many women identified as being at high genetic risk undergo prophylactic salpingo-oophorectomy, and careful histopathological examination of these specimens may identify occult carcinoma, frequently in the distal fallopian tube. In addition, serous cancer precursors, including tubal intraepithelial carcinoma, have been increasingly recognized in distal and fimbrial epithelium. Little has been documented to date of the histopathological features of the cancers associated with the hereditary nonpolyposis colon cancer syndrome, but it appears these ovarian cancers may include a variety of histologic types, and in contrast to the BRCA cancers, are low grade and early stage.

Key Features
HEREDITARY OVARIAN CARCINOMAS

1. Carcinomas associated with germline mutations of the tumor suppressor genes, *BRCA1* or *BRCA2*, are the commonest hereditary cancers of the ovary, fallopian tube, or peritoneum, and account for about 15% of all high-grade serous cancers.

2. Risk-reducing salpingo-oophorectomy specimens from mutation carriers must be carefully assessed following protocols optimizing the microscopic examination of tube, ovary, and peritoneum to facilitate detection of occult carcinomas and tubal intraepithelial carcinomas.

3. BRCA cancers are usually high-grade serous carcinomas and present at an advanced stage.

4. The second most frequent group of hereditary ovarian cancers are associated with the Lynch syndrome, and are typically well or moderately differentiated carcinomas diagnosed at an early stage.

OVERVIEW

Inherited susceptibilities account for at least 10% of ovarian cancers, and family history is the

[a] Department of Laboratory Medicine and Pathobiology, University of Toronto, Toronto, ON, Canada
[b] Department of Pathology, University Health Network, Eaton Wing, Room 11-444, 200 Elizabeth Street, Toronto, ON M5G 2C4, Canada
* Department of Pathology, University Health Network, Eaton Wing, Room 11-444, 200 Elizabeth Street, Toronto, ON M5G 2C4, Canada.
E-mail address: patricia.shaw@uhn.on.ca

Surgical Pathology 4 (2011) 461–478
doi:10.1016/j.path.2010.03.003
1875-9181/11/$ – see front matter © 2011 Elsevier Inc. All rights reserved.

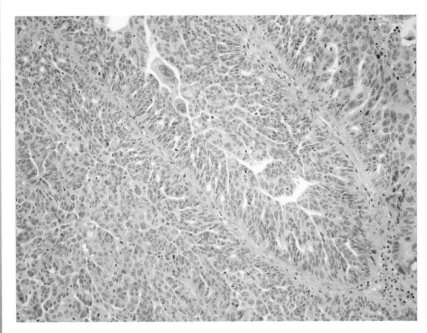

Fig. 1. This high-grade serous carcinoma in a *BRCA1* mutation carrier demonstrates characteristic histologic features, including intraglandular tufting, budding, and papillary formation producing slit-like spaces, marked nuclear pleomorphism with hyperchromasia, occasional tumor giant cells, and numerous mitotic figures. Scant fibrous tissue is seen in this example (original magnification ×100).

strongest known risk factor. The spectrum of hereditary carcinomas of the ovary, fallopian tube, and peritoneum includes at least 2 defined inherited genetic aberrations, associated with 3 syndromes:

1. "Site-specific" ovarian cancer
2. Hereditary breast-ovarian cancer syndrome (HBOC)
3. Lynch syndrome.

The first 2 syndromes are associated with inherited mutations in the oncosuppressor genes *BRCA1* and *BRCA2*, and account for 90% of hereditary ovarian carcinomas. The other 10% of hereditary cases are associated with mutations in the DNA mismatch repair genes, primarily *hMLH1*, *hMSH2*, and *hMSH6*. The HBOC includes cancers of the ovary, fallopian tube, and peritoneum with at least 13% of ovarian cancers, 17% of carcinomas of tubal origin, and up to 28% of

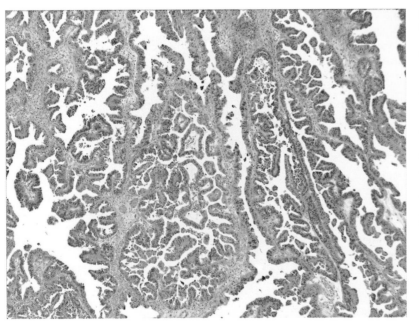

Fig. 2. The high-grade serous carcinomas found in mutation carriers have a similar spectrum of morphologic variations as is seen in sporadic high-grade serous carcinoma. In this example of carcinoma in a *BRCA1* mutation carrier, the architecture is prominently papillary with the formation of fibrovascular cores, with detachment of tumor cells, tufting, and budding clearly seen (original magnification ×50).

primary peritoneal carcinomas associated with inherited mutations of *BRCA1* or *BRCA2*.[1–3] To date, only carcinomas of the ovary, not tube or peritoneum, have been found in carriers of *hMLH1* or *hMSH2* mutations. The lifetime risk of a mutation carrier developing carcinoma varies with the mutation: up to 66% for *BRCA1*, 10% to 20% for *BRCA2*, and 3% to 12% for *MLH1/MSH2*.[4] Most hereditary cancers are diagnosed at a younger age than the sporadic counterparts; carriers of

BRCA1 mutations are diagnosed at a mean age of 51 years, *MLH1* carriers at 51 years, and *MSH2* carriers at 45 years, with *BRCA2* carriers diagnosed slightly later than the sporadic cancers, at 57 years.[5,6] Women who are known to carry a mutation of *BRCA1* or *BRCA2*, or have a strong family history indicative of HBOC syndrome are advised to undergo prophylactic salpingo-oophorectomy after the age of 35 years or after child-bearing is completed, and careful

Fig. 3. (A) In this example of serous carcinoma in a *BRCA1* mutation carrier, marked epithelial proliferation grow out from the surface of broad papillary cores, forming elongated thin papillae with prominent cellular detachment (original magnification ×50). (B) At higher magnification marked nuclear atypia, pleomorphism, and numerous mitoses including abnormal forms are seen (original magnification ×400).

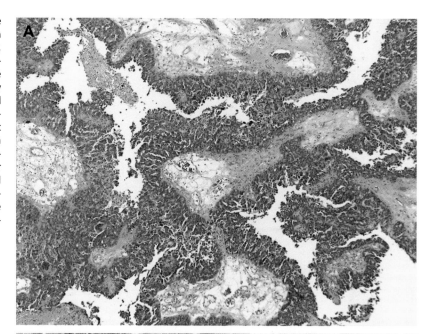

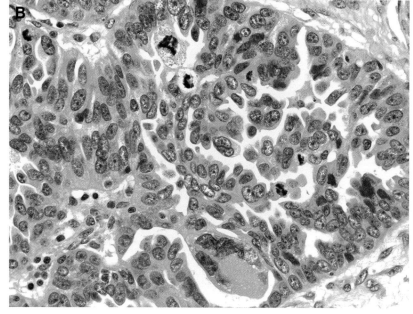

histopathological examination of these specimens has been key in improving our understanding of early lesions in *BRCA* mutation carriers.

CANCERS ASSOCIATED WITH MUTATIONS OF *BRCA1* OR *BRCA2*

The recognition that an ovarian cancer may be hereditary has important clinical and therapeutic implications for individual patients and their families, and the association with a family history does not always predict this: approximately 10% of ovarian cancer patients with *BRCA1/2* germline mutations have no known family history of breast or ovarian cancer.[5] The majority of BRCA cancers are diagnosed with peritoneal spread and extrapelvic disease. Epidemiologic data indicate cancers arising in *BRCA1/2* mutation carriers are invasive nonmucinous carcinomas, with serous carcinoma the predominant histotype.[1,5] However, there are few publications detailing the histopathological features, and results have been conflicting,

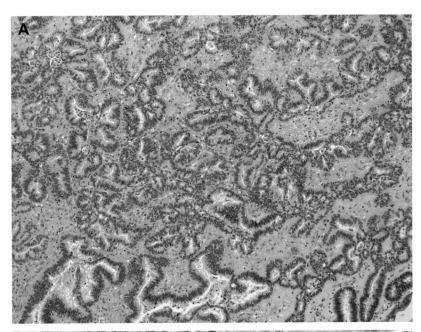

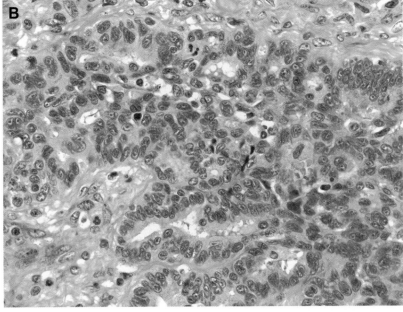

Fig. 4. (*A*) Some *BRCA* mutation associated tumors have less pronounced cellular stratification, with a glandular pattern, suggesting the diagnosis of endometrioid carcinoma (original magnification ×100). (*B*) In other areas of the tumor, marked nuclear hyperchromasia and pleomorphism are seen, characteristic of serous carcinoma (original magnification ×400).

reflecting interobserver differences in classifying poorly differentiated carcinomas. Thus a uniformly accepted histologic definition of "BRCAness" of ovarian carcinomas does not yet exist. Nevertheless, it is fairly certain that cancers of the gynecologic tract in *BRCA1* and *BRCA2* mutation carriers do not include borderline tumors, grade 1 carcinomas, or mucinous carcinomas. In addition, there is no reported histologic distinction between *BRCA1* and *BRCA2* carcinomas, although the number of reported BRCA2 tumors is small.

MICROSCOPIC FEATURES

Ovarian, tubal, and peritoneal cancers linked to *BRCA* mutations are poorly differentiated carcinomas with high-grade serous carcinoma the predominant histotype. Other histotypes that have been reported in BRCA mutation carriers are endometrioid, clear cell, transitional cell, undifferentiated, and malignant mixed mullerian tumor.[7,8] However, in one of the few blinded histologic reviews of mutation associated cancers, 100% of 32 *BRCA1* and *BRCA2* tumors were typed as high-grade serous carcinoma.[9] Using the Silverberg grading system, most of the carcinomas are grade 3, with a trend without statistical significance to a more solid architecture, and a higher mitotic count compared with sporadic tumors (**Fig. 1**).[9–11] It is the author's personal experience, on review of 45 *BRCA1*- and *BRCA2*-associated carcinomas, that all are high-grade serous carcinomas and, like the sporadic types,

they display similar morphologic variations to the sporadic carcinomas (**Figs. 2–6**).[12] The architectural pattern varies, although the majority has a mix of papillary and solid architecture. Occasionally tumors have a glandular pattern in some areas, reminiscent of an endometrioid pattern, but invariably the presence of marked nuclear atypia and numerous mitoses in the gland-forming areas are more in keeping with a diagnosis of serous type (see **Fig. 4**). Hobnailing may be present in tumors with a papillary architecture, with foci of cytoplasmic clearing, suggesting a clear cell component (see **Fig. 5**). Tumors with broad papillae covered in basophilic but markedly atypical tumor cells may suggest a diagnosis of transitional cell carcinoma (see **Fig. 6**).

Nuclear accumulation of p53 protein by immunohistochemistry is frequent in both *BRCA1*- and *BRCA2*-associated carcinomas, with intense positive nuclear staining in the majority of tumor cells present in approximately 70% of the carcinomas, a percentage similar to that found in sporadic high-grade serous carcinomas.[13] The characteristic p53 staining pattern corresponds to a high frequency of *p53* mutations in *BRCA1/2* associated cancers[14] and serous carcinomas.[15] Additional positive markers in the immunoprofile of *BRCA* cancers are CK7, WT-1, CA125, and estrogen receptor.

Classification of the carcinomas in patients treated with preoperative chemotherapy may present challenges in histotyping, but the correct diagnosis of serous carcinoma can be aided by

Fig. 5. A papillary pattern with hobnailing and occasional cytoplasmic clearing may suggest a diagnosis of clear cell carcinoma (original magnification ×50).

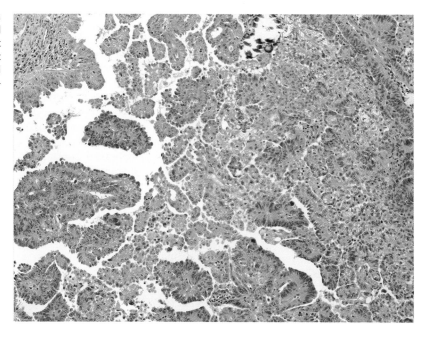

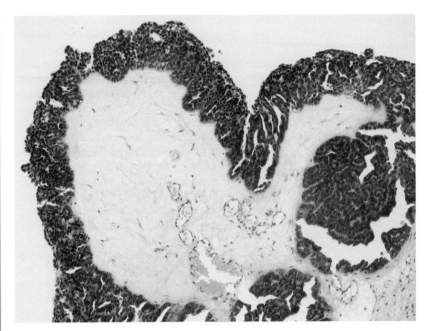

Fig. 6. This tumor has broad papillary cores covered in stratified tumor epithelium characterized by marked nuclear atypia and scant cytoplasm, with a pattern suggestive of transitional cell carcinoma (original magnification ×100).

the use of immunohistochemistry. Biomarkers that are frequently expressed in serous carcinomas, including WT-1, p53, CK7, CA125, and p16, tend to be stable before and after platinum-based treatment.[16]

Other histologic features, such as lymphovascular space invasion and necrosis, are not characteristic of *BRCA* cancers. In one small series of serous carcinomas with *BRCA* mutations, tumor-infiltrating lymphocytes (TIL) were seen, with CD8+ TILs present more frequently than CD3+ TILs, a finding that was associated with loss of BRCA protein in high-grade serous carcinomas, both by mutation and due to epigenetic loss; therefore, this finding is not specific to hereditary carcinomas.[17]

DIFFERENTIAL DIAGNOSIS

Mutation carriers are also at risk for breast cancer, usually triple negative carcinomas (negative expression of estrogen and progesterone receptors, and Her2-neu). Women with hereditary pelvic cancer may have a prior or concurrent history of breast carcinoma, and therefore recurrent/metastatic breast carcinoma may occasionally be included in the differential diagnosis.[18] Carriers of *BRCA2* mutations are also at risk for pancreatic carcinoma, and this may be included in the differential diagnosis of peritoneal carcinomatosis of uncertain origin. Ductal pancreatic carcinoma is another cancer type which, like serous carcinoma, is often associated with an elevated serum

CA125. The morphology of pancreatic carcinoma, including the characteristic well-differentiated architecture and high-grade nuclear atypia, may be sufficient to distinguish it from serous carcinoma. Unlike serous carcinoma, pancreatic carcinoma typically does not express WT-1 by immunohistochemistry, and may be positive for CK20 as well as carcinoembryonic antigen and CK7.

PROGNOSIS

BRCA1/BRCA2-associated cancers are high-grade, high-stage, and predominantly serous type—these are all features that are known adverse prognostic indicators. However, increasing evidence indicates that the 5-year survival in *BRCA1/2* mutation carriers is significantly greater than in noncarriers matched for other known prognostic, clinical, and demographic factors, and that the improved overall and treatment-free survivals may be due to increased sensitivity to platinum-based chemotherapy.[19,20] In addition, it has been shown that carcinomas with reduced levels of BRCA1 mRNA expression not only are associated with a significantly improved overall survival, with increased sensitivity to platinum derivatives, but also have reduced sensitivity to taxanes, indicating the possibility that BRCA1 protein expression may be a predictor of chemotherapy response.[21,22] A new family of drugs called PARP inhibitors are currently being studied in clinical trials, and these may offer an additional advantageous therapeutic approach to the medical management of carcinomas with BRCA deficiency.

OCCULT CANCERS IN *BRCA* MUTATION CARRIERS

Occult invasive carcinomas, defined as carcinomas diagnosed in the absence of preoperative clinical evidence of malignancy, that is, negative findings on physical examination, transvaginal ultrasound, and normal levels of serum CA125, are detected in 4% to 10% of prophylactic salpingo-oophorectomy specimens, and are poorly differentiated carcinomas with a predominant serous histotype.[23–26] Most occult carcinomas are detected by microscopic examination only, but occasional carcinomas are noted on macroscopic examination after resection, and have been as large as 5 cm. Pathologic staging of the

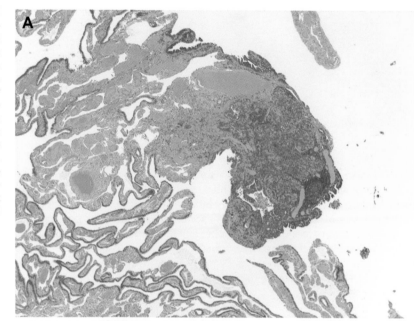

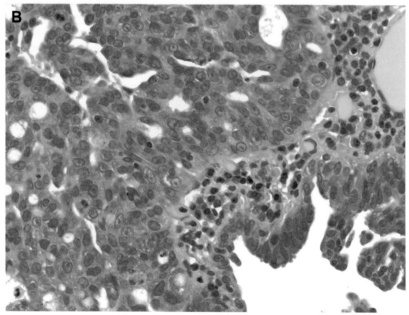

Fig. 7. (*A*) This fimbrial serous carcinoma measured only 1.6 mm, and was discovered only on microscopic examination (original magnification ×25). (*B*) On higher magnification, tubal intraepithelial carcinoma with an exophytic pattern is seen adjacent to the invasive component. Rounded spaces in the invasive carcinoma represent "cell dropout," not glandular spaces (original magnification ×400).

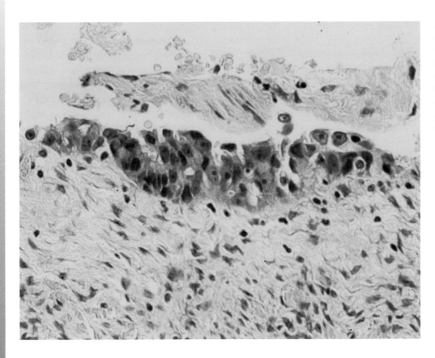

Fig. 8. Ovarian involvement may be limited to the ovarian surface, without significant ovarian stromal invasion. These foci may be metastases from occult tubal carcinomas (original magnification ×400).

occult carcinomas ranges from stage 0 to stage IIb, indicating a propensity for peritoneal spread despite the small volume of disease present.

The majority of the occult carcinomas involve the distal fallopian tube, usually the tubal fimbria, with occasional involvement of the adnexal peritoneum, and of the ovary alone (**Fig. 7**).[23,26] In one study of 159 consecutive risk-reducing salpingo-oophorectomies, the only case of carcinoma involving the ovary alone did not have complete histologic examination of fallopian tubes. It is, therefore, possible the ovarian surface deposits identified in this case were metastatic from an undiagnosed tubal primary (**Fig. 8**).[23] The occult cancer may also be found in adnexal peritoneum (**Fig. 9**).

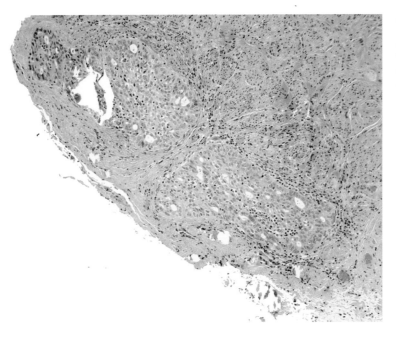

Fig. 9. An occult peritoneal high-grade serous carcinoma found on the fallopian tube. Occasional microcalcifications are present (original magnification ×100).

MICROSCOPIC FEATURES

Detailed microscopic descriptions of occult cancers in risk-reducing salpingo-oophorectomy (RRSO) specimens are scant in the literature. The majority are high-grade serous carcinomas, characterized by a predominant solid architecture, and range from 1 mm to 5 cm in maximum dimension. Cytoplasm is eosinophilic, with indistinct cell borders and occasional clear vacuoles. Slit-like spaces, or rounded spaces due to cell dropout, may be seen (see **Fig. 7**). Nuclei are typically pleomorphic, with irregularly cleared chromatin and frequently prominent single nucleoli. Mitoses including abnormal forms are easily recognized. On rare occasion microcalcifications are present (see **Fig. 9**). Scant collagen or fibrous tissue is seen within these small nodules of carcinoma. Tumor infiltrating lymphocytes are frequently present. Despite the small volume of carcinoma present, extratubal spread may be identified, usually characterized by microscopic surface deposits on the ipsilateral ovary (**Fig. 10**).

DIFFERENTIAL DIAGNOSIS

Resected ovaries in this patient population may rarely contain occult cancer metastatic from a breast primary. A small and high-grade metastatic breast carcinoma may be difficult to distinguish from an occult high-grade serous carcinoma. The breast carcinoma may express p53, CK7, and CA125, similar to the serous carcinoma; however, WT-1 and PAX8 by immunohistochemistry should be negative, and mammoglobin and GCDPF may be positive in the breast cancer.[18] Other possible mimics of occult carcinoma include stromal hyperthecosis, nodular hyperthecosis, adrenal rests, hilus cell nodules, and hilus cell hyperplasia. These lesions, however, should be readily differentiated from carcinomas based on benign morphology and the lack of an epithelial cell immunoprofile.[18]

RISK-REDUCING SALPINGO-OOPHORECTOMY

Primary prevention of carcinoma in women at high genetic risk involves RRSO. The surgery involves complete removal of ovarian tissue, requiring isolation of the ovarian blood supply in the retroperitoneal space, and removal of the entire fallopian tube with soft tissue. Some advocate the removal of the uterus as part of the prophylactic surgery, but removal of the interstitial portion of the tube, which is at low risk for carcinoma in this population, is likely not necessary. Hereditary carcinoma is rare in individuals younger than 30 years, but as many as 2% to 3% of *BRCA1*-associated carcinomas are diagnosed by age 40 years. RRSO is recommended to occur after completion of child-bearing, or after the age of 35 years.[27]

Because there is a significant incidence of occult carcinoma in RRSO specimens, the pathologist must be considered to have a key position in the multidisciplinary care of patients undergoing prophylactic surgery, and it is imperative that the reason for the surgery be communicated to the

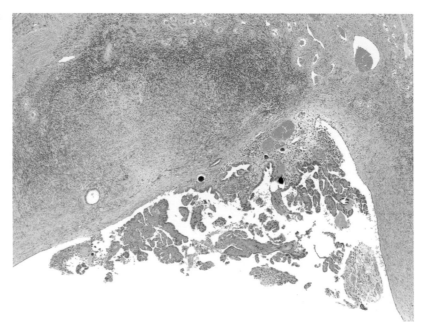

Fig. 10. A tumor deposit from an occult fimbrial carcinoma on the ipsilateral ovarian surface. No invasion of ovarian cortex is seen (original magnification ×50).

pathologist so the RRSO specimens are handled and processed to preserve the ovarian surface epithelium and the tubal fimbrial epithelium. Crum and colleagues have outlined a protocol for Sectioning and Extensively Examining the FIMbriated end of the fallopian tube (SEE-FIM), which optimizes the surface area of the high-risk epithelium available for microscopic analysis examination.[28] In brief, the tube and ovaries are fixed in formalin for at least several hours before handling. The fimbriated end is amputated and sectioned serially longitudinally to maximize histologic examination of fimbrial plicae. The remaining tube is serially sectioned at 2- to 3-mm intervals. All tissue is submitted for microscopic examination. There is no evidence to suggest that multiple levels are required for the detection of clinically significant lesions, but the sectioning protocol might include additional unstained sections adjacent to the hematoxylin-eosin–stained section, which may be used to further classify any lesion identified on histology.[29] Alternatively, immunohistochemistry, specifically p53 and MIB1, may be ordered on the high-risk epithelium, the fimbria, as the combination of these markers will highlight small lesions that may be overlooked on routine microscopy. This approach is not currently considered the standard of care, but has been used in the research setting.

Similarly, the ovaries must be handled with care to preserve the delicate covering of the surface. Intraoperative scrapings of the ovarian surface epithelium, sometimes included in research protocols, should be avoided in prophylactic specimens. Sectioning of the ovaries should occur only post fixation, and serial sections at 2- to 3-mm intervals are taken along the short axis of the ovary, perpendicular to the long axis, again maximizing microscopic examination of the ovarian tissue and surface.

TUBAL INTRAEPITHELIAL CARCINOMA

Careful examination of the fallopian tube epithelium in RRSO specimens has led to the identification of putative cancer precursors in mutation carriers, indicating that the origin of tubal, ovarian, and peritoneal serous cancer in high-risk women may be the epithelium of the distal tube.[28,30,31] Tubal intraepithelial carcinoma (TIC) is identified in as many as 8% of prophylactic salpingectomies, either alone or in association with an occult carcinoma.[32] TICs are also seen in tubes of patients undergoing debulking surgery with a diagnosis of advanced stage serous carcinoma and of primary peritoneal serous carcinoma.[33,34] When identified in the absence of invasive carcinomas, the fallopian tubes are normal on macroscopic

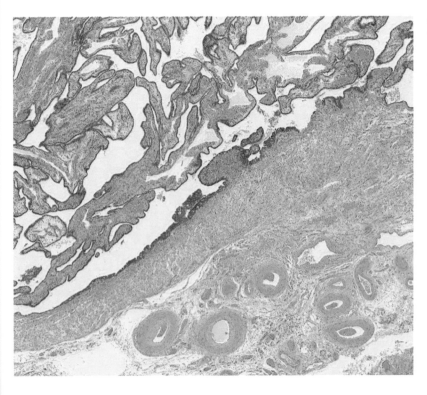

Fig. 11. A tubal intraepithelial carcinoma is recognized as a lesion at low magnification in a tube from a postmenopausal woman (original magnification ×50).

Fig. 12. A tubal intraepithelial carcinoma shows characteristic features of stratification, crowding, and nuclear pleomorphism. In addition, surface cells are beginning to detach (original magnification ×400).

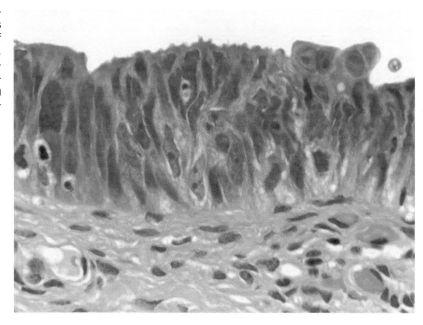

examination. TICs are usually identified in the distal tube, the fimbria, infundibulum, or distal ampulla. Rarely TICs are identified in the mid-isthmus, and are generally not seen in the proximal or intramural tube. TICs may be multifocal.[32]

MICROSCOPIC FEATURES

Recognizing significant epithelial lesions is usually possible at low power in post-menopausal fallopian tubes, because the uninvolved tubal epithelium is low columnar with little stratification (**Fig. 11**). TICs may, however, be more subtle in premenopausal patients, and normal epithelium has variable degrees of proliferation and stratification in the absence of a premalignant process.[35,36]

Microscopically, TIC is characterized by an increased nuclear/cytoplasmic ratio, nuclear pleomorphism, significant nuclear atypia with

Fig. 13. In this tubal intraepithelial carcinoma, atypical cells form tufts and slit-like spaces (original magnification ×400).

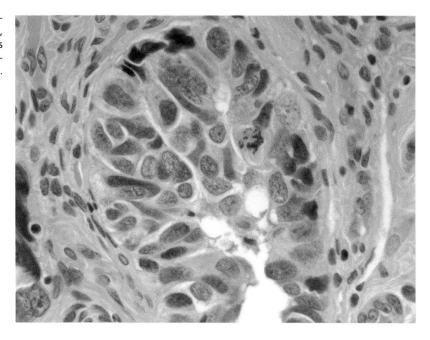

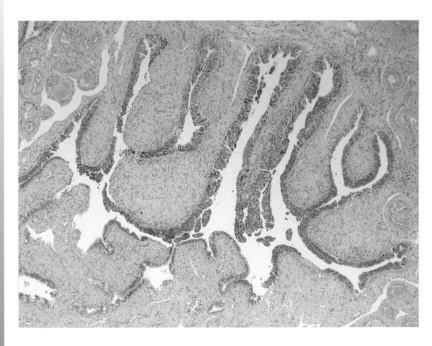

Fig. 14. A low-power magnification of a tubal intraepithelial carcinoma with cellular stratification, tufting, and small papillae projecting from the intraepithelial lesion, in the absence of stromal invasion (original magnification ×50).

hyperchromasia, loss of polarity and, usually, by cellular stratification. Mitoses are identified only occasionally, and nucleoli may be prominent. TICs are composed of cells without cilia, although occasional residual ciliated cells may be scattered through the lesion. Nuclear atypia, pleomorphism, crowding, and stratification are all features common to TICs. Occasional TICs also have cellular tufting, formation of slit-like spaces, and even detachment of surface cells, representing

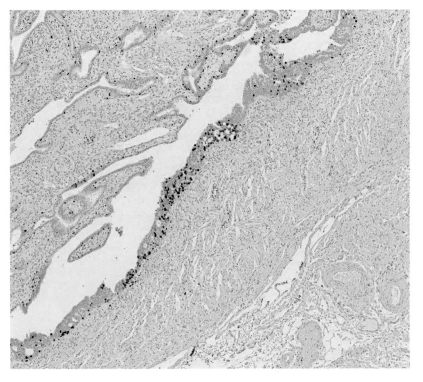

Fig. 15. A tubal intraepithelial carcinoma has increased cellular proliferation distinct from background tubal epithelium, as highlighted by immunohistochemistry for MIB1 (original magnification ×100).

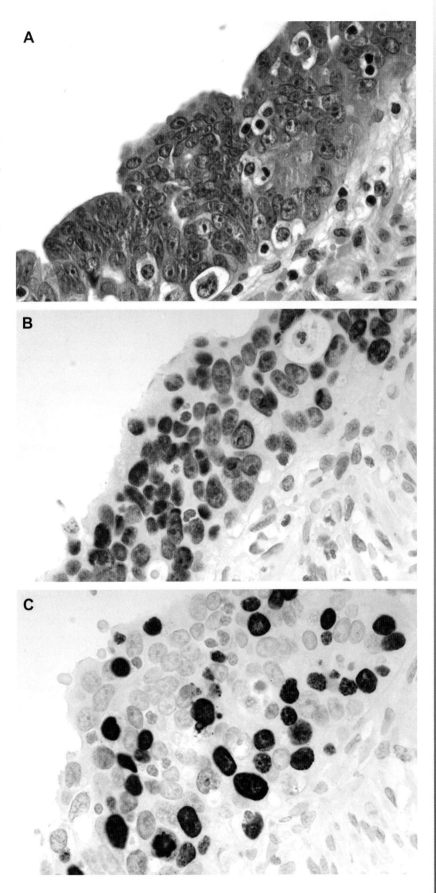

Fig. 16. A tubal intraepithelial carcinoma (*A*) with p53 nuclear overexpression (*B*) and increased MIB1 positivity (*C*) by immunohistochemistry (original magnification ×400). (*Reprinted from* Shaw PA, Rouzbahman M, Pizer ES, et al. Candidate serous cancer precursors in fallopian tube epithelium of BRCA1/2 mutation carriers. Mod Pathol 2009;22(9):1133–8; copyright 2009, Macmillan Publishers Ltd; with permission.)

an exophytic growth pattern in the absence of stromal invasion (**Figs. 12–14**).

Immunohistochemistry is useful, and may be necessary, to confirm a diagnosis of TIC. The increased proliferation can be confirmed by increased expression of Ki67, increased significantly compared with background epithelium, usually greater than 50% of the TIC cells somewhere in the lesion (**Fig. 15**). In addition, approximately 80% of TICs have diffuse nuclear overexpression of p53, although it should be noted that, as with the invasive high-grade serous carcinomas, p53 positivity by p53 is not a requirement for a diagnosis of TIC (**Fig. 16**). It should also be noted that the p53 positivity in these lesions, as in the cancers, is present in the majority of the nuclei. Scattered weak nuclear positivity is not a diagnostic pattern of staining in these lesions.

DIFFERENTIAL DIAGNOSIS

There are lesions that do not fulfill the histologic criteria for a diagnosis of malignancy, but do have atypia, stratification, p53 nuclear staining, and only marginally increased cell proliferation. The significance and the classification of these lesions is uncertain. The differential diagnosis of TIC may also include a benign entity, transitional cell metaplasia of the tubal epithelium. The lack of nuclear atypia, the lack of proliferation and the presence of nuclear grooves are features that readily distinguish this common entity from the malignant precursors.[37]

△△   *Differential Diagnosis*
     HEREDITARY OVARIAN CARCINOMAS

1. *BRCA*-associated cancers cannot be distinguished on histologic examination from sporadic high-grade serous carcinomas at present.

2. Like sporadic serous carcinomas, *BRCA*-associated serous carcinomas frequently overexpress p53, WT-1, and estrogen receptor on immunohistochemistry.

3. Occult *BRCA*-associated carcinomas within the ovary are uncommon, but when present, a diagnosis of metastatic breast carcinoma, also frequent in this patient population, should be excluded.

4. The use of immunohistochemistry for p53 and MIB1 may be needed to confirm a diagnosis of TIC, and distinguish it from a less clinically significant lesion.

PROGNOSIS

The clinical outcome of TICs diagnosed in the absence of invasive carcinoma and in the absence of peritoneal spread is not yet known. Adjuvant chemotherapy is usually not given based on a diagnosis of TIC alone, but it is imperative that the pathologist examine all resected tissues carefully to exclude the presence of microscopic peritoneal spread. It appears that some TICs may be capable of metastasizing in the absence of stromal invasion, and should therefore not always be considered as in situ lesions.

P53 SIGNATURE

Another lesion seen in the fallopian tubes of women with germline mutations is the p53 signature (**Fig. 17**).[30,31] As defined by Crum and colleagues, the p53 signature is a focus of at least 12 consecutive cells with intense nuclear staining with p53, but without other abnormal morphology or increased proliferation. Most lesions are small, but may extend to include hundreds of cells. p53 signatures may be multifocal and bilateral, and have the same distribution in the fallopian tube as TICs, with which they frequently coexist. The biologic significance of this lesion is uncertain, particularly as it is seen commonly in women at low genetic risk of carcinoma.[32] The p53 overexpression may coexist with *p53* mutations and evidence of DNA damage as documented by γ-H2AX immunohistochemistry, suggesting that the p53 signature may be a latent precursor of TIC and tubal serous carcinoma.[31] The p53 signature, however, should be considered as a benign nonneoplastic lesion.

CANCERS ASSOCIATED WITH THE LYNCH SYNDROME

More than 50% of women with Lynch syndrome present with a gynecologic cancer, usually endometrial cancer, as their first "sentinel" malignancy,[38] and inherited mutations in DNA mismatch repair genes account for approximately 2% of ovarian cancers. However, few reports delineate the histologic features of Lynch syndrome-associated ovarian carcinomas. In a registry of hereditary cancers, 25% of cases were reported as serous carcinomas, with the remaining 75% endometrioid or mixed cell types including clear cell and mucinous. Three of 8 cases were associated with endometriosis.[4] More than 90% of the tumors reported are carcinomas, with borderline tumors accounting for 4%. Most carcinomas are well to moderately differentiated, and 85% diagnosed at an early stage, stage I or II.[39] Nonepithelial tumors

Fig. 17. (*A*) p53 signatures have a lack of ciliated cells, but no significant atypia, stratification, or proliferation. p53 is overexpressed (*B*) but there is no increased MIB1 expression (*C*) by immunohistochemistry (original magnification ×400). (*Reprinted from* Shaw PA, Rouzbahman M, Pizer ES, et al. Candidate serous cancer precursors in fallopian tube epithelium of BRCA1/2 mutation carriers. Mod Pathol 2009;22(9): 1133–8; copyright 2009, Macmillan Publishers Ltd; with permission.)

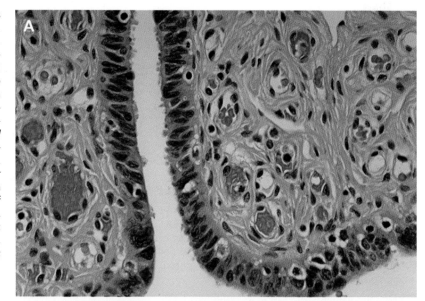

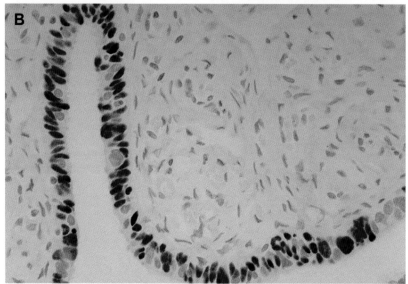

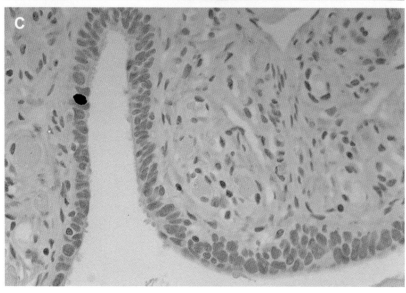

have also been reported, including granulosa cell tumor, dysgerminoma, sex cord tumor, and an endodermal sinus tumor.[39] It should be noted, however, that most reports of histologic type in Lynch syndrome families have not included an expert histologic review.

In a small series of Lynch syndrome-associated ovarian cancers with histologic review, 2 of 4 cases were clear cell carcinomas.[40] The possible predominance of clear cell type in tumors with microsatellite instability was also suggested in a study of ovarian cancers diagnosed in patients 50 years or younger.[41] This study did not assess germline mutations and only 2 of their 5 cases satisfied the Bethesda guidelines for the Lynch syndrome, but this does indicate that about 10% of ovarian carcinomas, and 17% of clear cell carcinomas, in women 50 years or younger have mismatch repair inactivation with loss of MSH2 and MLH6 protein expression by immunohistochemistry. Targeted testing of clear cell carcinomas with immunohistochemistry, particularly for MSH2 and MLH6, may be an important screening tool for Lynch syndrome.[41]

Interpretation of immunohistochemistry for the DNA-MMR proteins requires the presence of an internal positive control in the tissue section, and negative expression is defined as complete absence of nuclear staining in all tumor cells.[42] Occasionally, stains—often MLH1—are difficult to interpret or have focal weak staining, and should therefore be reviewed with experienced pathologists, or the stains repeated.[42]

It should be noted that immunohistochemistry for DNA-MMR proteins is not equivalent to testing for germline mutations. The predictive value of loss of MMR protein expression in ovarian cancer is not yet known, but in other cancers, such as endometrial cancer, absent MSH2 or MSH6 correlate highly with the presence of a germline mutation.[42] Regulatory and ethical issues need to be considered in performing immunohistochemistry for these markers, and these may vary from institution to institution. As a minimum, patients with abnormal results should be referred for genetic counseling.[42]

A small percentage of synchronous endometrial-ovarian cancers have either clinical or molecular evidence suggestive of Lynch syndrome.[43] Synchronous endometrial cancer and ovarian endometrioid carcinomas are common in young women, but these tumors do not appear to have MMR abnormalities.[44] In contrast, synchronous endometrial cancer and ovarian clear cell carcinoma may be part of the Lynch syndrome.[44]

Survival of patients with ovarian cancer associated with Lynch syndrome appears to be similar to that of sporadic cancers.[45]

Pitfalls
HEREDITARY OVARIAN CARCINOMAS

! *BRCA* associated serous carcinomas are high grade, and may be difficult to histotype as serous, particularly if the patient has been treated with preoperative chemotherapy.

! Occult carcinomas and TICs may be missed without optimized processing protocols for risk-reducing resection specimens.

! Rarely metastatic breast carcinoma may be found in resected ovaries of *BRCA* mutation carriers.

REFERENCES

1. Risch HA, McLaughlin JR, Cole DE, et al. Population BRCA1 and BRCA2 mutation frequencies and cancer penetrances: a kin-cohort study in Ontario, Canada. J Natl Cancer Inst 2006;98(23):1694–706.
2. Aziz S, Kuperstein G, Rosen B, et al. A genetic epidemiological study of carcinoma of the fallopian tube. Gynecol Oncol 2001;80(3):341–5.
3. Menczer J, Chetrit A, Barda G, et al. Frequency of BRCA mutations in primary peritoneal carcinoma in Israeli Jewish women. Gynecol Oncol 2003;88(1):58–61.
4. Lynch HT, Casey MJ, Snyder CL, et al. Hereditary ovarian carcinoma: heterogeneity, molecular genetics, pathology, and management. Mol Oncol 2009;3(2):97–137.
5. Risch HA, McLaughlin JR, Cole DE, et al. Prevalence and penetrance of germline BRCA1 and BRCA2 mutations in a population series of 649 women with ovarian cancer. Am J Hum Genet 2001;68(3):700–10.
6. Vasen HF, Stormorken A, Menko FH, et al. MSH2 mutation carriers are at higher risk of cancer than MLH1 mutation carriers: a study of hereditary nonpolyposis colorectal cancer families. J Clin Oncol 2001;19(20):4074–80.
7. Werness BA, Ramus SJ, Whittemore AS, et al. Histopathology of familial ovarian tumors in women from families with and without germline BRCA1 mutations. Hum Pathol 2000;31(11):1420–4.
8. Lakhani SR, Manek S, Penault-Llorca F, et al. Pathology of ovarian cancers in BRCA1 and BRCA2 carriers. Clin Cancer Res 2004;10(7):2473–81.
9. Shaw P, McLaughlin J, Zweemer R, et al. Histopathologic features of genetically determined ovarian cancer. Int J Gynecol Pathol 2002;21(4):407–11.
10. Shimizu Y, Kamoi S, Amada S, et al. Toward the development of a universal grading system for ovarian epithelial carcinoma: testing of a proposed

system in a series of 461 patients with uniform treatment and follow-up. Cancer 1998;82(5):893–901.

11. Silverberg SG. Histopathologic grading of ovarian carcinoma: a review and proposal. Int J Gynecol Pathol 2000;19(1):7–15.

12. Soslow RA. Histologic subtypes of ovarian carcinoma: an overview. Int J Gynecol Pathol 2008; 27(2):161–74.

13. Zweemer R, Shaw P, Verheijen R, et al. Accumulation of p53 protein is frequent in ovarian cancers associated with BRCA1 and BRCA2 germline mutations. J Clin Pathol 1999;52(5):372.

14. Rhei E, Bogomolniy F, Federici MG, et al. Molecular genetic characterization of BRCA1- and BRCA2-linked hereditary ovarian cancers. Cancer Res 1998;58:3193–6.

15. Salani R, Kurman RJ, Giuntoli R 2nd, et al. Assessment of TP53 mutation using purified tissue samples of ovarian serous carcinomas reveals a higher mutation rate than previously reported and does not correlate with drug resistance. Int J Gynecol Cancer 2008;18(3):487–91.

16. Miller K, Price JH, Dobbs SP, et al. An immunohistochemical and morphological analysis of post-chemotherapy ovarian carcinoma. J Clin Pathol 2008;61(5):652–7.

17. Clarke B, Tinker AV, Lee CH, et al. Intraepithelial T cells and prognosis in ovarian carcinoma: novel associations with stage, tumor type, and BRCA1 loss. Mod Pathol 2009;22(3):393–402.

18. Rabban JT, Barnes M, Chen LM, et al. Ovarian pathology in risk-reducing salpingo-oophorectomies from women with BRCA mutations, emphasizing the differential diagnosis of occult primary and metastatic carcinoma. Am J Surg Pathol 2009;33(8):1125–36.

19. Chetrit A, Hirsh-Yechezkel G, Ben-David Y, et al. Effect of BRCA1/2 mutations on long-term survival of patients with invasive ovarian cancer: the national Israeli study of ovarian cancer. J Clin Oncol 2008;26(1):20–5.

20. Tan DS, Rothermundt C, Thomas K, et al. "BRCAness" syndrome in ovarian cancer: a case-control study describing the clinical features and outcome of patients with epithelial ovarian cancer associated with BRCA1 and BRCA2 mutations. J Clin Oncol 2008;26(34):5530–6.

21. Quinn JE, James CR, Stewart GE, et al. BRCA1 mRNA expression levels predict for overall survival in ovarian cancer after chemotherapy. Clin Cancer Res 2007;13(24):7413–20.

22. Quinn JE, Carser JE, James CR, et al. BRCA1 and implications for response to chemotherapy in ovarian cancer. Gynecol Oncol 2009;113(1): 134–42.

23. Finch A, Shaw P, Rosen B, et al. Clinical and pathologic findings of prophylactic salpingo-oophorectomies in 159 BRCA1 and BRCA2 carriers. Gynecol Oncol 2006;100(1):58–64.

24. Rebbeck TR, Lynch HT, Neuhausen SL, et al. Prophylactic oophorectomy in carriers of BRCA1 or BRCA2 mutations. N Engl J Med 2002;346(21): 1616–22.

25. Kauff ND, Satagopan JM, Robson ME, et al. Risk-reducing salpingo-oophorectomy in women with a BRCA1 or BRCA2 mutation. N Engl J Med 2002; 346(21):1609–15.

26. Powell CB, Kenley E, Chen LM, et al. Risk-reducing salpingo-oophorectomy in BRCA mutation carriers: role of serial sectioning in the detection of occult malignancy. J Clin Oncol 2005;23(1):127–32.

27. Kauff ND, Barakat RR. Risk-reducing salpingo-oophorectomy in patients with germline mutations in BRCA1 or BRCA2. J Clin Oncol 2007;25(20):2921–7.

28. Medeiros F, Muto MG, Lee Y, et al. The tubal fimbria is a preferred site for early adenocarcinoma in women with familial ovarian cancer syndrome. Am J Surg Pathol 2006;30(2):230–6.

29. Rabban JT, Krasik E, Chen LM, et al. Multistep level sections to detect occult fallopian tube carcinoma in risk-reducing salpingo-oophorectomies from women with BRCA mutations: implications for defining an optimal specimen dissection protocol. Am J Surg Pathol 2009;33(12):1878–85.

30. Lee Y, Medeiros F, Kindelberger D, et al. Advances in the recognition of tubal intraepithelial carcinoma: applications to cancer screening and the pathogenesis of ovarian cancer. Adv Anat Pathol 2006;13(1):1–7.

31. Lee Y, Miron A, Drapkin R, et al. A candidate precursor to serous carcinoma that originates in the distal fallopian tube. J Pathol 2007;211(1):26–35.

32. Shaw PA, Rouzbahman M, Pizer ES, et al. Candidate serous cancer precursors in fallopian tube epithelium of BRCA1/2 mutation carriers. Mod Pathol 2009;22(9):1133–8.

33. Kindelberger DW, Lee Y, Miron A, et al. Intraepithelial carcinoma of the fimbria and pelvic serous carcinoma: evidence for a causal relationship. Am J Surg Pathol 2007;31(2):161–9.

34. Carlson JW, Miron A, Jarboe EA, et al. Serous tubal intraepithelial carcinoma: its potential role in primary peritoneal serous carcinoma and serous cancer prevention. J Clin Oncol 2008;26(25):4160–5.

35. Cheung AN, Young RH, Scully RE. Pseudocarcinomatous hyperplasia of the fallopian tube associated with salpingitis. A report of 14 cases. Am J Surg Pathol 1994;18(11):1125–30.

36. Yanai-Inbar I, Silverberg SG. Mucosal epithelial proliferation of the fallopian tube: prevalence, clinical associations, and optimal strategy for histopathologic assessment. Int J Gynecol Pathol 2000;19(2): 139–44.

37. Rabban JT, Crawford B, Chen LM, et al. Transitional cell metaplasia of fallopian tube fimbriae: a potential mimic of early tubal carcinoma in risk reduction salpingo-oophorectomies from women

With BRCA mutations. Am J Surg Pathol 2009;
33(1):111–9.

38. Lu KH, Broaddus RR. Gynecologic cancers in Lynch syndrome/HNPCC. Fam Cancer 2005;4(3):249–54.

39. Watson P, Butzow R, Lynch HT, et al. The clinical features of ovarian cancer in hereditary nonpolyposis colorectal cancer. Gynecol Oncol 2001;82(2): 223–8.

40. Bewtra C, Watson P, Conway T, et al. Hereditary ovarian cancer: a clinicopathological study. Int J Gynecol Pathol 1992;11(3):180–7.

41. Jensen KC, Mariappan MR, Putcha GV, et al. Microsatellite instability and mismatch repair protein defects in ovarian epithelial neoplasms in patients 50 years of age and younger. Am J Surg Pathol 2008;32(7):1029–37.

42. Garg K, Leitao MM Jr, Kauff ND, et al. Selection of endometrial carcinomas for DNA mismatch repair protein immunohistochemistry using patient age and tumor morphology enhances detection of mismatch repair abnormalities. Am J Surg Pathol 2009;33(6):925–33.

43. Soliman PT, Broaddus RR, Schmeler KM, et al. Women with synchronous primary cancers of the endometrium and ovary: do they have Lynch syndrome? J Clin Oncol 2005;23(36):9344–50.

44. Garg K, Shih K, Barakat R, et al. Endometrial carcinomas in women aged 40 years and younger: tumors associated with loss of DNA mismatch repair proteins comprise a distinct clinicopathologic subset. Am J Surg Pathol 2009;33(12): 1869–77.

45. Crijnen TE, Janssen-Heijnen ML, Gelderblom H, et al. Survival of patients with ovarian cancer due to a mismatch repair defect. Fam Cancer 2005; 4(4):301–5.

Index

Note: Page numbers of article titles are in **boldface** type.

A

Adenocarcinoma, low-grade endometrial, 161–185. See also *Low-grade endometrial adenocarcinoma.*

Adenocarcinoma in situ (AIS), cervical, 41–43
  biomarkers in, 46, 48
    reactive glandular atypia with inflammation in, 44–45, 48
    stratified mucin-producing intraepithelial lesion, 42–45
    variant, 42–48
    vs. glandular dysplasia, 45
    vs. tubal/tuboendometrial metaplasia, 45, 47

Adenocarcinoma of usual (HPV-associated) type, invasive cervical, prognosis for, 54–55
    vs. endometrial endometrioid, biomarkers in, 52–54
    immunohistochemical stains for, 54
  invasive endocervical, 48–49
    depth of invasion in, 50–51
    pattern of invasion in, 49–50
    villoglandular adenocarcinoma variant, 51
    vs. endometrial endometrioid, biomarkers in, 52–53

Appendiceal tumors involving ovary, differential diagnosis of, 302
  Krukenberg tumor and, 302–303
  markers for, 305–306
  microscopic and gross features of, 303–305
  pseudomyxoma peritonei and, 303

B

Breast carcinoma involving ovary,
  BRCA1/BRCA2 mutation in, risk for ovarian cancer and, 309
  ductal carcinoma, 309–310
  markers for, 310–311
  microscopic fatures of, 309–311

Brenner tumors, benign vs. borderline, 446–447
  differential diagnosis of, endometrioid carcinoma, 447
    squamous cell carcinoma, 447, 449
  gross features of, 446
    benign, 446
  malignant, 447, 449
  microscopic features of, 446–447
  types of, 446

C

Carcinoid tumors involving ovary, primary versus metastatic, 321

Cervical cancer, **1–11**

Cervical carcinoma, **1–11**
  clear cell, 62–64
  diagnosis of, cervical conization for, 2–3
    loop electrosurgical excision procedure in, 2
  epidemiology and etiology of, 1–2
  FIGO staging of, 3–4
  neoplastic lesions of, **17–86**
  pathologic reporting for, 1
  recurrence of, 9–11
    pelvic exenteration in, 9–10
    surgical approaches to, 11
  treatment of, stage IA1, 4–5
    stage IA2, 4–5
    stage IB1, 6–8
    stage IIA, 7–8
    stage IIB-IVA, 8–9
    surgical approaches to, 6

Cervical carcinoma involving ovary, markers for adenocarcinoma, 319
  microscopic and gross features of, 318–319

Cervix, adenocarcinoma in situ in, 41–48
  adenocarcinoma variants in, 55–71
    adenoid basal epithelioma/carcinoma, 67–69
    adenoid cystic carcinoma, 69–71
    clear cell, 61–65
    endometrioid, 55
    gastric type, 56–57, 59
    glassy cell, 67
    mesonephric, 60–61
    minimal deviation (adenoma malignum)/gastric type, 55
    minimal deviation type, 56, 57
      biomarkers for, 59
      lobular endocervical glandular hyperplasia and, 58
      prognosis for, 59–60
    serous carcinoma, 65–67
  glandular neoplasms of, 41–55
    adenocarcinoma in situ, 41–48
    invasive endocervical adenocarcinoma of usual type (HPV-associated), 48–55
  intraepithelial neoplasia, and invasive squamous carcinoma, 17
  intraepithelial neoplasia (spectrum of dysplasia and carcinoma in-situ), 17

Surgical Pathology 4 (2011) 479–486
doi:10.1016/S1875-9181(11)00009-2
1875-9181/11/$ – see front matter © 2011 Elsevier Inc. All rights reserved.

Moving?

Make sure your subscription moves with you!

To notify us of your new address, find your **Clinics Account Number** (located on your mailing label above your name), and contact customer service at:

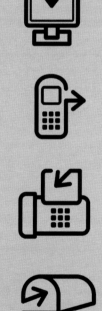

Email: journalscustomerservice-usa@elsevier.com

800-654-2452 (subscribers in the U.S. & Canada)
314-447-8871 (subscribers outside of the U.S. & Canada)

Fax number: 314-447-8029

Elsevier Health Sciences Division
Subscription Customer Service
3251 Riverport Lane
Maryland Heights, MO 63043

ELSEVIER

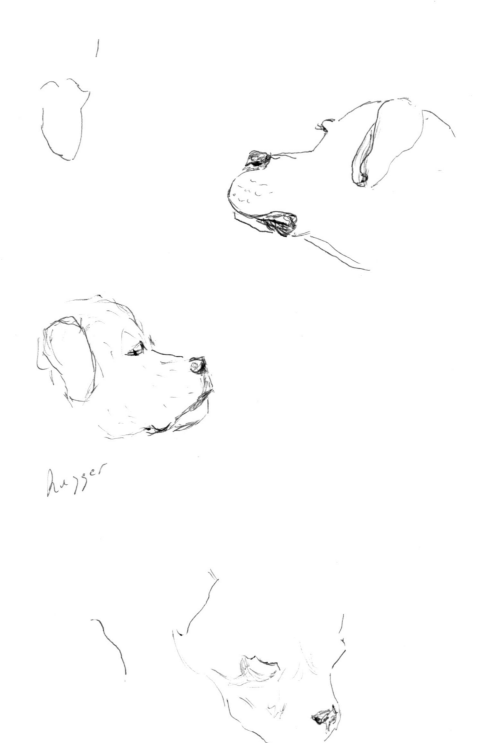

Rugger